Lecture Notes in Mathematics 2255

In recent years, the role of mathematics in the life sciences has evolved a long way from the role it played in the 1970's, in the early days of "biomathematics", and is a somewhat different one now, and its perception by the mathematical community is also different. We feel it is important for the Lecture Notes in Mathematics to reflect this and thus underline the immense significance of the life sciences as a field of application and interaction for mathematics in the 21st century.

We are particularly interested in going far beyond the traditional areas in which mathematics was applied to ecology, such as population dynamics, and would like to attract publications in areas such as cell growth, protein structures, physiology, vision, shape recognition & gestalt theory, neural dynamics, genomics, perhaps also some statistical aspects (this list is non-exhaustive).

More information about this series at http://www.springer.com/series/304

Tom Britton • Etienne Pardoux
Editors

Stochastic Epidemic Models with Inference

With Contributions by

Frank Ball, Tom Britton, Catherine Larédo, Etienne Pardoux,
David Sirl and Viet Chi Tran

Springer

Editors
Tom Britton
Department of Mathematics
Stockholm University
Stockholm, Sweden

Etienne Pardoux
Institut de Mathématiques de Marseille
Aix-Marseille Université
Marseille, France

ISSN 0075-8434 ISSN 1617-9692 (electronic)
Lecture Notes in Mathematics
ISSN 2524-6771 ISSN 2524-678X (electronic)
Mathematical Biosciences Subseries
ISBN 978-3-030-30899-5 ISBN 978-3-030-30900-8 (eBook)
https://doi.org/10.1007/978-3-030-30900-8

Mathematics Subject Classification (2010): 92D30, 62P10, 92B05, 60J85, 05C80, 62M05, 60J60, 62F12, 60J27

This Springer imprint is published by the registered company Springer Nature Switzerland AG
The registered company address is: Gewerbestrasse 11, 6330 Cham, Switzerland

Foreword

Epidemics and the spread of infectious diseases are a serious challenge in today's world, but especially in Africa, particularly following the recent Ebola outbreak. It is therefore easy to understand why there is a serious interest in mathematical models of epidemics in the African applied mathematics community.

The current volume is the late outcome of a two-week ICPAM/CIMPA school which took place from December 5 to December 16, 2015, in Ziguinchor, Senegal. The topic of the school was "Stochastic models of epidemics". The school consisted of four courses given by Tom Britton and Etienne Pardoux on homogeneous models, David Sirl on two-level mixing models, Viet Chi Tran on epidemics on graphs, and finally Catherine Larédo on statistics for epidemics models. Frank Ball could not attend the school but is a co-author with David Sirl in the current volume. The CIMPA school was co-organized by Alassane Diedhiou and Etienne Pardoux. After the school all lecturers (also including Frank Ball) were asked to write a chapter on their contributions to make up a short set of lecture notes. As it turned out, all contributions became longer than initially anticipated, and the four contributions are henceforth referred to as Parts I–IV, each part consisting of chapters and sections.

The CIMPA course was aimed at PhD students (and Post Docs) in the mathematical sciences, and we hence hope that (all or parts of) this volume can be used for PhD courses on the topic, either as a traditional PhD course or as an individual reading course. For this reason we have inserted Examples and Exercises (some with solutions) throughout the book.

We want to thank ICPAM/CIMPA, the Ministry of Higher Education of Senegal, the University of Ziguinchor, who supported our school, and the students, who made the event so unforgettable.

August 2019

Tom Britton, Stockholm
Alassane Diedhiou, Ziguinchor
Etienne Pardoux, Marseille

Preface

The aim of these Notes is to increase the reader's understanding of the spread of infectious diseases using mathematics, and in particular stochastic methods.

Needless to say, outbreaks of infectious diseases have had a huge impact on human society throughout history. During the 14th century, the black plague killed between 30% and 50% of Europe's population. In 1720 a plague epidemic removed almost half of the population of Marseille and a quarter of the population of Provence. In 1918–1919, the Spanish flu killed between 50 and 100 million people (3%–5% of the world's population!). Smallpox had existed for more than 3,000 years, killing many millions, before it was eradicated after a long and intense vaccination effort led by the WHO. More recently, some of the diseases causing most harm (casualties, suffering and/or economically) to humans have been HIV, influenza, foot and mouth disease, malaria and measles, and other diseases have caused unexpected dramatic outbreaks with a high mortality rate (e.g. SARS and most recently Ebola). In the future, endemic diseases will continue to be one the main causes of mortality, dramatic outbreaks of new and old infectious diseases are expected to continue to occur irregularly, the economic cost of disease outbreaks in domestic animal populations is expected to continue to increase, and the fear of large-scale treatment failure due to antibiotic resistance is becoming more and more realistic.

A paramount goal for public health is therefore to increase our understanding of how various infectious diseases spread in communities, with the goal of minimizing or even stopping their spread by various control measures (vaccination, quarantine, isolation, closing of schools, airports, ...). An important tool in this ambition is the use of mathematical models.

Mathematical modelling of infectious diseases has a long and successful history. The first such mathematical model was probably Bernoulli's model of smallpox [6], proposed in 1760. A little more than one hundred years ago, Sir Ronald Ross, a British medical doctor and Nobel laureate who contributed to the understanding of malaria, wrote: *"As a matter of fact all epidemiology, concerned as it is with variation of disease from time to time and from place to place, must be considered mathematically (...) and the mathematical method of treatment is really nothing but the application of careful reasoning to the problems at hand."* As a matter of fact, Ross deduced from mathematical arguments conclusions concerning malaria which his physician colleagues found hard to accept. Some other important mathematical epidemiological insights through history are: the notion of the *basic reproduction number* R_0 and its relation to the vaccination coverage v_c necessary to stop an outbreak (see e.g. Anderson and May [1]), the effect of local structures such as households on disease propagation (see e.g. Ball, Mollison and Scalia-Tomba [4]) and the insight that highly promiscuous individuals play a surprisingly dominant role for sexually transmitted diseases (see e.g. Pastor-Satorras and Vespignani [10]).

In the current Notes we study mathematical models for the spread of an infectious disease in a human population (it could of course also apply to an animal population, but we use terminology for humans). Learning this topic is also a good way to learn mathematics and mathematical modeling. Historically, deterministic models have received more attention, but our focus is on *stochastic models*. We believe that both deterministic and stochastic models have an important role to play; which model to use in a specific situation depends on the type of question asked, the type and complexity of the epidemic model, and whether or not there are data from which to infer model parameters.

We treat exclusively diseases that spread from person to person and hence we omit water-borne diseases or diseases that spread from food (e.g. Salmonella). For these diseases, individuals can often be classified as being susceptible (i.e. not yet infected) or infected, and if infected, an individual can either be latent (exposed but not yet infectious), infectious, or recovered and immune. For historical reasons, these states are categorized as susceptible (S), exposed (E), infectious (I) and recovered/immune (R). Susceptible individuals that become infected sequentially pass through the stages E, I and R (and possibly back to S again once immunity has waned). For simplicity, we call an individual in a given state susceptible, latent, infective or recovered, respectively. The type of model studied can then be expressed in terms of these abbreviations. For example, an SIR model has no latent (exposed) state and individuals remain recovered and immune forever, and in an SEIS model infected individuals are at first exposed, then infectious, after which they return to the susceptible state without being immune. Reality is of course not this simple: usually infectivity builds up gradually after having been latent for some time, and after some additional time infectivity drops down towards zero. Also, after having been immune for some time, this immunity gradually wanes and susceptibility picks up. In these Notes we mainly stick to the simplified situation where individuals have constant infectivity while being infectious, and complete immunity while recovered, possibly followed by complete susceptibility.

A very important factor for determining how a disease will spread in a community is how people mix. Individuals could either mix completely uniformly in the community, or, more likely, mix with household members, friends, work colleagues and neighbours at a higher rate than others. For sexually transmitted diseases, the relevant contacts depend on the sexual network of the community. It is not possible to say exactly which model to use for a given situation, but a general rule might be that the more highly infectious a disease is the better the simplifying approximation of assuming homogeneous mixing works. Thus, when considering measles and other childhood diseases (usually requiring only being in the same room for a substantial risk of getting infected) a homogeneous mixing model would work well, whereas for a sexually transmitted disease (where a very intimate contact is necessary, and even then there is only a small risk of transmission) conclusions made from a homogeneous mixing model would not be very reliable.

Another important factor affecting potential disease spread is whether individuals are similar (with respect to disease spreading) or not. For instance, individuals could vary in terms of their immune system, thus affecting their susceptibility to disease. Similarly, infected individuals could react differently, affecting how infectious they become, and they could differ in terms of how much they mix with others. These differences could either be known in advance and individuals classified accordingly (e.g. infants, schoolchildren and adults), or unknown – for example most diseases have both symptomatic and asymptomatic cases, often having different spreading potential.

Finally, the community under consideration could either be fixed or changing over time. Of course, no large community is completely constant over time, but if we consider a short-term outbreak, such as seasonal influenza, we may perhaps approximate the community as being fixed and constant. Similarly, if considering a short-term outbreak, what really is an SEIRS-disease can perhaps be approximated by the simpler SEIR model if immunity does not wane on the time horizon of the outbreak. For instance, individuals hardly ever catch influenza more than once during the *same* influenza season.

The idea behind this CIMPA-school, which carries over to the current volume, was to introduce stochastic models for the spread of infectious diseases and also some inference procedures for such models, and at the same time make use of various techniques from probability theory. The purpose of this volume is hence twofold: to help the reader learn about stochastic epidemic models (with inference) and, at the same time, enable them to see several probabilistic methods in use. The focus of the volume is on methodology, but in a few places there are connections to real-world epidemic outbreaks, in particular in Chapter 4 of Part III, where the spread of HIV in Cuba is analysed by means of a network epidemic model. In several other places we make connections to real-world problems without going into depth. The Notes aim to be self-contained and many of the most important results in the theory of stochastic epidemic models are derived. Needless to say, we also direct the reader to numerous articles where additional results are proven.

The contents of the different parts of the Notes can roughly be described as follows.

Part I, *Stochastic epidemic models in a homogeneous community*, written by the editors, sets the scene by defining and analysing some epidemic models in which all individuals are identical regarding social mixing and disease susceptibility and infectivity. This part looks at exact results for small communities, and large population approximations: laws of large numbers and central limit theorems for outbreaks in closed communities, but also endemic levels and extinction times (using large deviation techniques) for epidemics spreading in open (dynamic) populations.

Part II, *Stochastic SIR epidemic in structured populations*, is written by Frank Ball and David Sirl. In this part epidemic models are defined and analysed for communities that are not homogeneous, including household epidemic models, and general two-level mixing models containing both spreading at a local scale as well as at a global scale. The methods include branching processes, random graphs, the theory of susceptibility sets, laws of large numbers and central limit theorems.

Part III, *Stochastic epidemics in a heterogeneous community*, is written by Viet Chi Tran. This part is exclusively devoted to epidemic models on networks, and in particular on the configuration model network, and ends with an application to HIV in Cuba, which uses data from sexual contact questionnaires of diagnosed HIV patients. The methodology concerns the theory of random graphs and measure-valued processes for proving a law of large numbers.

Finally, Part IV, *Statistical inference for epidemic processes in a homogeneous community*, is written by Catherine Larédo, with a contribution by Viet Chi Tran in Chapter 4. Here the focus is on deriving inference procedures for the models described in earlier parts, in particular Part I, with extensive simulation studies illustrating the theory. The methodology involves classical likelihood theory, Bayesian inference, survival analysis and martingale theory, and computer intensive statistical techniques such as Approximate Bayesian Computation and Markov Chain Monte Carlo methods.

Most of the material in this volume has already appeared somewhere, but some aspects of the presentation, including a few technical results, are new compared to earlier publications. It is our belief that these Notes make up the most detailed *and* broad treatment of stochastic epidemic models ever published in one volume, covering both classical and new results and methods, from mathematical models to statistical procedures.

There are of course other books and lecture notes which treat similar questions and methods. We do not aim to give a complete list of such references, but instead give a subjectively chosen sample. One of the first books devoted to mathematical modelling of infectious diseases, mainly focussing on stochastic models, is Bailey's book [3], published in 1975. Note that this is the second edition of a book entitled *The mathematical theory of epidemics* published in 1957. In the 1980s, attention to mathematical epidemiology rose, at least partly due to the start of the HIV epidemic. The first book to focus on inference procedures for infectious diseases was Becker [5]. Another book from the same era which has had a huge impact is Anderson and May [1], which exclusively deals with deterministic models. Since then, there has been steady production of new research monographs, e.g. Andersson and Britton [2] also looking at inference methodology, Daley and Gani [7] focusing mainly on stochastic models, Keeling and Rohani [9] dealing also with animal populations, and Diekmann, Heesterbeek and Britton [8] covering both deterministic and stochastic modelling.

August 2019

Tom Britton, Stockholm
Etienne Pardoux, Marseille

References for the Preface

1. R.M. Anderson and R.M. May, *Infectious diseases of humans; dynamic and control*, Oxford: Oxford University Press, 1991.
2. H. Andersson and T. Britton, *Stochastic epidemic models and their statistical analysis*, Springer Lecture Notes in Statistics. New York: Springer Verlag, 2000.
3. N.T.J. Bailey, *The Mathematical Theory of Infectious Diseases and its Applications*, London: Griffin, 1975.
4. F.G. Ball, D. Mollison and G. Scalia-Tomba, Epidemics with two levels of mixing, *Ann. Appl. Prob.* **7**, 46–89, 1997.
5. N.G. Becker, *Analysis of Infectious Disease Data*, London: Chapman and Hall, 1989.
6. D. Bernoulli, Essai d'une nouvelle analyse de la mortalité causée par la petite vérole et des avantages de l'inoculation pour la prévenir, Mém. Math. Phys. Acad. Roy. Sci., Paris, 1–45, 1760.
7. D.J. Daley and J. Gani, *Epidemic Modelling: an introduction*, Cambridge University Press, Cambridge, 1999.
8. O. Diekmann, J.A.P. Heesterbeek and T. Britton, *Mathematical tools for understanding infectious disease dynamics*, Princeton UP, 2013.
9. M.J. Keeling and P. Rohani, *Modeling infectious diseases in humans and animals*, Princeton UP, 2008.
10. R. Pastor-Satorras and A. Vespignani, Epidemic spreading in scale-free networks, *Physical review letters* **86** (14), 3200, 2001.

Contents

Part I
Stochastic Epidemics in a Homogeneous Community

Tom Britton and Etienne Pardoux

Tom Britton, Stockholm
e-mail: tom.britton@math.su.se
Etienne Pardoux, Marseille
e-mail: etienne.pardoux@univ-amu.fr

Introduction

In this Part I of the lecture notes our focus lies exclusively on stochastic epidemic models for a homogeneously mixing community of individuals being of the same type. The important extensions allowing for different types of individuals and allowing for non-uniform mixing behaviour in the community is left for later parts in the Notes.

In Chapter 1, we present the stochastic SEIR epidemic model, derive some important properties of it, in particular for the beginning of an outbreak. Motivated by mathematical tractability rather than realism we then study in Chapter 2 the special situation where the model is Markovian, and derive additional results for this sub-model.

What happens later on in the outbreak will depend on our model assumptions, which in turn depend on the scientific questions. In Chapter 3 we focus on short-term outbreaks, when it can be assumed that the community is fixed and constant during the outbreak; we call these models closed models. In Chapter 4 we are more interested in long-term behaviour, and then it is necessary to allow for influx of new individuals and that people die, or to include return to susceptibility. Such so-called open population models are harder to analyse – for this reason we stick to the simpler class of Markovian models. In this chapter we consider situations where the deterministic model has a unique stable equilibrium, and use both the central limit theorem and large deviation techniques to predict the time at which the disease goes extinct in the population.

The Notes end with an extensive Appendix, giving some relevant probability theory used in the main part of the Notes and also solutions to most of the exercises being scattered out in the different chapters.

Chapter 1
Stochastic Epidemic Models

This first chapter introduces some basic facts about stochastic epidemic models. We consider the case of a closed community, i.e. without influx of new susceptibles or mortality. In particular, we assume that the size of the population is fixed, and that the individuals who recover from the illness are immune and do not become susceptible again. We describe the general class of stochastic epidemic models, and define the basic reproduction number, which allows one to determine whether or not a major epidemic may start from the initial infection of a small number of individuals. We then approximate the early stage of an outbreak with the help of a branching process, and from this obtain the distribution of the final size (i.e. the total number of individuals who ever get infected) in case of a minor outbreak. Finally we discuss the impact of vaccination.

The important problem of estimating model parameters from (various types of) data is left to Part IV of the current volume (also discussed in Chapter 4 of Part III). Here we assume the model parameters to be known.

1.1 The Stochastic SEIR Epidemic Model in a Closed Homogeneous Community

1.1.1 Model Definition

Consider a closed population of $N+1$ individuals (N is the number of initially susceptible). At any point in time each individual is either susceptible, exposed, infectious or recovered. Let $S(t)$, $E(t)$, $I(t)$ and $R(t)$ denote the numbers of individuals in the different states at time t (so $S(t)+E(t)+I(t)+R(t)=N+1$ for all t). The epidemic starts at $t=0$ in a specified state, often the state with one infectious individual, called the index case and thought of as being externally infected, and the rest being susceptible: $(S(0),E(0),I(0),R(0))=(N,0,1,0)$.

Definition 1.1.1. While infectious, an individual has infectious contacts according to a Poisson process with rate λ. Each contact is with an individual chosen uni-

T. Britton, E. Pardoux (eds.), *Stochastic Epidemic Models with Inference*,
Lecture Notes in Mathematics 2255, https://doi.org/10.1007/978-3-030-30900-8_1

formly at random from the rest of the population, and if the contacted individual is susceptible he/she becomes infected – otherwise the infectious contact has no effect. Individuals that become infected are first latent (called exposed) for a random duration L with distribution F_L, then they become infectious for a duration I with distribution F_I, after which they become recovered and immune for the remaining time. All Poisson processes, uniform contact choices, latent periods and infectious periods of all individuals are defined to be mutually independent.

The epidemic goes on until the first time τ when there are no exposed or infectious individuals, $E(\tau)+I(\tau)=0$. At this time no further individuals can get infected so the epidemic stops. The final state hence consists of susceptible and recovered individuals, and we let Z denote the *final size*, i.e. the number of infected (by then recovered) individuals at the end of the epidemic excluding the index case(s): $Z=R(\tau)-I(0)=N-S(\tau)$. The possible values of Z are hence $0,\dots,N$.

1.1.2 Some Remarks, Submodels and Model Generalizations

Quite often the rate of "infectious contacts" λ can be thought of as a product of a rate c at which the infectious individual has contact with others, and the probability p that such a contact results in infection given that the other person is susceptible, so $\lambda = cp$. As regards to the propagation of the disease it is however only the product λ that matters and since fewer parameters is preferable we keep only λ.

The rate of infectious contacts is λ, so the rate at which one infectious has contact with a specific other individual is λ/N since each contact is with a uniformly chosen other individual.

First we will look what happens in a very small community/group, but the main focus of these notes is for a large community, and the asymptotics are hence for $N\to\infty$. The parameters of the model, the infection rate λ, and the latent and infectious periods L and I, are defined independently of N, but the epidemic is highly dependent on N so when this needs to be emphasized we equip the corresponding notation with an N-index, e.g. $S^N(t)$ and τ^N which hence is not a power.

Some special cases of the model have received special attention in the literature. If both L and I are exponentially distributed (with rates ν and γ say), the model is Markovian which simplifies the mathematical analysis a great deal. This model is called the *Markovian SEIR*. If $L\equiv 0$ and $I\sim \text{Exp}(\gamma)$ then we have the *Markovian SIR* (whenever there is no latency period the model is said to be SIR) which is better known under the unfortunate name the *General stochastic epidemic*. Another special case of the stochastic SEIR model is where the infectious period I is non-random. Also here there is a underlying mathematical reason – when the duration of the infectious period is non-random and equal to ι say, then an infectious individual has infectious contacts with each other individual at rate λ/N during a non-random time implying that the number of contacts with different individuals are *independent*. Consequently, an infectious individual has infectious contacts with each other individual independently with probability $p=1-e^{-(\lambda/N)\iota}$, so the total number of contacts is Binomially distributed, and in the limit as $N\to\infty$ the number of infectious contacts an individual has is Poisson distributed with mean $\lambda\iota$. If further the latent period is long in comparison to the infectious period then it is possible to identify the infected individuals in terms of *generations*: the first generation are the index cases, the second generation those who were infected by the index case(s), and so one. When the model is described in this discrete time setting and individuals infect different individuals independently with probability p, this model is the well-known Reed–Frost model named after its inventors Reed and Frost.

The two most studied special cases are hence when the infectious period is exponentially distributed and when it is nonrandom. For real infectious diseases none of these two extremes apply, for influenza for example, the infectious period is believed to be about 4 days, plus or minus one or two days. If one has to choose between these choices a nonrandom infectious period is probably closer to reality.

The stochastic SEIR model in a closed homogeneous community may of course also be generalized towards more realism. Two such extensions have already been mentioned: allowing for individuals to die and new ones to be born, and allowing for some social structures. Some such extensions will be treated in the other articles of the current lecture notes but not here. But even when assuming a closed homogeneously mixing community of homogeneous individuals it is possible to make the model more realistic. The most important such generalization is to let the rate of infectious contact vary with time since infection. The current model assumes there are no infectious contacts during the latent state, and then, suddenly when the latent period ends, the rate of infectious contact becomes λ until the infectious period ends when it suddenly drops down to 0 again. In reality, the infectious rate is usually a function $\lambda(s)$ s time units after infection. In most situations $\lambda(s)$ is very small initially (corresponding to the latency period) followed by a gradual increase for some days, and then $\lambda(s)$ starts decaying down towards 0 which it hits when the individual has recovered completely (see Figure 1.1.1 for an example where infectivity starts growing after one day and is more or less over after one week). The

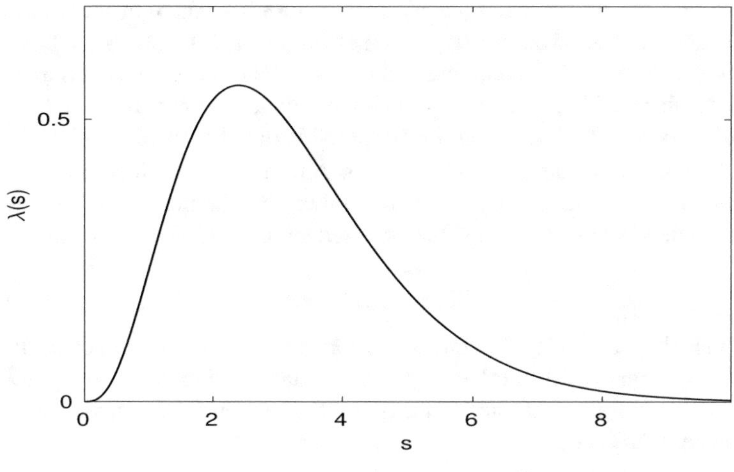

Fig. 1.1.1 Plot of a possible infectivity curve $\lambda(s)$. The time s denotes the time since infection in unit of days.

function $\lambda(s)$ could be the same for all individuals, or it may be random and hence a stochastic process, i.i.d. for different individuals. As regards to the temporal dynamics of the epidemic process, the functional form of $\lambda(s)$ is important, and also its random properties in case it is random. If one is only interested in the final size τ, it is however possible to show that all that affects the final size is the accumulated force of infection, i.e. the distribution of $\int_0^\infty \lambda(s)ds$. In particular, if we let λI in the stochastic SEIR model have the same distribution as $\int_0^\infty \lambda(s)ds$ in the more general model, then the two models have the same final size distribution. In that sense, the extended model can be included in the stochastic SEIR model.

1.1.3 Two Key Quantities: R_0 and the Escape Probability

The most important quantity for this, as well as most other epidemic models, is the *basic reproduction number* (sometimes "number" is replaced by "ratio") and denoted by R_0. In more complicated models its definition and interpretation are sometimes debated, but for the present model it is quite straightforward: R_0 denotes the mean number of infectious contacts a typical infected has during the early stage of an outbreak. As the population under consideration is becomes large, this number will coincide with the mean number of infections caused by a typical infected during the early stages of an outbreak. We derive an expression for R_0, but before that we should consider its important threshold value of 1. If $R_0 > 1$ this means that on average an infected infects more than one individual in the beginning of an epidemic. Then the index case on average is replaced by more than one infected, who in turn each are replaced by more than one infected and so on. This clearly suggests that a big community fraction can become infected. If on the other hand $R_0 \leq 1$, then the same reasoning suggests that there will never be a big community outbreak. Those results hold true which we prove in Section 1.2 (Corollaries 1.2.6 and 1.2.7).

In applications the basic reproduction number R_0 is a central quantity of interest. Many studies of disease outbreaks contain estimates of R_0 for a specific disease and community, together with modeling conclusions about preventive measures which, if put into place, will reduce the reproduction number R down to below the critical value of 1 when an outbreak is no longer possible (e.g. Fraser et al. [12]).

Let us now derive an expression for R_0. An infected individual has infectious contacts only when infectious, and when in this state the individual has infectious contacts at rate λ. This means that the expected number of infectious contacts equals

$$R_0 = \mathbb{E}(\lambda I) = \lambda \iota. \tag{1.1.1}$$

Sometimes the rate λ of having infectious contacts is replaced by an over-all rate of contact c multiplied by the probability p of a contact leading to infection, so $\lambda = cp$ and $R_0 = cp\iota$ (cf. the first lines of the above Subsection 1.1.2, Anderson and May [1] and Giesecke [14]).

Another key quantity appearing later several times is the probability for a given susceptible to escape getting infected from a specific infective. The instantaneous infectious force from the infective to this specific susceptible is λ/N, and the random duration of the infectious period is I. Conditional upon $I = x$, the escape probability is hence $e^{-(\lambda/N)x}$, and the unconditional probability to escape infection is therefore

$$\mathbb{P}(\text{escape infection from an infective}) = \mathbb{E}(e^{-\lambda I/N}) = \psi_I(-\lambda/N), \qquad (1.1.2)$$

where $\psi_I(b) = \mathbb{E}(e^{bI})$ is the moment generating function of the infectious period (so $\psi(-b)$ is the Laplace transform – in Part II in this volume the Laplace transform has a separate notation, ϕ, so $\phi(b) = \psi(-b)$).

Exercise 1.1.2. Consider the Markovian SEIR epidemic in which $\lambda = 1.8$, $\nu = 2$ and $\gamma = 1$ in a village of size $N = 100$, (parameters inspired by Ebola with weeks as time unit). Compute R_0 and the escape probability.

Exercise 1.1.3. Repeat the previous exercise, but now for the Reed–Frost epidemic with $\lambda = 1.8$, $L \equiv 2$ and $I \equiv \iota = 1$ in a village of size $N = 100$, (perhaps having more realistic distributions than in the previous exercise).

1.2 The Early Stage of an Outbreak

We now consider the situation where the community size N is large and study the stochastic SEIR epidemic in the beginning of an outbreak. By "beginning" we mean that less than $k = k(N)$ individuals have been infected. Recall from the model definition that infectious individuals have infectious contacts with others independently, each infective at rate λ. The dependence only appears because individuals can only get infected once, so if an individual has already received an infectious contact, then future infectious contacts with that individual no longer result in someone getting infected. However, in the beginning of an outbreak in a large community it is very unlikely that two infectives happen to have infectious contacts with the same individual. This suggests that during the early phase of an outbreak, infectives infect new individuals more or less independently. This implies that the number of infected can be approximated by a branching process in the beginning of an outbreak, where "being born" corresponds to having been infected, and "giving birth" corresponds to infecting someone. The current section is devoted to making this approximation rigorous, and thus obtaining asymptotic results for the epidemic in regards to having a minor versus a major outbreak. In the next section this approximation is exploited in order to determine the distribution of the final size in the case of a minor outbreak. If the epidemic takes off, which happens in the case of a major outbreak, then the approximation that individuals infect others independently breaks down. What happens in this situation is treated in later sections.

First we define the approximating branching process and derive some properties of it. After this we show rigorously that, as $N \to \infty$, the initial phase of the epidemic process converges to the initial phase of the branching process by using an elegant coupling technique.

The approximating branching process is defined similarly to the epidemic. A newborn individual is first unable to give birth to new individuals for a period with duration L (this period might be denoted childhood in the branching process setting). After this childhood, the individual enters the reproductive stage which last for I units of time. During this period individuals give birth to new individuals at rate λ (randomly in time according to a Poisson process with rate λ). Once the reproductive stage has terminated the individual dies (or at least cannot reproduce and hence plays no further role).

The number of offspring of an individual, X, depends on the duration of the reproductive stage I. Conditional upon $I = y$, the number of births follow the Poisson distribution $\mathrm{Poi}(\lambda y)$, so the unconditional distribution of number of offspring is mixed-Poisson, written as $X \sim \mathrm{MixPoi}(\lambda I)$, where I has distribution F_I.

If we forget calendar time, and simply study the number of individuals born in each generation, then our branching process is a Bienaymé–Galton–Watson process with offspring distribution being $\mathrm{MixPoi}(\lambda I)$. The mean number of children/offspring equals $m = \mathbb{E}(X) = \mathbb{E}(\mathbb{E}(X|I)) = \mathbb{E}(\lambda I) = \lambda \iota$.

Exercise 1.2.1. Compute the offspring distribution $\mathbb{P}(X = x)$ explicitly for the two cases: (i) where the infectious period is non-random, $I \equiv \iota$, corresponding to the continuous–time version of the Reed–Frost epidemic; and (ii) for the Markovian SEIR where I is exponential with mean ι.

We now show an elegant coupling construction which we will use to show that the epidemic and branching process have similar distributions in the beginning. To this end we define the approximating branching process as well as all epidemics, i.e. for each $N = 1, 2, \ldots$, on the same probability space. To this end, let $L_0, L_1, \ldots$ be i.i.d. latent periods having distribution F_L, and similarly let $I_0, I_1, \ldots$ be i.i.d. infectious periods having distribution F_I. Further, let $\xi_0(\cdot), \xi_1(\cdot), \ldots$ be i.i.d. Poisson processes having intensity λ, and let $U_1, U_2, \ldots$ be i.i.d. $U(0,1)$ random variables. All random variables and Poisson processes are assumed to be mutually independent. These will be used to construct the branching process as well as the stochastic SEIR epidemic for each N as follows.

Definition 1.2.2. The approximating branching process. At time $t = 0$ there is one new born ancestor having label 0. Let the ancestor have childhood length L_0 and reproductive stage for a duration I_0 (so the ancestor dies at time $L_0 + I_0$), during which the ancestor gives birth at the time points of the Poisson process $\xi_0(\cdot)$. If the jump times of this Poisson process are denoted $T_{0,1} < T_{0,2} < \ldots$ and X_0 denotes the number of jumps prior to I_0, then the ancestor gives birth at the time points $L_0 + T_{0,1}, \ldots, L_0 + T_{0,X_0}$ (the set is empty if $X_0 = 0$). The first born individual is given label 1, and having childhood period L_1, reproductive period I_1 and birth process $\xi_1(\cdot)$. This individual gives birth according to the same rules (starting the latency period at time $L_0 + T_{0,1}$), and the next individual born, either to individual 0 or 1, is given label 2 and variables L_2, I_2 and birth process $\xi_2(\cdot)$, and so on. This defines the branching process, and we let $L(t), I(t), R(t)$ respectively denote the numbers of individuals in the childhood state, in the reproductive state and dead, respectively, at time t. The total number of individuals born up to time t, excluding the ancestor/index case, is denoted by $Z(t) = L(t) + I(t) + R(t) - 1$ in the branching process, and the ultimate number ever born, excluding the ancestor, is denoted by Z which may be finite or infinite.

We now define the epidemic for any fixed N (in the epidemic childhood corresponds to latent and reproductive stage to being infectious). This is done similarly to the branching process with the exception that we now keep track of which individuals who get infected using the uniform random variables $U_1, U_2, \ldots$.

Definition 1.2.3. The stochastic SEIR epidemic with N initial susceptibles. We label the $N+1$ individuals $0, 1, \ldots, N$, with the index case having label 0 and the others being labelled arbitrarily. As for the branching process, the index case is given latency period L_0, infectious period I_0 and contact process $\xi_0(\cdot)$ and the epidemic is started at time $t = 0$. The infectious contacts of the index case occur at the time points $L_0 + T_{0,1}, \ldots, L_0 + T_{0,X_0}$. The first infectious contact is with individual $[U_1 N] + 1$, the integer part of NU_1 plus 1 (this picks an individual uniformly among $1, \ldots, N$). This individual, k say, then becomes infected (and latent) and is given latent period, infectious period and contact process L_1, I_1 and $\xi_1(\cdot)$. The next infectious contact (from either the index case or individual k) will be with individual $[U_2 N] + 1$. If the contacted person is individual k then nothing happens, but otherwise this new individual gets infected (and latent), and so on. Infectious contacts only result in infection if the contacted individual is still susceptible. When a contact is with an already infected individual the branching process has a birth whereas there is no infection in the epidemic – we say a "ghost" was infected when comparing with the branching process. Descendants of all ghosts are also ignored in the epidemic. The epidemic goes on until there are no latent or infectious individuals. This will happen within a finite time (bounded by $\sum_{j=0}^{N}(L_j + I_j)$). The final number of infected individuals excluding the index case is as before denoted $Z^N \in [0, \ldots, N]$. Similar to before we let $L^N(t), I^N(t), R^N(t)$ denote the numbers of latent, infectious and recovered individuals at time t, and now we can also define the number of susceptibles $S^N(t) = N + 1 - L^N(t) - I^N(t) - R^N(t)$.

In our model the index case cannot be contacted. This is of course unrealistic but simplifies notation. In the limit as N gets large this assumption has no effect. We now state two important results for these constructions of the branching process and epidemics.

Theorem 1.2.4. *The definition above agrees with the earlier definition of the Stochastic SEIR epidemic in a homogeneous community.*

Proof. The latent and infectious periods have the desired distributions, and an infective has infectious contacts with others at overall rate λ, and each time such a contact is with a uniformly selected individual as desired. □

We now prove that the branching process and the epidemic process (with population size N) are identical up to a time point which tends to infinity in probability as $N \to \infty$. To this end, we let M^N denote the number of infections prior to the first ghost (i.e. how many uniformly selected individuals $[U_k N]$ there were before someone was reselected. If this never happens we set $M^N = \infty$. Let T^N denote the time at which the first ghost appears (and if this never happens we also set $T^N = \infty$).

Theorem 1.2.5. *The branching process and N-epidemic agree up until T^N: $(L^N(t), I^N(t), R^N(t)) = (L(t), I(t), R(t))$ for all $t \in [0, T^N)$. Secondly, $T_N \to \infty$ and $M^N \to \infty$ in probability as $N \to \infty$.*

Proof. The first statement of the proof is obvious. The only difference between the epidemic and the branching process in our construction is that specific individuals are contacted in the epidemic, and up until the first time when some individual is contacted again, each infectious contact results in infection just as in the branching process.

As for the second part of the theorem we first compute the probability that M^N will tend to infinity, and then that the time T^N until the first ghost appears also tends to infinity. It is easy to compute $\mathbb{P}(M^N > k)$ since this will happen if and only if all the first k contacts are with distinct individuals:

$$\mathbb{P}(M^N > k) = 1 \times \frac{N-1}{N} \times \cdots \times \frac{N-k}{N} = \prod_{j=0}^{k} \left(1 - \frac{j}{N}\right).$$

(This formula is identical to the celebrated (...) birthday problem if $N+1 = 365$ and k is the size of the class.) For fixed k we see that this probability tends to 1 as $N \to \infty$. We can in fact say more. We have the following lower bound (which is easily proved by recurrence):

$$\mathbb{P}(M^N > k) = \prod_{j=0}^{k} \left(1 - \frac{j}{N}\right) \geq 1 - \sum_{j=1}^{k} \frac{j}{N} = 1 - \frac{(k+1)k}{2N}.$$

As a consequence, we see that $\mathbb{P}(M^N > k(N)) \to 1$ as long as $k = k(N) = o(\sqrt{N})$. In particular $M^N \to \infty$ in probability as $N \to \infty$. In what follows we write w.l.p. for "with large probability", meaning with a probability tending to 1 as $N \to \infty$. The consequence hence implies that all infectious contacts up to $k(N)$ will w.l.p. be with distinct individuals and thus will result in infections. So, up until $k(N)$ individuals have been infected, the epidemic can be approximated by a branching process for any $k(N) = o(\sqrt{N})$. Let $Z(t)$ denote the number of individuals born before t in the branching process (excluding the ancestor) and $Z^N(t) = N - S^N(t)$ the number of individuals that have been infected before t (excluding the index case) in the N-epidemic. Since the epidemic and branching process agree up until T^N it follows that $Z(t) = Z^N(t)$ for $t < T^N$. But, since $k(N) < M^N$ w.l.p. it follows that $\inf\{t; Z(t) = k(N)\} \leq T^N$ w.l.p. If the branching process is (sub)critical, then $Z(t)$ remains bounded as $t \to \infty$, so $T^N = +\infty$ w.l.p. Consider now the supercritical case. From Section A.1.2 (Proposition A.1.4) we know that $Z(t) = O_p(e^{rt})$ where the Malthusian parameter r solves the equation

$$\int_0^{\infty} e^{-rs} \lambda(s) ds = 1. \tag{1.2.1}$$

The function $\lambda(s)$ is the rate at which an individual gives birth s time units after being born, so $\lambda(s) = \lambda \mathbb{P}(\text{infectious at } s)$ and hence $\lambda(s) = \lambda \mathbb{P}(L < s < L+I)$ for our model. We thus have that $k(N) \leq ce^{rT^N}$ w.l.p., which implies that $T^N \geq \log k(N)/r - \log c$. So if for example $k(N) = N^{1/3}$, which clearly satisfies $k(N) = o(\sqrt{N})$, it follows that $T^N \to \infty$ in probability. □

Theorem 1.2.5 shows that the epidemic behaves like the branching process up to a time point tending to infinity as $N \to \infty$, and that the number of infections/births by then also tends to infinity. This implies that we can use theory for branching processes to obtain results for the early part of the epidemic. We state these important results in the following corollaries; the first corollary is for the subcritical and critical cases and the second corollary is for the supercritical case. Recall that $R_0 = \lambda \mathbb{E}(I)$, the basic reproduction number in the epidemic and the mean offspring number in the branching process.

Corollary 1.2.6. *If $R_0 \leq 1$, then $(L^N(t), I^N(t), R^N(t)) = (L(t), I(t), R(t))$ for all $t \in [0, \infty)$ w.l.p. As a consequence, $\mathbb{P}(Z^N = k) \to \mathbb{P}(Z = k)$ as $N \to \infty$, and in particular Z^N is bounded in probability.*

Proof. In Theorem 1.2.5 it was shown that the epidemic and branching process agree up until there has been M^N births, where $M^N > N^{1/3}$ w.l.p. for example. But from branching process theory (Proposition A.1.1) we know that this will happen with a probability tending to 0 with N when $R_0 \leq 1$, implying that $T^N = \infty$ w.l.p. □

Corollary 1.2.7. *If $R_0 > 1$, then for finite k: $\mathbb{P}(Z^N = k) \to \mathbb{P}(Z = k)$ as $N \to \infty$. Further, $\{Z^N \to \infty\}$ with the same probability as $\{Z = \infty\}$, which is the complement to the extinction probability, the latter being the smallest solution to the equation $z = g(z)$ described in Proposition A.1.1.*

Proof. Also this corollary is a direct consequence of Theorem 1.2.5 and properties of branching processes. If only k births occur, then there will be no ghost w.l.p., implying that the epidemic and the branching process agree forever w.l.p. On the other hand, the coupling construction showed that $M^N \to \infty$ on the other part of the sample space, and $Z \geq Z^N \geq M^N$ which completes the proof. □

The two corollaries state that the epidemic and branching process coincide forever as long as the branching process stays finite. If the branching process grows beyond all limits (only possible when $R_0 > 1$) then the epidemic and branching process will not remain identical even though also the epidemic tends to infinity with N. For any fixed N we have $0 \leq Z^N \leq N$ which clearly is different from $Z = \infty$ in that case. The distribution of Z^N on the part of the sample space where $Z^N \to \infty$ is treated below in Section 3.3.

The two corollaries show that the final number infected Z^N will be small with a probability equal to the extinction probability of the approximating branching process, and it will tend to infinity with the remaining (explosion) probability. In Section 3.3 we study the distribution of Z^N (properly normed) and then see that the distribution is clearly bimodal with one part close to 0 and the other part being $O(N)$. These two parts are referred to as *minor outbreak* and *major outbreak* respectively.

What happens during the early stage of an outbreak is particularly important when considering so-called *emerging epidemic outbreaks*. Then statistical inference based on this type of branching process approximation is often used. For example, in [38] a branching process approximation that is very similar to the SEIR branching process of Definition 1.2.2 is used for modelling the spread of Ebola during the early stage of the outbreak in West Africa in 2014.

Exercise 1.2.8. Use the branching process approximation of the current section to compute the probability of a major outbreak of the SEIR epidemic assuming that $I \equiv \iota$ (the continuous time Reed–Frost case), and $I \sim \text{Exp}(\gamma)$ (the Markovian SIR) with $\gamma = 1/\iota$. Only one of them will be explicit. Compute things numerically for $R_0 = 1.5$ and $\iota = 1$.

Exercise 1.2.9. Use the branching process approximation of the current section to compute the exponential growth rate r for the following two cases: $L \equiv 0$ and $I \equiv \iota$ (the continuous time Reed–Frost), and $L \equiv 0$ and $I \sim \text{Exp}(\gamma = 1/\iota)$ (the Markovian SIR). Compute r numerically for the two cases when $R_0 = 1.5$ and $\iota = \gamma = 1$.

1.3 The Final Size of the Epidemic in Case of No Major Outbreak

Let Z^N denote the final size of the epidemic (i.e. the total number of individuals that get infected during the outbreak) but now also including the initially infected individual. In the case of no major outbreak, if the total population size N is large enough, Z^N is well approximated by the total number of individuals in a branching process, as we saw in the previous section. Hence we consider Z as the total number of individuals ever born in a branching process (including the ancestor), where the number of offspring of the k-th individual is X_k. Let $X_1, X_2, \dots$ be i.i.d. $\mathbb{N}$-valued random variables. We start by establishing an identity which is an instance of Kemperman's formula, see e.g. Pitman [28] page 123.

Proposition 1.3.1. *For all $k \geq 1$,*

$$\mathbb{P}(Z = k) = \frac{1}{k}\mathbb{P}(X_1 + X_2 + \cdots + X_k = k - 1).$$

Proof. Consider the process of depth–first search of the genealogical tree of the infected individuals. This procedure can be defined as follows. The tree is explored starting from the root. Suppose we have visited k vertices. The next visit will be to the leftmost still unexplored son of this individual, if any; otherwise to the leftmost unexplored son of the most recently visited node among those having not yet visited son(s), see Figure 1.3.1. X_1 is the number of sons of the root, who is the first visited individual. X_k is the number of sons of the k-th visited individual. This exploration of the tree ends at step k if and only if $X_1 \geq 1$, $X_1 + X_2 \geq 2$, $X_1 + X_2 + X_3 \geq 3$, ... $X_1 + X_2 + \cdots X_{k-1} \geq k - 1$, and $X_1 + X_2 + \cdots + X_k = k - 1$. Let us rewrite those conditions. Define

$$Y_i = X_i - 1, \; i \geq 1,$$
$$S_k = Y_1 + Y_2 + \cdots + Y_k.$$

A trajectory $\{Y_i, \; 1 \leq i \leq k\}$ explores a tree of size k if and only if the following conditions are satisfied

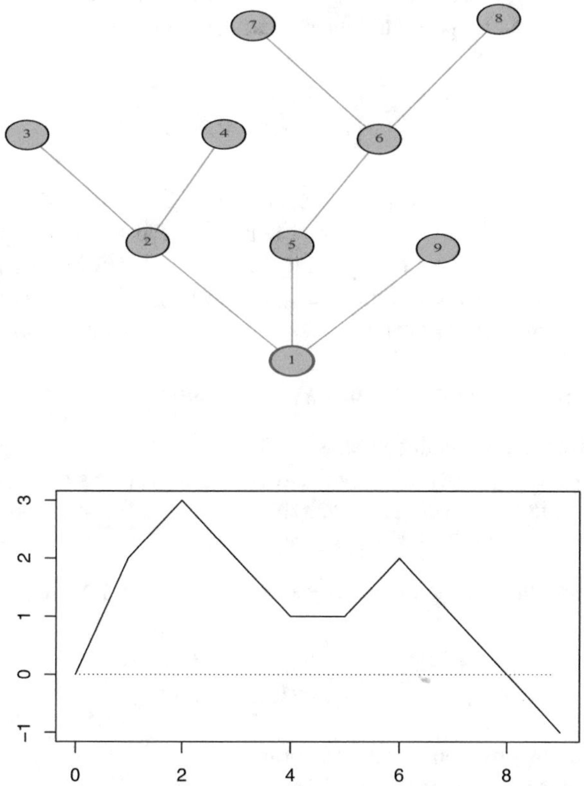

Fig. 1.3.1 Top: the tree. Bottom: the random walk S_k. Here $X_1 = 3, X_2 = 2, X_3 = 0, X_4 = 0, X_5 = 1,$ $X_6 = 2, X_7 = X_8 = X_9 = 0, Y_1 = 2, Y_2 = 1, Y_3 = Y_4 = -1, Y_5 = 0, Y_6 = 1, Y_7 = Y_8 = Y_9 = -1.$

$$(C_k) \quad S_0 = 0, S_1 \geq 0, S_2 \geq 0, \ldots, S_{k-1} \geq 0, S_k = -1.$$

Indeed, it is easy to convince oneself that it is the case if there is only one generation: if the ancestor has $k-1$ children, then $Y_1 = k-2$, and $Y_2 = \cdots = Y_k = -1$, hence (C_k) holds. If one attaches one generation trees to some of the leaves of the previous tree, then one replaces a unique -1 step by an excursion upwards which finishes at the same level as the replaced step. Iterating this procedure, we see that the exploration of a general tree with k nodes satisfies (C_k).

The statement of the proposition is equivalent to

$$\mathbb{P}(Z = k) = \frac{1}{k}\mathbb{P}(Y_1 + Y_2 + \cdots + Y_k = -1).$$

Denote by V_k the set of sequences of k integers ≥ -1 which satisfy conditions (C_k), and U_k the set of sequences of k integers ≥ -1 which satisfy the unique condition $S_k = -1$. We use circular permutations operating on the Y_i's. For $1 \leq i, \ell \leq k$, let

$$(i+\ell)_k = \begin{cases} i+\ell, & \text{if } i+\ell \leq k; \\ i+\ell-k, & \text{if } i+\ell > k. \end{cases}$$

For each $1 \leq \ell \leq k$, let $Z_i^\ell = Y_{(i+\ell)_k}$, $S_j^\ell = \sum_{i=1}^j Z_i^\ell$ for $1 \leq i \leq k$. Clearly $S_k^\ell = -1$ for all ℓ as soon as (C_k) is satisfied. On the other hand $S^k \equiv S$ is the only trajectory which satisfies conditions (C_k). The other S^ℓ hit the value -1 before rank k, see Figure 1.3.1. The Z^ℓ's are sequences of integers ≥ -1 of length k, whose sum equals -1. Finally to each element of V_k we have associated k distinct elements of U_k, all having the same probability.

Reciprocally, to one element S of $U_k \backslash V_k$, choosing $\ell = \underset{1\leq i\leq k}{\operatorname{argmin}} S_i$ and using the above transformation, we deduce that $S^\ell \in V_k$.

Finally, to each trajectory of V_k, we associate k trajectories of U_k, who all have the same probability, and which are such that the inverse transformation gives back the same trajectory of V_k. The result is proved. □

Note that from branching process theory (Proposition A.1.1), we have clearly

$$\sum_{k\geq 1} \mathbb{P}(Z=k) \begin{cases} = 1, & \text{if } \mathbb{E}R_0 \leq 1; \\ < 1, & \text{if } \mathbb{E}R_0 > 1, \end{cases}$$

which is not so obvious from the proposition.

We now deduce the exact law of Z from Proposition 1.3.1 in two cases which are probably the two most interesting cases for epidemics models. First we consider the case where the X_is are Poisson, which is the situation of the continuous time Reed–Frost model, where the infectious period is non-random. Second we consider the case where the X_is are geometric, which is the case in the Markovian model.

Example 1.3.2. Suppose that the joint law of the X_is is $\text{Poi}(\mu)$, with $0 < \mu < 1$. Then $X_1 + \cdots + X_k \sim \text{Poi}(k\mu)$, and consequently

$$\begin{aligned} \mathbb{P}(Z=k) &= \frac{1}{k}\mathbb{P}(X_1 + \cdots + X_k = k-1) \\ &= e^{-\mu k}\frac{(\mu k)^{k-1}}{k!}. \end{aligned}$$

This law of Z is called the Borel distribution with parameter μ. Note that

$$\begin{aligned} \mathbb{E}Z &= 1 + \mu + \mu^2 + \cdots \\ &= \frac{1}{1-\mu}. \end{aligned}$$

Example 1.3.3. Consider now the case where $X_i \sim \mathscr{G}(p)$, where we mean here that $\mathbb{P}(X_i = k) = (1-p)^k p$, $k = 0, 1, \ldots$. The law of $X_i + 1$ is the geometric distribution with parameter p whose support is $\mathbb{N}$, in other words $\mathbb{P}(X_i + 1 > k) = (1-p)^k$. Then $k + X_1 + \cdots + X_k$ follows the negative binomial distribution with parameters (k, p). Hence

$$\begin{aligned}\mathbb{P}(Z = k) &= \frac{1}{k}\mathbb{P}(k + X_1 + \cdots + X_k = 2k-1) \\ &= \frac{1}{k}\binom{2k-2}{k-1} p^k (1-p)^{k-1} \\ &= \frac{(2k-2)!}{k!(k-1)!} p^k (1-p)^{k-1}.\end{aligned}$$

In the case $p > 1/2$, $\mathbb{E}Z = (2p-1)^{-1}p$.

1.4 Vaccination

One important reason for modelling the spread of infectious diseases is to better understand effects of different preventive measures, such as for example vaccination, isolation and school closure. When a new outbreak occurs, epidemiologists (together with mathematicians and statisticians) estimate model parameters and then use these to predict effects of various preventive measures, and based on these predictions, health authorities decide upon which preventive measures to put in place, cf. [38].

We refer the reader to Part IV in this volume for estimation methods, but in the current section we touch upon the area of modeling prevention. Our focus is on vaccination, and we consider only vaccination prior to the arrival of an outbreak; the situation where vaccination (or other preventive measures) are put into place *during* the outbreak is not considered. “Vaccination” can be interpreted in a wider sense. From a mathematical and spreading point of view, the important feature is that the individual cannot spread the disease further, which could also be achieved by e.g. isolation or medication. Modelling effects of vaccination is also considered in Part II, Section 2.4, and in Part III, Section 2.6, in the current volume.

Suppose that a fraction v of the community is vaccinated prior to the arrival of the disease. We assume that the vaccine is perfect in the sense that it gives 100% protection from being infected and hence of spreading the disease (but see the exercise below). This implies that only a fraction $1-v$ are initially susceptible, and the remaining fraction v are immunized (as discussed briefly in Section 2.1). Hence we can neglect the latter fraction and consider only the initial susceptible part of the community of size $N' = N(1-v)$. However, it is not only the number of initially susceptibles that changes, the rate of having contact with initial susceptibles has also changed to $\lambda' = \lambda(1-v)$, since a fraction v of all contacts are “wasted” on vaccinated people. The spread of disease in a partly-vaccinated community can therefore be modelled using exactly the same SEIR stochastic model with the only difference being that we have a different population size N' and a different contact rate parameter λ'.

From this we conclude the new reproduction number, which we denote R_v to show the dependence on v, satisfies

$$R_v = \lambda' \mathbb{E}(I) = \lambda(1-v)\mathbb{E}(I) = (1-v)R_0.$$

As a consequence, a major outbreak in the community is not possible if $R_v \leq 1$, which (when $R_0 > 1$) is equivalent to $v \geq 1 - 1/R_0$. This limit, called the *critical vaccination coverage* and denoted

$$v_c = 1 - \frac{1}{R_0}, \tag{1.4.1}$$

is hence a very important quantity: if more than this fraction is vaccinated before an outbreak, then the whole community is protected from a major outbreak and not only the vaccinated, a situation called *herd immunity*. Equation (1.4.1) is well known among infectious disease epidemiologists (e.g. Giesecke [14]) and is used by public health authorities all over the world to determine the minimal yearly vaccination coverage in vaccination programs of childhood diseases.

If $v < v_c$ there is still a possibility of a major outbreak. The probability for such an outbreak is obtained using earlier results with λ replaced by $\lambda' = \lambda(1-v)$: the probability of a minor outbreak is the solution s_v to the equation $s = g_v(s)$, where $g_v(\cdot)$ is the probability generating function of $X_v \sim \text{MixPoi}(\lambda(1-v)I)$, the number of offspring (= new infections) in the case that a fraction v are immunized by vaccination.

In the case when there is a major outbreak, the relative size z_v of the outbreak (among the initially susceptible!) is given by the unique positive solution to the equation

$$1 - z = e^{-R_v z}, \text{ or equivalently } 1 - z = e^{-(1-v)R_0 z}, \tag{1.4.2}$$

this result is shown in later sections, cf. Equation (2.1.3). The community fraction getting infected is hence $(1-v)z_v$.

We summarize our result in the following theorem where we let Z_v^N denote the final number infected when a fraction v are vaccinated prior to the outbreak.

Theorem 1.4.1. *If $v \geq v_c = 1 - 1/R_0$, then $Z_v^N/N \to 0$ in probability. If $v < v_c = 1 - 1/R_0$, then $Z_v^N/N \Rightarrow Z_v^\infty$ which has a two-point distribution: $\mathbb{P}(Z_v^\infty = 0) = s_v$ and $\mathbb{P}(Z_v^\infty = (1-v)z_v) = 1 - s_v$, where s_v and z_v have been defined above.*

Exercise 1.4.2. Consider the Markovian SEIR epidemic with $\lambda = 2$, $L \sim \text{Exp}(2)$ and $I \sim \text{Exp}(1)$. Compute the critical vaccination coverage v_c. Compute also numerically the probability of a major outbreak, and the community-fraction that will get infected in the case of a major outbreak when $v = 0.333$.

Exercise 1.4.3. Suppose that the vaccine gives only partial protection to catching and spreading the disease. Suppose that the vaccine has the effect the risk of getting infected by a contact is only 20% of the risk of getting infected when not vaccinated, but that the vaccine has no effect on infectivity if the person gets infected (such a vaccine is said to be a "leaky vaccine" having 80% efficacy on susceptibility and 0% efficacy on infectivity). Compute the reproduction number R_v in the case that a fraction v is vaccinated with such a vaccine. (Another vaccine response model is "all-or-nothing" where a fraction is assumed to receive 100% effect and the remaining fraction receive no effect from vaccination, for example due to the cold chain being broken for a live vaccine.)

Chapter 2
Markov Models

This chapter describes the important class of Markov models. It starts with a presentation of the deterministic ODE models. We then formulate precisely the random Markov epidemic model as a Poisson process driven stochastic differential equation, and establish the law of large numbers (later referred to as LLN), whose limit is precisely the already described ODE model. The next section studies the fluctuations around this LLN limit, which is described by the central limit theorem. Finally we give a diffusion approximation result, i.e. a diffusion process (solution of a Brownian motion driven stochastic differential equation) which, again in the case of a large population, is a good approximation of our Poisson process driven model. One of the earliest references for those three approximation theorems is Kurtz [22]. See also chapter 11 of Ethier and Kurtz [11].

2.1 The Deterministic SEIR Epidemic Model

Before analysing the stochastic SEIR model assuming $N \to \infty$ in greater detail in the following subsections, we first derive heuristically a deterministic counterpart for the Markovian version and study some of its properties, which are relevant also for the asymptotic case of the stochastic model.

Consider the Markovian stochastic SEIR model. There are three types of events: a susceptible gets infected and becomes exposed, an exposed becomes infectious when the latent period terminates, and an infectious individual recovers and becomes immune. Since the model is Markovian all these events happen at rates depending only on the current state, and these rates are respectively given by: $\lambda S(t)I(t)/N$, $\nu E(t)$ and $\gamma I(t)$. When an infection occurs, the number of susceptibles decreases by 1 and the number of exposed increases by 1; when a latency period ends, the number of exposed decreases by 1 and the number of infectives increases by 1; and finally when there is a recovery, the number of infectives decreases by 1 and the number of recovered increases by 1. If we instead look at "proportions" (to simplify notation we divide by N rather than the more appropriate choice $N+1$), the corresponding changes are $-1/N$ and $+1/N$. This reasoning

T. Britton, E. Pardoux (eds.), *Stochastic Epidemic Models with Inference*,
Lecture Notes in Mathematics 2255, https://doi.org/10.1007/978-3-030-30900-8_2

justifies a deterministic model for proportions where one should think of an infinite population size allowing the proportions to be continuous. The deterministic SEIR epidemic $(s(t), e(t), i(t), r(t))$ is given by

$$s'(t) = -\lambda s(t)i(t),$$
$$e'(t) = \lambda s(t)i(t) - \nu e(t),$$
$$i'(t) = \nu e(t) - \gamma i(t),$$
$$r'(t) = \gamma i(t).$$

We start with all fractions being non-negative and summing to unity, which implies that $s(t) + e(t) + i(t) + r(t) = 1$ and all being nonnegative for all t. It is important to stress that this system of differential equations only approximates the *Markovian* SEIR model. If for example the latent and infectious stages are non-random, then a set of differential-delay equations would be the appropriate approximation. If these durations are random but not exponential one possible pragmatic assumption is to use a gamma distribution where the shape parameter is an integer (so it can be seen as a sum of i.i.d. exponentials). Then the deterministic approximation would be a set of differential equations where the state space has been expanded. Just like for the stochastic SEIR model, the deterministic model has to start with a positive fraction of exposed and/or infectives for anything to happen. Most often it is assumed that there is a very small fraction ε of latent and/or infectives.

The case where there is no latent period meaning that $\nu \to \infty$, the deterministic SIR epidemic (or deterministic general epidemic), sometimes called the Kermack–McKendrick equations, has perhaps received more attention in the literature:

$$\begin{cases} s'(t) = -\lambda s(t)i(t), \\ i'(t) = \lambda s(t)i(t) - \gamma i(t), \\ r'(t) = \gamma i(t). \end{cases} \tag{2.1.1}$$

This system of differential equations (and the SEIR system on the previous page) are undoubtedly the most commonly analysed epidemic models (e.g. Anderson and May [1]), and numerous related extended models, capturing various heterogeneous aspects of disease spreading, are published every year in mathematical biology journals.

The deterministic SEIR and SIR share the two most important properties in that they have the same basic reproduction number R_0 and give the same final size (assuming the initial number of infectives/exposed are positive but negligible in both cases), which we now show. In Figure 2.1.1 both the SEIR and SIR systems are plotted for the same values of $\lambda = 1.5$ and $\gamma = 1$ (so $R_0 = 1.5$), and with $\nu = 1$ in the SEIR system.

From the differential equations we see that $s(t)$ is monotonically decreasing and $r(t)$ monotonically increasing. The differential for $i(t)$ in the SIR model can be written $i'(t) = \gamma i(t)\left(\frac{\lambda}{\gamma}s(t) - 1\right)$. The initial value is $i(0) = \varepsilon \approx 0$ and $s(0) = 1 - \varepsilon \approx 1$. From this we see that for having $i'(0) > 0$ we need that $\lambda/\gamma > 1$. If this holds, $i(t)$ grows up until $s(t) < \gamma/\lambda$ after which $i(t)$ decays down to 0. If on the other

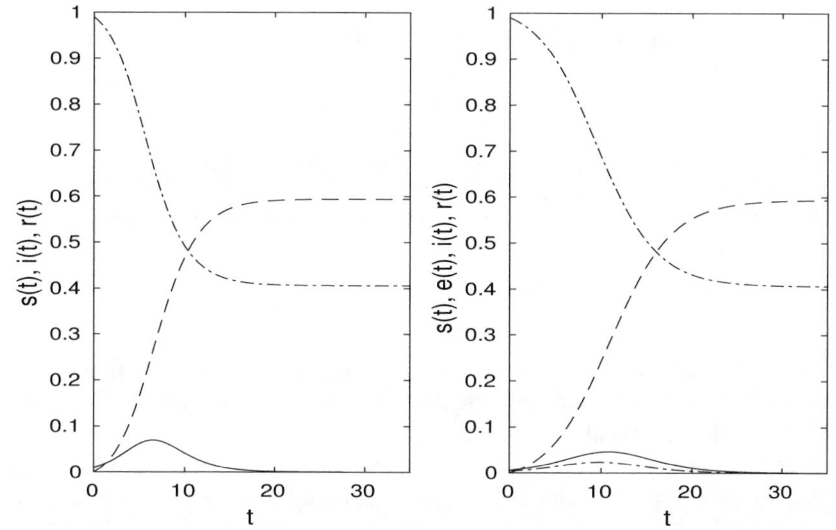

Fig. 2.1.1 Plot of the deterministic SIR (left) and SEIR (right) systems for $\lambda = 1.5$ and $\gamma = 1$, and with $\nu = 1$ in the SEIR model. The dash-dotted curve is the fraction of susceptibles, the solid curve the fraction of infectives, the dashed curve the fraction of recovered, and the lowest curve in the right figure is the fraction of exposed (latent).

hand $\lambda/\gamma \leq 1$, then $i(t)$ is decreasing from the start and since its initial value is $\varepsilon \approx 0$, nothing much will happen so $s(\infty) \approx s(0) \approx 1$ and $r(\infty) \approx r(0) = 0$. We hence see that also in the deterministic model, $R_0 = \lambda/\gamma$ plays an important role in that whether or not R_0 exceeds 1 determines whether there will be a substantial or a negligible fraction getting infected during the outbreak. Note that this is the same R_0 as for the Markovian SEIR epidemic. There the infectious period is exponentially distributed with parameter γ, so $\iota := E(I) = 1/\gamma$.

An important difference between deterministic and stochastic epidemic models lies in the initial values. Stochastic models usually start with a small *number* of infectious individuals (in the model of the current Notes we assumed one initial infective: $I(0) = 1$). This implies that the initial *fraction* of infectives tend to 0 as $N \to \infty$. In the deterministic setting we however have to assume a fixed and strictly positive fraction ε of initially infectives (if we start with a fraction 0 of infectives nothing happens in the deterministic model). This implicitly implies that the deterministic model starts to approximate the stochastic counterpart only when the number of infectives in the stochastic model has grown up to a *fraction* ε, so a number $N\varepsilon$. The earlier part of the stochastic model cannot be approximated by this deterministic model, and as we have seen it might in fact never reach this level (if there is only a minor outbreak).

In order to derive an expression for the ultimate fraction getting infected we use the differential for $s(t)$ (and below also the one for $r(t)$). Dividing by s and multiplying by dt gives the following differential: $ds/s = -\lambda i dt$. Integrating both sides and recalling that $R_0 = \lambda/\gamma$, we obtain

$$\begin{aligned}
\log s(t) - \log s(0) &= -\lambda \int_0^t i(t)dt \\
&= -R_0 \int_0^t r'(s)ds \\
&= -R_0(r(t) - r(0)) = -R_0 r(t).
\end{aligned}$$

And since $s(0) = 1 - \varepsilon \approx 1$ and $r(\infty) = 1 - s(\infty)$ we obtain the following equation for the final size $z = r(\infty) = 1 - s(\infty)$:

$$1 - z = e^{-R_0 z}. \tag{2.1.2}$$

In Section 3.3.1 we show that this final size equation coincides with that of the LLN limit of the final fraction getting infected in the stochastic model (cf. Equation (3.3.2), which is identical to (2.1.2)).

The equation always has a root at $z = 0$ corresponding to no (or minor) outbreak. It can be shown (cf. Exercise 2.1.1) that if and only if $R_0 > 1$ there is a second solution to (2.1.2), corresponding to the size of a major outbreak, and this solution z^* is strictly positive and smaller than 1. For a given value of $R_0 > 1$ the solution z^* has to be computed numerically. In Figure 2.1.2 the solution is plotted as a function of R_0.

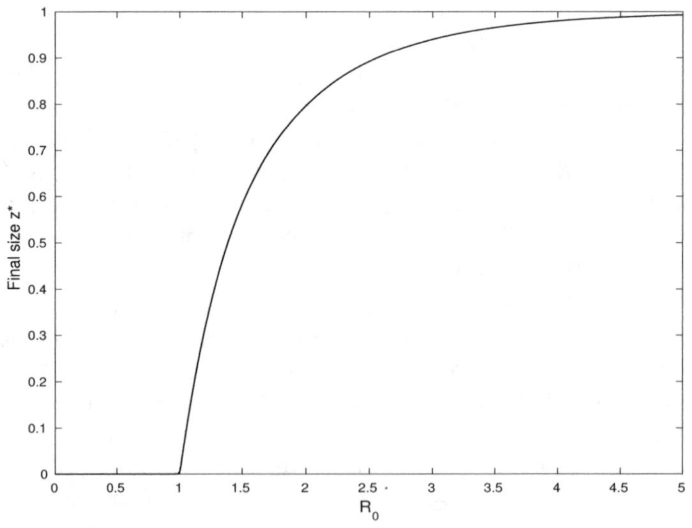

Fig. 2.1.2 Plot of the final size solution z^* to Equation (2.1.2) as a function of R_0.

It is important to point out that the final size equation (2.1.2) assumes that, at $t = 0$, all individuals (except the very few initially latent and infectives) are susceptible. If a fraction v is initially immune (perhaps due to natural immunity, or vaccination as described in Section 1.4) then $r(0) = v$ and $s(0) = 1 - v$, resulting in the equation

$$1 - z = e^{-R_0 z(1-v)}, \tag{2.1.3}$$

where its solution z_v now is interpreted as the fraction among the initially susceptible that get infected. The overall fraction getting infected is hence $z_v(1-v)$. Using the same argument as for the final size without immunity, we conclude that $z = 0$ is the only solution if $R_0(1-v) \leq 1$. This is equivalent to $v \geq 1 - 1/R_0$. If immunity was caused by vaccination, this hence suggests that a fraction exceeding $v_c = 1 - 1/R_0$ should be vaccinated; then there will be no outbreak! For this reason, the quantity $v_c = 1 - 1/R_0$ is often called the *critical vaccination coverage*, and if this coverage is reached, so-called *herd immunity* is achieved. Herd immunity implies that not only the vaccinated are protected, but so are also the unvaccinated, since the community is protected from epidemic outbreaks.

Exercise 2.1.1. Show that $z = 0$ is the only solution to (2.1.2) when $R_0 \leq 1$ and that there is a unique positive solution if $R_0 > 1$. (*Hint*: Study suitable properties of the function $f(z) = e^{-R_0 z} + z - 1$.)

Exercise 2.1.2. Compute the final size numerically for $R_0 = 1.5$ (e.g. influenza), $R_0 = 3$ (e.g. rubella) and $R_0 = 15$ (e.g. measles).

2.2 Law of Large Numbers

Consider a general compartmental model, which takes the form

$$\mathscr{Z}_t^N = z_N + \sum_{j=1}^{k} h_j P_j \left(\int_0^t \beta_{N,j}(s, \mathscr{Z}_s^N) ds \right),$$

where the P_js are mutually independent standard (i.e. unit rate) Poisson processes, and $\beta_{N,j}(t, \mathscr{Z}_t^N)$ is the rate of jumps in the direction h_j at time t, h_j being a d-dimensional vector. $\mathscr{Z}_t^N$ takes values in $\mathbb{Z}_+^d$. The i-th component of $\mathscr{Z}_t^N$ is the number of individuals in the i-th compartment at time t. N is a scale parameter. In the case of models with fixed total population size, $N = \sum_{i=1}^d Z_t^{N,i}$ is the total population at any time t. Note that the above formula for $\mathscr{Z}_t^N$ can be rewritten equivalently, following the comments at the end of Section A.2 in the Appendix below, as

$$\mathscr{Z}_t^N = z_N + \sum_{j=1}^{k} h_j \int_0^t \int_0^{\beta_{N,j}(s, \mathscr{Z}_s^N)} Q_j(ds, du),$$

where $Q_1, \ldots, Q_k$ are mutually independent Poisson random measures on $\mathbb{R}_+^2$, with mean measure $ds\,du$.

We now define

$$Z_t^N = N^{-1} \mathscr{Z}_t^N$$

the vector of rescaled numbers of individuals in the various compartments. In the case of a constant population size equal to N, the components of the vector Z_t^N are the proportions of the total population in the various compartments at time t. The equation for Z_t^N reads, with $x_N = N^{-1}z_N$,

$$Z_t^N = x_N + \sum_{j=1}^{k} \frac{h_j}{N} P_j \left(\int_0^t \beta_{N,j}(s, NZ_s^N) ds \right).$$

Example 2.2.1 (The SIR model).

One important example is that of the *SIR* model with constant population size. Suppose there is no latency period and that the duration of infection satisfies $I \sim \text{Exp}(\gamma)$. In that case, let $S(t)$, $I(t)$, and $R(t)$) denote respectively the number of susceptibles, infectives and recovered at time t.

In this model, two types of events happen:

1. infection of a susceptible (such an event decreases $S(t)$ by one, and increases $I(t)$ by one, so $h_1 = (-1,1,0)$); these events happen at rate
$$\beta_{N,1}(t, \mathscr{Z}_t) = \frac{\lambda}{N} S(t)I(t), \quad \text{where } \lambda = cp;$$
2. recovery of an infective (such an event decreases $I(t)$ by one, and increases $R(t)$ by one, so $h_2 = (0,-1,1)$); these events happen at rate
$$\beta_{N,2}(t, \mathscr{Z}_t) = \gamma I(t).$$

Hence we have the following equations, with $P_1(t)$ and $P_2(t)$ two standard mutually independent Poisson processes:

$$\begin{aligned} S(t) &= S(0) - P_1\left(\frac{\lambda}{N}\int_0^t S(r)I(r)dr\right), \\ I(t) &= I(0) + P_1\left(\frac{\lambda}{N}\int_0^t S(r)I(r)dr\right) - P_2\left(\gamma\int_0^t I(r)dr\right), \\ R(t) &= R(0) + P_2\left(\gamma\int_0^t I(r)dr\right). \end{aligned}$$

We can clearly forget about the third equation, since $R(t) = N - S(t) - I(t)$.

We now define $(S^N(t), I^N(t)) = (N^{-1}S(t), N^{-1}I(t))$. We have

$$\begin{aligned} S^N(t) &= S^N(0) - \frac{1}{N}P_1\left(N\lambda\int_0^t S^N(r)I^N(r)dr\right), \\ I^N(t) &= I^N(0) + \frac{1}{N}P_1\left(N\lambda\int_0^t S^N(r)I^N(r)dr\right) - \frac{1}{N}P_2\left(N\gamma\int_0^t I^N(r)dr\right). \end{aligned}$$

The above model assumes that λ and γ are constant, but in applications at least λ may depend upon t.

Example 2.2.2 (The SEIRS model with demography).

We now describe one rather general example. We add to the preceding example the state E and the fact that removed individuals lose their immunity at a certain rate, which gives the SEIRS model. In addition, we add demography. There is an influx of susceptible individuals at rate μN, and each individual, irrespective of its type, dies at rate μ. This gives the following stochastic differential equation

$$
\begin{aligned}
S(t) &= S(0) - P_{se}\left(\frac{\lambda}{N}\int_0^t S(r)I(r)dr\right) + P_{rs}\left(\rho\int_0^t R(r)dr\right) \\
&\quad + P_b(\mu N t) - P_{ds}\left(\mu\int_0^t S(r)dr\right), \\
E(t) &= E(0) + P_{se}\left(\frac{\lambda}{N}\int_0^t S(r)I(r)dr\right) - P_{ei}\left(\nu\int_0^t E(r)dr\right) \\
&\quad - P_{de}\left(\mu\int_0^t E(r)dr\right), \\
I(t) &= I(0) + P_{ei}\left(\nu\int_0^t E(r)dr\right) - P_{ir}\left(\gamma\int_0^t I(r)dr\right) - P_{di}\left(\mu\int_0^t I(r)dr\right), \\
R(t) &= R(0) + P_{ir}\left(\gamma\int_0^t I(r)dr\right) - P_{rs}\left(\rho\int_0^t R(r)dr\right) - P_{dr}\left(\mu\int_0^t R(r)dr\right).
\end{aligned}
$$

In this system, the various Poisson processes are standard and mutually independent. The indices should be self-explanatory. Note that the rate of births is $\mu \times N$ rather than $\mu\times$ the actual number of individuals in the population, in order to avoid the pitfalls of branching processes (either exponential growth or extinction). Also, the probability $S(t)/N(t)$ that an infective meets a susceptible (where $N(t)$ denotes the total population at time t) is approximated by $S(t)/N$ for the sake of mathematical simplicity. Note however that $\frac{N(t)}{N} \to 1$ a.s. as $N \to \infty$, see Exercise 4.1.1 below. The equations for the proportions in the various compartments read

$$
\begin{aligned}
S^N(t) &= S^N(0) - \frac{1}{N}P_{se}\left(N\lambda\int_0^t S^N(r)I^N(r)dr\right) + \frac{1}{N}P_{rs}\left(N\rho\int_0^t R^N(r)dr\right) \\
&\quad + \frac{1}{N}P_b(\mu N t) - \frac{1}{N}P_{ds}\left(\mu N\int_0^t S^N(r)dr\right), \\
E^N(t) &= E^N(0) + \frac{1}{N}P_{se}\left(N\lambda\int_0^t S^N(r)I^N(r)dr\right) \\
&\quad - \frac{1}{N}P_{ei}\left(\nu N\int_0^t E^N(r)dr\right) - \frac{1}{N}P_{de}\left(\mu N\int_0^t E^N(r)dr\right), \\
I^N(t) &= I^N(0) + \frac{1}{N}P_{ei}\left(\nu N\int_0^t E^N(r)dr\right) - \frac{1}{N}P_{ir}\left(N\gamma\int_0^t I^N(r)dr\right) \\
&\quad - \frac{1}{N}P_{di}\left(\mu N\int_0^t I^N(r)dr\right),
\end{aligned}
$$

$$R^N(t) = R^N(0) + \frac{1}{N}P_{ir}\left(N\gamma\int_0^t I^N(r)dr\right) - \frac{1}{N}P_{rs}\left(N\rho\int_0^t R^N(r)dr\right)$$
$$-\frac{1}{N}P_{dr}\left(\mu N\int_0^t R^N(r)dr\right).$$

Example 2.2.3 (A variant of the SEIRS model with demography).

In the preceding example, we decided to replace the true proportion of susceptibles by its approximation $S(t)/N$, in order to avoid complications. There is another option, which is to force the population to remain constant. The most natural way to achieve this is to assume that each death event coincides with a birth event. Every susceptible, exposed, infected, removed individual dies at rate μ. Each death is compensated by the birth of a susceptible. The equation for the evolution of $(S(t), E(t), I(t), R(t))$ reads

$$\begin{aligned}
S(t) = S(0) &- P_{se}\left(\frac{\lambda}{N}\int_0^t S(r)I(r)dr\right) + P_{rs}\left(\rho\int_0^t R(r)dr\right)\\
&+ P_{ds}\left(\mu\int_0^t S(r)dr\right) + P_{de}\left(\mu\int_0^t E(r)dr\right) + P_{di}\left(\mu\int_0^t I(r)dr\right)\\
&+ P_{dr}\left(\mu\int_0^t R(r)dr\right) - P_{ds}\left(\mu\int_0^t S(r)dr\right),\\
E(t) = E(0) &+ P_{se}\left(\frac{\lambda}{N}\int_0^t S(r)I(r)dr\right) - P_{ei}\left(\nu\int_0^t E(r)dr\right)\\
&- P_{de}\left(\mu\int_0^t E(r)dr\right),\\
I(t) = I(0) &+ P_{ei}\left(\nu\int_0^t E(r)dr\right) - P_{ir}\left(\gamma\int_0^t I(r)dr\right) - P_{di}\left(\mu\int_0^t I(r)dr\right),\\
R(t) = R(0) &+ P_{ir}\left(\gamma\int_0^t I(r)dr\right) - P_{rs}\left(\rho\int_0^t R(r)dr\right) - P_{dr}\left(\mu\int_0^t R(r)dr\right).
\end{aligned}$$

The equations for the proportions in the various compartments read

$$\begin{aligned}
S^N(t) = S^N(0) &- \frac{1}{N}P_{se}\left(N\lambda\int_0^t S^N(r)I^N(r)dr\right)\\
&+ \frac{1}{N}P_{rs}\left(N\rho\int_0^t R^N(r)dr\right) + \frac{1}{N}P_{ds}\left(N\mu\int_0^t S^N(r)dr\right)\\
&+ \frac{1}{N}P_{de}\left(N\mu\int_0^t E^N(r)dr\right) + \frac{1}{N}P_{di}\left(N\mu\int_0^t I^N(r)dr\right)\\
&+ \frac{1}{N}P_{dr}\left(N\mu\int_0^t R^N(r)dr\right) - \frac{1}{N}P_{ds}\left(N\mu\int_0^t S^N(r)dr\right),\\
E^N(t) = E^N(0) &+ \frac{1}{N}P_{se}\left(N\lambda\int_0^t S^N(r)I^N(r)dr\right) - \frac{1}{N}P_{ei}\left(N\nu\int_0^t E^N(r)dr\right)\\
&- \frac{1}{N}P_{de}\left(N\mu\int_0^t E^N(r)dr\right),
\end{aligned}$$

$$I^N(t) = I^N(0) + \frac{1}{N}P_{ei}\left(\nu\int_0^t E^N(r)dr\right) - \frac{1}{N}P_{ir}\left(\gamma\int_0^t I^N(r)dr\right)$$
$$- \frac{1}{N}P_{di}\left(N\mu\int_0^t I^N(r)dr\right),$$
$$R^N(t) = R^N(0) + \frac{1}{N}P_{ir}\left(N\gamma\int_0^t I^N(r)dr\right) - \frac{1}{N}P_{rs}\left(N\rho\int_0^t R^N(r)dr\right)$$
$$- \frac{1}{N}P_{dr}\left(N\mu\int_0^t R^N(r)dr\right).$$

In the three above examples, for each j, $\beta_{N,j}(t,Nz) = N\beta_j(t,z)$, for some $\beta_j(t,z)$ which does not depend upon N. We shall assume from now on that this is the case in our general model, namely that

$$\beta_{N,j}(t,Nz) = N\beta_j(t,z), \quad \text{for all } 1 \le j \le k,\ N \ge 1,\ z \in \mathbb{R}_+^d.$$

Remark 2.2.4. We could assume more generally that

$$\beta_{N,j}(t,Nz) = N\widetilde{\beta}_{N,j}(t,z), \ \text{ where } \widetilde{\beta}_{N,j}(t,z) \to \beta_j(t,z),$$

locally uniformly as $N \to \infty$.

Finally our model reads

$$Z_t^N = x_N + \sum_{j=1}^k \frac{h_j}{N}P_j\left(\int_0^t N\beta_j(s,Z_s^N)ds\right). \tag{2.2.1}$$

We note that in the first example above, $0 \le Z_j^N(t) \le 1$ for all $1 \le j \le k$, $t \ge 0$, $N \ge 1$. In the second example however, such a simple upper bound does not hold, but a much weaker assumption will suffice.

We assume that all β_j are locally bounded, which is clearly satisfied in all examples we can think of, so that for any $K > 0$,

$$C(T,K) := \sup_{1\le j\le k}\sup_{0\le t\le T}\sup_{|z|\le K}\beta_j(t,z) < \infty. \tag{2.2.2}$$

We first prove the Law of Large Numbers for Poisson processes.

Proposition 2.2.5. *Let $\{P(t),\ t \ge 0\}$ be a rate λ Poisson process. Then*

$$t^{-1}P(t) \to \lambda \ \ a.s.\ as\ t \to \infty.$$

Proof. Consider first for $n \in \mathbb{Z}_+$

$$n^{-1}P(n) = n^{-1}\sum_{i=1}^n [P(i) - P(i-1)]$$
$$\to \lambda \ \text{ a.s. as } n \to \infty$$

from the standard strong Law of Large Numbers, since the random variables $P(i) - P(i-1)$, $1 \le i \le n$ are i.i.d. Poisson with parameter λ. Now

$$t^{-1}P(t) = \frac{[t]}{t}[t]^{-1}P([t]) + t^{-1}\{P(t) - P([t])\},$$

$$\text{so } |t^{-1}P(t) - \lambda| \le \left|\frac{[t]}{t}[t]^{-1}P([t]) - \lambda\right| + t^{-1}\{P([t]+1) - P([t])\}.$$

But

$$t^{-1}\{P([t]+1) - P([t])\} = t^{-1}P([t]+1) - t^{-1}P([t])$$

is the difference of two sequences which converge a.s. towards the same limit, hence it converges to 0 a.s. □

Define the continuous time martingales (see Section A.4.2 in the Appendix) $M_j(t) = P_j(t) - t$, $1 \le j \le k$. We have

$$Z_t^N = x_N + \int_0^t b(s, Z_s^N)ds + \sum_{j=1}^k \frac{h_j}{N} M_j\left(\int_0^t N\beta_j(s, Z_s^N)ds\right),$$

where

$$b(t,x) = \sum_{j=1}^k h_j \beta_j(t,x).$$

Consider the k-dimensional process $\mathcal{M}^N(t)$ whose j-th component is defined as

$$\mathcal{M}_j^N(t) := \frac{1}{N} M_j\left(N\int_0^t \beta_j(r, Z_r^N)dr\right).$$

From the above, we readily deduce the following.

Proposition 2.2.6. *For any $K > 0$, let $\tau_K := \inf\{t > 0, |Z_t^N| \ge K\}$. As $N \to \infty$, for all $T > 0$, provided* (2.2.2) *holds,*

$$\sup_{0 \le t \le T \wedge \tau_K} |\mathcal{M}^N(t)| \to 0 \ a.s.$$

Proof. In order to simplify the notation we treat the case $d = 1$. It follows from (2.2.2) that, if $M(t) = P(t) - t$ and N is large enough,

$$\sup_{0 \le t \le T \wedge \tau_K} |\mathcal{M}^N(t)| \le \frac{1}{N} \sup_{0 \le r \le NTC(T,K)} |M(r)|.$$

From the previous proposition, for all $t > 0$,

$$\frac{P(Nt)}{N} \to t \quad \text{a.s. as } N \to \infty.$$

Note that we have pointwise convergence of a sequence of increasing functions towards a continuous (and of course increasing) function. Consequently from the second Dini Theorem (see e.g. pages 81 and 270 in Polya and Szegö [30]), this convergence is uniform on any compact interval, hence for all $T > 0$,

$$\frac{1}{N}\sup_{0\le r\le NTC(T,K)}|M(r)| \to 0 \text{ a.s.}$$

□

Concerning the initial condition, we assume that for some $x \in [0,1]^d$, $x_N = [Nx]/N$, where $[Nx]$ is of course a vector of integers. We can now prove the following theorem.

Theorem 2.2.7 (Law of Large Numbers). *Assume that the initial condition is given as above, that* $b(t,x) = \sum_{j=1}^k \beta_j(t,x)h_j$ *is locally Lipschitz as a function of* x*, locally uniformly in* t*, that* (2.2.2) *holds and that the unique solution of the ODE*

$$\frac{dz_t}{dt} = b(t,z_t), \quad z_0 = x$$

does not explode in finite time. Let Z_t^N *denote the solution of the SDE* (2.2.1). *Then* $Z_t^N \to z_t$ *a.s. locally uniformly in* t*, where* $\{z_t, t \ge 0\}$ *is the unique solution of the above ODE.*

Needless to say, our theorem applies to the general model (2.2.1). We shall describe below three specific models to which we can apply it. Note that if the initial fraction of infected is zero, then the fraction of infected is zero for all $t \ge 0$.

Proof. We have

$$Z_t^N = x_N + \int_0^t b(s,Z_s^N)ds + \sum_{j=1}^k h_j \mathscr{M}_j^N(t).$$

Let us fix an arbitrary $T > 0$. We want to show uniform convergence on $[0,T]$. Let $K := \sup_{0\le t\le T}|z_t| + C$, where $C > 0$ is arbitrary, and let $\tau_K = \inf\{t > 0, |Z_t^N| \ge K\}$. Since $b(t,\cdot)$ is locally Lipschitz,

$$c_{T,K} := \sup_{0\le t\le T, x\ne x', |x|,|x'|\le K} \frac{|b(t,x)-b(t,x')|}{|x-x'|} < \infty.$$

For any $0 \le t \le T$, if we define $Y_t^N = \sum_{j=1}^k h_j \mathscr{M}_j^N(t)$, we have

$$\begin{aligned}|Z_{t\wedge\tau_K}^N - z_{t\wedge\tau_K}| &\le |x_N - x| + c_{T,K}\int_0^{t\wedge\tau_K}|Z_s^N - z_s|ds + |Y_{t\wedge\tau_K}^N| \\ &\le \varepsilon_N \exp(c_{T,K}t),\end{aligned}$$

where $\varepsilon_N := |x_N - x| + \sup_{0\le t\le T\wedge\tau_K} |Y_t^N|$ and we have used Gronwall's Lemma 2.2.9 below. It follows from our assumption on x_N and Proposition 2.2.6 that $\varepsilon_N \to 0$ as $N \to \infty$. The result follows, since as soon as $\varepsilon_N \exp(c_{T,K}T) \le C$, $\tau_K \ge T$. □

Remark 2.2.8. Showing that a stochastic epidemic model (for population proportions) converges to a particular deterministic process is important also for applications. This motivates the use of deterministic models, which are easier to analyse, in the case of large populations.

Lemma 2.2.9 (Gronwall). *Let $a, b \ge 0$ and $\varphi : [0,T] \to \mathbb{R}$ be such that for all $0 \le t \le T$,*

$$\varphi(t) \le a + b\int_0^t \varphi(r)dr.$$

Then $\varphi(t) \le ae^{bt}$.

Proof. We deduce from the assumption that

$$e^{-bt}\varphi(t) - be^{-bt}\int_0^t \varphi(r)dr \le ae^{-bt},$$

or in other words

$$\frac{d}{dt}\left(e^{-bt}\int_0^t \varphi(r)dr\right) \le ae^{-bt}.$$

Integrating this inequality, we deduce

$$e^{-bt}\int_0^t \varphi(r)dr \le a\frac{1-e^{-bt}}{b}.$$

Multiplying by be^{bt} and exploiting again the assumption yields the result. □

Example 2.2.10 (The SIR model). It is clear that Theorem 2.2.7 applies to Example 2.2.1. The limit of $(S^N(t), I^N(t))$ is the solution $(s(t), i(t))$ of the ODE

$$\begin{aligned} s'(t) &= -\lambda s(t)i(t), \\ i'(t) &= \lambda s(t)i(t) - \gamma i(t). \end{aligned}$$

Example 2.2.11 (The SEIRS model with demography (continued)). Again Theorem 2.2.7 applies to Example 2.2.2. The limit of $(S^N(t), E^N(t), I^N(t), R^N(t))$ is the solution $(s(t), e(t), i(t), r(t))$ of the ODE

$$\begin{aligned} s'(t) &= \mu(1 - s(t)) - \lambda s(t)i(t) + \rho r(t), \\ e'(t) &= \lambda s(t)i(t) - (\nu + \mu)e(t), \\ i'(t) &= \nu e(t) - (\gamma + \mu)i(t), \\ r'(t) &= \gamma i(t) - (\rho + \mu)r(t). \end{aligned}$$

Note that of we define the total renormalized population as $n(t) = s(t) + e(t) + i(t) + r(t)$, then it is easy to deduce from the above ODE that $n'(t) = \mu(1 - n(t))$, consequently $n(t) = 1 + e^{-\mu t}(n(0) - 1)$. If $n(0) = 1$, then $n(t) \equiv 1$, and we can reduce the above model to a three-dimensional model (and to a two-dimensional model as in the previous example if we are treating the SIR or the SIRS model with demography).

We note that this "Law of Large Numbers" approximation is only valid when $s, i > 0$, i.e. when significant fractions of the population are infective and are susceptible, in particular at time 0. The ODE is of course of no help to compute the probability that the introduction of a single infective results in a major epidemic.

The vast majority of the literature on mathematical models in epidemiology considers ODEs of the type of equations which we have just obtained. The probabilistic point of view is more recent.

Exercise 2.2.12. Let us consider Ross's model of malaria, which we write in a stochastic form. Denote by $H(t)$ the number of humans (hosts) who are infected by malaria, and by $V(t)$ the number of mosquitos (vectors) who are infected by malaria at time t. Let N_H denote the total number of humans, and N_V denote the total number of mosquitos, which are assumed to be constant in time. The humans (resp. the mosquitos) which are not infected are all supposed to be susceptibles. Let $m = N_V/N_H$ and denote by a the mean number of bites of humans by one mosquito per time unit, p_{VH} the probability that the bite of a susceptible human by an infected mosquito infects the human, and by p_{HV} the probability that a susceptible mosquito gets infected while biting an infected human. We assume that the infected humans (resp. mosquitos) recover at rate γ (resp. at rate μ).

1. What is the mean number of bites that a human suffers per time unit?
2. Given 4 mutually independent standard Poisson processes $P_1(t), P_2(t), P_3(t)$ and $P_4(t)$, justify the following as a stochastic model of the propagation of malaria.

$$H(t) = H(0) + P_1\left(ap_{VH}\int_0^t V(s)\frac{N_H - H(s)}{N_H}ds\right) - P_2\left(\gamma\int_0^t H(s)ds\right)$$
$$V(t) = V(0) + P_3\left(amp_{HV}\int_0^t H(s)\frac{N_V - V(s)}{N_V}ds\right) - P_4\left(\mu\int_0^t V(s)ds\right).$$

3. Define now (with $N_H = N$, $N_V = mN$)

$$h_N(t) = \frac{H(t)}{N_H}, \quad v_N(t) = \frac{V(t)}{N_V}.$$

Write the equation for the pair $(h_N(t), v_N(t))$. Show that as $N \to \infty$, with m constant, $(h_N(t), v_N(t)) \to (h(t), v(t))$, the solution of Ross's ODE:

$$\frac{dh}{dt}(t) = ap_{VH}mv(t)(1 - h(t)) - \gamma h(t),$$
$$\frac{dv}{dt}(t) = ap_{HV}h(t)(1 - v(t)) - \mu v(t).$$

2.3 Central Limit Theorem

In the previous section we have shown that the stochastic process describing the evolution of the proportions of the total population in the various compartments converges, in the asymptotic of large population, to the deterministic solution of a system of ODEs. In the current section we look at fluctuations of the difference between the stochastic epidemic process and its deterministic limit.

We now introduce the rescaled difference between Z_t^N and z_t, namely

$$U_t^N = \sqrt{N}(Z_t^N - z_t).$$

We wish to show that U_t^N converges in law to a Gaussian process. It is clear that

$$U_t^N = \sqrt{N}(x_N - x) + \sqrt{N}\int_0^t [b(s,Z_s^N) - b(s,z_s)]ds + \sum_{j=1}^k h_j \widetilde{\mathcal{M}_j^N}(t),$$

where for $1 \le j \le k$,

$$\widetilde{\mathcal{M}_j^N}(t) = \frac{1}{\sqrt{N}} M_j\left(N\int_0^t \beta_j(r,Z_r^N)dr\right).$$

We certainly need to find the limit in law of the k dimensional process $\widetilde{\mathcal{M}_t^N}$, whose j-th coordinate is $\widetilde{\mathcal{M}_j^N}(t)$. We prove the following proposition below.

Proposition 2.3.1. *As $N \to \infty$,*

$$\{\widetilde{\mathcal{M}_t^N}, t \ge 0\} \Rightarrow \{\widetilde{\mathcal{M}_t}, t \ge 0\}$$

meaning weak convergence for the topology of locally uniform convergence, where for $1 \le j \le k$, $\widetilde{\mathcal{M}_j}(t) = \int_0^t \sqrt{\beta_j(s,z_s)}dB_j(s)$ and the processes $B_1(t), \ldots, B_k(t)$ are mutually independent standard Brownian motions.

Let us first show that the main result of this section is indeed a consequence of this proposition.

Theorem 2.3.2 (Central Limit Theorem). *In addition to the assumptions of Theorem 2.2.7, we assume that $x \to b(t,x)$ is of class C^1, locally uniformly in t. Then, as $N \to \infty$, $\{U_t^N, t \ge 0\} \Rightarrow \{U_t, t \ge 0\}$, where*

$$U_t = \int_0^t \nabla_x b(s,z_s)U_s ds + \sum_{j=1}^k h_j \int_0^t \sqrt{\beta_j(s,z_s)}dB_j(s),\ t \ge 0. \tag{2.3.1}$$

Proof. We shall fix an arbitrary $T > 0$ throughout the proof. Let $V^N(s) := \sqrt{N}[b(s,Z_s^N) - b(s,z_s)]$ and $\widetilde{\mathcal{N}_t^N} := \sum_{j=1}^k h_j \widetilde{\mathcal{M}_j^N}(t)$. We have

$$U_t^N = U_0^N + \int_0^t V^N(s)ds + \widetilde{\mathcal{N}_t^N}.$$

Let us admit for the moment the following lemma.

Lemma 2.3.3. *For each $N \geq 1$, $0 \leq t \leq T$ there exists a random $d \times d$ matrix A_t^N such that*

$$V_t^N = \nabla b(t, z_t) U_t^N + A_t^N U_t^N.$$

Moreover, $\sup_{0 \leq t \leq T} \|A_t^N\| \to 0$, *a.s., as* $N \to \infty$.

We clearly have

$$U_t^N = U_0^N + \int_0^t [\nabla b(s, z_s) + A_s^N] U_s^N ds + \widetilde{\mathscr{N}}_t^N.$$

It then follows from Gronwall's Lemma that

$$\sup_{0 \leq t \leq T} |U_t^N| \leq \left(|U_0^N| + \sup_{0 \leq t \leq T} |\widetilde{\mathscr{N}}_t^N| \right) \exp\left(\sup_{0 \leq t \leq T} \|\nabla b(t, z_t) + A_t^N\| \, T \right).$$

The right-hand side of this inequality is tight,[1] hence the same is true for the left-hand side. From this and Lemma 2.3.3 it follows that $R_t^N := A_t^N U_t^N$ tends to 0 in probability as $N \to \infty$, uniformly for $0 \leq t \leq T$. Consequently

$$U_t^N = \int_0^t \nabla_x b(s, z_s) U_s^N ds + W_t^N, \text{ where}$$

$$W_t^N = U_0^N + \int_0^t R_s^N ds + \widetilde{\mathscr{N}}_t^N.$$

The following two hold

1. $\sup_{0 \leq t \leq T} |U_0^N + \int_0^t R_s^N ds| \to 0$ in probability, and from Proposition 2.3.1 $\widetilde{\mathscr{N}}_t^N \Rightarrow \widetilde{\mathscr{N}}_t$, hence $W_t^N \Rightarrow \widetilde{\mathscr{N}}_t$ for the topology of uniform convergence on $[0, T]$.
2. The mapping $y \mapsto \Phi(y)$, which to $y \in C([0, T]; \mathbb{R}^d)$ associates $x \in C([0, T]; \mathbb{R}^d)$, the solution of the ODE

$$x(t) = \int_0^t \nabla b(s, z_s) x(s) ds + y(t),$$

is continuous.
Indeed, we can construct this mapping by first solving the ODE

$$\dot{z}(t) = \nabla b(t, z_t)[z(t) + y(t)], \quad z(0) = 0,$$

and then defining $x(t) = z(t) + y(t)$.

Since

$$U^N = \Phi(W^N),$$

the result follows from 1. and 2., and the fact that T is arbitrary. □

Proof of Lemma 2.3.3. For $1 \leq i \leq d, 0 \leq t \leq T$, define the random function $\rho_{i,t}(\theta) = b_i(t, z_t + \theta(Z_t^N - z_t))$, $0 \leq \theta \leq 1$. The mean value theorem applied to the function

[1] A sequence ξ_n of $\mathbb{R}_+$-valued random variables is tight if for any $\varepsilon > 0$, there exists an M_ε such that $\mathbb{P}(\xi_n > M_\varepsilon) \leq \varepsilon$, for all $n \geq 1$, see Section A.5 in the Appendix.

$\rho_{i,t}$ implies that for all $0 \le i \le d$, $0 \le t \le T$, there exists a random $0 < \bar{\theta}_{i,t} < 1$ such that

$$b_i(t, Z_t^N) - b_i(t, z_t) = \langle \nabla b_i(t, z_t + \bar{\theta}_{i,t}(Z_t^N - z_t)), Z_t^N - z_t \rangle.$$

Applying the same argument for all $1 \le i \le d$ yields the first part of the Lemma. Theorem 2.2.7 and the continuity in z of $\nabla b(t,z)$ uniformly in t imply that $\nabla b_i(t, z_t + \bar{\theta}_{i,t}(Z_t^N - z_t)) - \nabla b_i(t, z_t) \to 0$ a.s., uniformly in t, as $N \to \infty$. □

It remains to prove Proposition 2.3.1. Let us first establish a central limit theorem for standard Poisson processes. Let $\{P_j(t),\ t \ge 0\}_{1 \le j \le k}$ be k mutually independent standard Poisson processes and $M(t)$ denote the k-dimensional process whose j-th component is $P_j(t) - t$.

Lemma 2.3.4. *As $N \to \infty$,*

$$\frac{M(Nt)}{\sqrt{N}} \Rightarrow B(t),$$

where $B(t)$ is a k-dimensional standard Brownian motion (in particular $B(t) \sim \mathcal{N}(0, tI)$, with I the $d \times d$ identity matrix) and the convergence is in the sense of convergence in law in $D([0,+\infty); \mathbb{R}^k)$.

For a definition of the space $D([0,+\infty); \mathbb{R}^k)$ of the $\mathbb{R}^k$-valued càlàg functions of $t \in [0,\infty)$ and its topology, see section A.5 in the Appendix.

Proof. It suffices to consider each component separately, since they are independent. So we do as if $k = 1$. We first note that our process is a martingale, whose associated predictable increasing process is given by $\langle N^{-1/2}M(N\cdot), N^{-1/2}M(N\cdot)\rangle_t = t$. Hence it is tight.

Let us now compute the characteristic function of the random variable $N^{-1/2}M(Nt)$. We obtain

$$\mathbb{E}\left(\exp\left[iuN^{-1/2}M(Nt)\right]\right) = \exp\left(Nt\left[e^{i\frac{u}{\sqrt{N}}} - 1 - i\frac{u}{\sqrt{N}}\right]\right) \to \exp\left(-t\frac{u^2}{2}\right),$$

as $N \to \infty$. This shows that $N^{-1/2}M(Nt)$ converges in law to an $\mathcal{N}(0,t)$ r.v.

Now let $n \ge 1$ and $0 < t_1 < \cdots < t_n$. The random variables $N^{-1/2}M(Nt_1)$, $N^{-1/2}M(Nt_2) - N^{-1/2}M(Nt_1), \ldots, N^{-1/2}M(Nt_n) - N^{-1/2}M(Nt_{n-1})$ are mutually independent and, if $B(t)$ denotes a standard one dimensional Brownian motion, the previous argument shows that, with $M(0) = B(0) = 0$, for any $1 \le k \le n$, $N^{-1/2}(M(Nt_k) - M(Nt_{k-1})) \Rightarrow B(t_k) - B(t_{k-1})$. Thus, since the random variables $B(t_1), B(t_2) - B(t_1), \ldots, B(t_n) - B(t_{n-1})$ are mutually independent, we have shown that

$$\left(\frac{M(Nt_1)}{\sqrt{N}}, \frac{M(Nt_2) - M(Nt_1)}{\sqrt{N}}, \ldots, \frac{M(Nt_n) - M(Nt_{n-1})}{\sqrt{N}}\right)$$
$$\Rightarrow (B(t_1), B(t_2) - B(t_1), \ldots, B(t_n) - B(t_{n-1}))$$

as $N \to \infty$. This proves that the finite dimensional distributions of the process $N^{-1/2}M(Nt)$ converge to those of $B(t)$. Together with tightness, this shows the lemma. □

Proof of Proposition 2.3.1. With the notation of the previous lemma,

$$\mathscr{M}_j^N(t) = N^{-1/2} M_j\left(N\int_0^t \beta_j(s, Z_s^N)ds\right).$$

We write

$$\mathscr{M}_j^N(t) = N^{-1/2} M_j\left(N\int_0^t \beta_j(s, z_s)ds\right) + \widetilde{\mathscr{M}}_j^N(t),$$

where

$$\widetilde{\mathscr{M}}_j^N(t) = N^{-1/2} M_j\left(N\int_0^t \beta_j(s, Z_s^N)ds\right) - N^{-1/2} M_j\left(N\int_0^t \beta_j(s, z_s)ds\right).$$

For $C > 0$, let $\tau_{N,C} = \inf\{t > 0, |Z_t^N| > C\}$. We assume for a moment the identity

$$\mathbb{E}\left(\left|\widetilde{\mathscr{M}}_j^N(t\wedge\tau_{N,C})\right|^2\right) = \mathbb{E}\left(\int_0^{t\wedge\tau_{N,C}}\left|\beta_j(s, Z_s^N)ds - \int_0^t \beta_j(s, z_s)ds\right|\right). \quad (2.3.2)$$

The above right-hand side is easily shown to converge to 0 as $N\to\infty$. Jointly with Doob's inequality from Proposition A.4.8 in the Appendix, this shows that for all $T > 0$, $\varepsilon > 0$,

$$\begin{aligned}\mathbb{P}\left(\sup_{0\le t\le T}\left|\widetilde{\mathscr{M}}_j^N(t)\right| > \varepsilon\right) &\le \mathbb{P}(\tau_{N,C} < T) + \mathbb{P}\left(\sup_{0\le t\le T\wedge\tau_{N,C}}\left|\widetilde{\mathscr{M}}_j^N(t)\right| > \varepsilon\right)\\ &\le \mathbb{P}(\tau_{N,C} < T)\\ &\quad + \frac{4}{\varepsilon^2}\mathbb{E}\left(\int_0^{t\wedge\tau_{N,C}}\left|\beta_j(s, Z_s^N)ds - \int_0^t \beta_j(s, z_s)ds\right|\right).\end{aligned}$$

It follows from Theorem 2.2.7 that for $C > 0$ large enough, both terms on the right tend to 0, as $N\to\infty$. Consequently $\sup_{0\le t\le T}\left|\widetilde{\mathscr{M}}_j^N(t)\right| \to 0$ in probability as $N\to\infty$.

It remains to note that an immediate consequence of Lemma 2.3.4 is that

$$N^{-1/2} M_j\left(N\int_0^t \beta_j(s, z_s)ds\right) \Rightarrow B_j\left(\int_0^t \beta_j(s, z_s)ds\right)$$

in the sense of weak convergence in the space $D((0,+\infty);\mathbb{R})$, and the coordinates are mutually independent. However the two processes $B_j\left(\int_0^t \beta_j(s, z_s)ds\right)$ and $\int_0^t \sqrt{\beta_j(s, z_s)}dB_j(s)$ are two centered Gaussian processes which have the same covariance functions. Hence they have the same law.

We finally need to establish (2.3.2). Following the development in Section A.2 in the Appendix, we can rewrite the local martingale $\widetilde{\mathscr{M}}_j^N(t)$ as follows, forgetting the index j, and the time parameter of β for the sake of simplifying notations

$$\widetilde{\mathcal{M}}^N(t) = N^{-1/2}\int_0^t\int_0^\infty \mathbf{1}_{\{N\beta(z_s)\le u\le N\beta(Z^N_{s-})\}}\overline{Q}(ds,du) - N^{-1/2}\int_0^t\int_0^\infty \mathbf{1}_{\{N\beta(Z^N_{s-})\le u\le N\beta(z_s)\}}\overline{Q}(ds,du),$$

where $\overline{Q}(ds,du) = Q(ds,du) - dsdu$ and Q is a standard Poisson point measure on $\mathbb{R}^2_+$. Noting that the square of each jump of the above martingale equals N^{-1}, we deduce from Proposition A.4.9 in the Appendix that

$$\mathbb{E}\left(\left|\widetilde{\mathcal{M}}^N(t\wedge\tau_{N,C})\right|^2\right) = N^{-1}\mathbb{E}\int_0^{t\wedge\tau_{N,C}}\int_{N[\beta(Z^N_{s-}\wedge\beta(z_s)]}^{N[\beta(Z^N_{s-}\vee\beta(z_s)]} Q(ds,du)$$
$$= N^{-1}\mathbb{E}\int_0^{t\wedge\tau_{N,C}}\int_{N[\beta(Z^N_s\wedge\beta(z_s)]}^{N[\beta(Z^N_s\vee\beta(z_s)]} dsdu,$$

which yields (2.3.2). □

Example 2.3.5. The *SIR* model. It is clear that Theorem 2.3.2 applies to Example 2.2.1. If we define $\begin{pmatrix}U_t\\V_t\end{pmatrix} = \lim_{N\to\infty}\sqrt{N}\begin{pmatrix}S^N(t)-s(t)\\I^N(t)-i(t)\end{pmatrix}$, we have

$$U_t = -\lambda\int_0^t [i(r)U_r + s(r)V_r]\,dr - \int_0^t \sqrt{\lambda s(r)i(r)}dB_1(r),$$
$$V_t = \int_0^t [\lambda(i(r)U_r + s(r)V_r) - \gamma V_r]\,dr + \int_0^t \sqrt{\lambda s(r)i(r)}dB_1(r) - \int_0^t \sqrt{\gamma i(r)}dB_2(r).$$

Remark 2.3.6. Consider now the SIR model, started with a fixed small number of infectious individuals, all others being susceptible, so that $(S^N(0), I^N(0)) \to (1,0)$, as $N\to\infty$. The solution of the ODE from Example 2.2.10 starting from $(s(0), i(0)) = (1,0)$ is the constant $(s(t), i(t)) \equiv (1,0)$. So in that case the coefficients of the noise in the last example are identically 0, and, the initial condition of the stochastic model being deterministic, it is natural to assume that $(U_0, V_0) = (0,0)$. Then $(U_t, V_t) \equiv (0,0)$. Consequently Theorem 2.3.2 tells us that, as $N\to\infty$, for any $T > 0$,

$$\sqrt{N}\begin{pmatrix}S^N(t)-1\\I^N(t)-0\end{pmatrix} \to 0, \text{ in probability, uniformly w.r.t. } t\in[0,T].$$

In the case $R_0 > 1$, i.e. $\lambda > \gamma$, with positive probability the epidemic gets off. However, as we shall see in Section 3.4 below, this take time of the order of $\log(N)$, and there is no contradiction with the present result.

We close this section by a discussion of some of the properties of solutions of linear SDEs of the above type, following some of the developments in section 5.6 of Karatzas and Shreve [17]. Suppose that $\{A(t), t\ge 0\}$ and $\{C(t), t\ge 0\}$ are $d\times d$ matrix-valued measurable and locally bounded deterministic functions of t. With $\{B(t), t\ge 0\}$ being a d-dimensional Brownian motion, we consider the SDE

$$dX_t = A(t)X_t dt + C(t)dB_t, t \geq 0,$$

X_0 being a given d-dimensional Gaussian random vector independent of the Brownian motion $\{B(t)\}$. The solution to this SDE is the $\mathbb{R}^d$-valued process given by the explicit formula

$$X(t) = \Gamma(t,0)X_0 + \int_0^t \Gamma(t,s)C(s)dB_s,$$

where the $d \times d$ matrix $\Gamma(t,s)$ is defined for all $0 \leq s \leq t$ as follows. For each fixed $s \geq 0$, $\{\Gamma(t,s), t \geq s\}$ solves the linear ODE

$$\frac{d\Gamma(t,s)}{dt} = A(t)\Gamma(t,s), \quad \Gamma(s,s) = I,$$

where I denotes the $d \times d$ identity matrix. It follows that $\{X_t, t \geq 0\}$ is a Gaussian process, and for each $t > 0$, the mean and the covariance matrix of the Gaussian random vector X_t are given by (denoting by C^* the transpose of the matrix C)

$$\begin{aligned}
\mathbb{E}(X_t) &= \Gamma(t,0)\mathbb{E}(X_0), \\
\mathrm{Cov}(X_t) &= \Gamma(t,0)\mathrm{Cov}(X_0)\Gamma^*(t,0) + \int_0^t \Gamma(t,s)C(s)C^*(s)\Gamma^*(t,s)ds.
\end{aligned}$$

Assume now that $A(t) \equiv A$ and $C(t) \equiv C$ are constant matrices. Then $\Gamma(t,s) = \exp((t-s)A)$. If we define $V(t) := \mathrm{Cov}(X_t)$, we have that

$$V(t) = e^{tA}\left[V(0) + \int_0^t e^{-sA}CC^*e^{-sA^*}ds\right]e^{tA^*}.$$

If we assume moreover that all the eigenvalues of A have negative real parts, then it is not hard to show that as $t \to \infty$,

$$V(t) \to V := \int_0^\infty e^{sA}CC^*e^{sA^*}ds.$$

In that case the Gaussian law with mean zero and covariance matrix V is an invariant distribution of Gauss–Markov process X_t. This means in particular that if X_0 has that distribution, then the same is true for X_t for all $t > 0$. We now show the following result, which is often useful for computing the covariance matrix V in particular cases.

Lemma 2.3.7. *Under the above assumptions on the matrix A, V is the unique $d \times d$ positive semidefinite symmetric matrix which satisfies*

$$AV + VA^* + CC^* = 0.$$

Proof. Uniqueness follows from the fact that the difference $\bar{V}$ of two solutions satisfies $A\bar{V} + \bar{V}A^* = 0$. This implies that for all $x \in \mathbb{R}^d$, $\langle A\bar{V}x, x\rangle = 0$. Since none of the eigenvalues of A^* is zero, this implies that $\langle \bar{V}x, x\rangle = 0$ for all eigenvectors x of A^*, hence for all $x \in \mathbb{R}^d$. Since $\bar{V}$ is symmetric, this implies that $\bar{V} = 0$.

To show that V satisfies the wished identity, assume that the law of X_0 is Gaussian with mean 0 and Covariance matrix V. Then V is also the covariance matrix of X_t. Consequently

$$V = e^{tA} V e^{tA^*} + \int_0^t e^{(t-s)A} CC^* e^{(t-s)A^*} ds.$$

Differentiating with respect to t, and letting $t = 0$ yields the result. □

We leave the last result as an exercise for the reader.

Exercise 2.3.8. Consider again the case of time varying matrices $A(t)$ and $C(t)$. We assume that $A(t) \to A$ and $C(t) \to C$ as $t \to \infty$, and moreover that the real parts of all the eigenvalues of A are negative. Conclude that the law of X_t converges to the Gaussian law with mean 0 and covariance matrix V defined as above.

2.4 Diffusion Approximation

We consider again the vector of proportions in our model as

$$Z^N(t) = x + \frac{1}{N} \sum_{j=1}^{k} h_j P_j \left(\int_0^t N\beta_j(Z^N(s))ds \right). \tag{2.4.1}$$

From the strong law of large numbers, $\sup_{0 \le t \le T} \|Z^N(t) - z_t\| \to 0$ almost surely as $N \to \infty$, for all $T > 0$, where z_t solves the ODE

$$\dot{z}_t = b(z_t),\ z_0 = x; \ \text{ where } b(x) = \sum_{j=1}^{k} h_j \beta_j(x).$$

We now consider a diffusion approximation X_t^N of the above model, which solves the SDE

$$X_t^N = x + \int_0^t b(X_s^N)ds + \sum_{j=1}^{k} \frac{h_j}{\sqrt{N}} \int_0^t \sqrt{\beta_j(X_s^N)} dB_s^j,$$

where $B^1, \ldots, B^k$ are mutually independent standard Brownian motions. Let us define the Wasserstein-1 distance on the interval $[0,T]$ between two $\mathbb{R}^d$-valued processes U_t and V_t as

$$W_{1,T}(U,V) = \inf \mathbb{E}\left(\|U - V\|_T\right),$$

where, if $x : [0,T] \to \mathbb{R}^d$, $\|x\|_T = \sup_{0 \le t \le T} \|x(t)\|$, and the above infimum is over all couplings of the two processes $U(t)$ and $V(t)$, i.e. over all ways of defining jointly the two processes, while respecting the two marginal laws of U and V. We shall use the two following well–known facts about the Wasserstein distance: it is a distance (and satisfies the triangle inequality); if U_n is a sequence of random elements of $D([0,T];\mathbb{R}^d)$ which converges in law to a continuous process U, and is such that the sequence of random variables $\|U_n\|_T$ is uniformly integrable, then $W_{1,T}(U_n, U) \to 0$ as $n \to \infty$.

The aim of this section is to establish the following theorem.

Theorem 2.4.1. *For all $T > 0$, as $N \to \infty$,*

$$\sqrt{N} W_{1,T}(Z^N, X^N) \to 0,$$

or in other words, $W_{1,T}(Z^N, X^N) = o(N^{-1/2})$.

Proof. We have proved in Theorem 2.2.7 that $\sup_{0\le t\le T} \|Z_t^N - z_t\|_T \to 0$ almost surely, as $N \to \infty$, and moreover $\sqrt{N}(Z^N - z) \Rightarrow U$ as $N \to \infty$, where the above convergence holds for the topology of uniform convergence on the interval $[0,T]$, and U is the Gaussian process solution of the SDE

$$U_t = \int_0^t \nabla b(z_s) U_s ds + \sum_{j=1}^k h_j \int_0^t \sqrt{\beta_j(z_s)} dB_s^j.$$

It is not hard to prove the following.

Exercise 2.4.2. As $N \to \infty$, $\sup_{0\le t\le T} \|X_t^N - z_t\|_T \to 0$ almost surely, and moreover $\sqrt{N}(X^N - z) \Rightarrow U$.

We first note that from the triangle inequality

$$\begin{aligned} W_{1,T}(\sqrt{N}(Z^N - z), \sqrt{N}(X^N - z)) &\le W_{1,T}(\sqrt{N}(Z^N - z), U) \\ &\quad + W_{1,T}(\sqrt{N}(X^N - z), U) \\ &\to 0, \end{aligned}$$

as $N \to \infty$. Moreover

$$\begin{aligned} W_{1,T}(\sqrt{N}(Z^N - z), \sqrt{N}(X^N - z)) &= \inf_{\text{couplings}} \mathbb{E}\|\sqrt{N}(Z^N - z) - \sqrt{N}(X^N - z)\|_T \\ &= \inf_{\text{couplings}} \sqrt{N}\mathbb{E}\|(Z^N - z) - (X^N - z)\|_T \\ &= \inf_{\text{couplings}} \sqrt{N}\mathbb{E}\|Z^N - X^N\|_T \\ &= \sqrt{N} W_{1,T}(Z^N, X^N). \end{aligned}$$

Theorem 2.4.1 follows from the two last computations. □

Remark 2.4.3. If we combine the law of large numbers and the central limit theorem which have been established in the previous two sections, we conclude that $Z_t^N - z_t - N^{-1/2} U_t = \circ(N^{-1/2})$. In other words, if we replace Z_t^N by the Gaussian process $z_t + N^{-1/2} U_t$, the error we make, at least on any given finite time interval, is small compared to $N^{-1/2}$. The same is true for the diffusion approximation X_t^N.

Chapter 3
General Closed Models

In this chapter we go back to the general model, i.e. not assuming exponential latent and infectious periods implying that the epidemic process is Markovian. We consider models which are closed in the sense that there is no influx of new susceptibles during the epidemic. No birth, no immigration, and the removed individual are either dead or recovered, with an immunity which they do not lose in the considered time frame.

In this context, the epidemic will stop sooner or later. The questions of main interest are: the evaluation of the duration of the epidemic, and the total number of individuals which are ever infected. The first section gives exact results concerning the second issue in small communities. The rest of the chapter is concerned with large communities. We present the Sellke construction, and then use it to give a law of large number and a central limit theorem for the number of infected individuals. Finally we study the duration of the epidemic.

3.1 Exact Results for the Final Size in Small Communities

In earlier sections it is often assumed that the population size N is large. In other situations this is not the case, for example in planned infectious disease experiments in veterinary science the number of studied animals is of the order 5–20 (e.g. Quenee et al. [29]), and in such cases law of large numbers and central limit theorems have not yet kicked in, which motivates the current section about exact results in small populations.

It turns out that it is quite complicated to derive expressions for the distribution of the final size, even when N is quite small. The underlying reason for this is that there are many ways in which an outbreak can result in exactly k initially susceptible individuals getting infected. We illustrate this by computing the final size distribution $\{p_k^{(N)}\}$ for the Reed–Frost model for $N = 1$, 2 and 3. We then derive a recursive formula for the final outcome of the full model valid for general N and k (but numerically unstable for N larger than, say, 40).

T. Britton, E. Pardoux (eds.), *Stochastic Epidemic Models with Inference*,
Lecture Notes in Mathematics 2255, https://doi.org/10.1007/978-3-030-30900-8_3

Consider the Reed–Frost epidemic where the probability to infect a given susceptible equals $p\ (= 1-e^{-\lambda\iota/N})$. And let $N=1$, one susceptible and one infectious individual to start with. The possible values of Z are then 0 and 1, and obviously we have $p_0^{(1)} = \mathbb{P}(Z=0|N=1) = 1-p$ and $p_1^{(1)} = p$. For $N=2$ things are slightly more complicated. No one getting infected is easy: $p_0^{(2)} = (1-p)^2$, since both individuals have to escape infection from the index case. For $Z=1$ to occur, the index case must infect exactly one of the two remaining, but further, this individual must not infect the third person: $p_1^{(2)} = \binom{2}{1} p(1-p) * (1-p)$. Finally, the probability of $Z=2$ is of course the complimentary probability, but it can also be obtained by considering the two possibilities for this to happen: either the index case infects both, or else the index case infects exactly one of the two, and that individual in turn infects the remaining individual: $p_2^{(2)} = p^2 + 2p(1-p) * p$.

For $N=3$ initial susceptibles the situation becomes even more complicated. It is best to write down the different epidemic generation chains at which individuals get infected. We always have one index case. The chain in which the index case infects two individuals who in turn together infect the last individual, is denoted $1 \to 2 \to 1 \to 0$. The probability for such a chain can be computed sequentially for each generation keeping in mind: how many susceptibles there are at risk, how many that get infected and what is the risk of getting infected (the complimentary probability of escaping infection). The probability for the chain just mentioned is given by

$$\mathbb{P}(1 \to 2 \to 1 \to 0|N=3) = \binom{3}{2} p^2(1-p)^1 * (1-(1-p)^2).$$

The last factor comes from the final individual getting infected when there were two infected individuals in the previous generation (so the escape probability equals $(1-p)^2$). We hence see that the probability of a chain is the product of (different) binomial probabilities. The final size probabilities are then obtained by writing down the different possible chains giving the desired final outcome:

$$\begin{aligned}
p_0^{(3)} &= \mathbb{P}(1 \to 0) = (1-p)^3 \\
p_1^{(3)} &= \mathbb{P}(1 \to 1 \to 0) = \binom{3}{1} p(1-p)^2 * (1-p)^2 \\
p_2^{(3)} &= \mathbb{P}(1 \to 2 \to 0) + \mathbb{P}(1 \to 1 \to 1 \to 0) \\
&= \binom{3}{2} p^2(1-p) * ((1-p)^2) + \binom{3}{1} p(1-p)^2 * \binom{2}{1} p(1-p) * (1-p) \\
p_3^{(3)} &= \mathbb{P}(1 \to 3 \to 0) + \mathbb{P}(1 \to 2 \to 1 \to 0) + \mathbb{P}(1 \to 1 \to 2 \to 0) \\
&\qquad + \mathbb{P}(1 \to 1 \to 1 \to 1 \to 0) \\
&= \dots
\end{aligned}$$

Exercise 3.1.1. Compute $p_3^{(3)}$ explicitly by computing the probabilities of the different chains. Check that $\sum_{k=0}^{3} p_3^{(k)} = 1$ for any $p \in [0,1]$.

For general N it is possible to write down the outcome probability for a specific chain as follows. If we denote the number of susceptibles and infectives in generation k by (S_k, I_k), then the epidemic starts with $(S_0, I_0) = (s_0, i_0) = (N, 1)$. From a chain $1 \to i_1 \to \dots i_j \to 0$ (so $i_{j+1} = 0$) the number of susceptibles in generation k is also known from the relation $s_k = s_0 - \sum_{j=1}^{k} i_k$. We use this when we compute the binomial probabilities of a given generation of the chain, these binomial probabilities depend on: how many were at risk, how many infectives there were in the previous generation, and how many to be infected in the current. Finally, the probability of a chain is the product of the different binomial probabilities of the different generations. From this we obtain the following so called chain-binomial probabilities

$$\mathbb{P}(1 \to i_1 \to \dots i_j \to 0) = \prod_{k=1}^{j+1} \binom{s_{k-1}}{i_k} \left(1-(1-p)^{i_{k-1}}\right)^{i_k} \left((1-p)^{i_{k-1}}\right)^{s_{k-1}-i_k}.$$

As seen, these expression are quite long albeit explicit. However, computing the final outcome probabilities $p_N(k)$, $k = 0, \dots, N$, is still tedious since there are many different possible chains resulting in exactly k getting infected at the end of the epidemic. Further, things become even more complicated when considering different distributions of the infectious period than a constant infectious period as is assumed for the Reed–Frost epidemic model.

However, it is possible to derive a recursive formula for the final number infected $p_N(k)$, see e.g. Ball [5], which we now show. The derivation of the recursion of the final size uses two main ideas: a Wald's identity for the final size and the total infection pressure, and the exchangeability of individuals making it possible to express the probability of having k infections among the initially N susceptibles in terms of the probability of getting all k infected in the subgroup containing those k individuals and the index case, and the probability that the remaining $N-1-k$ individuals escape infection from that group.

Let us start with the latter. Fix N and write $\bar{\lambda} = \lambda/N$. As before we let Z^N denote the total number infected excluding the index case(s), explicitly showing the dependence on the number of initially susceptible N. Since individuals are exchangeable we can label the individuals according to the order in which they get infected. The index case is labelled 0, the individuals who get infected during the outbreak are labelled: $1, \dots, Z^N$, and those who avoid infection according to any order $Z^N+1, \dots, N$. With this labelling we define the total infection pressure A^N by

$$A^N = \bar{\lambda} \sum_{i=0}^{Z^N} I_i \tag{3.1.1}$$

i.e. the infection pressure, exerted on any individual, during the complete outbreak (sometimes referred to as the "total cost" or the "severity" of the epidemic).

As earlier we let $p_i^{(N)} = \mathbb{P}(Z^N = i)$ denote the probability that exactly k initial susceptibles out of N get infected during the outbreak. Reasoning in terms of subsets among the initial susceptibles as described earlier, and using the exchangeability of individuals, it can be shown ([5]) that for any $i \le k \le N$,

$$\frac{p_i^{(N)}}{\binom{N}{i}} = \frac{p_i^{(k)}}{\binom{k}{i}} \mathbb{E}\left(e^{-(N-k)A^k} | Z^k = i\right). \tag{3.1.2}$$

The equation is explained as follows. On the left-hand side is the probability that a specific group of size i (out of N) get infected and no one else. On the right-hand side this event is divided into two sub events.This is done by considering another group of size $k \geq i$, containing the earlier specified group of size i as a subset. The first factor is then the probability that exactly the subgroup of size i get infected within the bigger group of size k. The second factor, the expectation, is the probability that all individuals outside the bigger subgroup avoid getting infected. The notation A^k and Z^k hence denote the total pressure and final size starting with k susceptibles.

We use the following steps to show Wald's identity recalling that $\psi_I(b) = \mathbb{E}(e^{bI})$ is the moment generating function of the infectious period (so $\psi_I(-b)$ is the Laplace transform)

$$\begin{aligned} (\psi_I(-\theta\bar{\lambda}))^{k+1} &= \mathbb{E}\left[\exp\left(-\theta\bar{\lambda}\sum_{i=0}^{k} I_i\right)\right] \\ &= \mathbb{E}\left[\exp\left(-\theta\left(A^k + \bar{\lambda}\sum_{i=Z^k+1}^{k} I_i\right)\right)\right] \\ &= \mathbb{E}\left[e^{-\theta A^k}(\psi_I(-\theta\bar{\lambda})^{k-Z^k}\right]. \end{aligned}$$

The last identity follows since the $k - Z^k$ infectious periods $I_{Z^k+1}, \ldots I_k$, are mutually independent and also independent jointly of the total pressure A^k (which only depends on the first Z^k infectious periods and the contact processes of these individuals). If we now divide both sides by $(\psi_I(-\theta\bar{\lambda}))^{k+1}$ we obtain Wald's identity for Z^k and A^k:

$$\mathbb{E}\left(\frac{e^{-\theta A^k}}{(\psi_I(\theta\bar{\lambda}))^{1+Z^k}}\right) = 1, \qquad \theta \geq 0. \tag{3.1.3}$$

If we apply Wald's identity with $\theta = N - k$ and condition on the value of Z^k we get

$$\sum_{i=0}^{k} \frac{\mathbb{E}\left(e^{-(N-k)A^k} | Z^k = i\right)}{(\psi_I(-(N-k)\bar{\lambda}))^{i+1}} p_i^{(k)} = 1. \tag{3.1.4}$$

If we now use Equation (3.1.2) in the equation above we get

$$\sum_{i=0}^{k} \frac{\binom{k}{i} p_i^{(N)}}{\binom{N}{i}(\psi_I(-(N-k)\bar{\lambda}))^{i+1}} = 1.$$

Simplifying the equation, returning to $\lambda = \bar{\lambda}N$ and putting $p_k^{(N)}$ on one side, we obtain the recursive formula for the final size distribution $p_k^{(N)}, k = 0, \ldots, N$.

Theorem 3.1.2. *The exact final size distribution is given by the recursive formula*

$$p_k^{(N)} = \binom{N}{k}[\psi_I(-(N-k)\lambda/N)]^{k+1} - \sum_{i=0}^{k-1}\binom{N-i}{k-i}[\psi_I(-(N-k)\lambda/N)]^{k-i}p_i^{(N)}. \tag{3.1.5}$$

For example, solving Equation (3.1.5) for $k = 0$ (when the sum is vacuous) and then for $k = 1$ gives, after some algebra,

$$\begin{aligned}
p_0^{(N)} &= \psi_I(\lambda), \\
p_1^{(N)} &= N\psi_I\left(\frac{(N-1)\lambda}{N}\right) \\
&\quad \times \left[\left(\psi_I\left(\frac{(N-1)\lambda}{N}\right)\right) - \psi_I(\lambda)\right].
\end{aligned}$$

In order to compute $p_k^{(N)}$ using (3.1.5) it is required to sequentially compute $p_0^{(N)}$ up to $p_{k-1}^{(N)}$. Further, the formula is not very enlightening and it may be numerically very unstable when k (and hence $N \geq k$) is large. For this reason we devote the major part of these notes to approximations assuming N is large.

In Section 1.9 of Part II of this volume the exact results above are generalized to a model allowing for heterogeneous spreading, meaning that the transmission rate depends on the two individuals involved.

Exercise 3.1.3. Compute the final size distribution $\{p_k^{(N)}\}$ numerically using some suitable software for $N = 10,\ 50$ and 100, for $\lambda = 2$ and $I \equiv 1$ (the Reed–Frost model) and $I \sim \Gamma(3, 1/3)$ (having mean 1 and variance 1/3).

3.2 The Sellke Construction

We now present the Sellke construction (Sellke [36]), which is an ingenious way to define the epidemic outbreak in continuous time using two sets of i.i.d. random variables. This elegant construction is made use of in many new epidemic models, as proven by having more than 50 citations in the past decade.

We number the individuals from 0 to N: $0\ 1\ 2\ 3\ \ldots\ N$. Index 0 denotes the initially infected individual, and the individuals numbered from 1 to N are all susceptible at time 0.

Let

$Q_1, Q_2, \ldots, Q_N$ be i.i.d. random variables, with the law $\mathrm{Exp}(1)$;

$(L_0, I_0), (L_1, I_1), \ldots, (L_N, I_N)$ be i.i.d. random variables, with the law $\mathbb{P}_{(L,I)}$.

In the Markov model, L_i and I_i are independent, hence $\mathbb{P}_{(L,I)} = \mathbb{P}_L \otimes \mathbb{P}_I$,[2] where $\mathbb{P}_L$ is the law of the latency period and $\mathbb{P}_I$ that of the infectious period. But this need not be the case in more general non-Markov models.

Individual 0 has the latency period L_0 and the infectious period I_0. We denote below

$L(t)$ the number of individuals in state E at time t;
$I(t)$ the number of individuals in state I at time t.

Note that for each i, the two random variables L_i and I_i could be dependent, which typically is not the case in a Markov model.

We define the cumulative force of infection experienced by an individual, between times 0 and t as

$$\Lambda_C(t) = \frac{\lambda}{N}\int_0^t I(s)ds.$$

For $i = 1,\ldots,N$, individual i is infected at the time when $\Lambda_C(t)$ achieves the value Q_i (which might be considered as the "level of resistance to infection of individual i"). The j-th infected susceptible has the latency period L_j and the infectious period I_j. The epidemic stops when there is no individual in either the latent or infectious state, after which $\Lambda_C(t)$ does not grow any more, $\Lambda_C(t) = \Lambda_C(\infty)$. The individuals such that $Q_i > \Lambda_C(\infty)$ escape infection.

We put the Q_is in increasing order: $Q_{(1)} < Q_{(2)} < \cdots < Q_{(N)}$. It is the order in which individuals are infected in Sellke's model. Note that Sellke's model respects the durations of latency and infection. In order to show that Sellke's construction gives a process which has the same law as the process from Definition 1.1.1, it remains to verify that the rates at which infections happen are the correct ones.

In the initial model, we assume that each infectious meets other individuals at rate c. Since each individual has the same probability of being the one who is met, the probability that a given individual is that one is $1/N$. Hence the rate at which a given individual is met by a given infectious one is c/N. Each encounter between a susceptible and an infectious individual achieves an infection with probability p. Hence the rate at which a given individual is infected by a given infectious individual is λ/N, where we have set $\lambda = cp$. The rate at which an infectious individual infects susceptibles is then $\lambda S(t)/N$. Finally the epidemic propagates at rate $\lambda S(t)I(t)/N$.

Let us go back to Sellke's construction. At time t, $S(t)$ susceptibles have not yet been infected. Each of those corresponds to a $Q_i > \Lambda_C(t)$. At time t, the slope of the curve which represents the function $t \mapsto \Lambda_C(t)$ is $\lambda I(t)/N$. If $Q_i > \Lambda_C(t) = x$, then

$$\mathbb{P}(Q_i > x+y | Q_i > x) = e^{-y},$$

$$\text{hence } \mathbb{P}(Q_i > \Lambda_C(t+s) | Q_i > \Lambda_C(t)) = \exp\left(-\frac{\lambda}{N}\int_t^{t+s} I(r)dr\right)$$
$$= \exp\left(-\frac{\lambda}{N} I(t)s\right),$$

[2] This notation stands for the product of the two probability measures $\mathbb{P}_L$ and $\mathbb{P}_I$. The fact that the law of the pair is the product of the two marginals is equivalent to the fact that the two random variables L and I are independent.

if I is constant on the interval $[t, t+s]$. Consequently, conditionally upon $Q_i > \Lambda_C(t)$,

$$Q_i - \Lambda_C(t) \sim \text{Exp}\left(\frac{\lambda}{N} I(t)\right).$$

The same is true for all $S(t)$ of those Q_i which are $> \Lambda_C(t)$. The next individual to get infected corresponds to the minimum of those Q_i, hence the waiting time after t for the next infection follows the law $\text{Exp}\left(\frac{\lambda}{N} I(t)S(t)\right)$, if no removal of an infectious individual happens in the mean time, which would modify $I(t)$.

Thus in Sellke's construction, at time t the next infection comes at rate

$$\frac{\lambda}{N} I(t)S(t),$$

as in the model described above.

3.3 LLN and CLT for the Final Size of the Epidemic

Define, for $0 \leq w \leq N+1$, with the notation $[w]$ = integer part of w, and the convention that a sum over an empty index set is zero,

$$\mathscr{I}(w) = \frac{\lambda}{N} \sum_{i=0}^{[w]-1} I_i.$$

Note that $i = 0$ is the index of the initially infected individual, I_i denotes here the length of the infectious period of individual whose resistance level is $Q_{(i)}$ (who is not that of the i-th individual of the original list, but of the individual having the i-th smallest resistance).

$\mathscr{I}(w)$ is the infection pressure produced by the first $[w]$ infected individuals (including number 0). For any integer k, $\mathscr{I}$ is of course constant on the interval $[k, k+1)$. Define for $v > 0$ the number of individuals who do not resist to the infectious pressure v:

$$\overline{q}(v) = \sum_{i=1}^{N} \mathbf{1}_{\{Q_i \leq v\}}.$$

The total number of infected individuals in the epidemic is

$$\begin{aligned} Z &= \min\left\{k \geq 0;\ Q_{(k+1)} > \frac{\lambda}{N} \sum_{i=0}^{k} I_i\right\} \qquad (3.3.1) \\ &= \min\left\{k \geq 0;\ Q_{(k+1)} > \mathscr{I}(k+1)\right\} \\ &= \min\left\{w \geq 0;\ \overline{q}(\mathscr{I}(w+1)) = w\right\}. \end{aligned}$$

Suppose indeed that $Z = i$. Then according to (3.3.1),

$$\mathscr{I}(j) > Q_{(j)}, \ \text{hence } \overline{q}(\mathscr{I}(j)) \geq j, \quad \text{for all } j \leq i,$$

$$\text{and } \mathscr{J}(i+1) < Q_{(i+1)} \text{ hence } \overline{q}(\mathscr{J}(i+1)) < i+1.$$

In other words $Z = i$ if and only if i is the smallest integer such that

$$\overline{q}(\mathscr{J}(i+1)) < i+1, \text{ hence } \overline{q}(\mathscr{J}(i+1)) = i.$$

3.3.1 Law of Large Numbers

Let us index $\mathscr{J}$ and $\overline{q}$ by N, the population size, so that they become $\mathscr{J}_N$ and $\overline{q}_N$. We now define

$$\begin{aligned} \overline{\mathscr{J}}_N(w) &= \mathscr{J}_N(Nw) \\ \overline{\overline{q}}_N(v) &= \frac{\overline{q}_N(v)}{N}. \end{aligned}$$

It follows from the strong law of large numbers that as $N \to \infty$,

$$\begin{aligned} \overline{\mathscr{J}}_N(w) &\to \lambda \mathbb{E}(I) w = R_0 w \text{ almost surely, and} \\ \overline{\overline{q}}_N(v) &\to 1 - e^{-v} \text{ a.s.} \end{aligned}$$

Hence, with the notation $f \circ g(u) := f(g(u))$, as $N \to \infty$,

$$\overline{\overline{q}}_N \circ \overline{\mathscr{J}}_N(w) \to 1 - e^{-R_0 w}$$

a.s., uniformly on $[0,1]$ (the uniformity in w follows from the second Dini theorem, as in the proof of Proposition 2.2.6). We have (replacing now Z by Z^N)

$$\begin{aligned} \frac{Z^N}{N} &= \min\left\{\frac{w}{N} \geq 0;\ \overline{q}_N(\mathscr{J}_N(w+1)) = w\right\} \\ &= \min\left\{s \geq 0;\ \frac{1}{N}\overline{q}_N\left(\mathscr{J}_N\left(N\left(s + \frac{1}{N}\right)\right)\right) = s\right\} \\ &= \min\left\{s \geq 0;\ \overline{\overline{q}}_N\left(\overline{\mathscr{J}}_N\left(s + \frac{1}{N}\right)\right) = s\right\}. \end{aligned}$$

Recall from (1.1.1) that $R_0 = \lambda \iota$, where $\iota = \mathbb{E}(I)$. Note that when $R_0 > 1$, the equation

$$z = 1 - e^{-R_0 z} \tag{3.3.2}$$

(which is equation (2.1.2) from Section 2.1) has a unique solution $z^* \in (0,1)$ (besides the zero solution). Indeed, $f(z) = 1 - e^{-R_0 z}$ is concave, $f(1) < 1$, and $f'(0) = R_0$.

For the proof of the next theorem, we follow an argument from Andersson and Britton [2] (see also Ball and Clancy [6]).

Theorem 3.3.1. *If $R_0 \le 1$, then $Z^N/N \to 0$ a.s., as $N \to \infty$.*

If $R_0 > 1$, as $N \to \infty$, Z^N/N converges in law to the random variable ζ which is such that $\mathbb{P}(\zeta = 0) = z_\infty = 1 - \mathbb{P}(\zeta = z^*)$, where

z_∞, the probability of a minor outbreak (i.e. that the epidemic does not get off), is the solution in $(0,1)$ of (3.3.3) below, and z^* is the positive solution of (3.3.2).

Let us explain how one can characterize z_∞. It follows from Theorem 1.2.5 that the probability z_∞ that the epidemic does not get off equals the probability that the associated branching process goes extinct, which is the probability that the associated discrete time branching process (where we consider the infected by generation) goes extinct. According to Proposition A.1.1 from Appendix A, the probability that this happens is the solution in the interval $(0,1)$ of the equation $g(s) = s$, where g is the generating function of the random number ξ of individuals that one infected infects. As explained in Section 1.2, the law of ξ is MixPoi(λI), so if we denote by $\psi_I(\mu) = \mathbb{E}[\exp(-\mu I)]$ the Laplace transform of I, which is well defined for $\mu > 0$, then $g(s) = \psi_I(\lambda(1-s))$. Hence z_∞ is the unique solution in $(0,1)$ of the equation

$$\psi_I(\lambda(1-s)) = s\,. \tag{3.3.3}$$

Proof. If $R_0 \le 1$, then from Corollary 1.2.6, Z^N remains bounded, hence $Z^N/N \to 0$.

If $R_0 > 1$, then Z^N remains bounded with probability z_∞, which is the probability of extinction in the branching process which approximates the early stage of the epidemic. We now need to see what happens on the complementary event. For that sake, we first choose an arbitrary sequence of integers t_N, which satisfies both $t_N/N \to 0$ and $t_N/\sqrt{N} \to \infty$, as $N \to \infty$. We note that on the event $\{Z^N \le t_N\}$, each infective infects susceptibles at a rate which is bounded below by $\lambda_N = \lambda \frac{N+1-t_N}{N}$. Let $Z(\lambda_N, I)$ denote the total progeny of a single ancestor in a branching process, where each individual has children according to a rate λ_N Poisson process, during his life whose length is I. It is plain that for ant $t \in \mathbb{Z}_+$, and N large enough such that $t \le t_N$,

$$\mathbb{P}(B(\lambda, I) \le t) \le \mathbb{P}(Z^N \le t) \le \mathbb{P}(Z^N \le t_N) \le \mathbb{P}(B(\lambda_N, I) < \infty).$$

Define as in the statement $z_\infty = \mathbb{P}(B(\lambda, I) < \infty)$ the probability of extinction of the branching process approximating the early stage of the epidemic, and $z_{N,\infty} = \mathbb{P}(B(\lambda_N, I) < \infty)$. It is not hard to show that $z_{N,\infty} \to z_\infty$ as $N \to \infty$, as a consequence of the fact that $\lambda_N \to \lambda$ (since $t_N/N \to 0$). Hence for any $\varepsilon > 0$, we can choose t large enough such that $\mathbb{P}(B(\lambda, I) \le t) \le z_\infty - \varepsilon$, and N large enough such that $z_{N,\infty} \le z_\infty + \varepsilon$. We have shown that

$$\mathbb{P}(Z^N \le t_N) \to z_\infty, \quad \text{as } N \to \infty. \tag{3.3.4}$$

This shows that a.s. on the event that the epidemic goes off, Z^N tends to ∞ faster than t_N. We will next prove that

$$\lim_{c\to\infty} \lim_{N\to\infty} \mathbb{P}\left(\left\{t_N < Z^N < Nz^* - c\sqrt{N}\right\} \bigcup \left\{Z^N > Nz^* + c\sqrt{N}\right\}\right) = 0\,. \tag{3.3.5}$$

Recalling the last formula preceding the statement of the present theorem,

$$\left\{\frac{Z^N}{N} \in \left(t_N, z^* - \frac{c}{\sqrt{N}}\right) \bigcup \left(z^* - \frac{c}{\sqrt{N}}, 1\right]\right\}$$
$$\subset \left\{\exists s \in \left(t_N, z^* - \frac{c}{\sqrt{N}}\right) \bigcup \left(z^* - \frac{c}{\sqrt{N}}, 1\right]; \bar{\bar{q}}_N\left(\overline{\mathscr{I}}_N\left(s + \frac{1}{N}\right)\right) = s\right\}$$
$$\subset \left\{\sup_{0 \le s \le 1} \left|\bar{\bar{q}}_N\left(\overline{\mathscr{I}}_N\left(s + \frac{1}{N}\right)\right) - 1 + e^{-R_0 s}\right| > \frac{\phi(c)}{\sqrt{N}}\right\}, \tag{3.3.6}$$

where $\phi(c) \to \infty$, as $c \to \infty$, for N large enough. We have exploited the facts that $t_N/\sqrt{N} \to \infty$ as $N \to \infty$, and $f'(0) > 1$, $f'(z^*) < 1$. However, we shall see in the next subsection (see (3.3.7)) that

$$\left\{\sqrt{N}\left(\bar{\bar{q}}_N\left(\overline{\mathscr{I}}_N\left(s + \frac{1}{N}\right)\right) - 1 + e^{-R_0 s}\right), s \in [0,1]\right\}$$

converges weakly, for the sup–norm topology, to a centred Gaussian process with finite covariance, hence the limit as $N \to \infty$ of the probability of the event (3.3.6) tends to 0, as $c \to \infty$, which establishes (3.3.5). It is easily seen that the second part of the Theorem follows from the combination of (3.3.4) and (3.3.5). □

We see that z^* is the size, measured as the proportion of the total population, of a "significant" epidemic, if it takes off, which happens with probability $1 - z_\infty$.

We notice that z^* depends on the particular model only through the quantity R_0. In particular it depends on the law of the infectious period I only through its mean. In the case where both E and I are exponential random variables, we know from Section 2.2 that the model has a law of large numbers limit, which is a system of ODEs. The same value for z^* has been deduced from an analysis of this deterministic model in Section 2.1. The last theorem holds for a larger class of models.

3.3.2 Central Limit Theorem

From the classical CLT, as $N \to \infty$,

$$A_N(\omega) := \sqrt{N}(\overline{\mathscr{I}}_N(w) - R_0 w) = \frac{\lambda\sqrt{w}}{\sqrt{Nw}} \sum_{i=0}^{[Nw]} [I_i - \mathbb{E}(I_i)] + O(1/\sqrt{N})$$
$$\Rightarrow A(w),$$

where $A(w) \sim \mathscr{N}(0, p^2c^2\mathrm{Var}(I)w)$. One can in fact show that, as processes

$$\{\sqrt{N}(\overline{\mathscr{I}}_N(w) - R_0 w),\ 0 \le w \le 1\} \Rightarrow \{A(w),\ 0 \le w \le 1\}$$

for the topology of uniform convergence, where $\{A(w),\ 0 \le w \le 1\}$ is a Brownian motion (i.e. a centered Gaussian process with independent increments and continuous trajectories) such that $\mathrm{Var}(A(w)) = r^2 R_0^2 w$, where $r^2 = (\mathbb{E}I)^{-2}\mathrm{Var}(I)$. It is easy to show that for all $k \ge 1$, all $0 < w_1 < \cdots < w_k \le 1$, if we define $A_N(w) := \sqrt{N}(\overline{\mathscr{I}}_N(w) - R_0 w)$,

$$(A_N(w_1),\dots,A_N(w_k)) \Rightarrow (A(w_1),\dots,A(w_k)).$$

This means the convergence of the finite dimensional distributions. Combining this with the techniques exposed in Section A.5 of the Appendix yields the above functional weak convergence.

Consider now $\overline{\overline{q}}_N$. Again from the usual CLT,

$$\begin{aligned}B_N(v) &= \sqrt{N}(\overline{\overline{q}}_N(v) - [1-e^{-v}])\\ &= \frac{1}{\sqrt{N}}\sum_{i=1}^{N}\left[\mathbf{1}_{\{Q_i\le v\}} - (1-e^{-v})\right]\\ &\Rightarrow B(v),\end{aligned}$$

where $B(v) \sim \mathcal{N}(0, e^{-v}(1-e^{-v}))$. We have again a functional convergence, according to the Kolmogorov–Smirnov theorem, towards a time changed Brownian bridge. In simpler words, $\{B(v),\ v \ge 0\}$ is a centred Gaussian process with continuous trajectories whose covariance function is specified by the identity $\mathbb{E}[B(u)B(v)] = e^{-u\vee v} - e^{-(u+v)}$, where $u \vee v := \sup(u,v)$.

Let us now combine the two functional central limit theorems which we have just derived. We have

$$\begin{aligned}&\sqrt{N}\left(\overline{\overline{q}}_N(\overline{\mathscr{I}}_N(w)) - 1 + e^{-R_0 w}\right)\\ &\quad= \sqrt{N}(\overline{\overline{q}}_N(\overline{\mathscr{I}}_N(w)) - 1 + \exp(-\overline{\mathscr{I}}_N(w))) + \sqrt{N}\left(e^{-R_0 w} - e^{-\overline{\mathscr{I}}_N(w))}\right)\\ &\quad\sim B_N(\overline{\mathscr{I}}_N(w)) - R_0 e^{-R_0 w} A_N(w).\end{aligned}$$

Consequently

$$\sqrt{N}\left(\overline{\overline{q}}_N(\overline{\mathscr{I}}_N(w)) - 1 + e^{-R_0 w}\right) B(R_0 w) - R_0 e^{-R_0 w} A(w), \tag{3.3.7}$$

which is the functional central limit theorem which was used in the proof of Theorem 3.3.1.

Recall that the above Law of Large Numbers has been obtained by taking the limit in the equation

$$\overline{\overline{q}}_N\left(\overline{\mathscr{I}}_N\left(z+N^{-1}\right)\right) = z.$$

Making use of the above two CLTs, we get

$$\begin{aligned}z &= 1 - e^{-\overline{\mathscr{I}}_N(z+N^{-1})} + N^{-1/2}B_N(\overline{\mathscr{I}}_N(z+N^{-1}))\\ &= 1 - \exp\left(-R_0(z+N^{-1}) - N^{-1/2}A_N(z+N^{-1})\right)\\ &\quad + N^{-1/2}B_N\left(R_0(z+N^{-1}) + N^{-1/2}A_N(z+N^{-1})\right).\end{aligned}$$

Let $z = z^* + z_N N^{-1/2} + \mathrm{o}(N^{-1/2})$, where z^* satisfies $e^{-R_0 z^*} = 1 - z^*$. We obtain

$$\begin{aligned}
&z^* + z_N N^{-1/2} + \circ(N^{-1/2}) \\
&= 1 - \exp\left(-R_0 z^* - R_0 z_N N^{-1/2} - A_N(z^*) N^{-1/2} + \circ(N^{-1/2})\right) \\
&\quad + N^{-1/2} B_N(R_0 z^*) + \circ(N^{-1/2}) \\
&= 1 - e^{-R_0 z^*} + N^{-1/2} e^{-R_0 z^*} \left(R_0 z_N + A_N(z^*)\right) + N^{-1/2} B_N(R_0 z^*) + \circ(N^{-1/2}).
\end{aligned}$$

We simplify this relation by making use of the equation which specifies z^*. Multiplying the remaining terms by $N^{1/2}$, we deduce

$$[1 - (1 - z^*)R_0] z_N = B_N(R_0 z^*) + (1 - z^*) A_N(z^*) + \circ(1).$$

Hence $z_N \Rightarrow \Xi$, where (note that $e^{-R_0 z^*}(1 - e^{-R_0 z^*}) = z^*(1 - z^*)$)

$$\Xi \sim \mathcal{N}\left(0, \frac{z^*(1-z^*)}{(1-(1-z^*)R_0)^2}\left(1 + r^2(1-z^*)R_0^2\right)\right),$$

where we have exploited the independence of the two processes $A(\cdot)$ and $B(\cdot)$, which follows from that of the two collections of random variables $(I_i,\ i \geq 0)$ and $(Q_i,\ i \geq 1)$.

Finally we can conclude with the following theorem. We refer to Scalia-Tomba [32] and [33] for a more complete justification.

Theorem 3.3.2. *As $N \to \infty$, conditionally upon the event that the epidemic takes off, the law of $N^{-1/2}(ZN - Nz^*)$ converges towards the Gaussian distribution*

$$\mathcal{N}\left(0, \frac{z^*(1-z^*)}{(1-(1-z^*)R_0)^2}\left(1 + r^2(1-z^*)R_0^2\right)\right).$$

Exercise 3.3.3. Compute numerically the limiting mean and standard deviation of the final size Z^N in case of a major outbreak and $N = 1000$, $\lambda = 1.5$ and $\iota = 1$, for the following two situations. The first scenario is when $I \equiv 1$ (fixed infectious period), and the second when $I \sim \mathrm{Exp}(1)$ (Markovian SIR).

3.4 The Duration of the Stochastic SEIR Epidemic

Recall that $L^N(t)$ and $I^N(t)$ denote the numbers of latent and infectious individuals at time t respectively, and introduce $Z^N(t) = N - L^N(t) - I^N(t) - R^N(t)$ to denote the number of individuals who have been infected by time t (i.e. who are no longer susceptible). We now study how long it takes for the epidemic to first grow big, and then later to end, i.e. for the end of the epidemic we will study properties of $\tau^N = \inf\{t; L^N(t) + I^N(t) = 0\}$ as $N \to \infty$. It will only be a sketch since it is quite technical to prove the results rigorously. For detailed results we refer to Barbour [7]. From an applied point of view, this question has clear practical relevance, since for instance hospitals are on highest pressure when the epidemic peaks, and knowing how long until the outbreak is over indicates how long preventive measures should be enforced.

If the epidemic does not take off we know from branching process theory that the time to extinction is finite, so $\tau^N = O_p(1)$ on this part of the sample space ($O_p(1)$ denotes bounded in probability). We hence focus on the situation where the epidemic takes off resulting in a major outbreak, hence implicitly assuming that $R_0 > 1$.

We divide the duration of the whole epidemic τ^N into three parts: the beginning, the main part and the end of the epidemic. Pick $\varepsilon > 0$ small. Formally we define these parts by defining two intermediate times (inspired by Sir Winston Churchill): the end of the beginning $\tau^N_{Beg} = \inf\{t \le \tau^N; Z^N(t) \ge \varepsilon N\}$, and the beginning of the end $\tau^N_{End} = \inf\{t \le \tau^N; Z^N(t) \ge (1-\varepsilon)z^* N\}$, where z^* is the positive solution to the final size equation from Section 2.1. Each of these times are equal to τ^N in the case when the event never occurs.

With these definitions the beginning of the epidemic is the time interval $[0, \tau^N_{Beg})$, the main part $[\tau^N_{Beg}, \tau^N_{End})$ and the end part $[\tau^N_{End}, \tau^N]$.

During the beginning we can sandwich the epidemic between two branching processes. The upper bound is the branching process $Z(t)$ described in Section 1.2. Similarly, we can construct a lower bound using a very similar branching process $Z^-(t)$, the only difference being that the birth rate is $\lambda(1-\varepsilon)$ as opposed to λ for the upper branching process. This is true because before τ^N_{Beg} the rate of new infections in the epidemic equals $\lambda(1 - Z^N(t)/N)$ which lies between $\lambda(1-\varepsilon)$ and λ. Since $Z^-(t) \le Z^N(t) \le Z(t)$ for $t \le \tau^N_{Beg}$ it follows that $\tau^N_+ \le \tau^N_{Beg} \le \tau^N_-$, where $\tau^N_+ = \inf\{t; Z(t) \ge \varepsilon N\}$ and $\tau^N_- = \inf\{t; Z^-(t) \ge \varepsilon N\}$.

From Section A.1.2 we know the rate at which a branching process grows. More specifically, we know that when a branching process $Z'(t)$ takes off, it grows exponentially: $Z'(t) \sim e^{r't}$, where r' is the unique solution to $1 = \int_0^\infty e^{-r's}\lambda(s)ds = 1$, where $\lambda(s)$ is the average (expected) rate at which an individual gives birth at age s (cf. Equation (1.2.1)). For our two branching processes $Z(t)$ and $Z^-(t)$ we have $\lambda(s) = \lambda\mathbb{P}(L < s < L+I)$ and $\lambda^-(s) = \lambda(1-\varepsilon)\mathbb{P}(L < s < L+I)$ respectively. From this it follows that the exponential growth rates r and r^- can be made arbitrary close to each other by choosing ε small enough ($r^- = r(1+o(\varepsilon))$). The particular form of r and r^- depends on the distribution of L and I (see Exercise 3.4.2 below). Recall that $\tau^N_+ = \inf\{t; Z(t) \ge \varepsilon N\}$, so the fact that $Z(t) \sim e^{rt}$ implies that $\tau^N_+ = \frac{\log(\varepsilon N)}{r} + O_p(1)$. Similarly, $\tau^N_- = \frac{\log(\varepsilon N)}{r^-} + O_p(1)$. As a consequence, the two stopping times are arbitrary close to each other on the logarithmic scale. From this we have $\tau^N_{Beg} = \frac{\log(N)}{r}(1+o(\varepsilon)) + O_p(1)$.

We now turn to the duration of the main part of the epidemic: $\tau^N_{End} - \tau^N_{Beg}$ which is positive only if the epidemic takes off, which we hence condition upon. During this part of the epidemic, the Markovian SEIR epidemic can be approximated by the deterministic SEIR model. This means that for the Markovian SEIR model, the duration of the main part of the epidemic $\tau^N_{End} - \tau^N_{Beg}$ can be well approximated by the corresponding duration of the deterministic system $\tau^{Det}_{End} - \tau^{Det}_{Beg}$. The deterministic system is started at $\tau^{Det}_{Beg} = 0$ with initial conditions $(s(0), e(0), i(0), r(0)) = (1-\varepsilon, a\varepsilon, b\varepsilon, (1-a-b)\varepsilon)$ for some positive numbers a and b with $0 < a+b \le 1$ (there is no closed form expression for how the infected individuals are divided into exposed, infectives and recovereds). The system is then run until $\tau^{Det}_{End} =$

$\inf\{t; e(t)+i(t)+r(t) \geq (1-\varepsilon)z\}$. We know that $z(t) = e(t)+i(t)+r(t) \to z$ and $z(t)$ is monotonically increasing (since $s(t) = 1-z(t)$ is decreasing). This implies that $\tau_{End}^{Det} - \tau_{Beg}^{Det} = \tau_{Beg}^{Det}$ is just a constant for any fixed positive ε. It will depend slightly on a and b, but when ε is small the dependence is weak and there is a uniform bound. From this we conclude that the main part of the epidemic is bounded:

$$\tau_{End}^{N} - \tau_{Beg}^{N} = \tau_{Beg}^{Det} + o_p(\varepsilon) = O_p(1).$$

If the latent and infectious periods are not exponentially distributed, then the stochastic SEIR epidemic is not Markovian, and the deterministic approximating system is a difference-delay-system which we will not study more closely. The qualitative properties of this system coincide with those of the Markovian SEIR system; in particular, the duration of the main part is bounded in probability.

Just like the main part of the epidemic the duration of end of the epidemic, $\tau^N - \tau_{End}^N$ is only positive if the epidemic takes off, which we hence condition upon. At the beginning of the end part, the number of infected (either exposed, infectious or recovered) equals $Z^N(\tau_{End}^N) = (1-\varepsilon)z^*N$ and $S^N(\tau_{End}^N) = (1-z^*)N + \varepsilon z^*N$. Since ε is assumed to be small, infectious individuals give birth at rate $\lambda(1-z^*+\varepsilon z^*) \approx (1-z^*)$ during the rest of the epidemic (we know the final fraction infected converges to z^* in probability). Further, at the start of the beginning the fractions exposed and infectious will both close to that of the deterministic system which are both small, having size $c_E\varepsilon$ and $c_I\varepsilon$ say (cf. Figure 2.1.1 where it is seen that $e(t)$ and $i(t)$ are both small for large t). So, from the beginning of the end part, the epidemic behaves like a branching process with childhood duration L, adult duration I and birth rate $\lambda(1-z^*)$ during the adult life stage, and this part is started with $c_E\varepsilon N$ children (exposed) and $c_I\varepsilon N$ adults (infectious). The mean off-spring distribution for this branching process equals $\lambda\mathbb{E}(I)(1-z^*) = R_0(1-z)$ where z^* is the positive solution to $1-z = e^{R_0 z}$. It can be shown (cf. Exercise 3.4.1 below) that $R_0(1-z^*) < 1$ implying that the branching process is subcritical (otherwise the epidemic would not be on decline).

The duration $\tau^N - \tau_{End}^N$ of the end part can hence be approximated by the time until extinction of a subcritical branching process, starting with $c_E\varepsilon N$ children (exposed) and $c_I\varepsilon N$ adults (infectious). This branching process will have *negative* drift $r^* < 0$ being the solution to the corresponding equation $\int_0^\infty e^{-rs}\lambda(s)ds = 1$ where now $\lambda(s) = \lambda(1-z^*)\mathbb{P}(L < s < L+I)$. So, $E(t)+I(t) \sim (E(0)+I(0))e^{r^*t} = (c_E+c_I)\varepsilon N e^{r^*t}$. The time until this branching process goes extinct (i.e. $E(t)+I(t) < 1$) is hence of order $-\log((c_E+c_I)\varepsilon N)/r^* = -\log N/r^* + O_p(1)$.

To sum up, the duration of the epidemic $\tau^N = O_p(1)$ if the epidemic does not take off, whereas it has the following structure in case it does take off:

$$\tau^N = \tau_{Beg}^N + \left(\tau_{End}^N - \tau_{Beg}^N\right) + \left(\tau^N - \tau_{End}^N\right) = \frac{\log N}{r} + O_p(1) + \frac{-\log N}{r^*}. \tag{3.4.1}$$

Note that the last term is also positive since $r^* < 0$.

Exercise 3.4.1. Show that $R_0(1-z^*) < 1$ and compute it numerically for $R_0 = 1.5$.

Exercise 3.4.2. Consider the stochastic SEIR epidemic with infection rate $\lambda = 1.5$ per time unit. Compute the two leading terms of the duration of a major outbreak for the following three cases: $L \equiv 0$ and $I \sim \text{Exp}(1)$ (Markovian SIR), $L \equiv 0$ and $I \equiv 1$ (continuous time Reed–Frost), and $L \sim \text{Exp}(1)$ and $I \sim \text{Exp}(1)$ (Markovian SEIR).

Chapter 4
Open Markov Models

In this chapter, contrary to the situation considered in earlier chapters, we study models where there is a constant supply of susceptibles (either by births, immigration or loss of immunity of the removed individuals) giving rise to endemic type situations. We study how the random fluctuations in the model can drive the system out of the basin of attraction of the stable endemic equilibrium of the deterministic model, such that the disease goes extinct.

As we shall see in Section 4.1, in the case of a moderate population size, one may expect that the Gaussian fluctuations described by the central limit theorem are strong enough to stop the endemy in a SIR model with demography. For larger population sizes, following Freidlin and Wentzell [13], we describe in Section 4.2 how long it will take for the random perturbations to stop the endemy. We apply this approach successively to the SIRS, the SIS and the SIR model with demography. In the case of the SIS model, we compute explicitly the constant which appears in the Freidlin–Wentzell theory, see Proposition 4.2.29 below. This is unfortunately the only case where we have such a simple and explicit formula in terms of the coefficients of the model.

4.1 Open Populations: Time to Extinction and Critical Population Size

Up until now we have (mainly) considered the stochastic SEIR epidemic model in a fixed community of size N, where N has been assumed large (except in Section 3.1 when N was assumed small). This is of course an approximation of reality, but when considering outbreaks of a few months (e.g. influenza outbreaks) it seems like a fair approximation; recall that the time to extinction of our model was $O_p(\log N)$. For other diseases including childhood diseases, the disease is present in the community constantly – such diseases are said to be *endemic*. When trying to understand the behaviour of such diseases it is necessary to also allow people to die and new people entering the population (by birth or immigration). In the current section we do this and derive approximations for two important quantities: the time to extinction

T. Britton, E. Pardoux (eds.), *Stochastic Epidemic Models with Inference*,
Lecture Notes in Mathematics 2255, https://doi.org/10.1007/978-3-030-30900-8_4

of the endemic disease T_E^N, and the critical community size N_c. These two quantities have received much attention in the literature over the years. In particular, the critical community size N_c and how it depends on properties of the disease and the community have been studied both in the mathematical and applied communities (e.g. Lindholm and Britton [23] and Keeling and Grenfell [18]).

Let us first describe the population model, which is the simplest model for a population which fluctuates randomly in time with a mean size of N individuals, and where individuals have life time distribution with mean $1/\mu$ (cf. Example 2.2.2). The population $N(t)$ is defined to be a Markovian birth-death process with constant birth rate μN and linear death rate, all individuals dying at rate μ. This process $N(t)$ will fluctuate around N, a parameter we denote by the mean population size. If N is large, it is known that $N(t)$ will be approximately normally distributed with mean N and standard deviation proportional to $\sqrt{N}$, so for practical purposes we will later approximate $N(t)$ by N.

Exercise 4.1.1. Assuming that $N(0) = N$, write $N(t)$ as the solution of an SDE of the same form as the SDE appearing at the beginning of Section 2.2. Define $Q_t^N = N(t)/N$ and show that, as a consequence of Theorem 2.2.7, $Q_t^N \to 1$ a.s., locally uniformly in t. Then deduce from Theorem 2.3.2 that $\sqrt{N}(Q_t^N - 1)$ converges weakly, as $N \to \infty$, towards an Ornstein–Uhlenbeck process of the form

$$U_t = \sqrt{2\mu}\int_0^t e^{-\mu(t-s)}dB_s,$$

where B_t is a standard Brownian motion. Prove that $\mathbb{E}(U_t) = 0$ and $\mathrm{Var}(U_t) \to 1$ as $t \to \infty$. Deduce that for large N and t, $N(t)$ is approximately normally distributed with mean N and standard deviation proportional to $\sqrt{N}$.

For this population model, we assume that the Markovian SIR epidemic spreads (this can easily be extended to the Markovian SEIR model). By this we mean that individuals who get infected immediately become infectious and remain so for an Exp(γ) time, unless they happen to die before by chance. In the fixed population size model, the contact rate was λ which implied that it was λ/N to each specific individual. Now, in the open population model, we assume that the infection rate to a specific individual is unchanged, λ/N. More appropriate would perhaps have been to instead have $\lambda/N(t)$ but since $N(t) \approx N$ for all t we use the simpler choice λ/N. So, new individuals enter the community at constant rate μN and all individuals die, irrespective of being susceptible, infectious or recovered, at rate μ, susceptible individuals get infected at rate $\lambda I^N(t)/N$, and infectious individuals recover at rate γ. The rate at which susceptibles get infected and infected recover hence equals $\lambda I^N(t)S^N(t)/N$, and $\gamma I^N(t)$ respectively.

If we study the limiting deterministic system for the *fractions* in each state we get the following system of differential equations:

$$\begin{aligned}
s'(t) &= \mu - \lambda s(t)i(t) - \mu s(t), \\
i'(t) &= \lambda s(t)i(t) - \gamma i(t) - \mu i(t), \\
r'(t) &= \gamma i(t) - \mu r(t),
\end{aligned} \tag{4.1.1}$$

which is identical to those of Example 2.2.11 with $\rho = 0$ and $\nu = +\infty$. From this we can compute the endemic state where all derivatives are 0. First we note that the basic reproduction number R_0 (the expected number of infectious contact while infectious and alive) and the expected relative time of a life an individual is infected, ε, are given by

$$R_0 = \frac{\lambda}{\gamma + \mu} \qquad \varepsilon = \frac{1/(\gamma+\mu)}{1/\mu} = \frac{\mu}{\gamma+\mu}. \tag{4.1.2}$$

The rate of recovery γ is much larger than the death rate μ (52 compared to 1/75 for a one week infectious period and 75 year life length) so for all practical purposes the two expressions can be approximated by $R_0 \approx \lambda/\gamma$ and $\varepsilon \approx \mu/\gamma$.

If we solve the system of differential equations (4.1.1) by setting all derivatives equal to 0, and replace μ, λ and γ by the dimensionless quantities R_0 and ε (three parameters can be replaced by two because the unit of time for the rates is arbitrary and one rate can be set to unity), we obtain the endemic level which is given by

$$(\hat{s}, \hat{i}, \hat{r}) = \left(\frac{1}{R_0}, \varepsilon\left(1 - \frac{1}{R_0}\right), 1 - \frac{1}{R_0} - \varepsilon\left(1 - \frac{1}{R_0}\right)\right) \tag{4.1.3}$$

Exercise 4.1.2. Show that this is the endemic level, i.e. that the solution solves Equation (4.1.1) with all derivatives being 0.

This state is only meaningful if $R_0 > 1$ (otherwise some fraction is negative), so the endemic level only exists if $R_0 > 1$. Another solution to the equation system is of course the disease free equilibrium $(s,i,r) = (1,0,0)$. It is well known that when $R_0 > 1$ (which we from now on assume), then the endemic state is globally stable whereas the disease free state is locally unstable, meaning the system converges to the endemic level irrespective of starting value as long as $i(0) > 0$.

Using the theory of Section 2.2 it can be shown that the current Markov model (for an open population) converges to the above deterministic model as $N \to \infty$, if the starting point is such that the fraction initially infectious is strictly positive ($I^N(0)/N \to i(0) > 0$).

This suggests that the stochastic model (for the fractions in different states) can be approximated by the corresponding deterministic function

$$(S^N(t)/N, I^N(t)/N, R^N(t)/N) \approx (s(t), i(t), r(t))$$

which solves Equation (4.1.1) and having the same initial condition as the stochastic system. And, since we know that $(s(t),i(t),r(t)) \to (\hat{s},\hat{i},\hat{r})$ as $t \to \infty$ this suggests that $(S^N(t)/N, I^N(t)/N, R^N(t)/N) \approx (\hat{s},\hat{i},\hat{r})$ when N and t are large. This is indeed true in some sense, but it is only true depending on the relation between N and t. For any finite N, the stochastic epidemic, which fluctuates randomly around the endemic equilibrium, will eventually go extinct, meaning that for some random T_{Ext}^N

(the extinction time) it will happen that $I^N(T_{Ext}^N) = 0$. When this happens the rate of new infections is 0 so the stochastic epidemic will remain disease free ever after (and eventually all removed will have died so all individuals are susceptible. Using large deviation theory (cf. Section 4.2 below) it can be shown that the time to extinction grows exponentially with N, $T_{Ext}^N \approx e^{cN}$ for some $c > 0$ as $N \to \infty$.

On the other hand, for any arbitrary but fixed time horizon $[0, t_{\max}]$ the stochastic epidemic will converge to the deterministic process as $N \to \infty$. It also follows from Theorem 2.3.2 that the scaled process

$$\sqrt{N}(S^N(t)/N - s(t),\ I^N(t)/N - i(t),\ R^N(t)/N - r(t))$$

converges to an Ornstein–Uhlenbeck process $(\tilde{S}(t), \tilde{I}(t), \tilde{R}(t))$. This Ornstein–Uhlenbeck process is a Gaussian process with stationary distribution being Normally distributed. In particular, the variance of $\tilde{I}(t)$ in stationarity is well approximated by $1/R_0 - 1/R_0^2$, see Nåsell [24].

Exercise 4.1.3. Show this as a consequence of Theorem 2.3.2, Lemma 2.3.7, and Exercise 2.3.8

This suggests that $I^N(t)$ will be approximately Gaussian with mean $N\hat{i}$ and standard deviation $\sqrt{N/R_0}$ when N is large and t is moderately large (smaller than T_{Ext}^N but still large since we assume the Ornstein–Uhlenbeck is close to stationary).

From above we know that T_{Ext}^N will grow exponentially with N as $N \to \infty$. On the other hand, if N is small or moderate, the disease will go extinct very quickly, e.g. within a year. We now use the Gaussian approximation above to define a sort of threshold, the *critical population size* N_c, between these two scenarios (quick extinction and very long time before extinction). Of course, there is no unique exact such value, so it will involve some arbitrary choice(s).

Above we noted that $I^N(t)$ was approximately Gaussian with mean $N\hat{i}$ and standard deviation $\sqrt{N/R_0}$. If we want to be above the critical population size, then we want to avoid quick extinction for which it is necessary that this approximately Gaussian process avoids extinction for a fairly long time. Extinction occurs when $I^N(t) = 0$, and if we want to avoid this we want the value 0 to be far enough away from the mean, e.g. at least 3 standard deviations away. The choice 3 is of course arbitrary but if we instead choose 2 the *process* will hit 0 fairly quickly with large enough probability, and if we choose 4 it seems extremely unlikely that it will hit extinction within e.g. a life time, so 3 seems like a reasonable compromise when it is unlikely but not completely impossible. This choice then suggests that the threshold is for the case $N\hat{i} - 3\sqrt{N/R_0} = 0$. This is equivalent to $\sqrt{N} = 3/\hat{i}\sqrt{R_0}$, i.e. $N = 9/\hat{i}^2 R_0$. Inserting that $\hat{i} = \varepsilon(1 - 1/R_0)$ (remember that $\varepsilon = \mu/(\gamma + \mu)$ is the relative length of the infectious period compared to life-length), then we arrive at our definition of the *critical population size* N_c:

$$N_c = \frac{9}{\varepsilon^2 (1 - \frac{1}{R_0})^2 R_0}. \tag{4.1.4}$$

The conclusion is that, for a given infectious disease, i.e. given R_0 and ε, the disease will die out quickly in a community of size $N \ll N_c$ whereas it will persist for a very long time if $N \gg N_c$, during which the disease is endemic. As an illustration, consider measles prior to vaccination. If we assume that $R_0 \approx 15$ and the infectious period is 1 week (1/52 years) and life duration 75 years, implying that $\varepsilon \approx \frac{1/75}{1/(1/52)+1/75} \approx 1/3750$ we arrive at $N_c \approx 9(3750)^2/15 \approx 8 \cdot 10^6$. So, if the population is a couple of million (or less) the disease will go extinct quickly, whereas the disease will become endemic (for a very long time) in a population being larger than e.g. 20 million people. This confirms the empirical observation that measles was continuously endemic in UK whereas it died out quickly in Iceland (and was later reintroduced by infectious people visiting the country).

Exercise 4.1.4. Which parameter affects N_c the most? Compute N_c using the measles example but making R_0 50% bigger/smaller and the same for the duration of the infectious period (assuming we live equally long).

Exercise 4.1.5. Suppose that a vaccine giving 100% life long immunity is available, and that a fraction v of all infants are continuously vaccinated. How does this affect the critical community size, i.e. give an expression for N_c also containing v. (*Hint*: Vaccinating people affects both the relevant population size N_v, the non-vaccinated population, and the reproduction number R_v, but other than that nothing has changed.)

4.2 Large Deviations and Extinction of an Endemic Disease

4.2.1 Introduction

In Section 2.2, we have proved that, under appropriate conditions, the solution of the SDE

$$Z_t^N = x_N + \sum_{j=1}^{k} \frac{h_j}{N} P_j\left(N \int_0^t \beta_j(s, Z_s^N) ds\right) \tag{4.2.1}$$

converges a.s., locally uniformly in t, towards the unique solution of the ODE

$$\frac{dz_t}{dt} = b(t, z_t), \quad z_0 = x, \tag{4.2.2}$$

see Theorem 2.2.7, where $b(t,x) = \sum_{j=1}^{k} h_j \beta_j(t,x)$. Consequently the above SDE (4.2.1) can be considered for large N as a small random perturbation of the ODE (4.2.2). Small random perturbations of ODEs by Brownian motion have been studied by many authors, starting with Freidlin and Wentzell [13]. Our aim is to study the above type of random perturbations of an ODE like (4.2.2). The starting point is the estimation of a large deviation from the law of large numbers, which has been studied for our type of Poisson driven SDEs by Shwartz and Weiss [34]. The difficulty is the fact that some of the rates in the SDE (4.2.1) vanish when the solution hits part of the boundary. This makes the estimate a bit delicate, since the logarithms of the rates enter the rate function in our large deviations estimate. This situation has been addressed first by Shwartz and Weiss [35], but their assumptions are not quite satisfied in our framework. Recently Kratz and Pardoux [21] and Pardoux and Samegni-Kepgnou [26] have developed an approach to Large Deviations which is well adapted to the epidemics models which are considered in these Notes. In fact the main difficulty concerns the lower bound. In the following, we present a new approach to the lower bound, based upon a quasi–continuity result, Proposition 4.2.4 below, which mimics a similar result for Brownian motion driven SDEs due to Azencott [4]. The same approach, for other types of Poisson driven SDEs, will soon appear in Kouegou-Kamen and Pardoux [19], [20].

The main application we have in mind is to estimate the time needed for the small random perturbations to drive the system from a stable endemic equilibrium to the disease free equilibrium (i.e. extinction). This applies to the classical SIS and SIRS models, as well as to an SIR model with demography, as well as to models with vaccination and to models with several levels of susceptibility, thus predicting the time it will take for the random perturbation to end an endemic disease.

We rewrite our model as

$$Z_t^{N,x_N} = x_N + \sum_{j=1}^{k} h_j \int_0^t \int_0^{\beta_j(s,Z_{s-}^{N,x_N})} Q_j^N(ds,du),$$

where

$$Q_j^N(ds,du) = \frac{1}{N} Q_j(ds,Ndu),$$

and the Q_j's are i.i.d. Poisson random measures on $[0,T] \times \mathbb{R}_+$, with mean λ^2, the 2-dimensional Lebesgue measure.

(A.1) We shall assume in all of this section that the β_j's are locally Lipschitz with respect to x, uniformly for $t \in [0,T]$.

4.2.2 The Rate Function

We want to establish a large deviations principle for trajectories in the space $D([0,T];\mathbb{R}^d)$ of $\mathbb{R}^d$-valued right-continuous functions which have a left limit at any time $t \in (0,T]$. We shall also consider the sets $C([0,T];\mathbb{R}^d)$ of continuous functions from $[0,T]$ into $\mathbb{R}^d$, and the subset of absolutely continuous functions, which we will denote $\mathscr{AC}_{T,d}$. For any $\phi \in \mathscr{AC}_{T,d}$, let $\mathscr{A}_k(\phi)$ denote the (possibly empty) set of functions $c \in L^1(0,T;\mathbb{R}_+^k)$ such that $c_j(t) = 0$ a.e. on the set $\{t,\, \beta_j(\phi_t) = 0\}$ and

$$\frac{d\phi_t}{dt} = \sum_{j=1}^{k} c_j(t) h_j, \quad \text{t a.e.}$$

We define the rate function

$$I_T(\phi) := \begin{cases} \inf_{c \in \mathscr{A}_k(\phi)} I_T(\phi|c), & \text{if } \phi \in \mathscr{AC}_{T,A}; \\ \infty, & \text{otherwise,} \end{cases}$$

where as usual the infimum over an empty set is $+\infty$, and

$$I_T(\phi|c) = \int_0^T \sum_{j=1}^k g(c_j(t), \beta_j(\phi_t))dt$$

with $g(\nu, \omega) = \nu \log(\nu/\omega) - \nu + \omega$. We assume in the definition of $g(\nu, \omega)$ that for all $\nu > 0$, $\log(\nu/0) = \infty$ and $0\log(0/0) = 0\log(0) = 0$.

We consider I_T as a functional defined on the space $D([0,T];\mathbb{R}^d)$ equipped with Skorokhod's topology. We first give two other possible definitions of the functional I_T. Let $\ell : \mathbb{R}^{3d} \mapsto \mathbb{R}$ be defined as

$$\ell(x,y,\theta) = \langle y, \theta \rangle - \sum_{j=1}^k \beta_j(x)\left(e^{\langle h_j, \theta \rangle} - 1\right).$$

We define the map $L : \mathbb{R}^{2d} \mapsto (-\infty, +\infty]$ as

$$L(x,y) = \sup_{\theta \in \mathbb{R}^d} \ell(x,y,\theta).$$

We let

$$\hat{I}_T(\phi) = \int_0^T L(\phi_t, \dot{\phi}_t)dt.$$

It is not hard to see that the following is an equivalent definition of $\hat{I}_T(\phi)$:

$$\hat{I}_T(\phi) = \sup_{\theta \in C^1([0,T];\mathbb{R}^d)} \int_0^T \ell(\phi_t, \dot{\phi}_t, \theta_t)dt.$$

We first establish

Proposition 4.2.1. *For any $\phi \in D([0,T] : \mathbb{R}^d)$, $I_T(\phi) = \hat{I}_T(\phi)$.*

Proof. We note that if $y = \sum_{j=1}^k c_j h_j$ with some $c \in \mathbb{R}_+^k$,

$$\ell(x,y,\theta) = \sum_{j=1}^k \left[c_j\langle h_j, \theta\rangle - \beta_j(x)\left(e^{\langle h_j, \theta \rangle} - 1\right)\right].$$

But for any $1 \le j \le k$,

$$\begin{aligned} c_j\langle h_j, \theta\rangle - \beta_j(x)\left(e^{\langle h_j, \theta \rangle} - 1\right) &\le \sup_{r \in \mathbb{R}}[c_j r - \beta_j(x)(e^r - 1)] \\ &= c_j \log\left(\frac{c_j}{\beta_j(x)}\right) - c_j + \beta_j(x) \\ &= g(c_j, \beta_j(x)). \end{aligned}$$

The inequality $\hat{I}_T(\phi) \le I_T(\phi)$ for any $\phi \in D([0,T];\mathbb{R}^d)$ follows readily.

In order to prove the converse inequality, we fix $x, y \in \mathbb{R}^d$ such that $L(x,y) < \infty$ (otherwise there is nothing to prove). Let θ_n be a sequence in $\mathbb{R}^d$ such that

$L(x,y) = \lim_{n\to\infty} \ell(x,y,\theta_n)$. It is clear that for any $1 \le j \le k$ such that $\beta_j(x) > 0$, the sequence $\langle \theta_n, h_j \rangle$ is bounded from above. Hence we can and do assume that, after the extraction of a subsequence, for any $1 \le j \le k$ such that $\beta_j(x) > 0$, the sequence $e^{\langle \theta_n, h_j \rangle} \to s_j$, for some $s_j \ge 0$. Consequently, as $n \to \infty$,

$$\langle \theta_n, y \rangle \to L(x,y) + \sum_{j=1}^{k} \beta_j(x)\,(s_j - 1)\,. \tag{4.2.3}$$

Differentiating $\ell(x,y,\theta_n)$ with respect to its last variable, we get

$$\begin{aligned} \nabla_\theta \ell(x,y,\theta_n) &= y - \sum_{j=1}^{k} \beta_j(x) e^{\langle h_j, \theta_n \rangle} h_j \\ &\to y - \sum_{j=1}^{k} \beta_j(x) s_j h_j, \end{aligned}$$

as $n \to \infty$. But since θ_n is a maximizing sequence and the gradients converge, then since $L(x,y) < \infty$, their limit must be zero. Consequently

$$y = \sum_{j=1}^{k} \beta_j(x) s_j h_j\,.$$

Hence, with $c_j = \beta_j(x) s_j$, we have

$$\begin{aligned} \langle \theta_n, y \rangle &= \sum_{j=1}^{k} c_j \langle \theta_n, h_j \rangle \\ &\to \sum_{j=1}^{k} c_j \log(s_j), \end{aligned}$$

with the convention that $c_j \log(s_j) = 0$ if both $c_j = 0$ and $s_j = 0$. This, combined with (4.2.3), yields that

$$L(x,y) = \sum_{j=1}^{k} g(c_j, \beta_j(x))$$

which entails that $\hat{I}_T(\phi) \ge I_T(\phi)$. The proposition is established. □

We have the

Proposition 4.2.2. *For any $T > 0$, $\phi \in D([0,T];\mathbb{R}^d)$, $I_T(\phi) \ge 0$, and $I_T(\phi) = 0$ iff ϕ solves the ODE* (4.2.2).

Proof. It suffices to show that $L(x,y) \ge L(x, \sum_j \beta_j(x) h_j) = 0$, with strict inequality if $y \ne \sum_j \beta_j(x) h_j$. We first note that

$$L\left(x, \sum_j \beta_j(x) h_j\right) = \sup_\theta \left\{ \sum_j \beta_j(x)(\langle h_j, \theta \rangle - \exp\langle h_j, \theta \rangle + 1) \right\} = 0,$$

since $z - e^z + 1 \le 0$, with equality at $z = 0$. Let now y be such that $L(x,y) = 0$. Then

$$\langle y, \theta \rangle - \sum_j \beta_j(x)(\exp\langle h_j, \theta \rangle - 1) \le 0 \text{ for all } \theta \in \mathbb{R}^d.$$

Choosing $\theta = \varepsilon e_i$ (where e_i is the i-th basis vector of $\mathbb{R}^d$) yields

$$\varepsilon y_i \le \sum_j \beta_j(x)(\exp(\varepsilon h^i_j) - 1).$$

Dividing by ε, then letting $\varepsilon \to 0$ yields $y_i \le \sum_j \beta_j(x) h^i_j$, while the opposite inequality follows if we start with $\theta = -\varepsilon e_i$. The result follows. □

In the next statement, we use the notion of a lower semi-continuous real-valued function, which is defined in Definition A.7.1 below. In the proof we use the notion of an equicontinuous collection of functions, which is defined in Definition A.7.2.

Theorem 4.2.3. $\phi \to I_T(\phi)$ *is lower semi-continuous on* $D([0,T];\mathbb{R}^d)$, *and for any* R, $K > 0$, *the set* $\{\phi \in D([0,T];\mathbb{R}^d), \sup_{0\le t\le T} |\phi_t| \le R, I_T(\phi) \le K\}$ *is compact.*

Proof. The lower semicontinuity property is an immediate consequence of the fact that, from its second definition, $\hat{I}_T$ is a supremum over continuous functions. To finish the proof, it suffices from the Arzelà–Ascoli theorem (see e.g. Theorem 7.2 in Billingsley [8]) to show that the set of functions satisfying $\sup_{0\le t\le T} |\phi_t| \le R$ and $I_T(\phi) \le K$ is equicontinuous. It is clear that if $\bar{h} = \sup_{1\le j\le k} |h_j|$ and $\bar{\beta}_R = \sup_{1\le j\le k} \sup_{0\le t\le T, |x|\le R} \beta_j(t,x)$,

$$\begin{aligned} L(x,y) &\ge \ell\left(x, y, \frac{y \log(|y|)}{\bar{h}|y|}\right) \\ &\ge \frac{|y| \log(|y|)}{\bar{h}} - k\bar{\beta}_R |y|. \end{aligned}$$

Now let $0 \le s < t \le T$, with $t - s \le \delta$.

$$\begin{aligned} |\phi_t - \phi_s| &\le \int_s^t |\dot{\phi}_r| dr \\ &\le \delta^{-1/2} \int_s^t \mathbf{1}_{|\dot{\phi}_r| \le \delta^{-1/2}} dr + \int_s^t \mathbf{1}_{|\dot{\phi}_r| > \delta^{-1/2}} \frac{L(\phi_r, \dot{\phi}_r)}{L(\phi_r, \dot{\phi}_r)/|\dot{\phi}_r|} dr \\ &\le \delta^{1/2} + \frac{K}{f(\delta^{-1/2})}, \end{aligned}$$

where $f(a) = \inf_{|x|\le R, |y|\ge a} \frac{L(x,y)}{|y|}$. The result follows from the fact that from the above lower bound of $L(x,y)$, $f(a) \to \infty$, as $a \to \infty$. □

4.2.3 The Lower Bound

Let $\eta = (\eta_1, \ldots, \eta_k)$ be a vector of locally finite measures on $[0,T] \times \mathbb{R}_+$. We shall say that $\eta \in \mathscr{M}^k$. To $x \in \mathbb{R}^d$ and $\eta \in \mathscr{M}^k$, we associate $\Phi_t^x(\eta)$, solution (if it exists) of the ODE

$$\Phi_t^x(\eta) = x + \sum_{j=1}^{k} h_j \int_0^t \int_0^{\beta_j(s,\Phi_{s-}^x)} \eta_j(ds,du).$$

If $\eta_j(ds,du) = f_j(s,u)dsdu$, $1 \le j \le k$, the above ODE has at least one solution (possibly up to an explosion time, as the solution of an ODE with continuous coefficients). If moreover

$$\sup_{u \ge 0} f_j(\cdot,u) \in L^1[0,T],\ 1 \le j \le k,$$

then the above ODE has a unique solution (as the solution of an ODE with locally Lipschitz coefficients).

Let $\phi \in C([0,T];\mathbb{R}^d)$ be an absolutely continuous function. We define

$$K_\phi := \inf_{c \in \mathscr{A}_k(\phi)} \sum_{j=1}^{k} \int_0^T \frac{c_j(t)}{\beta_j(t,\phi_t)} dt. \tag{4.2.4}$$

To a pair (ϕ,c) with $c \in \mathscr{A}_k(\phi)$, we associate for $1 \le j \le k$ the measure $\eta_j(ds,du)$ with the density

$$f_j(s,u) = \frac{c_j(s)}{\beta_j(s,\phi_s)} \mathbf{1}_{[0,\beta_j(s,\phi_s)]}(u) + \mathbf{1}_{(\beta_j(s,\phi_s),+\infty)}(u).$$

Then, with $x = \phi_0$, $\phi_t = \Phi_t^x(\eta)$.

Moreover, given $\phi \in C([0,T];\mathbb{R}^d)$ and $L > 0$, we consider the set

$$A_{\phi,L} = \{(t,x),\ 0 \le t \le T,\ |x - \phi_t| \le L+1\},$$

and define

$$\overline{\beta}(\phi,L) = \sup_{1 \le j \le k} \sup_{(t,x) \in A_{\phi,L}} \beta_j(t,x).$$

We can now prove the following.

Proposition 4.2.4. *Let $T > 0$ be arbitrary. Given (ϕ,η) as above, such that in particular $K_\phi < \infty$, if $x_N = Z_0^N$, for any $R, L > 0$, there exists a $\delta, r > 0$ (depending upon K_ϕ) and N_0 such that whenever $|x - x_N| \le r$, $N \ge N_0$,*

$$\mathbb{P}\left(\|Z^N - \phi\|_T > L,\ d_{T,\overline{\beta}}(Q^N,\eta) \le \delta \right) \le e^{-NR},$$

where

$$d_{T,\overline{\beta}}(\nu,\eta) = \sum_{j=1}^{k} \sup_{0 \le t \le T, 0 \le u \le \overline{\beta}} |\nu_j([0,t] \times [0,u]) - \eta_j([0,t] \times [0,u])|,$$

and $\overline{\beta} := \overline{\beta}(\phi, L)$.

Proof. It is clear that

$$
\begin{aligned}
|Z_t^N - \phi_t| &\le |x_N - x| + \sum_{j=1}^k |h_j| \left| \int_0^t \int_0^{\beta_j(s, Z_{s-}^N)} [Q_j^N(ds, du) - \eta_j(ds, du)] \right| \\
&\quad + \sum_{j=1}^k |h_j| \left| \int_0^t \int_{\beta_j(s, Z_{s-}^N) \wedge \beta_j(s, \phi_s)}^{\beta_j(s, Z_{s-}^N) \vee \beta_j(s, \phi_s)} f_j(s, u) \vee 1 \, du ds \right| \\
&\le r + \sum_{j=1}^k |h_j| \left| \int_0^t \int_0^{\beta_j(s, Z_{s-}^N)} [Q_j^N(ds, du) - \eta_j(ds, du)] \right| \\
&\quad + \sum_{j=1}^k |h_j| C \int_0^t \left(\frac{c_j(s)}{\beta_j(s, \phi_s)} \vee 1 \right) |Z_s^N - \phi_s| ds,
\end{aligned}
$$

where C is an upper bound of the Lipschitz constants of the β_j's in $[0, T] \times [0, \overline{\beta}]$. Subdividing $[0, T]$ into $\left[\frac{T}{\rho}\right] + 1$ intervals of the form $[(i-1)\rho, i\rho \wedge T]$ and denoting

$$
\overline{\beta_j^i} := \sup_{(i-1)\rho \le s \le i\rho} \beta_j(s, Z_{s-}^{N, x^N}), \qquad \underline{\beta_j^i} := \inf_{(i-1)\rho \le s \le i\rho} \beta_j(s, Z_{s-}^{N, x^N}),
$$

we define the random sets

$$
A_j^{\rho, i} := [(i-1)\rho, i\rho] \times [0, \underline{\beta_j^i}], \quad B_j^{\rho, i} := [(i-1)\rho, i\rho] \times [\underline{\beta_j^i}, \overline{\beta_j^i}].
$$

For all i and j,

$$
\sum_{j=1}^k |Q_j^N(A_j^{\rho, i}) - \eta_j(A_j^{\rho, i})| \le 2 d_{T, \bar{\beta}}(Q^N, \eta), \; \sum_{j=1}^k |Q_j^N(B_j^{\rho, i}) - \eta_j(B_j^{\rho, i})| \le 4 d_{T, \bar{\beta}}(Q^N, \eta).
$$

Consequently for all $0 \le t \le T$, if $\bar{h} := \sup_{1 \le j \le k} |h_j|$, then on the event $\{d_{T, \overline{\beta}}(Q^N, \eta) \le \delta\}$,

$$
\begin{aligned}
&\sum_{j=1}^k |h_j| \left| \int_0^t \int_0^{\beta_j(s, Z^{N, s-})} [Q_j^N(ds, du) - \eta_j(ds, du)] \right| \\
&\le \bar{h} \sum_{j=1}^k \left(\sum_{i=1}^{\left[\frac{t}{\rho}\right]+1} \left| Q_j^N(A_j^{\rho, i}) - \eta_j(A_j^{\rho, i}) \right| + \sum_{i=1}^{\left[\frac{t}{\rho}\right]+1} \left\{ Q_j^N\left(B_j^{\rho, i}\right) + \eta_j\left(B_j^{\rho, i}\right) \right\} \right)
\end{aligned}
$$

$$\leq \bar{h}\sum_{j=1}^{k}\left(\sum_{i=1}^{\left[\frac{t}{\rho}\right]+1}\left|Q_j^N(A_j^{\rho,i})-\eta_j(A_j^{\rho,i})\right|+\sum_{i=1}^{\left[\frac{t}{\rho}\right]+1}\left|Q_j^N\left(B_j^{\rho,i}\right)-\eta_j\left(B_j^{\rho,i}\right)\right|\right.$$
$$\left.+2\sum_{i=1}^{\left[\frac{t}{\rho}\right]+1}\eta_j\left(B_j^{\rho,i}\right)\right)$$
$$\leq 6\left(\frac{t}{\rho}+1\right)\bar{h}\delta+2\bar{h}\sum_{j=1}^{k}\sum_{i=1}^{\left[\frac{t}{\rho}\right]+1}\eta_j\left(B_j^{\rho,i}\right).$$

It follows from the two above inequalities and Gronwall's Lemma that

$$\sup_{0\leq t\leq T}|Z_t^N-\phi_t|\leq\left(r+6\left(\frac{T}{\rho}+1\right)\bar{h}\delta+2\bar{h}\sum_{j=1}^{k}\sum_{i=1}^{\left[\frac{t}{\rho}\right]+1}\eta_j\left(B_j^{\rho,i}\right)\right)\exp\left[C(K_\phi+kT)\bar{h}\right]. \tag{4.2.5}$$

Since the $\left(B_j^{\rho,i}\right)_i$ are disjoints we have for all j

$$\sum_{i=1}^{\left[\frac{T}{\rho}\right]+1}\eta_j(B_j^{\rho,i})=\eta_j\left(\bigcup_{i=1}^{\left[\frac{T}{\rho}\right]+1}B_j^{\rho,i}\right)\leq\sum_{i=1}^{\left[\frac{T}{\rho}\right]+1}(\bar{\beta}_j^i-\underline{\beta}_j^i)\int_{(i-1)\rho}^{i\rho}\frac{c_j(s)}{\beta_j(\phi_s)}\vee 1\,ds$$
$$\leq\max_{1\leq i\leq\left[\frac{T}{\rho}\right]+1}\left(\overline{\beta_j^i}-\underline{\beta_j^i}\right)\int_0^T\frac{c_j(s)}{\beta_j(\phi_s)}\vee 1\,ds$$
$$\leq(K_\phi+T)\max_{1\leq i\leq\left[\frac{T}{\rho}\right]+1}\left(\overline{\beta_j^i}-\underline{\beta_j^i}\right).$$

We note that for every i,j

$$\overline{\beta_j^i}-\underline{\beta_j^i}\leq C\frac{X_i}{N}$$

where X_i is a Poisson random variable of mean $\rho N\bar{\beta}$. For any $a>0$, we have with $\bar{a}=\frac{a}{k(K_\phi+T)}$, using Cramér's Theorem A.3.1 for the fourth inequality,

$$\mathbb{P}\left[\sum_{j=1}^{k}\sum_{i=1}^{\left[\frac{T}{\rho}\right]+1}\eta_j(B_j^{\rho,i})>a\right]\leq k\max_j\mathbb{P}\left[\sum_{i=1}^{\left[\frac{T}{\rho}\right]+1}\eta_j(B_j^{\rho,i})>\frac{a}{k}\right]$$
$$\leq k\mathbb{P}\left[\max_{1\leq i\leq\left[\frac{T}{\rho}\right]+1}\frac{X_i}{N}>\bar{a}\right]$$

$$\leq k\mathbb{P}\left[\bigcup_{1\leq i\leq\left[\frac{T}{\rho}\right]+1}\left\{\frac{X_i}{N}>\bar{a}\right\}\right] \tag{4.2.6}$$

$$\leq k\left(\frac{T}{\rho}+1\right)\exp\left(-N\left[\bar{a}\log\frac{\bar{a}}{\rho\bar{\beta}}+\bar{a}-\rho\bar{\beta}\right]\right)$$

$$=\exp\left(-N\left[\bar{a}\log\frac{\bar{a}}{\rho\bar{\beta}}+\bar{a}-\frac{1}{N}\log\left(k\left[\frac{T}{\rho}+1\right]\right)-\rho\bar{\beta}\right]\right).$$

We choose $\rho=\sqrt{\delta}$. Let δ_0 be such that

$$6\left(T\sqrt{\delta_0}+\delta_0\right)\bar{h}\leq\frac{L}{3}\exp\left[-C(K_\phi+kT)\bar{h}\right],\ \text{and}$$

$$r=\frac{L}{3}\exp\left[-C(K_\phi+kT)\bar{h}\right],$$

$$a=\frac{L}{6\bar{h}}\exp\left[-C(K_\phi+kT)\bar{h}\right],$$

so that from (4.2.5),

$$\left\{\sum_{j=1}^{k}\sum_{i=1}^{\left[\frac{T}{\rho}\right]+1}\eta_j(B_j^{\rho,i})\leq a\right\}\subset\left\{\|Z^N-\phi\|_T\leq L\right\}. \tag{4.2.7}$$

$R>0$ being arbitrary, we now choose

$$\delta=\min\left\{\delta_0,\left(\frac{\bar{a}}{\bar{\beta}}\right)^2e^{-2R/\bar{a}},\frac{\bar{a}}{2\bar{\beta}}\right\},\ \text{and}$$

$$N_0=\left[\frac{2}{\bar{a}}\log\left(k\left[\frac{T}{\rho}+1\right]\right)\right].$$

The result follows from those choices, (4.2.6) and (4.2.7). □

Before we establish the lower bound, we need to formulate an assumption.

(A.2) We assume that for any $\phi\in C([0,T];\mathbb{R}^d)$ such that $I_T(\phi)<\infty$ and any $\varepsilon>0$, there exists a ϕ^ε such that $\phi_0^\varepsilon=\phi_0$, $K_{\phi^\varepsilon}<\infty$, $\|\phi-\phi^\varepsilon\|_T\leq\varepsilon$ and $I_T(\phi^\varepsilon)\leq I_T(\phi)+\varepsilon$.

Exercise 4.2.5. Consider the SIRS model with fixed population size, and let $A:=\{(x,y),0\leq x,0\leq y,x+y\leq 1\}$. Show that if $\phi\in C([0,T];A)$ hits the boundary, then for any $\varepsilon>0$, one can find ϕ^ε such that $\phi_0^\varepsilon=\phi_0$, $K_{\phi^\varepsilon}<\infty$, $\|\phi-\phi^\varepsilon\|\leq\varepsilon$ and $I_T(\phi^\varepsilon)\leq I_T(\phi)+\varepsilon$, where ϕ^ε can either remain in the interior of A, or else can hit the boundary.

We now have, with the notation $I_{T,x}(O)=\inf_{\phi\in O,\phi_0=x}I_T(\phi)$,

Theorem 4.2.6. *If the assumptions (A.1) and (A.2) are satisfied, then for any open subset $O \subset D([0,T];\mathbb{R}^d)$, if $x_N \to x$ as $N \to \infty$,*

$$\liminf_{N\to\infty} \frac{1}{N} \log \mathbb{P}\left(Z^{N,x_N} \in O\right) \geq -I_{T,x}(O).$$

Proof. It clearly suffices to treat the case where $I_{T,x}(O) < \infty$. Then for any $\varepsilon > 0$ there exists a $\phi \in O$ such that $\phi_0 = x$ and

$$I_T(\phi) \leq I_{T,x}(O) + \frac{\varepsilon}{4}.$$

It follows from assumption (A.2) that there exists a $\hat{\phi} \in O$ such that $\hat{\phi}_0 = \phi_0$, $K_{\hat{\phi}} < \infty$, $\|\hat{\phi} - \phi\|_T \leq \varepsilon$ and

$$I_T(\hat{\phi}) \leq I_T(\phi) + \frac{\varepsilon}{4}.$$

Now there exists a $c \in \mathscr{A}_k(\phi)$ such that $\sum_{j=1}^k \int_0^T \frac{c_j(t)}{\beta_j(t,\phi_t)} dt < \infty$, and

$$I_T(\hat{\phi}|c) \leq I_T(\hat{\phi}) + \frac{\varepsilon}{4}.$$

If ε has been chosen small enough, there exists an $L > 0$ be such that $\{\psi;\, \|\psi - \hat{\phi}\|_T < L\} \subset O$. From Proposition 4.2.4, if η^c denotes the vector of measures associated to c, $|x - x_N|$ is small enough and N large enough, for any $R > 0$, there exists a $\delta > 0$ such that with $\hat{\beta} = \overline{\beta}(\hat{\phi}, L)$,

$$\begin{aligned}
\mathbb{P}\left(Z^{N,x_N} \in O\right) &\geq \mathbb{P}\left(\|Z^{N,x_N} - \phi\|_T < L\right) \\
&\geq \mathbb{P}\left(d_{T,\hat{\beta}}(Q^N, \eta^c) < \delta\right) \\
&\qquad - \mathbb{P}\left(\|Z^{N,x_N} - \phi\|_T > L, d_{T,\hat{\beta}}(Q^N, \eta^c) < \delta\right) \\
&\geq \mathbb{P}\left(d_{T,\hat{\beta}}(Q^N, \eta^c) < \delta\right) - e^{-NR}.
\end{aligned} \tag{4.2.8}$$

Let us admit for a moment the next lemma.

Lemma 4.2.7. *There exists a sequence of partitions $\{A_n^i, 1 \leq i \leq a_n\}$ of $[0,T] \times [0,\hat{\beta}]$ such that $\sup_i \lambda^2(A_n^i) \to 0$ as $n \to \infty$, and a sequence $\delta_n \downarrow 0$ and n_0 such that for all $n \geq n_0$,*

$$\bigcap_{j=1}^{k} \bigcap_{i=1}^{a_n} \{Q_j^N(A_n^i) \in (\eta_j^c(A_n^i) - \delta_n, \eta_j^c(A_n^i) + \delta_n)\} \subset \{d_{T,\hat{\beta}}(Q^N, \eta^c) < \delta\}.$$

As a consequence of this lemma, making use of Cramér's Theorem A.3.1, for the second inequality,

$$
\begin{aligned}
&\liminf_{N\to\infty}\frac{1}{N}\log\mathbb{P}\left(d_{T,\hat\beta}(Q^N,\eta^c)<\delta\right)\\
&\quad\ge\sum_{j=1}^{k}\sum_{i=1}^{a_n}\liminf_{N\to\infty}\frac{1}{N}\log\mathbb{P}\left(Q_j^N(A_n^i)\in(\eta_j^c(A_n^i)-\delta_n,\eta_j^c(A_n^i)+\delta_n)\right)\\
&\quad\ge-\sum_{j=1}^{k}\sum_{i=1}^{a_n}\left(\eta_j^c(A_n^i)\log\frac{\eta_j^c(A_n^i)}{\lambda^2(A_n^i)}-\eta_j^c(A_n^i)+\lambda^2(A_n^i)\right)\\
&\quad\ge-\sum_{j=1}^{k}\int_0^T\int_0^{\bar\beta}\left[f_j^c(s,u)\log[f_j^c(s,u)]-f_j^c(s,u)+1\right]dsdu-\frac{\varepsilon}{4}\\
&\quad=-\sum_{j=1}^{k}\int_0^T\left[c_j(s)\log\frac{c_j(s)}{\beta_j(s,\phi_s)}-c_j(s)+\beta_j(s,\phi_s)\right]ds-\frac{\varepsilon}{4}\\
&\quad=-I_T(\hat\phi|c)-\frac{\varepsilon}{4}\\
&\quad\ge-I_{T,x}(O)-\varepsilon,
\end{aligned}
$$

where

$$
f_j^c(s,u)=\frac{c_j(s)}{\beta_j(s,\phi_s)}\mathbf{1}_{[0,\beta_j(s,\phi_s)]}(u)+\mathbf{1}_{(\beta_j(s,\phi_s),+\infty)}(u)
$$

and the second inequality holds true for n chosen large enough as a function of ε. We let $\varepsilon\to 0$, and to combine the resulting inequality with (4.2.8), hence

$$
\begin{aligned}
-I_{T,x}(O)&\le\liminf_{N\to\infty}\frac{1}{N}\log\left(\mathbb{P}\left(Z^{N,x_N}\in O\right)+e^{-NR}\right)\\
&\le\left(\liminf_{N\to\infty}\frac{1}{N}\log\mathbb{P}\left(Z^{N,x_N}\in O\right)\right)\vee(-R).
\end{aligned}
$$

The result finally follows by letting $R\to\infty$. □

We now need to pass to the

Proof of Lemma 4.2.7. For convenience, we replace the partition $\{A_n^i,\ 1\le i\le a_n\}$ by a partition $\{A_n^{i,j},\ 1\le i,j\le n\}$, which we construct as follows. We first choose $0=\beta_n^0<\beta_n^1<\cdots<\beta_n^n=\hat\beta$ such that

$$
\sup_{1\le j\le n}\eta^c([0,T]\times(\beta_n^{j-1},\beta_n^j])\le\frac{2}{n}\eta^c([0,T]\times[0,\hat\beta]).
$$

We next choose a sequence $0=t_n^0<t_n^1<\cdots t_n^n=T$ such that, if $A_n^{i,j}=(t_n^{i-1},t_n^i]\times(\beta_n^{j-1},\beta_n^j]$,

$$
\sup_{1\le i\le n}\eta^c(A_n^{i,j})\le\frac{2}{n}\eta^c([0,T]\times(\beta_n^{j-1},\beta_n^j])\le\frac{4}{n^2}\eta^c([0,T]\times[0,\hat\beta]):=\frac{C}{n^2}.
$$

For an arbitrary $0 \le t \le T$ and $0 \le \alpha \le \hat{\beta}$, we define the set

$$\partial_{t,\alpha} = \{t\} \times [0,\hat{\beta}] \cup [0,T] \times \{\alpha\},$$

which is the "boundary" of $[0,t] \times [0,\alpha]$. We note that $|\{i,j,\ A_n^{i,j} \cap \partial_{t,\alpha} \neq \emptyset\}| \le 2n$. We need to bound

$$\begin{aligned}
&\left| Q^N([0,t] \times [0,\alpha]) - \eta^c([0,t] \times [0,\alpha]) \right| \\
&\quad \le \sum_{i,j,\ A_n^{i,j} \subset [0,t]\times[0,\alpha]} \left| Q^N(A_n^{i,j}) - \eta^c(A_n^{i,j}) \right| + \sum_{i,j,\ A_n^{i,j} \cap \partial_{t,\alpha} \neq \emptyset} \left(Q^N(A_n^{i,j}) + \eta^c(A_n^{i,j}) \right) \\
&\quad \le n^2 \delta_n + 2n \left(\frac{2C}{n^2} + \delta_n \right) \\
&\quad \le \delta,
\end{aligned}$$

for all $n \ge n_0$, provided we choose first $n_0 \ge \frac{8C}{\delta}$, and then a sequence δ_n such that $\delta_n \le [2(n^2 + 2n)]^{-1} \delta$ for each $n \ge n_0$. □

We now establish a slightly stronger result. Here and below we shall use the following notation concerning the initial condition of Z^N. We fix $x \in \mathbb{R}^d$ and start Z^N from the point $Z_0^N = x_N$, where the i-th coordinate x_N^i of x_N is given by $x_N^i = \frac{[x^i N]}{N}$. Here we assume that the process Z^N lives in a closed subset $A \subset \mathbb{R}^d$. We shall need the following

Definition 4.2.8. We shall say that the compact set of initial conditions $\mathscr{K}$ is **adapted** to the open set of trajectories $O \subset D([0,T];A)$ if

1. $\mathscr{K} \subset \{\phi_0,\ \phi \in O\}$.
2. For any $\varepsilon > 0$, the following holds. For any $x \in \mathscr{K}$, there exists a $\phi^x \in O$ such that $\phi_0^x = x$, $I_T(\phi^x) \le I_{T,x}(O) + \varepsilon$ and moreover $\sup_{x \in \mathscr{K}} K_{\phi^x} < \infty$.

It follows readily from the proof of Theorem 4.2.6 that the following reinforced version holds.

Theorem 4.2.9. *For any open subset $O \subset D([0,T];A)$ and any compact subset $\mathscr{K}$ of initial conditions which is adapted to O,*

$$\liminf_{N\to\infty} \frac{1}{N} \log \inf_{x \in \mathscr{K}} \mathbb{P}(Z^{N,x_N} \in O) \ge - \sup_{x \in \mathscr{K}} I_{T,x}(O).$$

4.2.4 The Upper Bound

In this subsection, we shall again use the notation x_N for the vector whose i-th coordinate is given by $x_N^i = \frac{[x^i N]}{N}$. We want to prove that for any closed F, $F \subset D([0,T];\mathbb{R}^d)$,

$$\limsup_{N\to\infty} \log \mathbb{P}(Z^{N,x_N} \in F) \le -I_{T,x}(F). \tag{4.2.9}$$

Let us recall the concept of exponential tightness.

Definition 4.2.10. The sequence Z^N is said to be exponentially tight if for any $\alpha > 0$, there exists a compact K^α such that

$$\limsup_N \frac{1}{N} \log \mathbb{P}(Z^N \in K_\alpha^c) \le -\alpha.$$

We have the following lemma.

Lemma 4.2.11. *If* (4.2.9) *holds for any compact subset* $F = K \subset\subset D([0,T];A)$, *and* Z^N *is exponentially tight, then* (4.2.9) *holds for any closed subset* $F \subset D([0,T];A)$.

Proof. Let F be closed and $\alpha := I_{T,x}(F)$. We assume w.l.o.g. that $\alpha > 0$ (unless the conclusion below would be obvious). Let K_α be the compact set associated to α by Definition 4.2.10. It is clear that $F \cap K_\alpha$ is compact and $I_{T,x}(F \cap K_\alpha) \ge \alpha$. Hence from our assumption

$$\limsup_{N\to\infty} \frac{1}{N} \log \mathbb{P}(Z^N \in F \cap K_\alpha) \le -\alpha.$$

Also from the choice of K_α,

$$\limsup_{N\to\infty} \frac{1}{N} \log \mathbb{P}(Z^N \in K_\alpha^c) \le -\alpha.$$

But $\mathbb{P}(Z^N \in F) \le \mathbb{P}(Z^N \in F \cap K_\alpha) + \mathbb{P}(Z^N \in K_\alpha^c)$, hence

$$\log \mathbb{P}(Z^N \in F) \le \log 2 + \sup(\log \mathbb{P}(Z^N \in F \cap K_\alpha), \log \mathbb{P}(Z^N \in K_\alpha^c)),$$

and we clearly deduce that

$$\limsup_{N\to\infty} \frac{1}{N} \log \mathbb{P}(Z^N \in F) \le -\alpha,$$

as desired. □

Let us first establish

Theorem 4.2.12. *Let* $T > 0$ *and* $x \in \mathbb{R}^d$ *be fixed. Let* $x_N \to x$ *as* $N \to \infty$. *For any compact set* $K \subset D([0,T];\mathbb{R}^d)$,

$$\limsup_{N\to\infty} \frac{1}{N} \log \mathbb{P}\left(Z^{N,x_N} \in K\right) \le -I_{T,x}(K).$$

Proof. Recall the formula

$$\begin{aligned} I_T(\phi) &= \sup_{\theta \in C^1([0,T];\mathbb{R}^d)} \int_0^T \ell(\phi_t, \dot\phi_t, \theta_t)dt \\ &= \sup_{\theta \in C^1([0,T];\mathbb{R}^d)} \mathscr{L}(\phi, \theta), \end{aligned}$$

where

$$\mathscr{L}(\phi,\theta)=\langle\phi_T,\theta_T\rangle-\langle\phi_0,\theta_0\rangle-\int_0^T\langle\phi_t,\dot\theta_t\rangle dt-\sum_{j=1}^k\int_0^T\beta_j(\phi_t)\left[e^{\langle h_j,\theta_t\rangle}-1\right]dt.$$

For any $\theta\in C^1([0,T];\mathbb{R}^d)$, $0\le s<t\le T$, we define

$$M_{s,t}^{N,\theta}=\langle Z_t^{N,x_N},\theta_t\rangle-\langle Z_s^{N,x_N},\theta_s\rangle-\int_s^t\langle Z_r^{N,x_N},\dot\theta_r\rangle dr-\sum_{j=1}^k\int_s^t\langle h_j,\theta_r\rangle\beta_j(r,\mathbb{Z}_r^{N,x_N})dr,$$

$$\Xi_{s,t}^{N,\theta}=\exp\left(NM_{s,t}^{N,\theta}-N\sum_{j=1}^k\int_s^t\tau(\langle h_j,\theta_r\rangle)\beta_j(r,\mathbb{Z}_r^{N,x_N})dr\right),$$

where $\tau(a)=e^a-1-a$, are such that $M_{0,t}^{N,\theta}$ and $\Xi_{0,t}^{N,\theta}$ are local martingales, the second being also a supermartingale such that $\mathbb{E}[\Xi_{0,t}^{N,\theta}]\le 1$.

We assume that $I_{T,x}(K)>0$, since otherwise the result is trivial. We also assume that $I_{T,x}(K)<\infty$. The case $I_{T,x}(K)=\infty$ can be treated in a way which is very similar to what follows, and we will not repeat the argument. Since $\phi\mapsto I_T(\phi)$ is lower semicontinuous and $K_x=\{\phi\in K,\ \phi_0=x\}$ is compact, there exists a $\hat\phi\in K$ such that $\hat\phi_0=x$ and $I_T(\hat\phi)=I_{T,x}(K)$. Let now $\phi\in K_x$ be arbitrary. First assume that $I_T(\phi)<\infty$. Then there exists a $\theta_\phi\in C^1([0,T];\mathbb{R}^d)$ such that

$$I_T(\phi)\le\mathscr{L}(\phi,\theta_\phi)+\frac{\varepsilon}{2}.$$

Since $\psi\mapsto\mathscr{L}(\psi,\theta_\phi)$ is continuous on $D([0,T];\mathbb{R}^d)$ equipped with the Skorokhod topology, there exists a neighbourhood $\mathscr{V}_{\phi,\theta_\phi}(\varepsilon)$ of ϕ in $D([0,T];\mathbb{R}^d)$ such that for any $\psi\in\mathscr{V}_{\phi,\theta_\phi}(\varepsilon)$,

$$|\mathscr{L}(\phi,\theta_\phi)-\mathscr{L}(\psi,\theta_\phi)|\le\frac{\varepsilon}{2}.$$

Now

$$\begin{aligned}\mathbb{P}\left(Z^{N,x_N}\in\mathscr{V}_{\phi,\theta_\phi}(\varepsilon)\right)&=\mathbb{E}\left(\mathbf{1}_{Z^{N,x_N}\in\mathscr{V}_{\phi,\theta_\phi}(\varepsilon)}\right)\\&=e^{-N\mathscr{L}(\phi,\theta_\phi)}\mathbb{E}\left(e^{N\mathscr{L}(\phi,\theta_\phi)}\mathbf{1}_{Z^{N,x_N}\in\mathscr{V}_{\phi,\theta_\phi}(\varepsilon)}\right)\\&\le e^{-N[\mathscr{L}(\phi,\theta_\phi)-\frac{\varepsilon}{2}]}\mathbb{E}\left(e^{N\mathscr{L}(Z^{N,x_N},\theta_\phi)}\right)\\&\le e^{-N[\mathscr{L}(\phi,\theta_\phi)-\frac{\varepsilon}{2}]}\\&\le e^{-NI_T(\phi)+N\varepsilon},\end{aligned}\tag{4.2.10}$$

where the before last inequality follows the fact that $N\mathscr{L}(Z^{N,x_N},\theta_\phi)=\log(\Xi_T^{N,\theta_\phi})$ and $\mathbb{E}[\Xi_T^{N,\theta_\phi}]\le 1$.

The second case is the one where $I_T(\phi)=+\infty$. Then there exists $M>I_{T,x}(K)+1$ and $\theta_\phi\in C^1([0,T];\mathbb{R}^d)$ such that $\mathscr{L}(\phi,\theta_\phi)>M+\varepsilon$. From the same argument as above, we deduce that

$$\mathbb{P}\left(Z^{N,x_N} \in \mathscr{V}_{\phi,\theta_\phi}(\varepsilon)\right) \le e^{-NM}.$$

Let $K_x = \{\phi \in K, \phi_0 = x\}$. Since $K_x \subset \bigcup_{\phi \in K, \phi_0 = x} \mathscr{V}_{\phi,\theta_\phi}(\varepsilon)$ and K_x is compact, there exists $m = m(\varepsilon) \ge 1$ and $\phi_1, \ldots, \phi_m \in K_x$ where we assume that $\phi_1 = \hat{\phi}$, such that

$$K_x \subset \bigcup_{i=1}^{m} \mathscr{V}_{\phi_i,\theta_{\phi_i}}(\varepsilon).$$

Now there exists a finite set of functions $\{\phi_{m+1}, \ldots, \phi_{m+n}\} \subset K \backslash K_x$, such that

$$K \subset \bigcup_{i=1}^{m+n} \mathscr{V}_{\phi_i,\theta_{\phi_i}}(\varepsilon).$$

We choose ε small enough for $i \ge m+1$ such that $x \notin \mathscr{V}_{\phi,\theta_{\phi_i}}(\varepsilon)$. Then for N large enough, $\mathbb{P}(Z^{N,x_N} \in \mathscr{V}_{\phi_i,\theta_{\phi_i}}(\varepsilon)) = 0$ if $i \ge m+1$. Hence

$$\begin{aligned}
\limsup_{N\to\infty} \frac{1}{N} \log \mathbb{P}(Z^{N,x_N} \in K) &\le \limsup_{N\to\infty} \frac{1}{N} \log\left(\sum_{i=1}^{m+n} \mathbb{P}\left(Z^{N,x_N} \in \mathscr{V}_{\phi_i,\theta_{\phi_i}}(\varepsilon)\right)\right) \\
&\le \max_{1\le i\le m} \limsup_{N\to\infty} \frac{1}{N} \log \mathbb{P}\left(Z^{N,x_N} \in \mathscr{V}_{\phi_i,\theta_{\phi_i}}(\varepsilon)\right) \\
&\le -\inf_{1\le i\le m} I_T(\phi_i) + \varepsilon \\
&\le -I_{T,x}(K) + \varepsilon,
\end{aligned}$$

where we have used (4.2.10) in the third inequality. It remains to let $\varepsilon \to 0$. □

It remains to establish exponential tightness. Now we need to impose a growth condition on the β_j's. One natural assumption would be to assume that for some $C > 0$, all $1 \le j \le m$ and $x \in \mathbb{R}^d$, $\beta_j(t,x) \le C(1+|x|)$. However, this condition is not satisfied in most of our examples, because one of the β_j's is quadratic. We shall instead formulate an assumption which is satisfied in our epidemic models. We shall write $\mathbb{1}$ for the vector in $\mathbb{R}^d$ whose coordinates are all equal to 1, and we exploit the fact that for those j's such that β_j is quadratic, $\langle h_j, \mathbb{1}\rangle = 0$.

(A.3) We assume that for all starting points $x_N \in \mathbb{Z}_+^d/N$, Z^{N,x_N} takes its values in $\mathbb{R}_+^d$ a.s., and moreover that there exists a $C_\beta > 0$ such that for any $0 \le j \le k$ such that $\langle h_j, \mathbb{1}\rangle \ne 0$, $\beta_j(t,x) \le C_\beta(1+|x|)$, $0 \le t \le T$, $x \in \mathbb{R}^d$.

We now prove

Proposition 4.2.13. *Assume that Conditions (A.1) and (A.3) are satisfied. Let $T > 0$ and $x \in \mathbb{R}^d$ be given, as well as a sequence $x_N \to x$ as $N \to \infty$, such that for all $N \ge 1$, $x_N \in \mathbb{Z}_+^d/N$. Then for all $\xi > 0$,*

$$\lim_{\delta\downarrow 0}\limsup_{N\to\infty}\frac{1}{N}\log\mathbb{P}\left(\sup_{0\le s,t\le T,\ |t-s|\le\delta}\left|Z_t^{N,x_N}-Z_s^{N,x_N}\right|>\xi\right)=-\infty.$$

Proof. $\xi>0$ and $T>0$ will be fixed throughout this proof. Consider the stopping time

$$\sigma_R^{N,x_N}=\inf\{t\in[0,T],\ |Z_t^{N,x_N}|>R\}.$$

It is clear that

$$\mathbb{P}\left(\sup_{|t-s|\le\delta}\left|Z_t^{N,x_N}-Z_s^{N,x_N}\right|>\xi\right)\le\mathbb{P}\left(\sup_{|t-s|\le\delta}\left|Z^{N,x_N}_{t\wedge\sigma_R^{N,x_N}}-Z^{N,x_N}_{s\wedge\sigma_R^{N,x_N}}\right|>\xi\right)$$
$$+\mathbb{P}\left(\sigma_R^{N,x_N}<T\right).$$

We first consider the first term of the above right-hand side. For that purpose, we divide $[0,T]$ into subintervals of length δ, and let $\underline{i}(s)\le s<\bar{i}(s)$ denote the points of the grid nearest to s.

$$\begin{aligned}
&\mathbb{P}\left[\sup_{|s-t|\le\delta}\left|Z^{N,x_N}_{t\wedge\sigma_R^{N,x_N}}-Z^{N,x_N}_{s\wedge\sigma_R^{N,x_N}}\right|>\xi\right]\\
&=\mathbb{P}\left[\exists 0\le s<t\le T, t-s\le\delta,\ \left|Z^{N,x_N}_{t\wedge\sigma_R^{N,x_N}}-Z^{N,x_N}_{s\wedge\sigma_R^{N,x_N}}\right|>\xi\right]\\
&\le\mathbb{P}\left[\exists 0\le s<t\le T, t-s\le\delta,\left|Z^{N,x_N}_{t\wedge\sigma_R^{N,x_N}}-Z^{N,x_N}_{\underline{i}(s)}\right|+\left|Z^{N,x_N}_{\underline{i}(s)}-Z^{N,x_N}_{s\wedge\sigma_R^{N,x_N}}\right|>\xi\right]\\
&\le 2\left(\frac{T}{\delta}+1\right)\sup_{s\in[0,T]}\mathbb{P}\left[\sup_{t\in[s,s+2\delta[}\left|Z^{N,x_N}_{t\wedge\sigma_R^{N,x_N}}-Z^{N,x_N}_{s\wedge\sigma_R^{N,x_N}}\right|>\xi/2\right].
\end{aligned}$$

Let $\{\theta_i\,,1\le i\le d\}$ (resp. $\{\theta_i\,,d+1\le i\le 2d\}$) denote the standard basis of $\mathbb{R}^d_+$ (resp. of $\mathbb{R}^d_-$). Thus for every $\lambda>0$, assuming w.l.o.g. that $|z|$ stands here for $\sup_{1\le i\le d}|z_i|$,

$$\begin{aligned}
&\mathbb{P}\left[\sup_{t\in[s,s+2\delta[}\left|Z^{N,x_N}_{t\wedge\sigma_R^{N,x_N}}-Z^{N,x_N}_{s\wedge\sigma_R^{N,x_N}}\right|>\xi/2\right]\\
&\le\sum_{i=1}^{2d}\mathbb{P}\left[\sup_{t\in[s,s+2\delta[}\langle Z_t^{N,x_N}-Z_s^{N,x_N},\lambda\theta_i\rangle>\lambda\xi/2\right]\\
&\le\sum_{i=1}^{2d}\mathbb{P}\left[\sup_{t\in[s,s+2\delta[}\mathbf{M}^{N,\lambda\theta_i}_{(s,t)\wedge\sigma_R^{N,x_N}}+\sum_{j=1}^{k}\int_{s\wedge\sigma_R^{N,x_N}}^{t\wedge\sigma_R^{N,x_N}}\langle h_j,\lambda\theta_i\rangle\beta_j\left(r,Z_r^{N,x_N}\right)dr>\lambda\xi/2\right]\\
&\le\sum_{i=1}^{2d}\mathbb{P}\left[\sup_{t\in[s,s+2\delta[}\exp\left(N\mathbf{M}^{N,\lambda\theta_i}_{(s,t)\wedge\sigma_R^{N,x_N}}+N\sum_{j=1}^{k}\int_{s\wedge\sigma_R^{N,x_N}}^{t\wedge\sigma_R^{N,x_N}}\langle h_j,\lambda\theta_i\rangle\beta_j\left(r,Z_r^{N,x_N}\right)dr\right)>e^{N\lambda\xi/2}\right]
\end{aligned}$$

$$\leq \sum_{i=1}^{2d} \mathbb{P}\left[\sup_{t\in[s,s+2\delta[} \Xi^{N,\lambda\theta_i}_{(s,t)\wedge\sigma_R^{N,x_N}} > \exp\left(N\lambda\xi/2 - N\sum_{i=1}^{k}\left(e^{\langle h_j,\lambda\theta_i\rangle}-1\right)\int_{s\wedge\sigma_R^{N,x_N}}^{t\wedge\sigma_R^{N,x_N}} \beta_j(s,Z_r^{N,x_N})dr\right)\right]$$
$$\leq \sum_{i=1}^{2d} \mathbb{P}\left[\sup_{t\in[s,s+2\delta[} \Xi^{N,\lambda\theta_i}_{(s,t)\wedge\sigma_R^{N,x_N}} > \exp\left(N\lambda\xi/2 - 2\delta Nk\bar{\beta}_R e^{\lambda\bar{h}}\right)\right]$$
$$\leq 2d\exp\left(-N\lambda\xi/2 + 2\delta Nk\bar{\beta}_R e^{\lambda\bar{h}}\right),$$

where $\bar{\beta}_R = \sup_{1\leq j\leq k}\sup_{0\leq t\leq T,\,|x|\leq R}\beta_j(t,x)$. Optimizing over $\lambda > 0$ yields

$$\limsup_{N\to\infty}\frac{1}{N}\log\mathbb{P}\left[\sup_{|s-t|\leq\delta}\left|Z^{N,x_N}_{t\wedge\sigma_R^{N,x_N}} - Z^{N,x_N}_{s\wedge\sigma_R^{N,x_N}}\right| > \xi\right] \leq -\frac{\xi}{2\bar{h}}\left(\log\left(\frac{\xi\delta^{-1}}{4\bar{h}k\bar{\beta}_R}\right)-1\right).$$

Consequently for any fixed $R > 0$,

$$\lim_{\delta\to 0}\limsup_{N\to\infty}\frac{1}{N}\log\mathbb{P}\left[\sup_{|s-t|\leq\delta}\left|Z^{N,x_N}_{t\wedge\sigma_R^{N,x_N}} - Z^{N,x_N}_{s\wedge\sigma_R^{N,x_N}}\right| > \xi\right] = -\infty.$$

It remains to show that

$$\lim_{R\to\infty}\limsup_{N\to\infty}\frac{1}{N}\log\mathbb{P}\left(\sigma_R^{N,x_N} < T\right) = -\infty. \tag{4.2.11}$$

Combing the fact that for all $t\leq T$

$$\sup_{s\leq t}|Z_s^{N,x_N}| \leq \sup_{s\leq t}|\langle Z_s^{N,x_N},\mathbb{1}\rangle|$$

and that by Gronwall's Lemma 2.2.9, with $\bar{h} = \sup_{1\leq j\leq k}|h_j|$ and C_β the constant from assumption (A.3),

$$\sup_{s\leq t}|\langle Z_s^{N,x_N},\mathbb{1}\rangle| \leq \left(|\langle x,\mathbb{1}\rangle + k\bar{h}Ct + \sup_{s\leq t}|M_s^{N,\mathbb{1}}|\right)e^{k\bar{h}C_\beta t},$$

we deduce that

$$\sup_{s\leq t}|Z_s^{N,x_N}| \leq \left(|\langle x,\mathbb{1}\rangle| + k\bar{h}Ct + \sup_{s\leq t}|M_s^{N,\mathbb{1}}|\right)e^{k\bar{h}C_\beta t}. \tag{4.2.12}$$

By Itô's formula we have, with $\mathscr{M}_t^{N,\mathbb{1}}$ a local martingale, and defining $A_s^N := 1\vee(\sup_{0\leq r\leq s}|M_r^{N,\mathbb{1}}|$,

$$\left(M_t^{N,\mathbb{1}}\right)^{2N}$$
$$= N\sum_{j;\langle h_j,\mathbb{1}\rangle\neq 0}\int_0^t \beta_j(s,Z_s^{N,x_N})\left[\left(M_s^{N,\mathbb{1}}+\frac{\langle h_j,\mathbb{1}\rangle}{N}\right)^{2N} - \left(M_{s-}^{N,\mathbb{1}}\right)^{2N} - 2N(M_s^{N,\mathbb{1}})^{2N-1}\frac{\langle h_j,\mathbb{1}\rangle}{N}\right]ds + \mathscr{M}_t^{N,\mathbb{1}}$$

$$\leq NC_\beta\sum_j\frac{N(2N-1)}{N^2}\langle h_j,\mathbb{1}\rangle^2\int_0^t(1+|Z_s^{N,x_N}|)\left(|M_s^{N,\mathbb{1}}| + \frac{\langle h_j,\mathbb{1}\rangle}{N}\right)^{2N-2}ds + \mathscr{M}_t^{N,\mathbb{1}}$$

$$\leq NC_\beta C_T \left(1+\frac{\bar{h}}{N}\right)^{2N} \int_0^t \frac{1+|Z_s^{N,x_N}|}{A_s^N}(A_s^N)^{2N-1}ds + \mathscr{M}_t^{N,\mathbb{1}}$$

$$\leq NC_T' \int_0^t (A_s^N)^{2N} ds + \mathscr{M}_t^{N,\mathbb{1}}, \tag{4.2.13}$$

where we have used (4.2.12) and the inequality $a+b \leq a(1+b)$ for $a \geq 1$, $b \geq 0$. From Doob's inequality,

$$\mathbb{E}\left[\sup_{s\leq t\wedge\sigma_R^{N,x_N}} (M_s^{N,\mathbb{1}})^{2N}\right] \leq \left(\frac{2N}{2N-1}\right)^{2N} \mathbb{E}\left[(M_{t\wedge\sigma_R^{N,x_N}}^{N,\mathbb{1}})^{2N}\right]. \tag{4.2.14}$$

Since $\mathscr{M}_{t\wedge\sigma_R^{N,x_N}}^{N,\mathbb{1}}$ is a martingale, we can take the expectation in the inequality (4.2.13) at time $t\wedge\sigma_R^{N,x_N}$, and deduce from the resulting inequality, (4.2.14) and $\sup_{N\geq 1}\left(\frac{2N}{2N-1}\right)^{2N} < \infty$

$$\mathbb{E}\left[\sup_{s\leq t\wedge\sigma_R^{N,x_N}} (M_s^{N,\mathbb{1}})^{2N}\right] \leq NC_T'' \int_0^t \mathbb{E}\left[\left(A_{s\wedge\sigma_R^{N,x_N}}^N\right)^{2N}\right] ds.$$

Since for $a \geq 0$, $(1\vee a)^{2N} \leq 1+a^{2N}$, it follows that for all $0\leq t\leq T$,

$$\mathbb{E}\left[\left(A_{t\wedge\sigma_R^{N,x_N}}^N\right)^{2N}\right] \leq 1+NC_T'' \int_0^t \mathbb{E}\left[\left(A_{s\wedge\sigma_R^{N,x_N}}^N\right)^{2N}\right] ds.$$

Hence it follows from Gronwall's lemma that

$$\mathbb{E}\left[\sup_{t\leq T\wedge\sigma_R^{N,x_N}} (M_t^{N,\mathbb{1}})^{2N}\right] \leq \exp\left(C_T N T\right). \tag{4.2.15}$$

For any $0<\kappa<R$, denoting

$$C(R,\kappa) := (R-\kappa)e^{-k\bar{h}C_T T} - |\langle x,\mathbb{1}\rangle| - k\bar{h}C_T T,$$

we have

$$\limsup_{N\to+\infty}\frac{1}{N}\log\mathbb{P}\left[\sigma_R^{N,x_N}\leq T\right] \leq \limsup_{N\to+\infty}\frac{1}{N}\log\mathbb{P}\left[\sup_{t\leq T\wedge\sigma_R^{N,x_N}}|Z_t^{N,x}| > R-\kappa\right]$$

$$\leq \limsup_{N\to+\infty}\frac{1}{N}\log\mathbb{P}\left[\sup_{t\leq T\wedge\sigma_R^{N,x_N}}|M_t^{N,\mathbb{1}}| > C(R,\kappa)\right]$$

$$\leq \limsup_{N\to+\infty}\frac{1}{N}\log\mathbb{P}\left[\sup_{t\leq T\wedge\sigma_R^{N,x_N}}(M_t^{N,\mathbb{1}})^{2N} > [C(R,\kappa)]^{2N}\right]$$

$$\leq -2\log[C(R,\kappa)] + \limsup_{N\to+\infty} \frac{1}{N} \log \mathbb{E}\left[\sup_{t\leq T\wedge\sigma_R^{N,x_N}} \left(M_t^{N,\mathbb{1}}\right)^{2N}\right]$$
$$\leq -2\log[C(R,\kappa)] + CT,$$

where we have used (4.2.15) for the last inequality. We deduce (4.2.11) by letting R tend to $+\infty$. □

We shall also need the following lemma, where we use the notation

$$w'_{Z^N}(\delta) = \inf_{\{t_i\}} \max_{1\leq i\leq n} w_x([t_{i-1},t_i)),$$

with $w_x([t_{i-1},t_i)) = \sup_{t_{i-1}\leq s<t<t_i)} |x_t - x_s|$ and the infimum is taken over all sequences $0 = t_0 < t_1 < \ldots < t_n = T$ satisfying $\inf_{1\leq i\leq n}(t_i - t_{i-1}) \geq \delta$.

Lemma 4.2.14. *If Conditions (A.1) and (A.3) are satisfied, then for any $N \geq 1$, $\rho >$ 0,*

$$\lim_{\delta\to 0} \mathbb{P}(w'_{Z^N}(\delta) > \rho) = 0.$$

Proof. Since the space $D([0,T];\mathbb{R}^d)$ is separable and complete, the law of Z^N on this space is tight, see Theorem 1.3 in Billingsley [8], which implies the lemma, from Theorem 13.2 of the same reference. □

We can now deduce the following theorem from Proposition 4.2.13 and Lemma 4.2.14.

Theorem 4.2.15. *If Conditions (A.1) and (A.3) is satisfied, then the sequence $\{Z^{N,z_N}, N \geq 1\}$ is exponentially tight in $D([0,T];\mathbb{R}^d)$.*

Proof. Given $R > 0$ and a sequence $\{\delta_\ell > 0, \ell \geq 1\}$ the following is a compact subset of $D([0,T];\mathbb{R}^d)$ (see Theorem 12.3 in Billingsley [8]):

$$K_{R,\{\delta_\ell\}} = \{x, \|x\|_T \leq R\} \bigcap \bigcap_{\ell\geq 1} \{x, w'_x(\delta_\ell) \leq \ell^{-1}\}.$$

For any $\alpha > 0$, we need to find R_α and $\{\delta_\ell^\alpha, \ell \geq 1\}$ such that

$$\limsup_{N\to\infty} \frac{1}{N} \log \mathbb{P}\left(\{\|Z^{N,z_N}\|_T > R_\alpha\} \bigcup \bigcup_{\ell\geq 1} \{w'_{Z^N}(\delta_\ell^\alpha) > \ell^{-1}\} \right) \leq -\alpha. \quad (4.2.16)$$

It is not hard to find R_α such that $\mathbb{P}(\|Z^N\|_T > R_\alpha) \leq e^{-N\alpha}$, for all $N \geq 1$. Since $w'_x(\delta) \leq w_x(2\delta)$, it follows from Proposition 4.2.13 that for each $\ell \geq 1$, there exists a $\delta_\ell > 0$ such that

$$\limsup_{N\to\infty} \frac{1}{N} \log \mathbb{P}\left(w'_{Z^N}(\delta_\ell) > \ell^{-1}\right) \leq -(\alpha + \ell).$$

Consequently, there exists an N_ℓ such that for $N \geq N_\ell$,

$$\mathbb{P}\left(w'_{Z^N}(\delta_\ell) > \ell^{-1}\right) \le e^{-N(\alpha+\ell)}.$$

Combining this with Lemma 4.2.14, we deduce that there exists $0 < \delta_\ell^\alpha \le \delta_\ell$ such that for all $N \ge 1$,

$$\mathbb{P}\left(w'_{Z^N}(\delta_\ell^\alpha) > \ell^{-1}\right) \le e^{-N(\alpha+\ell)}.$$

It follows that for all $N \ge 1$,

$$\begin{aligned}\mathbb{P}\left(\{\|Z^{N,z_N}\|_T > R_\alpha\} \bigcup \bigcup \{w'_{Z^N}(\delta_\ell^\alpha) > \ell^{-1}\}\right) &\le e^{-N\alpha} \sum_{\ell \ge 0} e^{-N\ell} \\ &\le (1-e^{-N})^{-1} e^{-\alpha N},\end{aligned}$$

from which (4.2.16) follows. □

It is not hard to see that a combination of the exact same arguments as used in the proofs of Theorem 4.2.12, Proposition 4.2.13 and Theorem 4.2.15 yields the following result.

Theorem 4.2.16. *Assume that assumptions (A.1) and (A.3) are satisfied. Then for any closed subset $F \subset D([0,T];\mathbb{R}^d)$ and any compact $\mathscr{K} \subset \mathbb{R}^d$, we have*

$$\limsup_{N\to\infty} \frac{1}{N} \log \sup_{x\in\mathscr{K}} \mathbb{P}(Z^{N,x_N} \in F) \le -\inf_{x\in\mathscr{K}} I_{T,x}(F).$$

4.2.5 Time of Extinction in the SIRS Model

We shall denote by T^N_{Ext} the time of extinction of the disease, and we want to learn what large deviations can tell us about it. In order to simplify the presentation, we start with to the two most simple examples of the SIRS model and the SIS model. These are models with fixed population size N. We treat the SIRS model in this section, and the SIS model in the next one. In this section, we shall follow the arguments from Kratz and Pardoux [21], which itself follows closely the arguments in Dembo and Zeitouni [9].

The deterministic SIRS Model can be reduced to a 2-dimensional ODE for the pair $(s(t), i(t))$ which reads

$$\begin{cases} i'(t) = \lambda s(t)i(t) - \gamma i(t), \\ s'(t) = -\lambda s(t)i(t) + \rho(1-s(t)-i(t)). \end{cases} \tag{4.2.17}$$

This process lives in the compact set $A = A_{SIRS} = \{(x,y), 0 \le x,y, x+y \le 1\}$. Provided again $R_0 = \frac{\lambda}{\gamma} > 1$, there is a unique stable endemic equilibrium $(i^*, s^*) = \left(\frac{\rho}{\lambda}\frac{\lambda-\gamma}{\rho+\gamma}, \frac{\gamma}{\lambda}\right) \in A$, while the disease free equilibrium $(1,0)$ is unstable. Here $h_1 = \begin{pmatrix}-1\\1\end{pmatrix}$, $\beta_1(x,y) = \lambda xy$, $h_2 = \begin{pmatrix}0\\-1\end{pmatrix}$, $\beta_2(x,y) = \gamma y$, $h_3 = \begin{pmatrix}1\\0\end{pmatrix}$, $\beta_3(x,y) = \rho(1-x-y)$.

The stochastic process $(I^N(t), S^N(t))$ may hit $\{0\} \times [0,1]$, and then stays there for ever (this is how the disease goes extinct). On the other hand, if it hits $\partial A \backslash \{0\} \times [0,1]$, the process comes back to $\mathring{A}$. Similarly, starting form $\{0\} \times [0,1]$, the ODE stays there for ever (and converges to $(0,1)$), while starting from $\partial A \backslash \{0\} \times [0,1]$), it enters $\mathring{A}$ instantaneously. We thus define

$$T^N_{\text{Ext}} = \inf\{t \geq 0, I^N(t) = 0\}.$$

Unfortunately, the theory of Large Deviations will not give us directly results on T^N_{Ext}, but rather on

$$T^N_\delta = \inf\{t \geq 0, I^N(t) \leq \delta\}, \text{ for any } \delta > 0.$$

An ad hoc argument, which we shall present at the end, allows us to deduce the desired result concerning T^N_{Ext}. We are interested in the exit time from $A_\delta := \{(x,y) \in A, x \geq \delta\}$ through the boundary $\partial A_\delta := \{(x,y) \in A, x = \delta\}$.

We shall write $D_{T,A} := D([0,T];A)$. In order to formulate our results, we shall need the following notations (below z stands for (x,y))

$$\begin{aligned} V(z,z',T) &= \inf_{\phi \in D_{T,A}, \phi_0 = z, \phi_T = z'} I_T(\phi) \\ V(z,z') &= \inf_{T>0} V(z,z',T) \\ \overline{V}_\delta &= \inf_{z \in \partial A_\delta} V(z^*,z), \\ \overline{V} &= \inf_{z \in \{0\} \times [0,1]} V(z^*,z). \end{aligned}$$

We want to prove the

Theorem 4.2.17. *Let $T^{N,z}_{Ext}$ denote the extinction time in the SIRS model starting from $z_N = \frac{[zN]}{N}$. Given $\eta > 0$, for all $z \in A$,*

$$\lim_{N \to \infty} \mathbb{P}\big(\exp\{N(\overline{V} - \eta)\} < T^{N,z}_{Ext} < \exp\{N(\overline{V} + \eta)\}\big) = 1.$$

Moreover, for all $\eta > 0$, $z \in A$ and N large enough,

$$\exp\{N(\overline{V} - \eta)\} \leq \mathbb{E}(T^{N,z}_{Ext}) \leq \exp\{N(\overline{V} + \eta)\}.$$

We shall first establish

Proposition 4.2.18. *Given $\eta > 0$, for all $z \in \mathring{A}_\delta$,*

$$\lim_{N \to \infty} \mathbb{P}\big(\exp\{N(\overline{V}_\delta - \eta)\} < T^{N,z}_\delta < \exp\{N(\overline{V}_\delta + \eta)\}\big) = 1.$$

Moreover, for all $\eta > 0$, $z \in \mathring{A}_\delta$ and N large enough,

$$\exp\{N(\overline{V}_\delta - \eta)\} \leq \mathbb{E}(T^{N,z}_\delta) \leq \exp\{N(\overline{V}_\delta + \eta)\}.$$

Let us now formulate a set of assumptions which are satisfied in our case, under which we will prove Proposition 4.2.18. For that sake, we shall rewrite the ODE (4.2.17) as

$$\frac{dz_t}{dt} = b(z_t),\ z_0 = z. \tag{4.2.18}$$

Assumption 4.2.19.

(E1) z^* is the only stable equilibrium point of (4.2.18) in A_δ and the solution z_t^x of (4.2.18) satisfies, for all $z_0 = z \in A_\delta$,

$$z_t^z \in \mathring{A}_\delta \text{ for all } t > 0 \text{ and } \lim_{t\to\infty} z_t^z = z^*.$$

(E2) $\bar{V} < \infty$.

(E3) For all $\rho > 0$ there exist constants $T(\rho)$, $\varepsilon(\rho) > 0$ with $T(\rho), \varepsilon(\rho) \downarrow 0$ as $\rho \downarrow 0$ such that for all $z \in \partial A_\delta \cup \{z^*\}$ and all $x, y \in \overline{B(z,\rho)} \cap A$ there exists

$$\phi = \phi(\rho,x,y) : [0,T(\rho)] \mapsto A \text{ with } \phi_0 = x, \phi_{T(\rho)} = y \text{ and } I_{T(\rho)}(\phi) < \varepsilon(\rho).$$

(E4) For all $z \in \partial A_\delta$ there exists an $\eta_0 > 0$ such that for all $\eta < \eta_0$ there exists a $\tilde{z} = \tilde{z}(\eta) \in A \backslash A_\delta$ with $|z - \tilde{z}| > \eta$.

Note that the conditions $(E1)$ and $(E4)$ would not be satisfied if we replace A_δ by A.

The proof of Proposition 4.2.18 relies upon the following sequence of lemmas, whose proofs will be given below, after the proof of the proposition.

Lemma 4.2.20. *For any $\varepsilon > 0$, there exists a $\rho_0 > 0$ such that for all $\rho < \rho_0$,*

$$\sup_{z\in\partial A_\delta\cup\{z^*\}} \ \sup_{|z'-z|\vee|z''-z|\le\rho} \ \inf_{0\le T\le 1} V(z',z'',T) < \varepsilon.$$

Lemma 4.2.21. *For any $\eta > 0$, there exists a $\rho_0 > 0$ such that for all $\rho < \rho_0$, there exists a $T_0 < \infty$ such that*

$$\liminf_{N\to\infty} \frac{1}{N} \log \inf_{|z-z^*|\le\rho} \mathbb{P}(T_\delta^{N,z} \le T_0) \ge -(\bar{V} + \eta).$$

Let us define for some $\rho > 0$ small enough, $B_\rho := \overline{B(z^*,\rho)}$ and

$$\sigma_\rho^N = \inf\{t \ge 0, Z_t^N \in B_\rho \cup \{z, z_1 \le \delta\}\}.$$

Lemma 4.2.22. *If $\rho > 0$ is such that $B_\rho \subset \mathring{A}_\delta$, then*

$$\lim_{t\to\infty} \limsup_{N\to\infty} \frac{1}{N} \log \sup_{x\in A_\delta} \mathbb{P}(\sigma_\rho^{N,z} > t) = -\infty.$$

Lemma 4.2.23. *Let C be a closed subset of $A\backslash \overset{\circ}{A}_\delta$. Then*

$$\lim_{\rho\to 0}\limsup_{N\to\infty}\frac{1}{N}\log\sup_{2\rho\le|z-z^*|\le 3\rho}\mathbb{P}(Z^{N,z}_{\sigma^N_\rho}\in C)\le -\inf_{z'\in C}V(z^*,z').$$

Lemma 4.2.24. *If $\rho>0$ is such that $B_\rho\subset \overset{\circ}{A}_\delta$ and $z\in \overset{\circ}{A}_\delta$,*

$$\lim_{N\to\infty}\mathbb{P}(Z^{N,z}_{\sigma^N_\rho}\in B_\rho)=1.$$

Lemma 4.2.25. *For all $\rho, c>0$, there exists a constant $T=T(c,\rho)<\infty$ such that*

$$\limsup_{N\to\infty}\frac{1}{N}\log\sup_{z\in A_\delta}\mathbb{P}(\sup_{0\le t\le T}|Z^{N,z}_t-z|\ge\rho)\le -c.$$

We first give the

Proof of Proposition 4.2.18. STEP 1: UPPER BOUND OF T^N_δ We choose $\eta=\varepsilon/2$, and ρ, T_0 as in Lemma 4.2.21. By Lemma 4.2.22, for any arbitrarily fixed $a>0$, there exists a T_1 such that

$$\limsup_{N\to\infty}\frac{1}{N}\log\sup_{z\in A_\delta}\mathbb{P}(\sigma^{N,z}_\rho>T_1)<-2a<0.$$

Let $T=T_0+T_1$. There exists an $N_0\ge 1$ such that for all $N\ge N_0$,

$$\begin{aligned}q:=\inf_{z\in A_\delta}\mathbb{P}(T^{N,z}_\delta\le T)&\ge\inf_{z\in A_\delta}\mathbb{P}(\sigma^{N,z}_\rho\le T_1)\inf_{z\in B_\rho}\mathbb{P}(T^{N,z}_\delta\le T_0)\\&\ge e^{-N(\bar V_\delta+\eta)},\end{aligned}\tag{4.2.19}$$

since the second factor is bounded from below by say $e^{-N(\bar V_\delta+\eta/2)}$ from Lemma 4.2.21, and from the previous estimate, we deduce that for N large enough,

$$\begin{aligned}\inf_{z\in A_\delta}\mathbb{P}(\sigma^{N,z}_\rho\le T_1)&=1-\sup_{z\in A_\delta}\mathbb{P}(\sigma^{N,z}_\rho>T_1)\\&\ge 1-e^{-Na}\\&\ge e^{-N\eta/2}.\end{aligned}$$

Next, by the strong Markov property,

$$\begin{aligned}\mathbb{P}(T^{N,z}_\delta>(k+1)T)&=[1-\mathbb{P}(T^{N,z}_\delta\le(k+1)T|T^{N,z}_\delta>kT)]\mathbb{P}(T^{N,z}_\delta>kT)\\&\le(1-q)\mathbb{P}(T^{N,z}_\delta>kT).\end{aligned}$$

Iterating, we get

$$\sup_{z\in A_\delta}\mathbb{P}(T^{N,z}_\delta>kT)\le(1-q)^k.$$

Therefore

$$\sup_{z\in A_\delta} \mathbb{E}(T_\delta^{N,z}) \le T[1+\sum_{k=1}^{\infty} \sup_{z\in A_\delta} \mathbb{P}(T_\delta^{N,z} > kT)] \le T\sum_{k=0}^{\infty}(1-q)^k = \frac{T}{q},$$

so from (4.2.19),

$$\sup_{x\in A_\delta} \mathbb{E}[T_\delta^{N,z}] \le Te^{N(\bar{V}_\delta+\eta)}, \tag{4.2.20}$$

and the upper bound for $\mathbb{E}[T_\delta^{N,z}]$ follows. From Chebycheff,

$$\mathbb{P}(T_\delta^{N,z} \ge e^{N(\bar{V}_\delta+\varepsilon)}) \le e^{-N(\bar{V}_\delta+\varepsilon)}\mathbb{E}[T_\delta^{N,z}] \le Te^{-N\varepsilon/2},$$

which tends to 0 as $N\to\infty$, hence the upper bound for T_δ^N.

STEP 2: LOWER BOUND OF T_δ^N Let $\rho>0$ be small enough such that $B_{2\rho} := B(z^*,2\rho)\subset \mathring{A}_\delta$. We define a sequence of stopping times as follows. $\theta_0=0$ and for $m\ge 0$,

$$\begin{aligned}\tau_m &= \inf\{t\ge\theta_m,\, Z_t^N\in B_\rho\cup\{z,\, z_1\le\delta\}\},\\ \theta_{m+1} &= \inf\{t>\tau_m,\, Z_t^N\in(B_{2\rho})^c\},\end{aligned}$$

with the convention that $\theta_{m+1}=\infty$ in case $Z_{\tau_m}^N\in\{z,\, z_1\le\delta\}$.

In case $\bar{V}_\delta=0$, the lower bound is an easy consequence of Lemmas 4.2.24 and 4.2.25. So we assume from now on that $\bar{V}_\delta>0$ and fix $\varepsilon>0$ arbitrarily small. Since $\{z,\, z_1\le\delta\}$ is a closed set, from Lemma 4.2.23, for $\rho>0$ small enough,

$$\limsup_{N\to\infty}\frac{1}{N}\log\sup_{2\rho\le|z-z^*|\le3\rho}\mathbb{P}(Z_{\sigma_\rho^N}^{N,z}\in\{z,\, z_1\le\delta\})\le-\bar{V}_\delta+\frac{\varepsilon}{3}.$$

Now with $c=\bar{V}_\delta$, we let $T_0=T(c,\rho)$ be as in Lemma 4.2.25. Then there exists an N_0 such that for $N\ge N_0$, and all $m\ge1$,

$$\sup_{z\in A_\delta}\mathbb{P}(T_\delta^{N,z}=\tau_m)\le\sup_{2\rho\le|z-z^*|\le3\rho}\mathbb{P}(Z_{\sigma_\rho^N}^{N,z}\in\{z,\, z_1\le\delta\})\le e^{-N(\bar{V}_\delta-\varepsilon/2)},$$

while

$$\sup_{z\in A_\delta}\mathbb{P}_z(\theta_m-\tau_{m-1}\le T_0)\le\sup_{z\in A_\delta}\mathbb{P}(\sup_{0\le t\le T_0}|Z_t^{N,z}-z|\ge\rho)\le e^{-N(\bar{V}_\delta-\varepsilon/2)}.$$

The event $\{T_\delta^N\le kT_0\}$ implies that either one of the first $k+1$ events $\{T_\delta^N=\tau_m\}$ occurs, or else at least one of the first k excursions $[\tau_m,\tau_{m+1}]$ away from B_ρ is of length at most T_0. Consequently, from the two preceding estimates,

$$\begin{aligned}\mathbb{P}(T_\delta^N\le kT_0)&\le\sum_{m=0}^{k}\mathbb{P}(T_\delta^N=\tau_m)+\mathbb{P}(\min_{1\le m\le k}(\theta_m-\tau_{m-1})\le T_0)\\ &\le\mathbb{P}(T_\delta^N=\tau_0)+2ke^{-N(\bar{V}_\delta-\varepsilon/2)}.\end{aligned}$$

Choosing now $k = [T_0^{-1} e^{N(\bar{V}_\delta - \varepsilon)}] + 1$ yields

$$\mathbb{P}(T_\delta^N \le e^{N(\bar{V}_\delta - \varepsilon)}) \le \mathbb{P}(Z^N_{\sigma^N_\rho} \notin B_\rho) + 3T_0^{-1} e^{-N\varepsilon/2}.$$

By Lemma 4.2.24, the right-hand side tends to 0 as $N \to \infty$. We have completed the proof of the first statement in Proposition 4.2.18. This result combined with Chebycheff's inequality and (4.2.20) yields the second result. □

We now turn to the proofs of the lemmas.

Proof of Lemma 4.2.20. This lemma is a direct consequence of the assumption (E3). □

Proof of Lemma 4.2.21. We make use of Lemma 4.2.20 with $\varepsilon = \eta/4$ and choose $\rho < \rho_0$. Let $z \in B_\rho$. There exists a continuous path ψ^z such that $\psi^z_0 = z$, $\psi^z_{t_z} = z^*$ for some $t_z \le 1$ and $I_{t_z}(\psi^z) \le \eta/4$. From assumption $(E2)$, there exists a continuous path $\phi \in C([0,T_1];A)$ such that $\phi_0 = z^*$, $\phi_{T_1} = z' \in \partial A_\delta$, and $I_{T_1}(\phi) \le \bar{V} + \eta/4$. From Lemma 4.2.20, there exists a continuous path $\tilde{\psi}$ such that $\tilde{\psi}_0 = z'$ and $\tilde{\psi}_{s_{z'}} = z'' \in A \backslash A_\delta$, with $s_{z'} \le 1$, $I_{s_{z'}}(\tilde{\psi}) \le \eta/4$ and $d(z'', A_\delta) = \Delta > 0$, where $\Delta < \delta$. Finally let $\{\xi_t, 0 \le t \le 2 - t_z - s_{z'}\}$ be a solution of (4.2.18) starting from $\xi_0 = z''$. From Proposition 4.2.2, $I(\xi) = 0$. Concatenating the paths ψ^z, ϕ, $\tilde{\psi}$ and ξ, we obtain a path $\phi^z \in C([0,T_0];A)$ (with $T_0 = T_1 + 2$) starting from z, with $I_{T_0}(\phi^z) \le \bar{V} + 3\eta/4$. Let now

$$\Psi = \bigcup_{z \in B_\rho} \{\psi \in D([0,T_0];A),\, \|\psi - \phi^z\|_{T_0} < \Delta/2\}.$$

Ψ is an open subset of $D([0,T_0];A)$, such that B_ρ is adapted to Ψ in the sense of Definition 4.2.8. Hence we can make use of Theorem 4.2.9, hence

$$\begin{aligned}
\liminf_{N \to \infty} \frac{1}{N} \log \inf_{z \in B_\rho} \mathbb{P}(Z^{N,z} \in \Psi) &\ge -\sup_{z \in B_\rho} \inf_{\phi \in \Psi, \phi_0 = z} I_{T_0}(\phi) \\
&\ge -\sup_{z \in B_\rho} I_{T_0}(\phi^z) \\
&> -(\bar{V} + \eta).
\end{aligned}$$

The results follows from this and $\{Z^N \in \Psi\} \subset \{T_\delta^N \le T_0\}$. □

Proof of Lemma 4.2.22. Since $\sigma_\rho^{N,z} = 0$ if $z \in B_\rho$, it suffices to restrict ourselves to $z \in A_\delta \backslash B_\rho$. For each $t > 0$, we define the closed set

$$\Psi_t := \{\phi \in D([0,t];A),\, \phi_s \in \overline{A_\delta \backslash B_\rho} \text{ for all } 0 \le s \le t\},$$

so that $\{\sigma_\rho^{N,z} > t\} \subset \{Z^{N,z} \in \Psi_t\}$. Hence by Theorem 4.2.16,

$$\limsup_{N \to \infty} \frac{1}{N} \log \sup_{z \in \overline{A_\delta \backslash B_\rho}} \mathbb{P}(\sigma_\rho^{N,z} > t) \le -\inf_{\phi \in \Psi_t} I_t(\phi).$$

It then suffices to show that

$$\inf_{\phi\in\Psi_t} I_t(\phi) \to \infty \text{ as } t \to \infty. \tag{4.2.21}$$

Starting from any $z \in \overline{A_\delta \backslash B_\rho}$, the solution z_t^z of (4.2.18) hits $\mathring{B}_{\rho/2}$ in finite time T_z which is upper semicontinuous (recall Definition A.7.1) in z, so by compactness $T := \sup_{z\in\overline{A_\delta\backslash B_\rho}} T_z < \infty$, and $z_\cdot \notin \Psi_T$ as soon as $z_\cdot$ solves (4.2.18).

Now if (4.2.21) does not hold, there would exist $M > 0$ and for each $n \geq 1$ $\phi_n \in \Psi_{nT}$ such that $I_{nT}(\phi_n) \leq M$ or all $n \geq 1$. Now if $\phi_{n,k}(t) = \phi_n(kT+t)$, $0 \leq t \leq T$, $0 \leq k \leq n-1$, we have that

$$n \min_{0\leq k\leq n-1} I_T(\phi_{n,k}) \leq \sum_{k=0}^{n-1} I_T(\phi_{n,k}) = I_{nT}(\phi_n) \leq M.$$

Hence we would produce a sequence $\psi_n \in \Psi_T$ such that $I_T(\psi_n) \to 0$ as $n \to \infty$. From Theorem 4.2.3, the sequence ψ_n belongs to a compact set, and I_T is lower semicontinuous (recall Definition A.7.1), so that along a subsequence, $\psi_n \to \psi^*$, where $\psi^* \in \Psi_T$ and $I_T(\psi^*) \leq \liminf_n I_T(\psi_n) = 0$, and those two last statements are contradictory from Proposition 4.2.2 and the fact that Ψ_T contains no solution of (4.2.18). □

Proof of Lemma 4.2.23. We need only consider the case $\inf_{z\in C} V(z^*,z) > 0$, since in the other case the result is trivial. So we can choose $\varepsilon > 0$ such that

$$V_C^\varepsilon := \left(\inf_{z\in C} V(z^*,z) - \varepsilon\right) \wedge \varepsilon^{-1} > 0.$$

By Lemma 4.2.20, there exists a $\rho_0 > 0$ such that for all $0 < \rho < \rho_0$,

$$\sup_{z\in\overline{B_{3\rho}\backslash B_{2\rho}}} V(z^*,z) < \varepsilon,$$

hence

$$\inf_{z'\in\overline{B_{3\rho}\backslash B_{2\rho}},z\in C} V(z',z) \geq \inf_{z\in C} V(z^*,z) - \sup_{z'\in\overline{B_{3\rho}\backslash B_{2\rho}}} V(z^*,z') > V_C^\varepsilon.$$

For $T > 0$, consider the closed set $\Phi^T \subset D([0,T];A)$ defined as

$$\Phi^T = \{\phi \in D([0,T];A),\, \phi_t \in C \text{ for some } 0 \leq t \leq T\}.$$

For $z' \in \overline{B_{3\rho}\backslash B_{2\rho}}$,

$$\mathbb{P}(Z^{N,z'}_{\sigma_\rho^N} \in C) \leq \mathbb{P}(\sigma_\rho^{N,z'} > T) + \mathbb{P}(Z^{N,z'} \in \Phi^T). \tag{4.2.22}$$

We next bound from above the two terms of the last right-hand side. Concerning the second term,

$$\inf_{\phi \in \Phi^T, \phi_0 \in \overline{B_{3\rho} \backslash B_{2\rho}}} I_T(\phi) \geq \inf_{z' \in \overline{B_{3\rho} \backslash B_{2\rho}}, z \in C} V(z', z) \geq V_C^\varepsilon.$$

Hence from Theorem 4.2.16,

$$\limsup_{N \to \infty} \frac{1}{N} \log \sup_{z' \in \overline{B_{3\rho} \backslash B_{2\rho}}} \mathbb{P}(Z^{N,z'} \in \Phi^T) \leq -V_C^\varepsilon.$$

For the first term, we deduce from Lemma 4.2.22 that for some $T_0 > 0$, all $T \geq T_0$,

$$\limsup_{N \to \infty} \frac{1}{N} \log \sup_{z' \in \overline{B_{3\rho} \backslash B_{2\rho}}} \mathbb{P}(\sigma_\rho^{N,z'} > T) < -V_C^\varepsilon.$$

(4.2.22) together with the last two estimates produces an inequality which, after letting $\varepsilon \to 0$, yields the result. □

Proof of Lemma 4.2.24. z_t^z denoting the solution of (4.2.18) starting from $z \in \mathring{A}_\delta$, let $T_\rho = \inf\{t > 0, z_t^z \in B_{\rho/2}\}$. From (E1) it follows that $T_\rho < \infty$ and $\Delta := \inf_{0 \leq t \leq T_\rho} d(z_t^z, \partial A_\delta) > 0$. Consequently

$$\mathbb{P}\left(Z_{\sigma_\rho^N}^{N,z} \notin B_\rho\right) \leq \mathbb{P}\left(\sup_{0 \leq t \leq T_\rho} |Z_t^{N,z} - z_t^z| \geq \frac{\Delta \wedge \rho}{2}\right),$$

which tends to 0 as $N \to \infty$ from Theorem 2.2.7. Q.E.D. □

Proof of Lemma 4.2.25. Let $\rho, c > 0$ be fixed. For $T > 0$, $N \geq 1$ and $z \in A_\delta$,

$$\begin{aligned}\mathbb{P}\left(\sup_{0 \leq t \leq T} |Z_t^{N,z} - z| \geq \rho\right) &= \mathbb{P}\left(\sup_{0 \leq t \leq T} \left|\sum_j h_j P_j\left(N \int_0^t \beta_j(Z_s^{;x}) ds\right)\right| \geq \rho\right) \\ &\leq \mathbb{P}\left(\sum_j P_j(N\bar{\beta}T) \geq N\rho\bar{h}^{-1}\right) \\ &\leq k\mathbb{P}(P(N\bar{\beta}T) \geq N\rho\bar{h}^{-1}k^{-1}).\end{aligned}$$

Now from Cramér's Theorem A.3.1

$$\limsup_{N \to \infty} \frac{1}{N} \log \sup_{z \in A_\delta} \mathbb{P}(\sup_{0 \leq t \leq T} |Z_t^{N,z} - z| \geq \rho) \leq -\frac{\rho}{\bar{h}k} \log\left(\frac{\rho}{\bar{h}k\bar{\beta}T}\right) + \frac{\rho}{\bar{h}k} - \bar{\beta}T,$$

and the absolute value of the right-hand side can be made arbitrarily large by choosing T arbitrarily small. □

It remains finally to turn to the

Proof of Theorem 4.2.17. Since $V_\delta \uparrow V$ as $\delta \downarrow 0$, it is clear that the lower bounds for T_{Ext}^N and its expectation follow from Proposition 4.2.18. It remains to establish the upper bound. Analyzing carefully the proof of the upper bound, we notice that the key step, which relies upon Lemmas 4.2.21 and 4.2.22 whose proof do not extend to our new situation, is the derivation of the inequality (4.2.19). The upper bound both for the time of exit and its expectation are a direct consequence of (4.2.19), without any further reference to those assumptions which are not valid any more. We fix $\eta > 0$. Let $t > 0$ be arbitrary. From Lemma 4.2.26 below, if $c_t := \log\left(\frac{\lambda-\gamma e^{(\gamma-\lambda)t}}{\gamma-\gamma e^{(\gamma-\lambda)t}}\right)$,

$$\inf_{z\in A\backslash A_\delta} \mathbb{P}(T^{N,z}_{Ext} \le t) \ge e^{-\lceil N\delta\rceil c_t} \ge e^{-N(\delta+N_0^{-1})c_t}, \tag{4.2.23}$$

provided $N \ge N_0$. Choose N_0 large enough and $\delta > 0$ small enough such that $(\delta + N_0^{-1})c_t \le \eta/2$. From (4.2.19), there exists a $T_\delta > 0$ such that, possibly increasing N_0 if necessary, if $N \ge N_0$,

$$\inf_{z\in A_\delta} \mathbb{P}(T^{N,z}_{\delta} \le T_\delta) \ge e^{-N(\bar{V}_\delta+\eta/2)} \ge e^{-N(\bar{V}+\eta/2)}. \tag{4.2.24}$$

We deduce from (4.2.23), (4.2.24) and the strong Markov property that, with $T = T_\delta + t$,

$$\inf_{z\in A} \mathbb{P}(T^{N,z}_{Ext} \le T) \ge e^{-N(\bar{V}+\eta)},$$

which is the wished extension of (4.2.19). □

Lemma 4.2.26. *For any $t > 0$, if $c_t := \log\left(\frac{\lambda-\gamma e^{(\gamma-\lambda)t}}{\gamma-\gamma e^{(\gamma-\lambda)t}}\right)$,*

$$\inf_{z\in A\backslash A_\delta} \mathbb{P}(T^{N,z}_{Ext} < t) \ge \exp\{-\lceil N\delta\rceil c_t\}.$$

Proof. Since $z \in A\backslash A_\delta$ implies that $z_1 \le \delta$, the first component of the process $NZ^{N,x}(t)$ is dominated by the process

$$\lceil N\delta\rceil + P_1\left(N\lambda\int_0^t Z_1^{N,z}(s)ds\right) - P_1\left(N\gamma\int_0^t Z_1^{N,z}(s)ds\right),$$

which is a continuous time binary branching process with birth rate λ and death rate γ. This process goes extinct before time t with probability

$$\left(\frac{\gamma-\gamma e^{(\gamma-\lambda)t}}{\lambda-\gamma e^{(\gamma-\lambda)t}}\right)^{\lceil N\delta\rceil},$$

as can be seen by combining formula (1) from section III.4 of Athreya and Ney [3] with the formula in section 5 for $F(0,t)$ in the birth and death case. The result follows readily. □

We shall need below the following additional results.

Proposition 4.2.27. *Under the assumptions of Proposition 4.2.18, if $C \subset \partial A_\delta$ is a closed set such that $V_C := \inf_{z\in C} V(z^*,z) > \bar{V}_\delta$, then for any $z \in \mathring{A}_\delta$, all $\varepsilon > 0$ small enough*

$$\lim_{N\to\infty} \mathbb{P}(d(Z^{N,z_N}_{T^N_\delta}, C) \le \varepsilon) = 0.$$

Proof. Fix $\eta < (V_C - \bar{V}_\delta)/3$. From Lemma 4.2.23, for $\varepsilon > O$ small enough, there exists a $\rho > 0$ small enough and N_0 large enough such that for all $N \geq N_0$,

$$\sup_{2\rho \leq |z-z^*| \leq 3\rho} \mathbb{P}(d(Z^{N,z_N}_{\sigma^N_\rho}, C) \leq \varepsilon) \leq e^{-N(V_C-\eta)}.$$

Let $c = V_C - \eta$ and $T_0 = T(c,\rho)$ given by Lemma 4.2.25. Then, increasing N_0 if necessary, we deduce from that Lemma that for any $N \geq N_0$, $\ell \geq 1$,

$$\mathbb{P}(\tau_\ell \leq \ell T_0) \leq \ell \sup_{z \in A_\delta} \mathbb{P}\left(\sup_{0 \leq t \leq T_0} |Z^{N,z_N}_t - z| \geq \rho \right) \leq \ell e^{-N(V_C-\eta)}.$$

For all $z \in B_\rho$, $\ell \geq 1$,

$$\begin{aligned}
&\mathbb{P}(d(Z^{N,z_N}_{T^N_\delta}, C) \leq \varepsilon) \\
&\leq \mathbb{P}(T^{N,z}_\delta > \tau_\ell) + \sum_{m=1}^{\ell} \mathbb{P}(T^{N,z}_\delta > \tau_{m-1}) \mathbb{P}(d(Z^{N,z_N}_{\tau_m}, C) \leq \varepsilon | T^{N,z}_\delta > \tau_{m-1}) \\
&\leq \mathbb{P}(T^{N,z}_\delta > \ell T_0) + \mathbb{P}(\tau_\ell \leq \ell T_0) \\
&\quad + \sum_{m=1}^{\ell} \mathbb{P}(T^{N,z}_\delta > \tau_{m-1}) \mathbb{E}[\mathbb{P}(d(Z^{N,Z^N_{\theta_m}}_{\sigma^N_\rho}, C) \leq \varepsilon | T^{N,z}_\delta > \tau_{m-1}] \\
&\leq \mathbb{P}(T^{N,z}_\delta > \ell T_0) + \mathbb{P}(\tau_\ell \leq \ell T_0) + \ell \sup_{2\rho \leq |z-z^*| \leq 3\rho} \mathbb{P}(d(Z^{N,z_N}_{\sigma^N_\rho}, C) \leq \varepsilon) \\
&\leq \mathbb{P}(T^{N,z}_\delta > \ell T_0) + 2\ell e^{-N(V_C-\eta)}.
\end{aligned}$$

Increasing further N_0 if necessary, we have that (4.2.20) holds for some $T > 0$ and all $N \geq N_0$. We choose $\ell = \left\lceil e^{N(\bar{V}_\delta + 2\eta)} \right\rceil$, hence from our choice of η,

$$\limsup_{N\to\infty} \sup_{z \in B_\rho} \mathbb{P}(d(Z^{N,z_N}_{T^N_\delta}, C) \leq \varepsilon) \leq \limsup_{N\to\infty} \left(\frac{T}{\ell T_0} e^{N(\bar{V}_\delta + \eta)} + 2\ell e^{-N(V_C-\eta)} \right) = 0.$$

It remains to combine Lemma 4.2.24 and the inequality

$$\mathbb{P}(d(Z^{N,z_N}_{T^N_\delta}, C) \leq \varepsilon) \leq \mathbb{P}(Z^{N,z_N}_{\sigma^N_\rho} \notin B_\rho) + \sup_{y \in B_\rho} \mathbb{P}(d(Z^{N,y_N}_{T^N_\delta}, C) \leq \varepsilon).$$

□

The proof of the next important result is a bit lengthy, and we refer to Pardoux and Samegni-Kepgnou [27] for it.

Corollary 4.2.28. *If $C \subset \{z, z_1 = 0\}$ is such that $V_C := \inf_{z \in C} V(z^*, z) > \bar{V}$, then for any $z \in \mathring{A}$,*

$$\lim_{N\to\infty} \mathbb{P}(Z^{N,z_N}_{T^N_{Ext}} \in C) = 0.$$

4.2.6 Time of Extinction in the SIS Model

While the above results are rather precise, it is frustrating that it does not seem possible to express the important constant $\overline{V}$ explicitly in terms of the few constants of the model. One can only do a numerical evaluation of $\overline{V}$. We now simplify the problem, and consider the SIS model, where when an infectious individual cures, he immediately becomes susceptible again: there is no immunity. The advantage of this simplified model is that it can be written in dimension one and, as we shall see now, we can deduce from the Pontryagin maximum principle, see Section A.6 in the Appendix, a very simple explicit formula for $\overline{V}$.

The deterministic SIS model can be reduced to the following one-dimensional equation for the proportion of infected individuals

$$\dot{x}_t = \lambda x_t(1-x_t) - \gamma x_t.$$

Here the process lives in the interval $A_{SIS} = [0,1]$. Provided $R_0 = \frac{\lambda}{\gamma} > 1$, there is a unique stable endemic equilibrium $x^* = 1 - \frac{\gamma}{\lambda} \in (0,1)$, while the disease free equilibrium $x^0 = 0$ is unstable. Here $h_1 = 1$, $\beta_1(x) = \lambda x(1-x)$, $h_2 = -1$, $\beta_2(x) = \gamma x$.

We assume that $\lambda > \gamma$, i.e. $R_0 > 1$. As the reader can easily verify, Theorem 4.2.17 applies to this situation, and now $\overline{V}$ is the minimal value of the following control problem. With the notations of Section A.6 below, we are in the situation $d=1$, $k=2$, $\beta_1(x) = \lambda x(1-x)$, $\beta_2(x) = \gamma x$, $B = \begin{pmatrix}1 & -1\end{pmatrix}$. The identity (A.6.1) reads here

$$\lambda x_t(1-x_t)(1-e^{p_t}) + \gamma x_t(1-e^{-p_t}) = 0.$$

Hence either $p_t = 0$, or else $p_t = \log\frac{\gamma}{\lambda(1-x_t)}$. It is easy to convince oneself that $p_t = 0$ does not produce a control which does the wished job. Hence $p_t = \log\frac{\gamma}{\lambda(1-x_t)}$, $\hat{u}_1(t) = e^{p_t}\beta_1(x_t) = \gamma x_t$, $\hat{u}_2(t) = e^{-p_t}\beta_2(x_t) = \lambda x_t(1-x_t)$. The optimal trajectory reads

$$\dot{x}_t = \gamma x_t - \lambda x_t(1-x_t). \tag{4.2.25}$$

From the right-hand side of the identity (A.6.2),

$$\begin{aligned}
\overline{V} &= \int_0^{\hat{T}} [\gamma x_t - \lambda x_t(1-x_t)] \log\frac{\gamma}{\lambda(1-x_t)} dt \\
&= \int_0^{\hat{T}} \log\frac{\gamma}{\lambda(1-x_t)} \dot{x}_t dt \\
&= \int_0^{\frac{\lambda-\gamma}{\lambda}} \log\frac{\gamma}{\lambda(1-x)} dx \\
&= \log\frac{\lambda}{\gamma} - 1 + \frac{\gamma}{\lambda}.
\end{aligned}$$

Finally

Proposition 4.2.29. *We have the identities*

$$\overline{V} = \log R_0 - 1 + R_0^{-1}, \quad e^{N\overline{V}} = R_0^N e^{-N(R_0-1)/R_0}.$$

Combining this result with Theorem 4.2.17 adapted to the SIS model yields the following.

Corollary 4.2.30. *Suppose that* $R_0 > 1$ *and define*

$$T_{Ext}^{N,z} = \inf\{t > 0,\ Z_t^{N,z} = 0\}.$$

Then for any $0 < z \le 1$*, and* $c > 1$*,*

$$\lim_{N\to\infty} \mathbb{P}\left((R_0/c)^N e^{-N(R_0-1)/R_0} < T_{Ext}^{N,z} < (cR_0)^N e^{-N(R_0-1)/R_0} \right) = 1,$$

$$\text{and } (R_0/c)^N e^{-N(R_0-1)/R_0} \le \mathbb{E}(T_{Ext}^{N,z}) \le (cR_0)^N e^{-N(R_0-1)/R_0}$$

for N large enough.

Remark 4.2.31. In fact, the pair $(\hat{u}_1(t), \hat{u}_2(t))$ is not an optimal control for the above control problem. Such an optimal control does not exist! The optimal trajectory, which is the original ODE time reversed, would take an infinite time to leave x^*, and an infinite time to reach 0. However, our $(\hat{u}_1(t), \hat{u}_2(t))$ is the limit of a minimizing sequence obtained by choosing a suboptimal control to drive the system from x^* to $x^* - \delta$, then the optimal control to drive the system from $x^* - \delta$ to δ, and finally a suboptimal control to drive the system from δ to 0. $\log \frac{\lambda}{\gamma} - 1 + \frac{\gamma}{\lambda}$ is indeed the minimal cost. Note that $\hat{T} = +\infty$.

4.2.7 Time of Extinction in the SIR Model with Demography

We now turn to the SIR model with demography, which is the model which has been formally presented in Example 2.2.2, but where we let $\nu = +\infty$ (we suppress the stage E between S and I), and $\gamma = 0$ (there is no loss of immunity). The limiting ODE reads

$$\begin{aligned}
\dot{x}_t &= \lambda x_t y_t - \gamma x_t - \mu x_t, \\
\dot{y}_t &= -\lambda x_t y_t + \mu - \mu y_t.
\end{aligned}$$

We assume that $\lambda > \gamma + \mu$, in which case there is a unique stable endemic equilibrium, namely $z^* = (x^*, y^*) = (\frac{\mu}{\gamma+\mu} - \frac{\mu}{\lambda}, \frac{\gamma+\mu}{\lambda})$. The extinction in such a model has been studied using the Central Limit Theorem for moderate population size in Section 4.1. We now finally apply Large Deviations to this model. In this model, $Z_t^N = (I_t^N, S_t^N)$ lives in all of $\mathbb{R}_+^2$. We note that in the proof of Proposition 4.2.18, the compactness of the set of possible values for Z_t^N has played a crucial role, especially in the proof of Lemma 4.2.22. However, if we define for each $R > 0$

$$T_{\text{Ext}}^{N,R} = T_{\text{Ext}}^{N} \wedge \sigma_R^N,$$

where $\sigma_N^R = \inf\{t > 0, I_t^N + S_t^N \geq R\}$, it is clear that we have reduced our situation to a bounded state space, and the exact same proofs leading to Proposition 4.2.18 and Theorem 4.2.17, which easily adapted to this new situation. Moreover, we have the

Lemma 4.2.32. *As $R \to \infty$, $V_R := \inf_{z=x+y\geq R} V(z^*, z) \to \infty$.*

Proof. We use the Pontryagin maximum principle and refer to the notations in Section A.6. Here $d = 2$ and $k = 5$, $B = \begin{pmatrix} 1 & -1 & -1 & 0 & 0 \\ -1 & 0 & 0 & 1 & -1 \end{pmatrix}$, $\beta_1(x,y) = \lambda xy$, $\beta_2(x,y) = \gamma x$, $\beta_3(x,y) = \mu x$, $\beta_4(x,y) = \mu$, $\beta_5(x,y) = \mu y$. The forward-backward ODE system reads

$$\begin{aligned}
\dot{x}_t &= \lambda x_t y_t e^{p_t - q_t} - (\gamma+\mu)x_t e^{-p_t}, \quad x_0 = \frac{\mu}{\gamma+\mu} - \frac{\mu}{\lambda} \\
\dot{y}_t &= -\lambda x_t y_t e^{p_t - q_t} + \mu e^{q_t} - \mu y_t e^{-q_t}, \quad y_0 = \frac{\gamma+\mu}{\lambda} \\
\dot{p}_t &= \lambda y_t + \gamma + \mu - \lambda y_y e^{p_t - q_t} - \gamma e^{-p_t} - \mu e^{-p_t}, \\
\dot{q}_t &= \lambda x_t + \mu - x_t e^{p_t - q_t} - \mu e^{-q_t}, \quad p_{\hat{T}} = q_{\hat{T}}.
\end{aligned}$$

Condition (A.6.1) at time $\hat{T}$ together with the condition $p_{\hat{T}} = q_{\hat{T}}$ allows us to conclude that

$$p_{\hat{T}} = q_{\hat{T}} = \log\left(R + \frac{\gamma}{\mu}x\right).$$

It is clear that $\dot{p}_{\hat{T}} > \dot{q}_{\hat{T}}$. In fact it is not hard to show that, as long as $p_t \geq 0$, $p_t < q_t$. However, $\dot{p}_t \leq \lambda y_t + \gamma + \mu \leq \lambda R + \gamma + \mu$. Let $a = \frac{1}{2}\frac{\log R}{\lambda R + \gamma + \mu}$. For any $\hat{T} - a \leq t \leq \hat{T}$, $p_t \geq \log(R + \frac{\gamma}{\mu}x_{\hat{T}}) - \frac{1}{2}\log R \geq \frac{1}{2}\log R > 0$. Next we notice that $\dot{x}_t + \dot{y}_t \leq \mu e^{q_t}$. As long as $\hat{T} - a \leq t \leq \hat{T}$, we both have that $p_t \leq q_t$ and $q_t \geq 0$, hence $\dot{q}_t \geq 0$, and $0 < q_t \leq q_{\hat{T}} = \log\left(R + \frac{\gamma}{\mu}x_{\hat{T}}\right)$. Consequently $\dot{x}_t + \dot{y}_t \leq \mu\left(R + \frac{\gamma}{\mu}x_{\hat{T}}\right) \leq (\gamma+\mu)R$. Finally, for $\hat{T} - a \leq t \leq \hat{T}$, $x_t + y_t \geq R - \frac{(\gamma+\mu)R\log R}{2(\lambda R+\gamma+\mu)} \geq \frac{1}{2}R$, for R large enough.

We can now lowed bound V_R. We use the expression on the left of (A.6.2) for the instantaneous cost. We have

$$\begin{aligned}
V_R &= \int_0^{\hat{T}} \Big[\lambda x_t y_t (1 - e^{p_t - q_t} + (p_t - q_t)e^{p_t - q_t}) + (\mu+\gamma)x_t(1 - e^{-p_t} - p_t e^{-p_t}) \\
&\qquad + \mu(1 - e^{q_t} + q_t e^{q_t}) + \mu y_t(1 - e^{-q_t} - q_t e^{-q_t})\Big] dt \\
&\geq \int_{\hat{T}-a}^{\hat{T}} \mu(x_t + y_t)\inf\{1 - e^{-p_t} - p_t e^{-p_t}, 1 - e^{-q_t} - q_t e^{-q_t}\} dt \\
&\geq \frac{\mu}{8}\frac{R\log R}{\lambda R + \mu + \gamma} \\
&\to +\infty,
\end{aligned}$$

as $R \to \infty$. □

It follows from Corollary 4.2.28 that as soon as $V_R > \hat{V}$, the probability that Z^N exits the truncated domain through the "extinction boundary" $\{z^1 = 0\}$ goes to 1 as $N \to \infty$. Also, for fixed N, $\mathbb{P}(T^N_{\text{Ext}} < \sigma^N_R) \to 1$, as $R \to \infty$.

Theorem 4.2.33. *Let $T^{N,z}_{Ext}$ denote the extinction time in the N–SIR model with demography starting from $z_N = \frac{[zN]}{N}$. Given $\eta > 0$, for all $z \in \mathbb{R}^2_+$ with $z_1 > 0$,*

$$\lim_{N\to\infty} \mathbb{P}\big(\exp\{N(\overline{V} - \eta)\} < T^{N,z}_{Ext} < \exp\{N(\overline{V} + \eta)\}\big) = 1.$$

Moreover, for all $\eta > 0$, $z \in \mathbb{R}^2_+$ with $z_1 > 0$ and N large enough,

$$\exp\{N(\overline{V} - \eta)\} \le \mathbb{E}(T^{N,z}_{Ext}) \le \exp\{N(\overline{V} + \eta)\}.$$

Appendix

This Appendix presents several mathematical notions, mostly from the theory of stochastic processes, as well as a couple of notions related to continuity of real-valued functions, which are used in the previous chapters. Most proofs are given. Otherwise we refer to existing monographs.

A.1 Branching Processes

We present the basic facts about branching processes, which are useful in these Notes. We give most of the proofs. Those which are missing can be found in classical monographs on branching processes, see e.g. Athreya and Ney [3] or Jagers [16], unless we give a precise reference in the text.

A.1.1 Discrete Time Branching Processes

Consider an ancestor (at generation 0) who has ξ_0 children, such that

$$\mathbb{P}(\xi_0 = k) = q_k,\ k \ge 0 \quad \text{and} \sum_{k\ge 0} q_k = 1.$$

Define $m = \mathbb{E}[\xi_0] = \sum_{k\ge 1} k\, q_k$ and $g(s) = \mathbb{E}\left[s^{\xi_0}\right]$.

Each child of the ancestor belongs to generation 1. The i-th of those children has himself $\xi_{1,i}$ children, where the random variables $\{\xi_{k,i},\ k \ge 0, i \ge 1\}$ are i.i.d., all having the same law as ξ_0. If we define X_n as the number of individuals in generation n, we have

$$X_{n+1} = \sum_{i=1}^{X_n} \xi_{n,i}.$$

We have $g(0) = q_0$, $g(1) = 1$, $g'(1) = m$, $g'(s) > 0$, $g''(s) > 0$, for all $0 \le s \le 1$ (we assume that $q_0 > 0$ and $q_0 + q_1 < 1$). Let us compute the generating function of X_n:

$g_n(s) = \mathbb{E}[s^{X_n}]$.

$$\begin{aligned} g_n(s) &= \mathbb{E}\left[s^{\sum_{i=1}^{X_{n-1}} \xi_{n-1,i}}\right] \\ &= \mathbb{E}\left[\mathbb{E}\left[s^{\sum_{i=1}^{X_{n-1}} \xi_{n-1,i}} \middle| X_{n-1}\right]\right] \\ &= \mathbb{E}\left[g(s)^{X_{n-1}}\right] \\ &= g_{n-1} \circ g(s). \end{aligned}$$

If we iterate this argument, we obtain

$$g_n(s) = g \circ \cdots \circ g(s),$$

and also

$$\begin{aligned} \mathbb{P}(X_n = 0) &= g^{\circ n}(0) \\ &= g\left[g^{\circ(n-1)}(0)\right]. \end{aligned}$$

Hence if $z_n = \mathbb{P}(X_n = 0)$, $z_n = g(z_{n-1})$, and $z_1 = q_0$. We have $z_n \uparrow z_\infty$, where $z_\infty =$

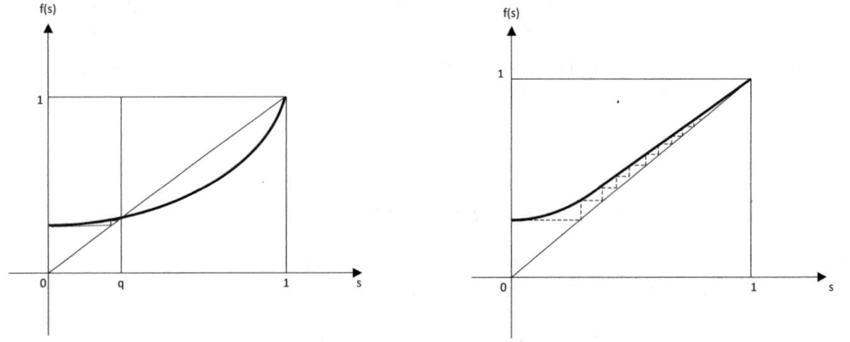

Fig. A.1.1 Graphs of g in case $m > 1$ (left) and in case $m \le 1$ (right). The successive heights of the dashed line are the successive values of $\mathbb{P}(X_n = 0)$.

$\mathbb{P}(X_n = 0$ from some $n)$. The proof of the following Proposition is essentially clear from Figure A.1.1.

Proposition A.1.1. *If $m \le 1$, then $\mathbb{P}(X_n = 0) \to 1$ as $n \to \infty$, and $z_\infty = 1$.*

If $m > 1$, $\mathbb{P}(X_n = 0) \to z_\infty = q$ as $n \to \infty$, where q is the smallest solution of the equation $z = g(z)$.

Note that on the event $\cup_{n=0}^{\infty}\{X_n = 0\}$, which has probability one in the first case, the population goes extinct after a finite number of generations, and the total progeny is finite.

In the second case, with probability $1 - z_\infty$, the branching process does not go extinct.

Let us show that $W_n = m^{-n} X_n$ is a martingale.

$$\begin{aligned}\mathbb{E}(W_{n+1}|X_n) &= m^{-n}\mathbb{E}\left(m^{-1}\sum_1^{X_n}\xi_{n,i}|X_n\right)\\ &= m^{-n}X_n\\ &= W_n.\end{aligned}$$

One can show that $W_n \to W$ a.s. as $n \to \infty$, and moreover, provided $\sum_{j\geq 1} q_j j \log j < \infty$,

$$\mathbb{E}[W] = 1, \text{ and } \mathbb{P}(W > 0) = \mathbb{P}(\{\text{the branching process does not go extinct}\}).$$

In the case $\sum_{j\geq 1} q_j j \log j = \infty$, then $\mathbb{P}(W = 0) = 1$.

A.1.2 Continuous Time Branching Processes

We shall consider only binary continuous time branching processes, i.e. where at most one child is born at a given time. This process starts with a single ancestor born at time $t = 0$. This ancestor is characterized by a pair $(L_0, \{N_0(t),\ t \geq 0\})$, where L_0 is the life length of the ancestor, and $N_0(t)$ is the number of children of the ancestor born on the time interval $[0,t]$. We assume that $N_0(\infty) = N_0(L_0)$, that is the ancestor does not give birth to offspring after his death. We now assume that the individuals are numbered in the order of their birth. To the individual i is attached a pair $(L_i, \{N_i(t)\})$, such that the sequence of pairs $\{(L_i, \{N_i(t)\})\}_{i\geq 0}$ is i.i.d. If the individual i is born at time B_i, the offspring of individual i are born at the jump times of the process $\{N_i(t - B_i),\ B_i \leq t \leq B_i + L_i\}$. Note that since B_i depends only upon the pairs $\{(L_j, \{N_j(t)\})\}_{0\leq j<i}$, B_i and $(L_i, \{N_i(t)\})$ are independent.

Let X_t denote the number of individuals in the population alive at time t. This process is Markovian if and only if the law of the pair $(L_i, N_i(t))$ is such that L_i and $\{N_i(t),\ t \geq 0\}$ are independent, L_i is an exponential random variable with parameter d, and $N_i(t)$ is a rate b Poisson process. We first assume that we are in this situation. We shall denote by X_t^k the number of descendants at time t of k ancestors at time 0. The branching property implies that $\{X_t^k,\ t \geq 0\}$ is the sum of k independent copies of $\{X_t,\ t \geq 0\}$. We have the following result.

Proposition A.1.2. *The generating function of the process X is given by*

$$\mathbb{E}\left(s^{X_t^k}\right) = \psi_t(s)^k,\ s \in [0,1],\ k \geq 1,$$

where

$$\frac{\partial \psi_t(s)}{\partial t} = \Phi(\psi_t(s)), \quad \psi_0(s) = s,$$

and the function Φ is defined by

$$\Phi(s) = d(1-s) + b(s^2 - s)$$
$$= (b+d)(h(s) - s), \; s \in [0,1],$$

where h is the generating function of the probability measure $\frac{d}{b+d}\delta_0 + \frac{b}{d+b}\delta_2$.

Proof. The process X_t is a continuous time $\mathbb{Z}_+$-valued jump Markov process. Denote by Q its infinitesimal generator. The non-zero elements of the n-th row of Q are given by

$$Q_{n,m} = \begin{cases} nd, & \text{if } m = n-1, \\ -n(b+d), & \text{if } m = n; \\ nb, & \text{if } m = n+1. \end{cases}$$

Define $f : \mathbb{N} \to [0,1]$ by $f(k) = s^k$, $s \in [0,1]$. Then $\psi_t(s) = P_t f(1) := \mathbb{E}[f(X_t^1)]$ (we use the unusual notation $X^1 = X$ to stress the fact that the process starts from $X_0 = 1$). It follows from the backward Kolmogorov equation for the process X (see e.g. Theorem 3.2, Chapter 7 in Pardoux [25]) that

$$\frac{dP_t f(1)}{dt} = (QP_t f)(1)$$
$$\frac{\partial \psi_t(s)}{\partial t} = Q_{1,0} + Q_{1,1}\psi_t(s) + Q_{1,2}\psi_t(s)^2$$
$$= d - (b+d)\psi_t(s) + b\psi_t(s)^2$$
$$= \Phi(\psi_t(s)).$$

□

Corollary A.1.3. *We have*

$$\mathbb{E}[X_t^k] = ke^{rt}, \quad \textit{where } r = b - d.$$

Proof. Differentiating with respect to s the above equation for $\psi_t(s)$ yields

$$\frac{\partial}{\partial t}\left(\frac{\partial}{\partial s}\psi_t(s)\right) = \Phi'(\psi_t(s))\frac{\partial}{\partial s}\psi_t(s)$$
$$= (b+d)(h'(s) - 1)\frac{\partial}{\partial s}\psi_t(s).$$

The last equation at $s = 1$ yields

$$\frac{d}{dt}\mathbb{E}[X_t] = r\mathbb{E}[X_t],$$

where $X_t = X_t^1$. The result follows for $k = 1$, and then the general case, since the mean number of offspring of k ancestors equals k times the mean number of offspring of one ancestor. □

The quantity r is often referred to as the Malthusian parameter. It is the mean number of births minus the mean number of death per unit time. Another important quantity is the mean number of offspring of each individual, which is equal to $m = b/d$. The process X_t^k is said to be subcritical if $m < 1$, i.e. $r < 0$. In that case $X_t^k \to 0$ in $L^1(\Omega)$, and it is easy to show that $X_t^k = 0$ for t large enough. This last conclusion holds in the critical case ($m = 1$, i.e. $r = 0$) as well. In those two cases, the total progeny is finite a.s. We now study the large time behaviour of X_t^k in the supercritical case. In the next proposition, we again write X_t for X_t^1.

Proposition A.1.4. *If $m > 1$, or equivalently $r > 0$, there exists a non-negative random variable W such that $X_t \sim We^{rt}$ almost surely, as $t \to \infty$. Moreover $\{W = 0\} = \{\exists t > 0$ such that $X_t = 0\}$ and*

$$\mathbb{P}(W = 0) = \mathbb{P}(\{\exists t > 0 \text{ such that } X_t = 0\}) = \frac{d}{b}.$$

Proof. The first part of the result follows readily from the fact that $e^{-rt}X_t$ is a positive martingale, which converges a.s. to a limit W as $t \to \infty$. Moreover it is not hard to show that $\sup_{t>0} \mathbb{E}[e^{-2rt}(X_t)^2] < \infty$, hence the convergence holds in $L^1(\Omega)$, so $\mathbb{E}[W] = 1$. Now clearly $\{\exists t > 0 \text{ s.t. } X_t = 0\} \subset \{W = 0\}$. If we start with k ancestors, the limiting W is clearly the sum of k i.i.d. copies of W when starting with one ancestor, and $\mathbb{P}_k(W = 0) = (\mathbb{P}_1(W = 0))^k$. It is now easy to deduce that

$$\mathbb{P}_1(W = 0|X_t) = \mathbb{P}_1(W = 0))^{X_t}.$$

Taking the expectation in this identity and writing $q = \mathbb{P}_1(W = 0)$, we obtain $q = \mathbb{E}[q^{X_t}]$. Differentiating that identity at $t = 0$ and taking advantage of Proposition A.1.2, we deduce that q solves $bq^2 - (b+d)q + d = 0$. Moreover since $\mathbb{E}(W) = 1$, $q < 1$, hence $q = d/b$. Finally $\mathbb{P}(X_t = 0) = \psi_t(0)$ is the solution of the ODE $\dot{x}(t) = bx(t)^2 - (b+d)x(t) + d$, $x(0) = 0$. It is clear that as $t \to \infty$, $\psi_t(0)$ increases to the smallest solution of the equation $bs^2 - (b+d)s + d = 0$, again d/b. □

We now consider non-Markovian continuous time binary branching processes. The non-Markovian continuous time branching processes which we have described at the beginning of this section are called Crump–Mode–Jagers processes. Now the law of the pairs $(L_i, \{N_i(t)\})$ can be quite general. For the application to epidemics models, we can consider the case where L_i and $\{N_i(t)\}$ are independent, N_i being a Poisson process, but the law of L_i is no longer exponential. We denote again by $m = \mathbb{E}[N_0(L_0)]$ the mean number of offspring of each individual. Of course, the process is subcritical, critical, or supercritical according as $m < 1$, $m = 1$ or $m > 1$. We denote again by X_t the number of individuals alive at time t. We define $F(t) = \mathbb{E}[N(t)]$ and $G(t) = \mathbb{P}(L \le t)$. We assume that F is non-lattice, and $F(0^+) < 1$. Doney [10] showed the following two results.

Proposition A.1.5. *If $1 < m < \infty$, then there exists a unique $r > 0$ such that*

$$\int_0^\infty e^{-rt} F(dt) = 1$$

and $\mathbb{E}[X_t] \sim ae^{rt}$, where

$$0 < a = \frac{\int_0^\infty (1-G(t))e^{-rt}dt}{\int_0^\infty te^{-rt}F(dt)} < \infty.$$

Again r is called the Malthusian parameter. In the next statement, we use the notation

$$Y = \int_0^\infty e^{-rt}N(dt).$$

It is clear that

$$\mathbb{E}[Y] = \int_0^\infty e^{-rt}F(dt) = 1.$$

Theorem A.1.6. *Suppose that* $1 < m < \infty$. *Then, as* $t \to \infty$

$$\frac{X_t}{\mathbb{E}[X_t]} \to W \quad \textit{in law}.$$

W is not identically 0 *if and only if* $\mathbb{E}[Y\log(Y)] < \infty$, *in which case* $\mathbb{E}[W] = 1$ *and* $\mathbb{P}(W = 0) = \mathbb{P}(\{\exists t > 0 \text{ s.t. } X_t = 0\})$. *Moreover, the law of W has an atom at* 0 *and is absolutely continuous on* $(0,\infty)$.

A.2 The Poisson Process and Poisson Point Process

The Poisson process is central in this whole volume. Let $\lambda > 0$ be given. A rate λ Poisson (counting) process is defined as

$$P_t = \sup\{k \geq 1,\ T_k \leq t\},$$

where $0 = T_0 < T_1 < T_2 < \cdots < T_k < \cdots < \infty$, the random variables $\{T_k - T_{k-1},\ k \geq 1\}$ being independent and identically distributed, each following the law $\text{Exp}(\lambda)$. We have

Proposition A.2.1. *For all* $n \geq 1$, $0 < t_1 < t_2 < \cdots < t_n$, *the random variables* $P_{t_1}, P_{t_2} - P_{t_1}, \ldots, P_{t_n} - P_{t_{n-1}}$ *are independent, and for all* $1 \leq k \leq n$, $P_{t_k} - P_{t_{k-1}} \sim$ *Poi*$[\lambda(t_k - t_{k-1})]$.

Proof. Let us first prove that for all $t, s > 0$,

$$\mathbb{P}(P_{t+s} - P_t = 0 | P_t = k, T_1, T_2, \ldots, T_k) = \exp(-\lambda s).$$

Indeed

$$\begin{aligned}
\mathbb{P}(P_{t+s} - P_t = 0 | P_t = k, T_1, T_2, \ldots, T_k) \\
&= \mathbb{P}(T_{k+1} > t+s | P_t = k, T_k) \\
&= \mathbb{P}(T_{k+1} - T_k > t+s-T_k | T_{k+1} - T_k > t - T_k > 0) \\
&= \mathbb{P}(T_{k+1} - T_k > s) \\
&= \exp(-\lambda s).
\end{aligned}$$

Let now $n \geq 1$. For $1 \leq i \leq n$, we define $X_{n,i} = \mathbf{1}_{\{P_{t+is/n} - P_{t+(i-1)s/n} \geq 1\}}$, and finally $S_n = X_{n,1} + X_{n,2} + \cdots + X_{n,n}$. It follows from the first part of the proof that conditionally upon $\sigma\{P_r,\ 0 \leq r \leq t\}$, the random variables $X_{n,1}, X_{n,2}, \ldots, X_{n,n}$ are i.i.d., each Bernoulli with parameter $1 - e^{-\lambda s/n}$. Then conditionally upon $\sigma\{P_r,\ 0 \leq r \leq t\}$, S_n is binomial with parameters $(n, 1 - e^{-\lambda s/n})$. But $S_n \to P_{t+s} - P_t$ a.s. as $n \to \infty$, while its conditional law given $\sigma\{P_r,\ 0 \leq r \leq t\}$ converges towards the Poisson distribution with parameter λs, according to the following lemma. The proposition follows. □

We have used the following well-known result. Recall the notation $\text{Bin}(n,p)$ for the binomial law with parameters n and p, where $n \geq 1$ and $0 < p < 1$.

Lemma A.2.2. *For all $n \geq 1$, let U_n be a $Bin(n, p_n)$ random variable. If $np_n \to \lambda$ as $n \to \infty$, with $\lambda > 0$, then U_n converges in law towards $Poi(\lambda)$.*

A Poisson process will be called standard if its rate is 1. If P is a standard Poisson process, then $\{P(\lambda t),\ t \geq 0\}$ is a rate λ Poisson process.

We will also use the following

Exercise A.2.3. Let $\{P_t,\ t \geq 0\}$ be a rate λ Poisson process, and $\{T_k,\ k \geq 1\}$ the random points of this Poisson process, i.e. for all $t > 0$, $P_t = \sup\{k \geq 1,\ T_k \leq t\}$. Let $0 < p < 1$. Suppose that each T_k is selected with probability p, not selected with probability $1-p$, independently from the others. Let P'_t denote the number of selected points on the interval $[0,t]$. Then $\{P'_t,\ t \geq 0\}$ is a rate λp Poisson process.

A rate λ Poisson process ($\lambda > 0$) is a counting process $\{R_t,\ t \geq 0\}$ such that $R_t - \lambda t$ is a martingale. Let $\{P(t),\ t \geq 0\}$ be a standard Poisson process (i.e. with rate 1). Then $P(\lambda t) - \lambda t$ is martingale, and it is not hard to show that $\{P(\lambda t),\ t \geq 0\}$ is a rate λ Poisson process. Let now $\{\lambda(t),\ t \geq 0\}$ be a measurable and locally integrable $\mathbb{R}_+$-valued function. Then the process $\{R_t := P\left(\int_0^t \lambda(s)ds\right),\ t \geq 0\}$ is called a rate $\lambda(t)$ Poisson process. Clearly $R_t - \int_0^t \lambda(s)ds$ is a martingale.

We now want to consider the case where λ is random. For that purpose, it is convenient to give an alternative definition of the above process R_t.

Consider a standard Poisson random measure Q on $\mathbb{R}_2^+$, which is defined as follows. M is the counting process associated to a random cloud of points in $\mathbb{R}_+^2$. One way to construct that cloud of points is as follows. We can consider $\mathbb{R}_+^2 = \cup_{i=1}^\infty A_i$, where the A_i's are disjoint squares with Lebesgue measure 1. Let K_i, $i \geq 1$ be i.i.d. mean one Poisson random variables. Let $\{X_j^i,\ j \geq 1, i \geq 1\}$ be independent random points of $\mathbb{R}_+^2$, which are such that for any $i \geq 1$, the X_j^i's are uniformly distributed in A_i. Then

$$Q(dx) = \sum_{i=1}^{\infty} \sum_{j=1}^{K_i} \delta_{X_j^i}(dx).$$

$\lambda(t)$ denoting a positive-valued measurable function, the above $\{R_t,\ t \geq 0\}$ has the same law as

$$R_t = \int_0^t \int_0^{\lambda(s)} Q(ds, du).$$

Now let $\{\lambda(t),\ t \geq 0\}$ be an $\mathbb{R}_+$-valued stochastic process, which is assumed to be predictable, in the following sense. Let for $t \geq 0$,

$$\mathscr{F}_t = \sigma\{Q(A),\ A \text{ Borel subset of } [0,t] \times \mathbb{R}_+\},$$

and consider the σ-algebra of subset of $[0,\infty) \times \Omega$ generated by the subsets of the form $\mathbf{1}_{(s,t]}\mathbf{1}_F$, where $0 \le s < t$ and $F \in \mathscr{F}_s$, which is called the predictable σ-algebra. Note that if X_t is $\mathscr{F}_t$-progressively measurable and left-continuous, then it is predictable. If X_t is progressively measurable and right-continuous, then X_{t-} is predictable.

We assume moreover that $\mathbb{E}\int_0^t \lambda(s)ds < \infty$ for all $t > 0$. We now define the process R_t as above:

$$R_t = \int_0^t \int_0^{\lambda(s)} Q(ds,du).$$

We have (see the next subsection for the definition of a martingale)

Lemma A.2.4. *$R_t - \int_0^t \lambda(s)ds$ is a martingale.*

Proof. For any $\delta > 0$, let

$$R_t^\delta = \int_0^t \int_0^{\lambda(s-\delta)} Q(ds,du),$$

where $\lambda(s) = 0$ for $s < 0$. It is not hard to show that $R_t^\delta - \int_0^t \lambda(s-\delta)ds$ is a martingale which converges in $L^1(\Omega)$ to $R_t - \int_0^t \lambda(s)ds$. Indeed, it suffices to show that if $0 < s < t$ with $t - s \le \delta$, the restriction of the random measure M to $(s,t] \times (0,+\infty)$ is independent of $\{\lambda(r-\delta),\ s < r \le t\}$, which is $\mathscr{F}_s$ measurable hence

$$\mathbb{E}^{\mathscr{F}_s}(R_t^\delta - R_s^\delta) = \mathbb{E}^{\mathscr{F}_s}\int_s^t \lambda(r-\delta)dr.$$

The result follows. □

The process R_t is sometimes called "a doubly stochastic Poisson process" or a Cox process. Of course the increments of R_t are not Poisson distributed. If we let $\sigma(t) = \inf\{r > 0,\ \int_0^r \lambda(s)ds > t\}$, we have that $P(t) := R_{\sigma(t)}$ is a standard Poisson process, and it is clear that $R_t = P\left(\int_0^t \lambda(s)ds\right)$.

In particular, the process which counts the new infections, which appears in Section 2.2, takes the form

$$P\left(\frac{\lambda}{N}\int_0^t I(r)S(r)dr\right) = \int_0^t \int_0^\infty \mathbf{1}_{u \le \frac{\lambda}{N}I(r-)S(r-)} Q(ds,du).$$

If we let $\overline{Q}(ds,du) = Q(ds,du) - ds \times du$ and $M(t) := P(t) - t$, it is clear that, as a consequence of the above Lemma, we have

Corollary A.2.5. *Define $M(\cdot)$ by*

$$\begin{aligned} M\left(\frac{\lambda}{N}\int_0^t I(r)S(r)dr\right) &= \int_0^t \int_0^\infty \mathbf{1}_{u \le \frac{\lambda}{N}I(r-)S(r-)} \overline{Q}(ds,du) \\ &= \int_0^t \int_0^\infty \mathbf{1}_{u \le \frac{\lambda}{N}I(r-)S(r-)} Q(ds,du) - \frac{\lambda}{N}\int_0^t I(r)S(r)dr. \end{aligned}$$

Then $M(t)$ is a martingale (see Definition A.4.7 below).

Note that $\int_0^t I(r-)S(r-)dr = \int_0^t I(r)S(r)dr$ since the two integrands coincide dr a.e. since they differ on each interval $[0,t]$ at most at finitely many points. We use the second formulation, since it is simpler.

A.3 Cramér's Theorem for Poisson Random Variables

In order to explain what Large Deviations is about, let us first establish Cramér's Theorem, in the particular case of Poisson random variables. Let $X_1, X_2, \ldots, X_n, \ldots$ be mutually independent Poi(μ) random variables. The Law of Large Numbers tells us that

$$\frac{1}{N}\sum_{i=1}^{N} X_i \to \mu \quad \text{a.s. as } N \to \infty.$$

Let us first define, for $X \sim \text{Poi}(\mu)$ the logarithm of its Laplace transform

$$\Lambda(\lambda) = \log \mathbb{E}[\exp(\lambda X)] = \mu(e^{\lambda} - 1),$$

and the Fenchel–Legendre transform of the latter

$$\Lambda^*(x) = \sup_{\lambda \in \mathbb{R}} \{\lambda x - \Lambda(\lambda)\} = x \log\left(\frac{x}{\mu}\right) - x + \mu.$$

Note that the minimum of Λ^* is achieved at $x = \mu$, and Λ^* is zero at that point.

Let ν_N denote the law of the random variable $\frac{1}{N}\sum_{i=1}^{N} X_i$. We can now state Cramér's theorem.

Theorem A.3.1. *Let $F \subset \mathbb{R}$ be a closed set.*

$$\textit{For any } N \geq 1,\ \nu_N(F) \leq \exp\left(-N \inf_{x \in F} \Lambda^*(x)\right).$$

$$\textit{Hence } \limsup_{N \to \infty} \frac{1}{N} \log \nu_N(F) \leq -\inf_{x \in F} \Lambda^*(x).$$

Let $G \subset \mathbb{R}$ be an open set.

$$\textit{For any } N \geq 1,\ \nu_N(G) \geq \exp\left(-N \inf_{x \in G} \Lambda^*(x)\right).$$

$$\textit{Hence } \liminf_{N \to \infty} \frac{1}{N} \log \nu_N(G) \geq -\inf_{x \in G} \Lambda^*(x).$$

Proof. FIRST STEP. PROOF OF THE UPPER BOUND Let $X_1, X_2, \ldots, X_n, \ldots$ be mutually independent Poi(μ) random variables. For $\sigma > \mu$, we want to estimate

$$\mathbb{P}\left(\frac{1}{N}\sum_{i=1}^{N} X_i \geq \sigma\right),$$

which is the probability of a Large Deviation from the LLN, since we know that for large N, $\frac{1}{N}\sum_{i=1}^{N} X_i \simeq \mu$.

For any $\lambda > 0$, using Chebycheff's inequality,

$$\begin{aligned}\mathbb{P}\left(\frac{1}{N}\sum_{i=1}^{N} X_i \geq \sigma\right) &= \mathbb{P}\left(\exp\left\{\lambda\left(\sum_{i=1}^{N} X_i - N\sigma\right)\right\} \geq 1\right)\\ &\leq \mathbb{E}\exp\left\{\lambda\left(\sum_{i=1}^{N} X_i - N\sigma\right)\right\}\\ &= \exp[-N(\lambda\sigma - \Lambda(\lambda)] .\end{aligned}$$

The best possible upper bound is then (since with $\sigma > \mu$, $\Lambda^*(\sigma)$ is obtained by taking the supremum over $\lambda > 0$)

$$\begin{aligned}\mathbb{P}\left(\frac{1}{N}\sum_{i=1}^{N} X_i \geq \sigma\right) &\leq e^{-N\Lambda^*(\sigma)}\\ &= \exp\left[-N\left(\sigma\log\left(\frac{\sigma}{\mu}\right) - \sigma + \mu\right)\right].\end{aligned}$$

Similarly, if $\sigma < \mu$, for any $\lambda < 0$,

$$\begin{aligned}\mathbb{P}\left(\frac{1}{N}\sum_{i=1}^{N} X_i \leq \sigma\right) &\leq \mathbb{E}\exp\left\{\lambda\left(\sum_{i=1}^{N} X_i - N\sigma\right)\right\}\\ &= \exp[-N(\lambda\sigma - \Lambda(\lambda)] .\end{aligned}$$

Since with $\sigma < \mu$, $\Lambda^*(\sigma)$ is obtained by taking the supremum over $\lambda < 0$, the above computation leads again to

$$\mathbb{P}\left(\frac{1}{N}\sum_{i=1}^{N} X_i \leq \sigma\right) \leq \exp\left[-N\left(\sigma\log\left(\frac{\sigma}{\mu}\right) - \sigma + \mu\right)\right].$$

It is not hard to see that the upper bound follows from the two above estimates.

SECOND STEP. PROOF OF THE LOWER BOUND For any $\delta > 0$,

$$\nu_N((-\delta,\delta)) \geq \nu_N(\{0\}) = e^{-N\mu}, \quad \text{hence } \frac{1}{N}\log\nu_N((-\delta,\delta)) \geq -\mu = -\Lambda^*(0).$$

Since transforming X into $Y = X - x$ results in Λ and Λ^* being transformed into $\Lambda_Y(\lambda) = \Lambda(\lambda) - \lambda x$ and $\Lambda_Y^*(\cdot) = \Lambda^*(\cdot + x)$, the above yields that for all $x > 0$,

$$\frac{1}{N}\log\nu_N((x-\delta, x+\delta)) \geq -\Lambda^*(x).$$

The lower bound follows readily. □

A.4 Martingales

A.4.1 Martingales in Discrete Time

$(\Omega, \mathscr{F}, \mathbb{P})$ being our standing probability space, let be given an increasing sequence $\{\mathscr{F}_n,\ n \geq 0\}$ of sub-σ-algebras of $\mathscr{F}$.

Definition A.4.1. A sequence $\{X_n,\ n \geq 0\}$ of random variables is called a martingale if

1. For all $n \geq 0$, X_n is $\mathscr{F}_n$-measurable and integrable,
2. For all $n \geq 0$, $\mathbb{E}(X_{n+1}|\mathscr{F}_n) = X_n$ a. s.

A sub-martingale is a sequence which satisfies the first condition and $\mathbb{E}(X_{n+1}|\mathscr{F}_n) \geq X_n$. A super-martingale is a sequence which satisfies the first condition and $\mathbb{E}(X_{n+1}|\mathscr{F}_n) \leq X_n$.

It follows readily from Jensen's inequality for conditional expectations the

Proposition A.4.2. *If $\{X_n,\ n \geq 0\}$ is a martingale, and $\varphi : \mathbb{R} \to \mathbb{R}$ is a convex function such that $\varphi(X_n)$ is integrable for all $n \geq 0$, then $\{\varphi(X_n),\ n \geq 0\}$ is a sub-martingale.*

We shall need the notion of stopping time

Definition A.4.3. A stopping time τ is an $\mathbb{Z}_+ \cup \{+\infty\}$-valued random variable which satisfies $\{\tau = n\} \in \mathscr{F}_n$, for all $n \geq 0$.

We also let

$$\mathscr{F}_\tau = \{B \in \mathscr{F},\ B \cap \{\tau = n\} \in \mathscr{F}_n,\ \forall n \in \mathbb{Z}_+\}.$$

We have Doob's optional sampling theorem:

Theorem A.4.4. *If $\{X_n,\ n \geq 0\}$ is a martingale (resp. a sub-martingale), and τ_1, τ_2 two stopping times s.t. $\tau_1 \leq \tau_2 \leq N$ a.s., then X_{τ_i} is $\mathscr{F}_{\tau_i}$ measurable and integrable, $i = 1, 2$, and moreover*

$$\mathbb{E}(X_{\tau_2}|\mathscr{F}_{\tau_1}) = X_{\tau_1}$$
$$(\textit{resp.}\ \ \mathbb{E}(X_{\tau_2}|\mathscr{F}_{\tau_1}) \geq X_{\tau_1}).$$

Proof. For all $A \in \mathscr{B}$, $n \geq 0$,

$$\{X_{\tau_i} \in A\} \cap \{\tau_i = n\} = \{X_n \in A\} \cap \{\tau_i = n\} \in \mathscr{F}_n,$$

and moreover

$$|X_{\tau_i}| \leq \sum_{k=1}^{N} |X_k|,$$

which establishes the first part of the statement.

Let $A \in \mathscr{F}_{\tau_1}$. Then

$$A \cap \{\tau_1 < k \leq \tau_2\} = A \cap \{\tau_1 \leq k-1\} \cap \{\tau_2 \leq k-1\}^c \in \mathscr{F}_{k-1}.$$

Indeed, we have

$$A \cap \{\tau_1 \leq k-1\} = \cup_{j=1}^{k-1} A \cap \{\tau_1 = j\} \in \mathscr{F}_{k-1}, \text{ and } \{\tau_2 \leq k-1\}^c \in \mathscr{F}_{k-1}.$$

Let $\Delta_k = X_k - X_{k-1}$. We have, with $A \in \mathscr{F}_{\tau_1}$,

$$\begin{aligned}\int_A (X_{\tau_2} - X_{\tau_1}) d\mathbb{P} &= \int_A \sum_{k=1}^n \mathbf{1}_{\{\tau_1 < k \leq \tau_2\}} \Delta_k d\mathbb{P} \\ &= \sum_{k=1}^n \int_{A \cap \{\tau_1 < k \leq \tau_2\}} \Delta_k d\mathbb{P} \\ &= 0\end{aligned}$$

or else ≥ 0, depending upon whether $\{X_n,\ n \geq 0\}$ is a martingale or a sub-martingale. □

We have a first Doob's inequality

Proposition A.4.5. *If $X_1, \ldots, X_n$ is a sub-martingale, then for all $\alpha > 0$,*

$$\mathbb{P}\left(\max_{1 \leq i \leq n} X_i \geq \alpha\right) \leq \frac{1}{\alpha} \mathbb{E}(X_n^+).$$

Proof. Define the stopping time $\tau = \inf\{0 \leq k \leq n,\ X_k \geq \alpha\}$ and let $M_k = \max_{1 \leq i \leq k} X_i$. We have

$$\{M_n \geq \alpha\} \cap \{\tau \leq k\} = \{M_k \geq \alpha\} \in \mathscr{F}_k.$$

Hence $\{M_n \geq \alpha\} \in \mathscr{F}_\tau$. From the optional sampling Theorem,

$$\begin{aligned}\alpha \mathbb{P}(M_n \geq \alpha) &\leq \int_{\{M_n \geq \alpha\}} X_\tau d\mathbb{P} \\ &\leq \int_{\{M_n \geq \alpha\}} X_n d\mathbb{P} \\ &\leq \int_{\{M_n \geq \alpha\}} X_n^+ d\mathbb{P} \\ &\leq \mathbb{E}(X_n^+).\end{aligned}$$

□

We have finally a second Doob's inequality

Proposition A.4.6. *If $M_1, \ldots, M_n$ is a martingale, then*

$$\mathbb{E}\left[\sup_{0 \leq k \leq n} |M_k|^2\right] \leq 4\mathbb{E}\left[|M_n|^2\right].$$

Proof. Let $X_k = |M_k|$. From Proposition A.4.2, $X_1, \ldots, X_n$ is a sub-martingale. It follows from the proof of Proposition A.4.5 that, with the notation $X_k^* = \sup_{0 \leq k \leq n} X_k$,

$$\mathbb{P}(X_n^* > \lambda) \leq \frac{1}{\lambda}\mathbb{E}\left(X_n \mathbf{1}_{X_n^* > \lambda}\right).$$

Consequently

$$\begin{aligned}
\int_0^\infty \lambda \mathbb{P}(X_n^* > \lambda) d\lambda &\leq \int_0^\infty \mathbb{E}\left(X_n \mathbf{1}_{X_n^* > \lambda}\right) d\lambda \\
\mathbb{E}\left(\int_0^{X_n^*} \lambda d\lambda\right) &\leq \mathbb{E}\left(X_n \int_0^{X_n^*} d\lambda\right) \\
\frac{1}{2}\mathbb{E}\left[|X_n^*|^2\right] &\leq \mathbb{E}(X_n X_n^*) \\
&\leq \sqrt{E(|X_n|^2)}\sqrt{E(|X_n^*|^2)},
\end{aligned}$$

from which the result follows. □

A.4.2 Martingales in Continuous Time

We are now given an increasing collection $\{\mathscr{F}_t,\ t \geq 0\}$ of sub-σ-algebras in continuous time.

Definition A.4.7. A process $\{X_t,\ t \geq 0\}$ is called a martingale if

1. for all $t \geq 0$, X_t is $\mathscr{F}_t$-measurable and integrable;
2. for all $0 \leq s < t$, $\mathbb{E}(X_t|\mathscr{F}_s) = X_s$ a. s.

A sub-martingale is a process which satisfies the first condition and $\mathbb{E}(X_t|\mathscr{F}_s) \geq X_s$. A super-martingale is a process which satisfies the first condition and $\mathbb{E}(X_t|\mathscr{F}_s) \leq X_s$.

Suppose $\{M_t,\ t \geq 0\}$ is a right-continuous martingale. For any $n \geq 1$, $0 = t_0 < t_1 < \cdots < t_n$, $(M_{t_0}, M_{t_1}, \ldots, M_{t_n})$ is a discrete time martingale, to which Proposition A.4.6 applies. Since

$$\sup_{0 \leq s \leq t} |M_s| = \sup_{\text{Partitions of } [0,t]} \sup_{1 \leq k \leq n} |M_{t_k}|,$$

Proposition A.4.6 implies readily

Proposition A.4.8. *If $\{M_t,\ t \geq 0\}$ is a right-continuous martingale,*

$$\mathbb{E}\left[\sup_{0 \leq s \leq t} |M_s|^2\right] \leq 4\mathbb{E}\left[|M_t|^2\right].$$

We now establish a particular (essentially obvious) instance of Itô's formula. Recall that an $\mathbb{R}$-valued function of t has locally bounded variations if and only if it is the difference of an increasing and a decreasing function. This class of functions excludes all non-zero continuous martingales, e.g. Brownian motion. But all processes considered in these Notes, except for the limit in the functional central limit theorem, are locally of bounded variations. Given such a locally bounded variation right-continuous 1-dimensional process X_t, we define the bracket $[X,X]_t = \sum_{0\le s\le t} |\Delta X_s|^2$, where $\Delta X_s = X_s - X_{s-}$ is the jump of X at time s. It follows from the fact that X has bounded variation on any compact interval that the set $\{s \ge 0, \Delta X_s \ne 0\}$ is at most countable, hence the above sum makes sense. If X and Y are two processes of the above type, then

$$[X,Y]_t = \sum_{0\le s\le t} \Delta X_s \Delta Y_s = \frac{1}{2}\left([X+Y,X+Y]_t - [X,X]_t - [Y,Y]_t\right).$$

Now we have what we call Itô's formula. If X_t and Y_t are right-continuous and have left limits at any t, have bounded variations on any compact interval, then for any $t > 0$,

$$X_t Y_t = X_0 Y_0 + \int_0^t X_{s-} dY_s + \int_0^t Y_{s-} dX_s + [X,Y]_t. \tag{A.4.1}$$

In case all jumps of X and Y are isolated, which is the only situation treated in these Notes, the result follows clearly by analyzing the evolution of both sides of the identity between the jumps, and at the jump times. The result in the more general situation is easily deduced by approximation.

If M_t is a right-continuous $\mathbb{R}$-valued martingale with locally bounded variation, we define as above its quadratic variation as

$$[M,M]_t = \sum_{0\le s\le t} |\Delta M_s|^2,$$

and $\langle M,M\rangle_t$ as the unique increasing predictable process such that $[M,M]_t - \langle M,M\rangle_t$ is a martingale. Note that both $M_t^2 - [M,M]_t$ and $M_t^2 - \langle M,M\rangle_t$ are martingales. Consequently, we have in particular

Proposition A.4.9. *Let M_t be a square–integrable right-continuous $\mathbb{R}$-valued martingale with finite variation such that $M_0 = 0$. Then for all $t > 0$,*

$$\mathbb{E}\left(M_t^2\right) = \mathbb{E}\left(\sum_{0\le s\le t} |\Delta M_s|^2\right).$$

A.5 Tightness and Weak Convergence in Path Space

In these Notes we consider continuous time processes with values in $\mathbb{R}^d$. Most of our processes are discontinuous. Their trajectories belong to the set $D([0,+\infty);\mathbb{R}^d)$ of functions which are right continuous and have left limits at any point $t \in [0,+\infty)$. It is not very convenient to use the topology of locally uniform convergence on this set, since we would like for instance the two Heaviside type functions $\mathbf{1}_{[1,+\infty)}(t)$ and $\mathbf{1}_{[1+\varepsilon,+\infty)}(t)$ to be close for ε small. The Skorokhod topology essentially says that two functions are close if after a time change which is close to the identity, they are (at least locally) close in the supremum topology. The only weak convergence (i.e.

convergence in law) results we consider in these Notes are convergence results towards a continuous process. In this case, convergence in the sense of the Skorokhod topology is equivalent to locally uniform convergence.

Note also that weak convergence of a sequence of processes X^n towards X is equivalent to the two following facts:

1. The sequence $\{X^n\}_{n\geq 1}$ is tight, as a sequence of random elements of $D([0,+\infty);\mathbb{R}^d)$ equipped with the Skorokhod topology.
2. For any $k \geq 1$, $0 \leq t_1 < t_2 < \cdots < t_k$, $(X^n_{t_1},\dots,X^n_{t_k}) \Rightarrow (X_{t_1},\dots,X_{t_k})$, in the sense of weak convergence in $\mathbb{R}^{d\times k}$.

If only 2 is satisfied, then one has convergence in the sense of finite-dimensional distributions.

What do we mean by tightness? A sequence $\{X_n\}_{n\geq 1}$ of random variables with values in a topological space S is said to be tight if for any $\varepsilon > 0$, there exists a compact set $K \subset S$ such that $\mathbb{P}(X_n \in K) \geq 1-\varepsilon$ for all $n \geq 1$.

Consider the product X_nY_n, where X_n and Y_n are real-valued. If one of the two sequences is tight and the other tends to 0 in probability, then $X_nY_n \to 0$ in probability. This easy result is used in the proof of Theorem 2.3.2.

In the proof of Lemma 2.3.4, we use the following argument: a sequence of continuous time martingales M^n_t satisfying $M^n_0 = 0$ is tight as soon as the associated sequence of predictable increasing processes $\langle M^n, M^n\rangle_t$ is C–tight, in the sense that both it is tight, and any weak limit of a converging sub–sequence is continuous, see e.g. Theorem VI.4.13 in Jacod and Shiryaev [15]. In the situation of Lemma 2.3.4, $\langle M^n, M^n\rangle_t = t$ which is C–tight, since it does not depend upon n and is continuous.

A.6 Pontryagin's Maximum Principle

In this section, we present the Pontryagin maximum principle in optimal control, which is useful in order to compute or give some estimates for the exponent in the asymptotic evaluation of the time to extinction derived from large deviation theory. We refer the reader for a more general presentation, proofs and references to Trélat [37] and Pontryagin et al. [31].

The quantity of interest, denoted by $\overline{V}$ in Section 4.2.5 and the following pages, is the value function of an optimal control problem which is of the following type. $x \in C([0,\infty);\mathbb{R}^d)$ solves the controlled ODE

$$\dot{x}_t = Bu_t, \quad x_0 = x^*,$$

where B is a $d\times k$ matrix, and $u \in L^1([0,\infty);\mathbb{R}^k_+)$ is to be chosen together with the final time T such as to minimize a cost functional

$$C(u) = \sum_{j=1}^{k} \int_0^T g(u_j(t), \beta_j(x_t))dt,$$

while the following constraint must be satisfied: $x_T \in M_1$, where M_1 is some affine subspace of $\mathbb{R}^d$. The function g is the one which appears in Section 4.2.2, namely $g(a,b) = a\log(a/b) - a + b$, while the β_j's are some mappings from $\mathbb{R}^d$ into $\mathbb{R}_+$, which, like the matrix B, depend upon the particular model we consider. Note that in our case all entries of B are either 1, 0, or -1.

We associate to this optimal control problem a Hamiltonian which takes the form

$$H(x,p,u) = \langle p, Bu \rangle - \sum_{j=1}^{k} g(u_j, \beta_j(x)),$$

where $p \in C([0,T];\mathbb{R}^d)$ is the adjoint state. The next statement constitutes Pontryagin maximum principle, applied to our particular situation.

Theorem A.6.1. *If $(\hat{u}, \hat{T})$ is an optimal pair, then there exists an adjoint state, such that the following is satisfied*

$$\begin{aligned} \dot{x}_t &= B\hat{u}_t, \quad x_0 = x^*, \; x_{\hat{T}} \in M_1, \\ \dot{p}_t &= \sum_{j=1}^{k} \left[\nabla\beta_j(x_t) - \hat{u}_j(t) \frac{\nabla\beta_j(x_t)}{\beta_j(x_t)} \right], \quad p_{\hat{T}} \perp M_1, \\ H(x_t, p_t, \hat{u}_t) &= \max_{v \in \mathbb{R}^k_+} H(x_t, p_t, v) = 0, \quad 0 \le t \le \hat{T}. \end{aligned}$$

Of course, the first equation could be of the more general form $\dot{x} = f(x,u)$. The general form of the adjoint equation reads $\dot{p} = -\nabla_x H$. The Hamiltonian is zero at time $\hat{T}$ since the final time is not fixed and there is no final cost. The Hamiltonian is constant along the optimal trajectory because none of the coefficients depends upon t.

Since $u \to (B^*p)_j u - g(u, \beta_j(x))$ is concave, the maximum is the zero of its derivative if it is non-negative. Hence

$$\hat{u}_j = e^{(B^*p)_j} \beta_j(x),$$

and the two above equations can be written as

$$\dot{x}_t = \sum_{j=1}^{k} e^{(B^*p_t)_j} \beta_j(x_t) h_j, \quad \dot{p}_t = \sum_{j=1}^{k} (1 - e^{(B^*p_t)_j}) \nabla\beta_j(x_t),$$

and the Hamiltonian along the optimal trajectory reads

$$H(x_t, p_t, \hat{u}_t) = \sum_{j=1}^{k} \beta_j(x_t)(e^{(B^*p_t)_j} - 1) = 0. \tag{A.6.1}$$

Finally the instantaneous cost takes the form

$$\sum_{j=1}^{k}\left(1-e^{(B^*p_t)_j}+(B^*p_t)_j e^{(B^*p_t)_j}\right)\beta_j(x_t)=\sum_{j=1}^{k}(B^*p_t)_j e^{(B^*p_t)_j}\beta_j(x_t), \qquad (A.6.2)$$

where this identity follows from (A.6.1).

A.7 Semi- and Equicontinuity

Let $\mathscr{X}$ be a metric space, equipped with a distance d, and f be a mapping from $\mathscr{X}$ into $\mathbb{R}\cup\{-\infty,\infty\}$.

Definition A.7.1. f is said to be lower (resp. upper) semi-continuous if for any $x_0 \in \mathscr{X}$,

$$\liminf_{x\to x_0} f(x) \ge f(x_0) \quad (\text{resp. } \limsup_{x\to x_0} f(x) \le f(x_0)).$$

Clearly f is continuous if and only if it is both lower and upper semi-continuous.

A lower (resp. upper) semi-continuous $(-\infty,\infty]$-valued (resp. $[-\infty,\infty)$-valued) function achieves its minimum (resp. maximum) on a compact subset of $\mathscr{X}$.

The pointwise supremum (resp. infimum) of a collection of continuous functions is lower (resp. upper) semi-continuous.

Let now $\{f_i,\ i\in I\}$ be a collection of elements of $C(\mathscr{X})$ (i.e. of continuous functions from $\mathscr{X}$ into $\mathbb{R}$), where I is an arbitrary index set.

Definition A.7.2. The collection $\{f_n,\ n\ge 1\}$ is said to be equicontinuous if for any $x_0\in\mathscr{X}$, $\sup_{i\in I}|f_i(x)-f_i(x_0)|\to 0$, as $x\to x_0$. The same collection is said to be uniformly equicontinuous if $\sup_{i\in I}\sup_{d(x,y)\le\delta}|f_i(x)-f_i(y)|\to 0$, as $\delta\to 0$.

Note that when $\mathscr{X}$ is compact, equicontinuity and uniform equicontinuity are equivalent.

A.8 Solutions to Selected Exercises

Solution to Exercise 1.1.2. $R_0=\lambda E(I)=\lambda/\gamma=1.8$. The escape probability from a given under infected individual equals $E(e^{-\lambda I/N})=\gamma/(\gamma+\lambda/N)$, since $\psi_I(-\lambda/N)=\gamma/(\gamma+\lambda/N)$ when $I\sim \text{Exp}(\gamma)$. For $\lambda=1.8,\ \gamma=1,\ N=100$ we get 0.9823.

Solution to Exercise 1.1.3. For the Reed–Frost epidemic we hence have the same $R_0 = \lambda E(I) = 1.8$. As for the escape probability we get

$$P(\text{avoid infection from an infective}) = e^{-\lambda \iota/N} = 0.9822.$$

The escape probabilities are not identical, but very similar for the two models.

Solution to Exercise 1.2.1. If $I \equiv 1$, then $X \sim \text{Poi}(R_0)$. If $I \sim \text{Exp}(1/\iota)$, then $X \sim \text{MixPoi}(\lambda I)$. So

$$P(X=k) = \int_0^\infty P(X=k|I=s)e^{-s/\iota}/\iota ds = (R_0/(R_0+1))^k(1/(R_0+1)),$$

so $X \sim \text{Geo}(p = 1/(R_0+1))$.

Solution to Exercise 1.2.8. The probability of a minor outbreak corresponds to the probability of extinction in the approximating branching process. This probability q was derived in Section A.1 by conditioning on the number k infected in the first generation, the offspring distribution: if k get infected these all start new independent branching processes so the probability that all go extinct equals q^k. The general equation is hence

$$q = \sum_{k=0}^{\infty} q^k P(X=k).$$

The offspring distribution X depends on the infectious period distribution I. Given that $I = s$, X has a Poisson distribution with mean λs, so $X \sim \text{MixPoi}(\lambda I)$. In situation 2 (cont-time R-F) $I \equiv 1$ so $X \sim \text{Poi}(\lambda = 1.5)$. This gives the following equation

$$q = \sum_{k=0}^{\infty} q^k \frac{\lambda^k e^{-\lambda}}{k!} = \ldots = e^{-R_0(1-q)} = e^{-1.5(1-q)}.$$

If this equation is solved numerically it gives the result that $q = 1 - 0.583 = 0.417$. So for the Reed–Frost case the probability of a major outbreak, equals 0.583.

As for the Markovian SIR, where $I \sim \text{Exp}(1)$ we get

$$\begin{aligned} P(X=k) &= \int_0^\infty P(X=k|I=s)f_I(s)ds \\ &= \int_0^\infty \frac{(\lambda s)^k e^{-\lambda s}}{k!} e^{-s} ds = \cdots = \frac{1}{1+\lambda}\left(\frac{\lambda}{1+\lambda}\right)^k \end{aligned}$$

i.e. the geometric distribution, which should not come as a surprise (each time, the event is either infection or recovery, and the latter has probability $1/(\lambda+1)$). We then get

$$q = \sum_{k=0}^{\infty} q^k P(X=k) = q^k \left(\frac{\lambda}{\lambda+1}\right)^k \frac{1}{\lambda+1} = \frac{1}{1+(1-q)\lambda}.$$

As a consequence, the probability of a minor outbreak for the Markovian SIR hence equals $q = 1/\lambda = 1/R_0 = 1/1.5 = 0.67$. The probability of a major outbreak is hence only 0.33. The randomness of the infectious period hence reduces the risk for a major outbreak. It can actually be proven that having a constant infectious period maximizes the outbreak probability among all distributions of the infectious period.

Solution to Exercise 1.2.9. The exponential growth rate (or decay rate if $R < 1$) r is the solution to Equation (1.2.1), where $h(s)$ is the average rate of infectious contacts s units after infection: $h(s) = \lambda P(L \le s \le L+I)$. For the Markovian SIR (for which $L \equiv 0$ and $I \sim \text{Exp}(\gamma = 1/\iota)$) we hence have $h(s) = \lambda e^{-s/\iota} = 1.5e^{-s}$, and the solution equals $r = \lambda - 1/\iota$ For $R_0 = 1.5$ and $\gamma = \iota = 1$ this gives the exponential growth rate $r = 0.5$.

For the continuous time Reed–Frost model we have $h(s) = \lambda 1_{(s<\iota)}$. The equation then becomes $\int_0^\iota e^{-rs}\lambda ds = \frac{\lambda}{r}(1-e^{-r\iota}) = 1$. The equation is hence $r/\lambda = 1-e^{-(r/\lambda)R_0}$. When $R_0 = 1.5$ we numerically get $r/\lambda = 0.583$, so $r = 0.874$ for the continuous time Reed–Frost model. This epidemic hence grows quicker than the Markovian SIR epidemic with the same parameters. The main reason for this is that even if the two infectious periods have equal mean $\iota = 1$, the average time of the infectious contacts are not the same. For the Reed–Frost the mean time to a randomly selected infectious contact (the mean of the generation time distribution) is of course 0.5 (the generation time distribution is uniform on $[0, 1]$, whereas for the Markovian SIR it equals 1 (the generation time distribution is Exp(1)).

For the third case, with exponentially distributed latency and infectious periods, we have $h(s) = P(L < s < L+I) = \frac{\lambda\nu}{\gamma-\nu}(e^{-\nu s} - e^{-\gamma s})$. Solving $\int_0^\infty e^{-rs}h(s)ds = 1$ gives the solution

$$r = \sqrt{\nu(\lambda-\gamma) + \left(\frac{\gamma+\nu}{2}\right)^2} - \frac{\gamma+\nu}{2} \approx 0.2247.$$

Of course, adding a latency period before the infectious period will reduce the growth rate r of the epidemic.

Solution to Exercise 1.4.2. $v_c = 1 - 1/R_0 = 0.5$. When $v = 0.33$, z_v solves the equation $1 - z_v = e^{-(1-v)R_0 z_v}$, and the numerical solution equals $z_v = 0.4544$. The over-all fraction infected is hence $(1-v)z_v = 0.3029$. As for the probability of a major outbreak we have that for the Markovian SIR $P(\text{major outbreak}) = 1 - 1/R_v = 0.25$, since $R_v = (1-v)R_0 = 0.67 \cdot 2 = 1.33$.

Solution to Exercise 1.4.3. The new rate at which an infectious individual makes infectious contacts when $v = 33\%$ are vaccinated is $\lambda' = \lambda p v + \lambda(1-v)$ where $p = 0.2$ (this is true irrespective of whether the infector was vaccinated or not). Since the average infectious period equals $E(I) = 1$ we have $R_v = \lambda' E(I) = 1.467$ (instead of $R_0 = 2$ when no one is vaccinated).

Solution to Exercise 2.1.2. $R_0 = 1.5$: 0.583, $R_0 = 3$: 0.940, $R_0 = 15$: 1.000 (of course not exactly, but to this precision).

Solution to Exercise 3.1.1.

$$p_3^{(3)} = p^3 + \binom{3}{2} p^2(1-p) * (1-(1-p)^2) \\ + \binom{3}{1} p(1-p)^2 * p^2 + \binom{3}{1} p(1-p)^2 * \binom{2}{1} p(1-p) * p.$$

Solution to Exercise 3.3.3 The limiting mean equals Nz where z solves $1-z=e^{-R_0 z}$ so with $R_0 = \lambda\iota = 1.5$ we get $z = 0.583$ and the limiting mean equals 583 for both scenarios. The limiting variance of Z^N equals $N\frac{z(1-z)(1+r^2(1-z)R_0^2)}{(1-(1-z)R_0)^2}$, where r is the coefficient of variation of the infectious period. For the Reed–Frost case with non-random infectious period we have $r = 0$ implying that the limiting variance equals 1737, so the standard deviation equals 41.7, so one can expect that the final size will be somewhere in the interval 583 ± 80 with about 95% probability. The Markovian SIR has exponential infectious period which has $r = 1$ giving a variance of 3367 and standard deviation 58.0. So, the fact that the infectious period is exponential as compared to fixed makes the standard deviation of the final size increase by close to 50%.

Solution to Exercise 3.4.1. The numerical values are: the final size equals $z = 0.583$ and $R_0(1-z) = 0.626 < 1$.

Solution to Exercise 3.4.2. Computing the two leading terms is equivalent to computing r and r^*. For the Markovian SIR we have $r = 0.5$ and $r^* = -0.3742$, for the continuous time Reed–Frost we get $r = 0.8742$ and $r^* = -0.8741$, and for the Markovian SEIR we have $r = 0.2247$ and $r^* = -0.2089$.

Solution to Exercise 4.1.3. Denoting by $U(t)$ the vector of the Gaussian fluctuations around $\begin{pmatrix} s(t) \\ i(t) \end{pmatrix}$, deduce from Theorem 2.3.2 that this vector solves the linear SDE

$$U(t) = \int_0^t A(r)U(r)dr + \int_0^t C(r)dB_r,$$

where $B(t)$ is a standard five-dimensional Brownian motion and

$$A(t) = \mu \begin{pmatrix} -1 - \frac{R_0}{\varepsilon} i(t) & -\frac{R_0}{\varepsilon} s(t) \\ \frac{R_0}{\varepsilon} i(t) & \varepsilon^{-1}(R_0 s(t) - 1) \end{pmatrix},$$

$$C(t) = \mu \begin{pmatrix} \sqrt{\mu} & -\sqrt{\frac{\mu R_0}{\varepsilon} s(t) i(t)} & -\sqrt{\mu s(t)} & 0 \\ 0 & \sqrt{\frac{\mu R_0}{\varepsilon} s(t) i(t)} & 0 & -\sqrt{\frac{\mu}{\varepsilon} i(t)} \end{pmatrix}.$$

Show that, as $t \to \infty$,

$$A(t) \to \mu \begin{pmatrix} -R_0 & -1/\varepsilon \\ R_0 - 1 & 0 \end{pmatrix}, \; C(t)C^*(t) \to \frac{\mu}{R_0} \begin{pmatrix} 2R_0 & -(R_0-1) \\ -(R_0-1) & 2(R_0-1) \end{pmatrix}.$$

Show that the eigenvalues of $A = \lim_{t \to \infty} A(t)$ are complex, as soon as $\varepsilon < 4/R_0$, and that the real parts of those eigenvalues are negative. Conclude from a combination of Exercise 2.3.8 and Lemma 2.3.7 that the covariance matrix of the stationary distribution of $U(t)$ reads

$$\begin{pmatrix} \frac{1}{R_0} + \frac{1}{\varepsilon R_0^2} & -\frac{1}{R_0} \\ -\frac{1}{R_0} & \frac{1}{R_0} - \frac{1}{R_0^2} + \varepsilon \end{pmatrix}.$$

Conclude by taking into account that we expect to have $\varepsilon << R_0^{-1}$.

Solution to Exercise 4.1.4. The relative length of the infectious period ε affects the critical community size N_c much more than R_0 does, since it is squared in the approximation of N_c. As an illustration, if the infectious period is doubled (with half infectivity per unit of time thus keeping R_0 fixed) N_c will decrease by a factor 4, whereas if the basic reproduction number is doubled (keeping everything else fixed) only decreases N_c by a factor close to 2.

Solution to Exercise 4.1.5. There are two effects of this vaccination strategy. The first is that vaccinated individuals can be ignored, so the relevant population (of unvaccinated people) is now $N^{(unvacc)} = N(1-v)$. Secondly, since infected individuals have contact with both types of individuals, the rate of having contact with the population of interest is reduced to $\lambda(1-v)$ implying that the reproduction number is changed to $R_v = R_0(1-v)$. The critical population size of unvaccinated people $N_c^{(unvacc)}$ is then simply obtained in the same way, but for these new parameters, so

$$N_c^{(unvacc)} = \frac{9}{\varepsilon^2(1-\frac{1}{R_v})^2 R_v} = \frac{9}{\varepsilon^2(1-\frac{1}{(1-v)R_0})^2(1-v)R_0}.$$

However, a more interesting quantity is the critical community size counting all individuals, hence also vaccinated. Since $N = N^{(unvacc)}(/1-v)$, the critical community size for a population in which a fraction v of the new-born are continuously being vaccinated is given by

$$N_c^{(v)} = \frac{9}{(1-v)^2\varepsilon^2(1-\frac{1}{(1-v)R_0})^2 R_0}.$$

By numerical studies it is easily shown that the critical community size grows very big with v, also agreeing with empirical evidence since e.g. measles is no longer endemic in England (or anywhere else in the world having high vaccination coverage).

References for Part I

1. R.M. Anderson and R.M. May, *Infectious diseases of humans; dynamic and control*, Oxford: Oxford University Press, 1991.
2. H. Andersson and T. Britton, *Stochastic epidemic models and their statistical analysis*, Springer Lecture Notes in Statistics. New York: Springer Verlag, 2000.
3. K.B. Athreya and P.E. Ney, *Branching Processes*, Grundlehren der Mathematischen Wissenschaften **196**, Springer, 1972. Reprinted in 2004 by Dover.
4. R. Azencott, Grandes déviations et applications. (French) *Eighth Saint Flour Probability Summer School - 1978*, pp. 1-176, Lecture Notes in Math. **774**, Springer, Berlin, 1980.
5. F.G. Ball, A unified approach to the distribution of total size and total area under the trajectory of infectives in epidemic models, *Adv. Appl. Prob.* **18**, 289-310, 1986.
6. F.G. Ball and D. Clancy, The final size and severity of a generalised stochastic multitype epidemic model, *Adv. Appl. Prob.* **25**, 721–736, 1993.
7. A.D. Barbour, The duration of the closed stochastic epidemic, *Biometrika* **62**, 477–482, 1975.
8. P. Billingsley, *Convergence of Probability Measures*, 2d ed., J. Wiley & Sons, Inc., 1999.
9. A. Dembo and O. Zeitouni, *Large deviations, techniques and applications*, 2nd ed., Applications of Mathematics **38**, Springer, 1998.
10. R.A. Doney, A limit theorem for a class of supercritical branching processes, *J. Appl. Prob.* **9**, 707–724, 1972.
11. S.N. Ethier and T.G. Kurtz, *Markov Processes, Characterization and Convergence*, J. Wiley & Sons, Inc., 1986.
12. C. Fraser, C.A. Donnelly, S. Cauchemez, W.P. Hanage, M.D. Van Kerkhove, T.D Hollingsworth, J. Griffin, R.F. Baggaley, H.E. Jenkins, E.J. Lyons, et al., Pandemic Potential of a Strain of Influenza A (H1N1): Early Findings, *Science*, **324**: 1557–1561, 2009.
13. M. Freidlin and A. Wentzell, *Random perturbations of dynamical systems*, 3d ed., Grundlehren des Mathematischen Wissenschaften **260**, Springer, 2012.
14. J. Giesecke, *Modern infectious disease epidemiology, 3rd Ed*, London: CRC Press, 2017.
15. J. Jacod and A. Shiryaev, *Limit Theorems for Stochastic Processes*, Grundlehren des Mathematischen Wissenschaften **288**, Springer, 1987.
16. P. Jagers, *Branching Processes with Biological Applications*, J. Wiley & Sons, Ltd., 1975.
17. I. Karatzas and S. Shreve, *Brownian motion and stochastic calculus*, 2d ed. 1991, Springer Verlag, 1988.
18. M.J. Keeling and B.T. Grenfell, Disease extinction and community size: modeling the persistence of measles, *Science* **275**(5295): 65–67, 1997.
19. B. Kouegou-Kamen and E. Pardoux, Large deviations of the small jumps asymptotic of the moving-optimum model, to appear.
20. B. Kouegou-Kamen and E. Pardoux, Large deviations for jump Markov processes : the lower bound, to appear.
21. P. Kratz and E. Pardoux, Large deviations for infectious diseases, Chapter 7 of *Séminaire de Probabilités XLIX*, Lecture Notes in Math. **2215**, pp. 221–327, 2018.

22. T.G. Kurtz, Strong approximation theorems for density dependent Markov chains, *Stochastic Processes and their Applications*, **6**(3): 223–240, 1978.
23. M. Lindholm and T. Britton, Endemic persistence or disease extinction: the effect of population separation into subcommunities, *Theor. pop. biol.*, **72**: 253–263, 2007.
24. I. Nåsell, On the time to extinction in recurrent epidemics, *J.R. Statist. Soc. B* **61**(2): 309–330, 1999.
25. E. Pardoux, *Markov processes and Applications*, J. Wiley, 2008.
26. E. Pardoux and B. Samegni-Kepgnou, Large deviation principle for Epidemic models, *J. Applied Probab.* **54** 905–920, 2017.
27. E. Pardoux and B. Samegni-Kepgnou, Large deviation of the exit measure through a characteristic boundary for a Poisson driven SDE, http://arxiv.org/abs/1808.04991, submitted 2018.
28. J. Pitman, *Combinatorial Stochastic Processes*, Ecole d'Eté de Probabilité de Saint-Flour XXXII - 2002, Lecture Notes in Mathematics **1875**, Springer Verlag, 2006.
29. L.E. Quenee, N.A. Ciletti, D. Elli, T.M. Hermanas and O. Schneewind, Prevention of pneumonic plague in mice, rats, guinea pigs and non-human primates with clinical grade rV10, rV10-2 or F1-V vaccines, *Vaccine* **29**(38): 6572–6583, 2011.
30. G. Polya and G. Szegö, *Problems and Theorems in Analysis I*, Springer Verlag, Berlin, Heidelberg, 1978.
31. L.S. Pontryagin, V.G. Boltyanskii, R.V. Gamkrelidze, E.F. Mishchenko, *The mathematical theory of optimal processes*, Transl. by K.N. Trirogoff; ed. by L.W. Neustadt, John Wiley & Sons, 1962.
32. G. Scalia-Tomba, Asymptotic final size distribution for some chain-binomial processes, *Adv. Appl. Prob.* **17** 477–495, 1985.
33. G. Scalia-Tomba, On the asymptotic final size distribution of epidemics in heterogeneous populations, in *Stochastic processes in epidemic theory*, J.P. Gabriel, C. Lefèvre and P. Picard, *Lecture notes in Biomathematics* **86**, 189–196, 1990.
34. A. Shwartz and A. Weiss, *Large Deviations for Performance Analysis*, Chapman Hall, London, 1995.
35. A. Shwartz and A. Weiss, Large deviations with diminishing rates, *Mathematics of Operations Research* **30** 281–310, 2005.
36. T. Sellke, On the asymptotic distribution of the size of a stochastic epidemic, *J. Appl. Prob.* **20**: 390–394, 1983.
37. E. Trélat, *Contrôle optimal, Théorie et Applications*, 2d ed. Vuibert, 2008.
38. WHO Ebola Response Team, Ebola virus disease in West Africa – the first 9 months of the epidemic and forward projections, *New Engl. J. Med.* **371**: 1481–1495, 2014.

Part II
Stochastic SIR Epidemics in Structured Populations

Frank Ball and David Sirl

Frank Ball, Nottingham
e-mail: Frank.Ball@nottingham.ac.uk
David Sirl, Nottingham
e-mail: david.sirl@nottingham.ac.uk

Introduction

Introducing further structure to the population model underlying an epidemic model is an important step towards having models which better capture real-world observations and data. Whilst the homogenously mixing assumption in force in Part I of this volume facilitates good qualitative predictions of many real-world infectious diseases, there are clearly many applied situations where it will not be applicable. There are several possible mechanisms through which such additional structure can be incorporated into our models. We might classify individuals as being one of a few different types (capturing for example some age structure of the population), and allow the distribution of infectious periods to depend on the type of the individual concerned and infection rates to depend on the types of the individuals involved. This leads to multitype analogues of the models, methods and results in Part I. One might want to introduce some sort of network structure to the model to capture population inhomogeneities that manifest in social networks, as in Part III. We consider structured populations, which include some notion of a 'local' contact. This local structure may try to capture (a simplification of) spatial structure, like animals in adjacent pens on a farm, or some less explicitly spatial element such as households or workplaces/schools in a human population.

In this part we work towards developing and analysing a general SIR epidemic model with two levels of mixing, called local and global, where global means in accordance with homogeneous mixing and local is quite flexible but permits the capturing of the aforementioned behaviour where individuals have more frequent contact with a specific (usually small) subset of the population.

In Chapter 1 we present results about epidemics in homogenously mixing populations which we shall use in the sequel. Then in Chapter 2 we study the households model, a prototypical (and historically important) example of the two level structure that we seek to describe. In Chapter 3 we present the major contribution to this Part, the development and analysis of the general two-level mixing model and application to several examples.

Chapter 1
Single Population Epidemics

In order to determine asymptotic properties of the final outcome of a stochastic SIR epidemic in a structured population, such as one partitioned into households, as the population size $N \to \infty$, *exact* results concerning the final outcome of a stochastic SIR epidemic in a homogeneously mixing population are required. These results are concerned with the distribution of the *total size* (number of initial susceptibles ultimately infected) and *severity* (sum of the infectious periods of all infected individuals) of an epidemic. In the literature, the severity of an epidemic is sometimes called the area under the trajectory of infectives. In this chapter, we give a self-contained derivation of these properties for the standard SIR epidemic model (see Section 1.1), which is a special case of the stochastic SEIR model described in described in Section 1.1 of Part I, obtained when the latent periods are all zero.

The main result (Theorem 1.7.2 in Section 1.7) is an expression for the joint generating function Laplace transform of (S, T_A), where S is the number of susceptibles remaining at the end of the epidemic and T_A is the severity of the epidemic. Corresponding results for S and T_A separately were first obtained by Ball [6], using a Wald's identity; see Section 3.1 of Part I. The joint generating function Laplace transform of (S, T_A) was first derived in Picard and Lefèvre [57], using martingales and optional stopping. These authors introduced a more general class of epidemics, namely *collective Reed–Frost* models (see Section 1.7) and exploited a non-standard family of polynomials, first introduced by Gontcharoff [35], to derive their results in this setting in an elegant and systematic fashion. In Ball [7], the author showed that the factorial moments of S are intimately related to the concept of a *susceptibility set* (see Section 1.5) and used that connection to give a simple, probabilistically illuminating proof of the joint generating function Laplace transform of (S, T_A), and of its extension to include other final state random variables, for collective Reed–Frost epidemics. (Final state random variables, defined in Ball and O'Neill [18], are sums over all infected individuals of random quantities associated with an individual.)

The presentation here is based on that in Ball [7] but restricted to the standard SIR epidemic model. The rest of the chapter is structured as follows. The standard SIR epidemic is described in Section 1.1 and its random graph representation is given in Section 1.2. The arguments make considerable use of *symmetric sampling schemes* and *Gontcharoff polynomials*, which are introduced in Sections 1.3 and 1.4,

T. Britton, E. Pardoux (eds.), *Stochastic Epidemic Models with Inference*,
Lecture Notes in Mathematics 2255, https://doi.org/10.1007/978-3-030-30900-8_5

respectively, together with some of their properties which are required in the sequel. Susceptibility sets are introduced in Section 1.5 and used in Section 1.6 to derive the probability generating-function of S. The joint generating function Laplace transform of (S, T_A) is derived in Section 1.7. When analysing the final outcome of the households model, we need to extend these results to a model in which susceptibles can also be infected externally; this is done in Section 1.8. All the results can be extended to multitype SIR epidemics in which the population is partitioned into groups that are homogeneous but different from each other (see Picard and Lefèvre [57] and Ball [7]) but we do not consider that extension in detail here. A result concerning the mean final size of a multitype SIR epidemic model, required for the analysis of vaccination schemes in the households model in Section 2.4, is given in Section 1.9.

1.1 Standard SIR Epidemic Model

In this section we introduce the standard SIR epidemic model, see Andersson and Britton [4, Chapter 2], for the spread of an SIR epidemic in a closed, homogeneously mixing population. (As noted above, the standard SIR epidemic model is a special case of the stochastic SEIR model described in Section 1.1 of Part I.) Suppose that initially there are n susceptibles and a infectives. The infectious periods of different infectives are i.i.d. (independent and identically distributed) according to a non-negative random variable I, having an arbitrary but specified distribution. An infective recovers at the end of its infectious period, after which it is immune to further infection. During its infectious period, an infective contacts any given individual in the population at the points of a homogeneous Poisson process having rate λ (see Appendix A.2 of Part I). If a contacted individual is susceptible then it becomes infected and is immediately able to infect other individuals. Thus there is no exposed (or latent) period. If a contacted individual is infective or recovered then nothing happens. All infectious periods and Poisson processes governing contacts are mutually independent. The epidemic ceases when there is no infective present in the population. We denote this model by $E_{n,a}(\lambda, I)$.

1.2 Random Graph Representation of Epidemic

We now describe a random directed graph representation of the epidemic $E_{n,a}(\lambda, I)$. Label the n susceptibles $1, 2, \ldots, n$ and the a initial infectives $-(a-1)$, $-(a-2), \ldots, 0$. Let $I_{-(a-1)}, I_{-(a-2)}, \ldots, I_n$ be i.i.d. copies of I. For $i = -(a-1), -(a-2), \ldots, 0$, the infectious period of the initial infective i is given by I_i. For $i = 1, 2, \ldots, n$, if individual i is infected in the epidemic then its infectious period is given by I_i. Consider two distinct individuals, i and j say. Suppose that i is infective and j is susceptible. Ignoring for the moment the fact that i has a finite infectious period, let W_{ij} be the time elapsing after i's infection before i first makes contact with j. Such contacts occur at the points of a Poisson process having rate λ, so $W_{ij} \sim \text{Exp}(\lambda)$, where $\text{Exp}(\lambda)$ denotes an exponential random variable with rate λ (and mean λ^{-1}). Further, when the infectious period of i is taken into account, i contacts j if and only if $W_{ij} \leq I_i$.

Let $V = \{-(a-1), -(a-2), \dots, n\}$ denote the set of all individuals in the population. Let $I_{-(a-1)}, I_{-(a-2)}, \dots, I_n$ and W_{ij} $(i, j \in V, i \neq j)$ be independent random variables, distributed as above. Let $\mathscr{G}_E$ be the directed random graph with vertex set V in which for any $(i, j) \in V^2$, with $i \neq j$, there is a directed edge from i to j if and only if $W_{ij} \leq I_i$, i.e. if and only if i tries to infect j if i becomes infected. (The infection fails if j is not susceptible.) For $i, j \in V$, write $i \rightsquigarrow j$ if and only if there is a chain of directed edges in $\mathscr{G}_E$ from i to j, with the convention that $i \rightsquigarrow i$.

Let $\mathscr{I}_0^{\text{inf}} = \{-(a-1), -(a-2), \dots, 0\}$ and $\mathscr{S}_0^{\text{sus}} = \{1, 2, \dots, n\}$ denote the sets of vertices in V corresponding respectively to initial infectives and initial susceptibles in $E_{n,a}(\lambda, I)$. (The superscripts ^{inf} and ^{sus} are not really necessary; we use them to help distinguish between $\mathscr{I}$ and $\mathscr{S}$.) Note that for $j \in \mathscr{S}_0^{\text{sus}}$, the initial susceptible j is infected by the epidemic if and only if there exists a chain of directed arcs from a member of $\mathscr{I}_0^{\text{inf}}$ to j, so the set of initial susceptibles who are infected by the epidemic is given by $\{j \in \mathscr{S}_0^{\text{sus}} : i \rightsquigarrow j \text{ for some } i \in \mathscr{I}_0^{\text{inf}}\}$. The total size of the epidemic, i.e. the number of initial susceptibles that are infected by the epidemic is given by $|\{j \in \mathscr{S}_0^{\text{sus}} : i \rightsquigarrow j \text{ for some } i \in \mathscr{I}_0^{\text{inf}}\}|$, where for a set, A say, $|A|$ denotes the number of elements it contains, i.e. its cardinality.

Remark 1.2.1 (Real time epidemic). The graph $\mathscr{G}_E$ is sufficient to determine which susceptibles are infected by the epidemic but it does not contain the temporal development of the epidemic. The latter can be recovered by weighting each directed edge $i \to j$ in $\mathscr{G}_E$ by W_{ij}. (Note that if $W_{ij} > I_i$ then the directed edge $i \to j$ is not present in $\mathscr{G}_E$.) Suppose that the epidemic starts with the initial infectives all becoming infected at time $t = 0$. For any chain of directed edges in $\mathscr{G}_E$, let the weight of that chain be given by the sum of the weights of its directed edges. Then, for $j \in \mathscr{S}_0^{\text{sus}}$, if j is infected by the epidemic, its time of infection is given by the minimum of the weights of all chains from any individual in $\mathscr{I}_0^{\text{inf}}$ to j.

Remark 1.2.2 (SEIR model). Suppose that an exposed period is incorporated into the model. More specifically, suppose that after infection an infected individual has an exposed period with length distributed according to a random variable L, having an arbitrary but specified distribution. Let $L_{-(a-1)}, L_{-(a-2)}, \dots, L_n$ be i.i.d. copies of L that are also independent of $I_{-(a-1)}, I_{-(a-2)}, \dots, I_n$ and W_{ij} $(i, j \in V, i \neq j)$. For $i = -(a-1), -(a-2), \dots, n$, if individual i is infected then its exposed period is given by L_i. The model then becomes the stochastic SEIR model studied in Section 1.1 of Part I. Note that the presence/absence of directed edges in $\mathscr{G}_E$ is independent of $L_{-(a-1)}, L_{-(a-2)}, \dots, L_n$, so the distribution of the final outcome of the epidemic is invariant to the distribution of L and is the same as that of the corresponding SIR epidemic $E_{n,a}(\lambda, I)$. If desired, the temporal development of the SEIR epidemic can be obtained by weighting each directed edge $i \to j$ in $\mathscr{G}_E$ by $L_i + W_{ij}$.

Remark 1.2.3 (Constant infectious period). Note that if the infectious period is constant, say $\mathbb{P}(I = \mu_I) = 1$ for some $\mu_I \in (0,\infty)$ (see the Reed–Frost model discussed in Section 1.1.2 of Part I), then the directed edges in $\mathscr{G}_E$ are present independently with probability $p = 1 - \mathrm{e}^{-\lambda\mu_I}$. Further, in constructing the final outcome $\{j \in \mathscr{S}_0^{\text{sus}} : i \rightsquigarrow j \text{ for some } i \in \mathscr{I}_0^{\text{inf}}\}$ of the epidemic, for any $i \neq j$ use is made of at most one of the pair of possible edges $i \to j$ and $j \to i$. (For example, if i infects j then whether or not j tries to infect i is immaterial as i has already been infected.) It follows that if I is constant then the directed graph can be replaced by an undirected graph, in which for any pair of vertices (i, j) an edge between them is present with probability p, independently for different pairs, i.e. by the Erdös–Rényi random graph $\mathrm{ER}(N, p)$ on $N = n+a$ vertices (see Definition 1.2.2 in Part III).

1.3 Symmetric Sampling Procedures

This short section contains a summary of results concerning *symmetric sampling procedures* which are required in the sequel, together with proofs. It is based on Section 1 of Martin-Löf [49].

Consider a fixed finite population $\mathscr{N}$ of size N. For definiteness, let $\mathscr{N} = \{1,2,\ldots,N\}$. Let X be a random subset of $\mathscr{N}$. We allow the possibility that X is the empty set $\emptyset$. In an epidemic setting, $\mathscr{N}$ could be the set of susceptible individuals at the start of an epidemic and X the subset consisting of those individuals that are still susceptible at the end of the epidemic.

For $A \subseteq \mathscr{N}$, let $p_A = \mathbb{P}(X = A)$ and $r_A = \mathbb{P}(X \supseteq A)$. For $i \in \mathscr{N}$, let

$$\chi_i = 1_{\{i \in X\}} = \begin{cases} 1 & \text{if } i \in X, \\ 0 & \text{if } i \notin X. \end{cases}$$

Note that

$$X \supseteq A \iff i \in X \text{ for all } i \in A,$$

so

$$r_A = \mathbb{E}\left[\prod_{i \in A} \chi_i\right] \qquad (A \subseteq \mathscr{N}).$$

Similarly, for $A \subseteq \mathscr{N}$,

$$\begin{aligned} p_A &= \mathbb{E}\left[\prod_{i \in A} \chi_i \prod_{j \in A^c} (1 - \chi_j)\right] \\ &= \mathbb{E}\left[\prod_{i \in A} \chi_i \sum_{C \subseteq A^c} \prod_{j \in C} (-\chi_j)\right] && (1.3.1) \\ &= \sum_{A \subseteq B \subseteq \mathscr{N}} (-1)^{|B|-|A|} r_B. && (1.3.2) \end{aligned}$$

A *symmetric sampling procedure* is one in which, for all $A \subseteq \mathscr{N}$, p_A depends only on the size $|A| = a$ of A. Thus,

$$p_A = \frac{p_a}{\binom{N}{a}},$$

where $p_a = \mathbb{P}(|X| = a)$. It follows that r_A also depends only on a, so we can write $r_A = r_a$ and, using (1.3.2),

$$p_a = \binom{N}{a} \sum_{b=a}^{N} (-1)^{b-a} \binom{N-a}{N-b} r_b \qquad (a = 0, 1, \dots, N). \tag{1.3.3}$$

The following lemma gives a very simple expression for the factorial moments of the number of objects sampled in a symmetric sampling procedure. For $s, k \in \mathbb{Z}_+$, let $s_{[k]} = s(s-1)\dots(s-k+1)$ denote a falling factorial, with the convention that $s_{[0]} = 1$.

Lemma 1.3.1. *For a symmetric sampling procedure,*

$$\mathbb{E}\left[|X|_{[k]}\right] = N_{[k]} r_k \qquad (k = 0, 1, \dots).$$

Proof. For $k = 0, 1, \dots,$

$$\begin{aligned}
\mathbb{E}\left[|X|_{[k]}\right] &= \sum_{a=k}^{N} a_{[k]} p_a \\
&= \sum_{a=k}^{N} a_{[k]} \binom{N}{a} \sum_{b=a}^{N} (-1)^{b-a} \binom{N-a}{N-b} r_b \qquad \text{(using (1.3.3))} \\
&= \sum_{b=k}^{N} \frac{N_{[b]} r_b}{(b-k)!} \sum_{a=k}^{b} (-1)^{b-a} \binom{b-k}{a-k} \\
&= \sum_{b=k}^{N} \frac{N_{[b]} r_b}{(b-k)!} \sum_{i=0}^{b-k} (-1)^{b-k-i} \binom{b-k}{i} \\
&= \sum_{b=k}^{N} \frac{N_{[b]} r_b}{(b-k)!} \delta_{bk} \\
&= N_{[k]} r_k,
\end{aligned}$$

as required. (In the above $\delta_{bk} = 1$ if $b = k$ and 0 if $b \neq k$). □

We now introduce some more notation. Let $\phi_I(\theta) = \mathbb{E}[\exp(-\theta I)]$ $(\theta \geq 0)$ be the Laplace transform of I, so $\phi_I(-\theta)$ is the moment-generating function of I. For $k = 0, 1, \dots,$ let $q_k = \phi_I(k\lambda)$. Thus $q_0 = 1$ and, for $k = 1, 2, \dots,$ q_k is the probability that a given infective fails to contact anyone in a given set of k susceptibles during its infectious period.

Exercise 1.3.2. In the standard SIR epidemic model $E_{n,a}(\lambda, I)$, let S_1 be the number of susceptibles that escape direct infection from the a initial infectives. Thus in terms of the random graph $\mathcal{G}_E$,

$$S_1 = |\mathcal{S}_1^{\text{sus}}|, \text{ where } \mathcal{S}_1^{\text{sus}} = \mathcal{S}_0^{\text{sus}} \setminus \{i \in \mathcal{S}_0^{\text{sus}} : j \to i \text{ for at least one } j \in \mathcal{I}_0^{\text{inf}}\}.$$

Let $P_{n,a}(k) = \mathbb{P}(S_1 = k)$ $(k = 0, 1, \ldots n)$.

(a) Show that

$$\sum_{i=k}^{n} i_{[k]} P_{n,a}(k) = n_{[k]} q_k^a \qquad (k = 0, 1, \ldots, n); \tag{1.3.4}$$

see the equation after (2.6) in Picard and Lefèvre [57].

The triangular system of linear equations (1.3.4) determine $P_{n,a}(k)$ $(k = 0, 1, \ldots n)$ in reverse order.

(b) Show that

$$P_{n,a}(k) = \binom{n}{k} \sum_{i=k}^{n} (-1)^{i-k} \binom{n-k}{i-k} q_k^a \qquad (k = 0, 1, \ldots, n). \tag{1.3.5}$$

1.4 Gontcharoff Polynomials

This section contains some results on *Gontcharoff polynomials* (Gontcharoff [35]) required in the sequel, together with proofs. It is based on Section 2 of Lefèvre and Picard [46].

Definition 1.4.1. Given a sequence $U = u_0, u_1, \ldots$ of real numbers, the Gontcharoff polynomials attached to U, viz. $G_0(x \mid U), G_1(x \mid U), \ldots$, are defined recursively by

$$\sum_{i=0}^{k} \frac{u_i^{k-i}}{(k-i)!} G_i(x \mid U) = \frac{x^k}{k!} \qquad (k = 0, 1, \ldots). \tag{1.4.1}$$

Remark 1.4.2. Note that $G_0(x \mid U) \equiv 1$ and $G_k(x \mid U)$ is a polynomial of degree k in x.

Property 1.4.3. For $i, j = 0, 1, \ldots,$

$$G_i^{(j)}(u_j \mid U) = \delta_{ij}, \tag{1.4.2}$$

where $G_i^{(j)}(x \mid U)$ denotes the jth derivative of $G_i(x \mid U)$. Moreover, this property characterises the family of polynomials.

Proof. We prove (1.4.2) by induction on i. First note that (1.4.2) holds when $i = 0$. Suppose that (1.4.2) holds for $i = 0, 1, \ldots, k-1$. Clearly $G_k^{(j)}(x \mid U) \equiv 0$ for $j > k$ and, differentiating (1.4.1) k times, $G_k^{(k)}(x \mid U) \equiv 1$. Also, for $j = 0, 1, \ldots, k-1$, differentiating (1.4.1) j times gives

$$\begin{aligned}
G_k^{(j)}(u_j \mid U) &= \frac{u_j^{k-j}}{(k-j)!} - \sum_{i=j}^{k-1} \frac{u_i^{k-i}}{(k-i)!} G_i^{(j)}(u_j \mid U) \\
&= \frac{u_j^{k-j}}{(k-j)!} - \sum_{i=j}^{k-1} \frac{u_i^{k-i}}{(k-i)!} \delta_{ij} \qquad \text{(inductive hypothesis)} \\
&= 0,
\end{aligned}$$

and (1.4.2) holds for $i = k$. Thus the first part follows by induction.

To prove the second part, let $R_i(x)$ be any polynomial of degree i in x. Then we may write

$$R_i(x) = \sum_{l=0}^{i} a_l G_l(x \mid U), \tag{1.4.3}$$

so, using (1.4.2),

$$R_i^{(j)}(u_j) = \sum_{l=0}^{i} a_l \delta_{lj} = a_j \qquad (j = 0, 1, \ldots). \tag{1.4.4}$$

Thus, if $R_i(x)$ satisfies (1.4.2), then $a_j = \delta_{ij}$ $(j \in \mathbb{Z}_+)$, so $R_i(x) = G_i(x \mid U)$, as required. □

Property 1.4.4. For $i = 0, 1, \ldots$, any polynomial $R_i(x)$ of degree i in x admits an Abel expansion

$$R_i(x) = \sum_{l=0}^{i} R_i^{(l)}(u_l) G_l(x \mid U) \tag{1.4.5}$$

with respect to the family $G_0(x \mid U), G_1(x \mid U), \ldots$.

Proof. This follows immediately from (1.4.3) and (1.4.4). □

Property 1.4.5. For $0 \le j \le i$,

$$G_i^{(j)}(x \mid U) = G_{i-j}(x \mid E^j U),$$

where $E^j U$ is the sequence $u_j, u_{j+1}, \ldots$.

Proof. For $0 \le j \le i$, $G_i^{(j)}(x \mid U)$ is a polynomial of degree $i - j$, so letting $R_{i-j}(x) = G_i^{(j)}(x \mid U)$ and using (1.4.5) with U replaced by $E^j U$ yields

$$\begin{aligned}
G_i^{(j)}(x \mid U) &= \sum_{l=0}^{i-j} G_i^{(j+l)}(u_{j+l} \mid U) G_l(x \mid E^j U) \\
&= \sum_{l=0}^{i-j} \delta_{i,j+l} G_l(x \mid E^j U) \qquad \text{(using (1.4.2))} \\
&= G_{i-j}(x \mid E^j U).
\end{aligned}$$

□

Property 1.4.6. For $a, b \in \mathbb{R}$,

$$G_i(ax+b \mid aU+b) = a^i G_i(x \mid U) \quad (i = 0, 1, \ldots),$$

where $aU+b$ denotes the sequence $au_0+b, au_1+b, \ldots$.

Proof. Note that $G_i(ax+b \mid aU+b)$ is a polynomial of degree i in x, so letting $R_i(x) = G_i(ax+b \mid aU+b)$ and using (1.4.5) gives

$$\begin{aligned} G_i(ax+b \mid aU+b) &= \sum_{l=0}^{i} a^l G_i^{(l)}(au_l+b \mid aU+b) G_l(x \mid U) \\ &= \sum_{l=0}^{i} a^l \delta_{il} G_l(x \mid U) \qquad \text{(using (1.4.2))} \\ &= a^i g_i(x \mid U). \end{aligned}$$

□

1.5 Susceptibility Sets

In this section we introduce the concept of a *susceptibility set*, which will prove useful in determining properties of the final outcome of the epidemic $E_{n,a}(\lambda, I)$, and derive the probability distribution of the size of a susceptibility set, which admits a simple expression in terms of Gontcharoff polynomials.

Recall from Section 1.2 the random directed graph $\mathscr{G}_E$, defined on the vertex set V. For $A \subseteq V$, the *susceptibility set* $\mathscr{S}_A$ of A is defined by

$$\mathscr{S}_A = \{j \in V \setminus A : j \rightsquigarrow i \text{ for some } i \in A\}, \tag{1.5.1}$$

with the convention that $\mathscr{S}_\emptyset = \emptyset$. Note that $A \subseteq \mathscr{S}_A$.

Remark 1.5.1. Recall that $\mathscr{I}_0^{\text{inf}}$ and $\mathscr{S}_0^{\text{sus}}$ denote respectively the sets of initial infectives and susceptibles. If $A \subseteq \mathscr{S}_0^{\text{sus}}$, so A consists entirely of initial susceptibles, then all members of A avoid infection if and only if $\mathscr{S}_A \cap \mathscr{I}_0^{\text{inf}} = \emptyset$, hence the terminology.

Before proceeding, we need some more notation. Let $S_A = |\mathscr{S}_A|$ denote the size of $\mathscr{S}_A$. Note that, for $A \subseteq V$, the distribution of S_A depends on A only through its size $|A|$. Suppose that $|V| = N$ and $|A| = j$, where $0 \le j \le N$, and write $\mathbb{P}_{jN}(S_A = l)$ for the probability that $\mathscr{S}_A$ is of size l ($l = j, j+1, \ldots, N$). Recall from page 129 that $q_k = \phi_I(k\lambda)$ ($k = 0, 1, \ldots$).

Lemma 1.5.2. *For $N = 0, 1, \ldots$ and $j = 0, 1, \ldots, N$,*

$$\mathbb{P}_{jN}(S_A = l) = (N-j)_{[l-j]} G_{l-j}(1 \mid E^j U) q_l^{N-l} \quad (l = j, j+1, \ldots, N), \tag{1.5.2}$$

where the sequence U is given by $u_k = q_k$ ($k = 0, 1, \ldots$).

Proof. Fix $0 \le j \le N$. For this proof only, give the elements of V the labels $1,2,\dots,N$. Let $\mathbf{0}$ denote the empty set and, for $i = 1,2,\dots,N$, let $\mathbf{i}$ denote the set $\{1,2,\dots,i\}$. Without loss of generality, take $A = \mathbf{j}$. For $l = j, j+1,\dots,N$, by symmetry, $\mathscr{S}_A \setminus A$ is equally likely to be any of the $\binom{N-j}{l-j}$ subsets of $V \setminus A$ having size $l-j$ so, in an obvious notation,

$$\mathbb{P}_{jN}(S_A = l) = \binom{N-j}{l-j} \mathbb{P}_{jN}(\mathscr{S}_A = \mathbf{l}) \quad (l = j, j+1,\dots,N). \tag{1.5.3}$$

For $l = j, j+1,\dots,N$, the susceptibility set $\mathscr{S}_A$ can be constructed by first constructing the susceptibility set of A among $\mathbf{l}$, to yield $\mathscr{S}_{A,\mathbf{l}}$ say, and then constructing the susceptibility set of $\mathscr{S}_{A,\mathbf{l}}$ among V. (For $A \subseteq B \subseteq V$, the susceptibility set of A among B is given by (1.5.1) with V replaced by B.) In particular, $\mathscr{S}_A = \mathbf{l}$ if and only if $\mathscr{S}_{A,\mathbf{l}} = \mathbf{l}$ and none of the $N-l$ individuals in $\mathbf{N} \setminus \mathbf{l}$ contact any member of $\mathbf{l}$. The probability of the latter event is q_l^{N-l}, since each of the $N-l$ individuals in $\mathbf{N} \setminus \mathbf{l}$ must not make contact with a set of l individuals and individuals make contacts independently. Moreover, the latter event is independent of the event $\mathscr{S}_{A,\mathbf{l}} = \mathbf{l}$, again because individuals make contacts independently. Thus,

$$\mathbb{P}_{jN}(\mathscr{S}_A = \mathbf{l}) = \mathbb{P}_{jl}(\mathscr{S}_A = \mathbf{l}) q_l^{N-l} \quad (l = j, j+1,\dots,N), \tag{1.5.4}$$

whence, using (1.5.3) and noting that $\mathbb{P}_{jl}(S_A = l) = \mathbb{P}_{jl}(\mathscr{S}_A = \mathbf{l})$,

$$\mathbb{P}_{jN}(S_A = l) = \binom{N-j}{l-j} \mathbb{P}_{jl}(S_A = l) q_l^{N-l} \quad (l = j, j+1,\dots,N). \tag{1.5.5}$$

Now $\sum_{l=j}^{N} P_{jN}(S_A = l) = 1$ so, using (1.5.5),

$$\sum_{l=j}^{N} \binom{N-j}{l-j} \mathbb{P}_{jl}(S_A = l) q_l^{N-l} = 1,$$

whence, letting $i = l - j$,

$$\sum_{i=0}^{N-j} \frac{q_{i+j}^{N-j-i}}{(N-j-i)!} \frac{\mathbb{P}_{j,j+i}(S_A = j+i)}{i!} = \frac{1}{(N-j)!} \quad (N = j, j+1,\dots).$$

Thus, by Definition 1.4.1,

$$\mathbb{P}_{j,j+i}(S_A = j+i) = i! G_i(1 \mid E^j U) \qquad (j,i = 0,1,\dots)$$

and the lemma follows using (1.5.5). □

Remark 1.5.3. If I is constant, so the directed edges in $\mathscr{G}_E$ are present independently, then if $j = a$ and $N = n + a$, the distribution of $S_A - a$ is the same as that of the total size of $E_{n,a}(\lambda, I)$, i.e. the number of susceptibles ultimately infected in the epidemic. If I is not constant, then a similar argument to the proof of Lemma 1.5.2 but for the total size of the epidemic $E_{n,a}(\lambda, I)$ breaks down at (1.5.4) because the event that an epidemic, E' say, among a sub-population of susceptibles fully infects that sub population is *not* independent of the infectious periods of infectives in E'.

1.6 Total Size

Consider the epidemic $E_{n,a}(\lambda, I)$ and let S be the number of susceptibles that remain uninfected at the end of the epidemic.

Lemma 1.6.1. *For* $j = 0, 1, \ldots,$

$$\mathbb{E}[S_{[j]}] = \sum_{i=0}^{n} n_{[i]} q_i^{n+a-i} G_i^{(j)}(1 \mid U), \tag{1.6.1}$$

where U is given by $u_k = q_k$ $(k = 0, 1, \ldots)$.

Proof. Fix $j \in \{1, 2, \ldots, n\}$ and let A be any fixed set of j initial susceptibles. The set of initial susceptibles that remain uninfected at the end of the epidemic is a symmetric sampling procedure on $\mathscr{S}_0^{\mathrm{sus}} = \{1, 2, \ldots, n\}$ so, by Lemma 1.3.1,

$$\mathbb{E}[S_{[j]}] = n_{[j]} \mathbb{P}(A \text{ avoids infection}), \tag{1.6.2}$$

where $\{A \text{ avoids infection}\}$ is the event that all members of A avoid infection by the epidemic. To calculate the probability $\mathbb{P}(A \text{ avoids infection})$, we condition on the size S_A of the susceptibility set $\mathscr{S}_A$ of A among the initial susceptibles $\mathscr{S}_0^{\mathrm{sus}}$. Note that A avoids infection if and only if all a initial infectives fail to contact anyone in $\mathscr{S}_A$ (see Remark 1.5.1). Thus, for $i = j, j+1, \ldots, n$,

$$\mathbb{P}(A \text{ avoids infection} | S_A = i) = q_i^a.$$

Hence, using (1.6.2),

$$\begin{aligned} \mathbb{E}[S_{[j]}] &= n_{[j]} \sum_{i=j}^{n} \mathbb{P}_{j,n}(|S_A| = i) q_i^a \\ &= n_{[j]} \sum_{i=j}^{n} (n-j)_{[i-j]} G_{i-j}(1 \mid E^j U) q_i^{n-i+a}, \end{aligned} \tag{1.6.3}$$

using Lemma 1.5.2 with $N = n$. Now $n_{[j]}(n-j)_{[i-j]} = n_{[i]}$ and, by Property 1.4.5 on page 131, $G_{i-j}(1 \mid E^j U) = G_i^{(j)}(1 \mid U)$, so (1.6.3) yields

$$\begin{aligned} \mathbb{E}[S_{[j]}] &= \sum_{i=j}^{n} n_{[i]} G_i^{(j)}(1 \mid U) q_i^{n+a-i} \\ &= \sum_{i=0}^{n} n_{[i]} G_i^{(j)}(1 \mid U) q_i^{n+a-i}, \end{aligned}$$

since $G_i^{(j)}(1 \mid U) = 0$ for $j > i$ as $G_i(x \mid U)$ is a polynomial of degree i in x. Thus (1.6.1) holds for $j = 1, 2, \ldots, n$.

Recall that $u_0 = 1$. Thus, using Property 1.4.3 on page 130 and $n_{[0]} = 1$, both sides of (1.6.1) are 1 when $j = 0$. Finally, both sides of (1.6.1) are clearly 0 when $j > n$. □

Let $f_{n,a}(x) = \mathbb{E}[x^S]$ $(x \in \mathbb{R})$ denote the probability-generating function of S.

Theorem 1.6.2. *For $n, a = 0, 1, \ldots,$*

$$f_{n,a}(x) = \sum_{i=0}^{n} n_{[i]} q_i^{n+a-i} G_i(x \mid U) \quad (x \in \mathbb{R}), \tag{1.6.4}$$

where U is given by $u_k = q_k$ $(k = 0, 1, \ldots)$.

Proof. Note that $f_{n,a}^{(j)}(1) = \mathbb{E}[S_{[j]}]$ $(j = 0, 1, \ldots)$ and $f_{n,a}(x)$ is a polynomial of degree n in x. Thus the Taylor expansion of $f_{n,a}(x)$ about $x = 1$ is exact, so

$$\begin{aligned}
f_{n,a}(x) &= \sum_{j=0}^{\infty} \frac{(x-1)^j}{j!} f_{n,a}^{(j)}(x) \\
&= \sum_{j=0}^{\infty} \frac{(x-1)^j}{j!} \mathbb{E}[S_{[j]}] \\
&= \sum_{j=0}^{\infty} \frac{(x-1)^j}{j!} \sum_{i=0}^{n} n_{[i]} q_i^{n+a-i} G_i^{(j)}(1 \mid U) \qquad \text{(using Lemma 1.6.1)} \\
&= \sum_{i=0}^{n} n_{[i]} q_i^{n+a-i} \sum_{j=0}^{\infty} \frac{(x-1)^j}{j!} G_i^{(j)}(1 \mid U) \\
&= \sum_{i=0}^{n} n_{[i]} q_i^{n+a-i} G_i(x \mid U).
\end{aligned}$$

□

Let $Z = n - S$ be the total size of the epidemic $E_{n,a}(\lambda, I)$, i.e. the number of initial susceptibles that are infected by the epidemic, and let $\mu_{n,a} = \mathbb{E}[Z]$. Now $\mu_{n,a} = n - f_{n,a}^{(1)}(1)$, so the following corollary follows immediately by differentiating (1.6.4) and using Property 1.4.5 on page 131.

Corollary 1.6.3. *For $n, a = 0, 1, \ldots,$*

$$\mu_{n,a} = n - \sum_{i=1}^{n} n_{[i]} q_i^{n+a-i} G_{i-1}(1 \mid U'),$$

where U' is given by $u'_k = q_{k+1}$ $(k = 0, 1, \ldots)$.

1.7 Total Size and Severity

The *severity* T_A of the epidemic $E_{n,a}(\lambda, I)$ is the sum of the infectious periods of all individuals infected in it, including the initial infectives. We need some properties of the joint distribution of (S, T_A) when analysing the households model in Section 2.2 below.

Let

$$\phi_{n,a}(x,\theta) = \mathbb{E}\left[x^S \exp(-\theta T_A)\right] \qquad (x \in \mathbb{R}, \theta \geq 0)$$

be the joint generating function Laplace transform of (S, T_A). We derive $\phi_{n,a}(x,\theta)$ by first proving a relationship between $\phi_{n,a}(x,\theta)$ and the probability-generating function of S for an epidemic with modified parameters (see Lemma 1.7.1 below). Some more notation is required.

Recall that $q_k = \phi_I(k\lambda)$ is the probability that a given infective fails to infect anyone in a given set of k susceptibles. Let I denote the infectious period of this infective and A_k denote the event that it fails to contact anyone in the set of k susceptibles. Let

$$q_k(\theta) = \mathbb{E}\left[\mathrm{e}^{-\theta I} 1_{A_k}\right] \qquad (k = 1, 2, \ldots; \theta \geq 0)$$

and $q_0(\theta) = \phi_I(\theta)$. Now, given I, the infective infects susceptibles independently, each with probability $1 - \mathrm{e}^{-\lambda I}$, so

$$\begin{aligned} q_k(\theta) &= \mathbb{E}\left[\mathrm{e}^{-\theta I} \mathbb{P}(A_k | I)\right] \\ &= \mathbb{E}\left[\mathrm{e}^{-\theta I} \mathrm{e}^{-k\lambda I}\right] \\ &= \phi_I(\theta + \lambda k). \end{aligned}$$

Note that the probability-generating function $f_{n,a}(x)$, and hence the distribution of the total size T, depends on λ and the distribution of I only through the escape probabilities $q_0, q_1, \ldots, q_n$. It is possible to define a more general SIR epidemic model, the *collective Reed–Frost epidemic* (Lefèvre and Picard [46]), via such escape probabilities. In this model infectives behave independently and the set of people contacted by a given infective is a symmetric sampling procedure on the individuals in the population, defined through the escape probabilities $q_0, q_1, \ldots$. The model is equivalent to the generalized Reed–Frost model defined in Martin-Löf [49]. The collective Reed–Frost model is more general than the standard SIR epidemic model as the q_ks need not take the form $q_k = \phi_I(k\lambda)$ $(k = 0, 1, \ldots)$ but note that some conditions need to be imposed on the q_ks so that, for each n, $q_0, q_1, \ldots, q_n$ corresponds to a symmetric sampling procedure; specifically, for each n, the p_a obtained by setting $N = n$ and $r_b = q_b$ $(b = 0, 1, \ldots, N)$ in (1.3.3) must satisfy $p_a \in [0, 1]$. See Lefèvre and Picard [47] for further discussion.

Note also that all of the above proofs extend immediately to the more general collective Reed–Frost epidemic. Let Q denote the sequence $q_0, q_1, \ldots$. We now write the probability-generating function $f_{n,a}(x)$ as $f_{n,a}(x; Q)$ to show explicitly its dependence on Q. The following lemma provides a simple way of deriving the joint generating function Laplace transform $\phi_{n,a}(x,\theta)$ of (S, T_A).

Lemma 1.7.1. *For* $n, a = 0, 1, \ldots,$

$$\phi_{n,a}(x,\theta) = (q_0(\theta))^{n+a} f_{n,a}(x/q_0(\theta)); \tilde{Q}(\theta)) \quad (\theta \in \mathbb{R}_+),$$

where $\tilde{Q}(\theta)$ *is given by* $\tilde{q}_k(\theta) = q_k(\theta)/q_0(\theta)$ $(k = 0, 1, \ldots)$.

Proof. The result is seen easily if $a = 0$, so suppose $a > 0$ and consider the epidemic $E_{n,a}(\lambda, I)$. Fix on an initial infective, i^* say, and let I denote its infectious period. In view of the random graph $\mathcal{G}_E$ defined in 1.2, we can construct a realisation of the final outcome of $E_{n,a}(\lambda, I)$ by first considering the set of susceptibles contacted by i^*, suppose there are Z_0 such susceptibles, and then considering the epidemic among the remaining $n - Z_0$ susceptibles with $a - 1 + Z_0$ initial infectives. Thus,

$$\phi_{n,a}(x,\theta) = \sum_{k=0}^{n} \mathbb{E}[\mathrm{e}^{-\theta I} 1_{\{Z_0 = k\}}] \phi_{n-k,a+k-1}(x,\theta). \tag{1.7.1}$$

Let

$$p_k^{(n)}(\theta) = \frac{\mathbb{E}[\mathrm{e}^{-\theta I} 1_{\{Z_0=k\}}]}{q_0(\theta)} \qquad (k = 0, 1, \ldots, n).$$

Note that $p_k^{(n)}$ $(k = 0, 1, \ldots, n)$ is the probability mass function of the number of objects that are *not* sampled in the symmetric sampling scheme induced by $\tilde{q}_k(\theta)$ $(k = 0, 1, \ldots, n)$. Let

$$\psi_{n,a}(x,\theta) = \phi_{n,a}(x,\theta)/(q_0(\theta))^{n+a} \qquad (n, a = 0, 1, \ldots). \tag{1.7.2}$$

If $n = 0$ then $S = 0$ and T_A is the sum of a i.i.d. copies of I, so $\phi_{0,a}(x,\theta) = \phi_I(\theta)^a$, whence $\psi_{0,a}(x,\theta) = 1$. If $a = 0$ then $S = n$ and $T_A = 0$, so $\phi_{n,0}(x,\theta) = x^n$, whence $\psi_{n,0}(x,\theta) = \left(\frac{x}{q_0(\theta)}\right)^n$. Thus, using (1.7.1), $\psi_{n,a}(x,\theta)$ $(n, a = 0, 1, \ldots)$ are determined by

$$\psi_{n,a}(x,\theta) = \sum_{k=0}^{n} p_k^{(n)}(\theta) \psi_{n-k,a+k-1}(x,\theta) \quad (n = 0, 1, \ldots; a = 1, 2, \ldots), \tag{1.7.3}$$

$$\psi_{0,a}(x,\theta) = 1 \quad (a = 0, 1, \ldots), \tag{1.7.4}$$

$$\psi_{n,0}(x,\theta) = \left(\frac{x}{q_0(\theta)}\right)^n \quad (n = 0, 1, \ldots). \tag{1.7.5}$$

Conditioning on Z_0 as above shows that $f_{n,a}(x) = f_{n,a}(x; \tilde{Q}(0)$ $(n, a = 0, 1, \ldots)$ are determined by

$$f_{n,a}(x) = \sum_{k=0}^{n} p_k^{(n)}(0) f_{n-k,a+k-1}(x) \quad (n = 0, 1, \ldots; a = 1, 2, \ldots), \tag{1.7.6}$$

$$f_{0,a}(x) = 1 \quad (a = 0, 1, \ldots), \tag{1.7.7}$$

$$f_{n,0}(x) = x^n \quad (n = 0, 1, \ldots). \tag{1.7.8}$$

The solutions of (1.7.3)–(1.7.5) and (1.7.6)–(1.7.8) are unique, so

$$\psi_{0,a}(x,\theta) = f_{n,a}(x/q_0(\theta); \tilde{Q}(\theta)),$$

and the lemma follows using (1.7.2). □

Theorem 1.7.2. *For $n,m = a,1,\ldots,$*

$$\phi_{n,a}(x,\theta) = \sum_{i=0}^{n} n_{[i]} (q_i(\theta))^{n+a-i} G_i(x \mid U(\theta)) \quad (x \in \mathbb{R},\ \theta \in \mathbb{R}_+),$$

where $U(\theta)$ is given by $u_k(\theta) = q_k(\theta)$ $(k = 0,1,\ldots)$.

Proof. By Lemma 1.7.1 and Theorem 1.6.2,

$$\phi_{n,a}(x,\theta) = (q_0(\theta))^{n+a} \sum_{i=0}^{n} n_{[i]} \left(\frac{q_i(\theta)}{q_0(\theta)}\right)^{n+a-i} G_i\left(\frac{x}{q_0(\theta)} \,\middle|\, \frac{1}{q_0(\theta)} U(\theta)\right)$$

and the result follows since

$$G_i\left(\frac{x}{q_0(\theta)} \,\middle|\, \frac{1}{q_0(\theta)} U(\theta)\right) = \frac{1}{(q_0(\theta))^i} G_i(x \mid U(\theta))$$

by Property 1.4.6 on page 132. □

1.8 Epidemics with Outside Infection

When we study the final outcome of a major outbreak for the households model in Section 2.3 below we need the following extension of the standard SIR epidemic $E_{n,a}(\lambda, I)$, which was introduced by Addy et al. [1] and we denote by $\tilde{E}_{n,a}(\lambda, I, \pi)$. The definition of $\tilde{E}_{n,a}(\lambda, I, \pi)$ is the same as $E_{n,a}(\lambda, I)$ except susceptibles can also be infected externally, i.e. from outside of the population. Specifically, each susceptible avoids external infection during the course of the epidemic independently with probability π. Let $\tilde{S}$ and $\tilde{T}_A$ denote respectively the number of initial susceptibles that ultimately remain uninfected and the severity of $\tilde{E}_{n,a}(\lambda, I, \pi)$. (As in Section 1.7, the severity $\tilde{T}_A$ includes the infectious period of any initial infective.) Let

$$\tilde{\phi}_{n,a}(x,\theta) = \mathbb{E}\left[x^{\tilde{S}} \exp(-\theta \tilde{T}_A)\right] \qquad (x \in \mathbb{R}, \theta \geq 0)$$

be the joint generating function Laplace transform of $(\tilde{S}, \tilde{T}_A)$.

Theorem 1.8.1. *For $n,a = 0,1,\ldots,$*

$$\tilde{\phi}_{n,a}(x,\theta) = \sum_{i=0}^{n} n_{[i]} (q_i(\theta))^{n+a-i} \pi^i G_i(x \mid U(\theta)) \quad (x \in \mathbb{R},\ \theta \in \mathbb{R}_+), \qquad (1.8.1)$$

where $U(\theta)$ is given by $u_k(\theta) = q_k(\theta)$ $(k = 0,1,\ldots)$.

Proof. The final outcome $(\tilde{S}, \tilde{T}_A)$ of $\tilde{E}_{n,a}(\lambda, I, \pi)$ can be constructed by first deciding which of the n initial susceptibles are infected externally, suppose there are Y

of them, and then considering the final outcome of a standard SIR epidemic with initially $a+Y$ infectives and $n-Y$ susceptibles. Hence, $(\tilde{S},\tilde{T}_A)$ has the same distribution as (S,T_A) for the epidemic $E_{n-Y,a+Y}(\lambda,I)$, where $Y \sim \text{Bin}(n,1-\pi)$. (A formal proof can be obtained by considering the random directed graph $\mathscr{G}_E$ associated with $E_{n,a}(\lambda,I)$.) Thus,

$$\begin{aligned}\tilde{\phi}_{n,a}(x,\theta) &= \sum_{k=0}^{n}\binom{n}{k}(1-\pi)^k\pi^{n-k}\phi_{n-k,a+k}(x,\theta)\\ &= \sum_{k=0}^{n}\binom{n}{k}(1-\pi)^k\pi^{n-k}\sum_{i=0}^{n-k}(n-k)_{[i]}q_i(\theta)^{n+a-i}G_i(x\mid U(\theta)),\end{aligned}$$

by Theorem 1.7.2. Now $\binom{n}{k}(n-k)_{[i]} = n_{[i]}\binom{n-i}{k}$, so changing the order of summation in the above equation yields

$$\tilde{\phi}_{n,a}(x,\theta) = \sum_{i=0}^{n} n_{[i]}q_i(\theta)^{n+a-i}\pi^i G_i(x\mid U(\theta))\sum_{k=0}^{n-i}\binom{n-i}{k}(1-\pi)^k\pi^{n-i-k}.$$

The theorem follows since $\sum_{k=0}^{n-i}\binom{n-i}{k}(1-\pi)^k\pi^{n-i-k} = 1$. □

For computational purposes, it is usually simpler to use the expression for $\tilde{\phi}_{n,a}(x,\theta)$ given by (1.8.1) in Theorem 1.8.1, rather than the other expressions in the proof of the theorem. Often, it is the moments of $(\tilde{S},\tilde{T}_A)$ of that are of interest. For example, in the households model, the mean of $\tilde{Z} = n-\tilde{S}$ (i.e. the total size of $\tilde{E}_{n,a}(\lambda,I,\pi)$) is required to determine the fraction of the population that are infected by a major outbreak (see Section 2.3 below) and the second moments of $(\tilde{Z},\tilde{T}_A)$ are required for an associated central limit theorem (cf. Section 3.4.2 below). These can be obtained by suitable differentiation of (1.8.1), as we now describe for the mean $\tilde{\mu}_{n,a} = \mathbb{E}[\tilde{Z}]$. Differentiating (1.8.1) partially with respect to x, setting $(x,\theta)=(1,0)$ and using Property 1.4.5 on page 131 yields immediately the following corollary.

Corollary 1.8.2. *For $n,a = 0,1,\ldots,$*

$$\tilde{\mu}_{n,a} = n - \sum_{i=1}^{n} n_{[i]}q_i^{n+a-i}\pi^i G_{i-1}(1\mid U'),$$

where U' is given by $u'_k = q_{k+1}$ $(k=0,1,\ldots)$.

For $n=0,1,\ldots$ and $i=0,1,\ldots,n$, let $\tilde{P}_i^{(n)} = \mathbb{P}(\tilde{Z}=i)$. The following corollary gives a triangular system of linear equations for $\tilde{P}_i^{(n)}$ $(i=0,1,\ldots,n)$, first given in Addy et al. [1]. These equations provide a simple way of computing the total size distribution of $\tilde{E}_{n,a}(\lambda,I,\pi)$, though numerical instability problems can occur even for moderately sized n.

Corollary 1.8.3. *For $n=0,1,\ldots,$*

$$\sum_{i=0}^{k}\binom{n-i}{k-i}\tilde{P}_i^{(n)}\Big/\left(q_{n-k}^{a+i}\pi^{n-k}\right) = \binom{n}{k} \qquad (k=0,1,\ldots,n). \tag{1.8.2}$$

Proof. Fix $l \in \{0,1,\ldots,n\}$. Let U be given by $u_k = q_k$ $(k=0,1,\ldots)$. Differentiating both sides of (1.8.1) partially l times with respect to x, setting $\theta = 0$ and noting that $U(0) = U$ and $G_i^{(l)}(x \mid U) = 0$ for $i < l$, gives

$$\mathbb{E}\left[\tilde{S}_{[l]} x^{\tilde{S}-l}\right] = \sum_{i=l}^{n} n_{[i]} q_i^{n+a-i} \pi^i G_i^{(l)}(x \mid U). \tag{1.8.3}$$

Setting $x = q_l$ in (1.8.3) and using Property 1.4.3 on page 130 yields

$$\mathbb{E}\left[\tilde{S}_{[l]} q_l^{\tilde{S}-l}\right] = n_{[l]} q_l^{n+a-l} \pi^l. \tag{1.8.4}$$

Note, for $j = 0,1,\ldots,n$, that $\tilde{S} = j$ if and only if $\tilde{Z} = n-j$. Thus, (1.8.4) implies

$$\sum_{j=l}^{n} \tilde{P}_{n-j}^{(n)} j_{[l]} q_l^j = n_{[l]} \pi^l q_l^{n+a}. \tag{1.8.5}$$

Substituting $i = n-j$ in (1.8.5) and dividing both sides by $l! q_l^{n+a} \pi^l$ gives

$$\sum_{i=0}^{n-l} \tilde{P}_i^{(n)} \binom{n-i}{l} / \left(q_l^{a+i} \pi^l\right) = \binom{n}{l}$$

and (1.8.2) follows on setting $k = n-l$. □

Remark 1.8.4 (Computing mean and distribution of total size). Setting $\pi = 1$ in Corollary 1.8.2 yields an expression for the mean total size of the standard SIR epidemic $E_{n,a}(\lambda, I)$ (cf. Lemma 1.6.1). Setting $\pi = 1$ in Corollary 1.8.3 yields a triangular system of linear equations that determines the total size distribution of $E_{n,a}(\lambda, I)$ (see, for example, Ball [6, equation (2.5)]). As indicated above, this system can be numerically unstable for even moderately sized n. See House et al. [41] for further discussion and also for alternative methods of computing the total size distribution.

1.9 Mean Final Size of a Multitype Epidemic

In this appendix we describe the multitype SIR model and the result about its mean final size that is necessary for the calculation of μ_{nv} (and thus R_v) with any vaccine action model other than all-or-nothing. The result follows from Theorem 3.5 of Ball [6] or Corollary 4.4 of Picard and Lefèvre [57] (who do not and do, respectively, frame their results in terms of multivariate Gontcharoff polynomials that we use here). The model and result are a natural extension of the model in Section 1.1 and Corollary 1.6.3 in Section 1.6. Further explanation of and references relating to multitype SIR epidemics can be found in Andersson and Britton [4, Chapter 6].

We shall need the following notation, which although a little cumbersome at first sight allows Proposition 1.9.1 to be written in essentially the same form as its single-type version Corollary 1.6.3. The symbols $\mathbb{Z}_+$ and $\mathbb{R}_+$ denote the non-negative integers and reals, respectively. For vectors $\mathbf{x} = (x_1, x_2, \ldots, x_m)$ and $\mathbf{y} = (y_1, y_2, \ldots, y_m)$ in $\mathbb{R}^m$, we define $\mathbf{xy} = \prod_{i=1}^m x_i y_i$ and $\mathbf{x}^{\mathbf{y}} = \prod_{i=1}^m x_i^{y_i}$. We write $\mathbf{x} \le \mathbf{y}$ if $x_i \le y_i$ $(i = 1, 2, \ldots, m)$ and $\mathbf{x} < \mathbf{y}$ if, in addition, $x_i < y_i$ for at least one i. For $n, k \in \mathbb{Z}_+$, the falling factorial $n!/(n-k)!$ is denoted by $n_{[k]}$. For $\mathbf{n}, \mathbf{k} \in \mathbb{Z}_+^m$, we define $\mathbf{n}_{[\mathbf{k}]} = \prod_{i=1}^m n_{i[k_i]}$. For $\mathbf{i}, \mathbf{j} \in \mathbb{Z}_+^m$, we write $\sum_{\mathbf{k}=\mathbf{i}}^{\mathbf{j}}$ for $\sum_{k_1=i_1}^{j_1} \sum_{k_2=i_2}^{j_2} \cdots \sum_{k_m=i_m}^{j_m}$. We take $\mathbf{0}$ and $\mathbf{1}$ to be vectors with all entries 0 and 1 respectively.

Consider a single-household SIR epidemic model with m types of individuals, labelled $1, 2, \ldots, m$. Suppose that, for $i = 1, 2, \ldots, m$, there are initially a_i infectives and n_i susceptibles of type i, and let $\mathbf{a} = (a_1, a_2, \ldots, a_m)$ and $\mathbf{n} = (n_1, n_2, \ldots, n_m)$. For $i = 1, 2, \ldots, m$, the infectious periods of type-i infectives are each distributed according to a random variable $I^{(i)}$ with Laplace transform $\phi_I^{(i)}(\theta) = \mathbb{E}[\mathrm{e}^{-\theta I^{(i)}}]$. For $i, j = 1, 2, \ldots, m$, the individual-to-individual infection rate from a given type-i infective to a given type-j susceptible is λ_{ij}. As in Section 1.1, such infections are governed by Poisson processes, and all Poisson processes and infectious periods are mutually independent.

Writing Z_i for the number of type-i individuals that are recovered at the end of the epidemic, our aim is to calculate $\boldsymbol{\mu}_{\mathbf{n},\mathbf{a}}(\Lambda)$, the vector with components $\mu_{\mathbf{n},\mathbf{a},i}(\Lambda) = \mathbb{E}[Z_i]$. Our expression for $\boldsymbol{\mu}_{\mathbf{n},\mathbf{a}}(\Lambda)$ is given in terms of multivariate Gontcharoff polynomials, first studied by Lefèvre and Picard [46], which we now define. Let $\mathbf{U} = (\mathbf{u}_{\mathbf{j}} \in \mathbb{R}^m : \mathbf{j} \in \mathbb{Z}_+^m)$ be a collection of real numbers. The Gontcharoff polynomials associated with $\mathbf{U}$, denoted $(G_{\mathbf{k}}(\mathbf{x} \mid \mathbf{U}), \mathbf{k} \in \mathbb{Z}_+^m, \mathbf{x} \in \mathbb{R}^m)$, are defined recursively by

$$\sum_{\mathbf{j}=\mathbf{0}}^{\mathbf{k}} \mathbf{k}_{[\mathbf{j}]} \mathbf{u}_{\mathbf{j}}^{\mathbf{k}-\mathbf{j}} G_{\mathbf{j}}(\mathbf{x} \mid \mathbf{U}) = \mathbf{x}^{\mathbf{k}} \quad (\mathbf{k} \ge \mathbf{0}). \tag{1.9.1}$$

Note that $G_{\mathbf{0}}(\mathbf{x} \mid \mathbf{U}) \equiv 1$ and that $G_{\mathbf{k}}(\mathbf{x} \mid \mathbf{U})$ is a polynomial of degree $k_1, k_2, \ldots, k_m$ in the variables $x_1, x_2, \ldots, x_m$, respectively, depending only on $(\mathbf{u}_{\mathbf{j}} : \mathbf{j} < \mathbf{k})$.

Proposition 1.9.1. *For* $\mathbf{n}, \mathbf{a} \ge \mathbf{0}$,

$$\boldsymbol{\mu}_{\mathbf{n},\mathbf{a}} = \mathbf{n} - \sum_{\mathbf{i}=\mathbf{1}}^{\mathbf{n}} \mathbf{n}_{[\mathbf{i}]} \mathbf{q}_{\mathbf{i}}^{\mathbf{n}+\mathbf{a}-\mathbf{i}} G_{\mathbf{i}-\mathbf{a}}(\mathbf{1} \mid \mathbf{U}'),$$

where $\mathbf{U}'$ *is given by* $\mathbf{u}'_{\mathbf{k}} = \mathbf{q}_{\mathbf{k}+\mathbf{a}}$ $(\mathbf{k} \ge \mathbf{0})$, *with the i-th component of the vector* $\mathbf{q}_{\mathbf{j}} = (\phi_I^{(i)}(\sum_{k=1}^m \lambda_{ik} j_k), i = 1, 2, \ldots, m)$ *being the probability that a type-i individual fails to contact a given set of* $\mathbf{j} = (j_1, j_2, \ldots, j_m)$ *individuals of the various types (cf. the notation for the single-type case in Section 1.5).*

As noted above, this result in terms of Gontcharoff polynomials is due to Lefèvre and Picard [46]. A proof using multitype analogues of the methods of the rest of this chapter may be obtained from Ball [7]: the proposition above follows from the first display in the proof of Theorem 4.1 of that paper in precisely the same way as Corollary 1.6.3 follows from Lemma 1.6.1 in Section 1.6.

Chapter 2
The Households Model

In this chapter we give a short and informal introduction to the *households model*, a key example (both historically and in applications) of the kind of two-level mixing models that are the focus of this Part. It is based mainly on Ball et al. [14] and Ball and Lyne [13]. Early work on epidemic models incorporating household-like structure includes Bartoszyński [23] and Becker and Deitz [25], but Ball et al. [14] gives the first treatment of the households model as discussed in this chapter. We first motivate and define the model in Section 2.1. In Section 2.2 we look at the early stages of an epidemic, deriving a threshold parameter which determines whether a major outbreak affecting a non-negligible proportion of the population is possible when there are few initial cases and a method of calculating the probability of such a major outbreak. Then in Section 2.3 we consider the final outcome of a major outbreak, focusing mainly on the expected proportion of the population infected. Lastly we consider the impact of vaccination on the epidemic, including consideration of the question of which individuals to target with a limited quantity of vaccine in order to 'control' the epidemic as effectively as possible.

2.1 Introduction and Definition

A natural first step in the direction of including more realistic structure in the population model of homogeneous mixing is to allow for *households*: mutually exclusive and collectively exhaustive (and usually relatively small) groups of individuals who interact more frequently with other individuals in the same group than they do with other members of the population. This applies to human populations, but similar groupings are also natural in other situations, for example cages/sheds in poultry farms or pens/fields on sheep/cattle farms. Additionally, there are outbreak control measures associated with households and similar structures (such as schools and workplaces) and epidemic data are often collected at the household level (or at least with some information about household structure). As we shall see, households models are also reasonably mathematically tractable and so can be quite readily interpreted and understood.

T. Britton, E. Pardoux (eds.), *Stochastic Epidemic Models with Inference*,
Lecture Notes in Mathematics 2255, https://doi.org/10.1007/978-3-030-30900-8_6

We define the stochastic SIR households model (or just 'the households model' for brevity) as follows. The closed, finite population is partitioned into m households, of which m_n are of size n, for $n = 1,2,\ldots,n_{\max}$. We therefore have $m = \sum_{n=1}^{n_{\max}} m_n$ and there are a total of $N = \sum_{n=1}^{n_{\max}} nm_n$ individuals in the population. We write $\alpha_n = m_n/m$ for the proportion of households that are of size n and $\tilde{\alpha}_n = nm_n/N$ ($= n\alpha_n/\mu_H$, where $\mu_H = \sum_{i=1}^{n_{\max}} i\alpha_i$ is the mean household size) for the proportion of individuals that belong to a household of size n. Our results are valid asymptotically as the number of households, m, (and the population size N too) tends to infinity. Note that the quantities above should in principle be indexed by m, e.g. $m_n^{(m)}$, $\alpha_n^{(m)}$, etc.; we avoid this wherever possible, but if necessary use superscript '(m)' in this way for clarity. (Since our results relate to the asymptotic $m \to \infty$ framework this does not often arise; we think of these quantities as being equal to their asymptotic values for all m.) We assume for simplicity of exposition in this less formal chapter that the household size is bounded, i.e. $n_{\max} < \infty$; however essentially all the results we state in this chapter carry over to the case of unbounded household sizes so long as the asymptotic mean household size $\mu_H = \lim_{m\to\infty} \mu_H^{(m)} = \lim_{m\to\infty} \sum_{n=1}^{\infty} nm_n^{(m)}/N^{(m)}$ is finite.

The epidemic begins with some individuals becoming infective at time $t = 0$, with the rest of the population assumed to be susceptible. The infectious periods of infective individuals are each distributed according to a random variable I with an arbitrary but specified distribution. During its infectious period, an infective individual makes *local* or *within-household* contacts with each susceptible in its household at the points of Poisson processes of rate λ_L and it also makes *global* contacts with each individual in the population at the points of Poisson processes of rate λ_G/N. A susceptible that is contacted immediately becomes infective; contacts have no effect on non-susceptible individuals. An infective becomes recovered at the end of its infectious period. All Poisson processes and infectious periods are assumed mutually independent. The epidemic ceases when there is no infection remaining in the population.

Note that the above assumptions about global contact are equivalent to an infective making global contacts at rate λ_G, with the individual contacted by each such contact being chosen independently and uniformly from the population. These assumptions also imply that global contacts may be with an individual in the same household as the infector, or may even be 'self-contacts' where the contact is with the same individual as made the contact. However both of these happen with probability tending to 0 in our asymptotic setting.

Our model assumes that there is no latent period where an individual has been infected but is not yet infectious, i.e. a susceptible becomes infective as soon as it is contacted. However, our focus will be on the final outcome of the epidemic, so including a latent period in the model has no effect on our results (cf. Remark 1.2.2 on page 127). In fact the final outcome properties of closed SIR epidemic models of this kind are invariant to very general assumptions about a latent period. Many of the results we present depend on the number of initial infectives only very weakly: so long as there are few such initial infectives then their number and position in the population relative to each other affects the chance of a large outbreak but not whether such an outbreak is possible nor the final outcome in the event that a large outbreak does occur.

The focus of our analysis is the final outcome of the epidemic: which individuals become infected during the course of the epidemic and are therefore in the recovered state when it ceases. The main quantity of interest is the final size, the number (or proportion) of initially susceptible individuals that are ultimately recovered. We also examine questions about the final outcome associated with the household structure. For example, if we expect half the population to become infected then is it likely to be that every household has roughly half of its residents infected, or might half of the households be completely infected and the other half unaffected?

Since the model and results in this chapter fit into the more general framework of Chapter 3 (though there we assume that all households are of the same size to simplify the exposition), in this chapter we provide only enough details and heuristic justifications to illustrate the main ideas. This more concrete model provides a good reference point for the later more general theory.

2.2 Early Stages

If we seek to approximate the early stages of the households model using discrete generation-based arguments along the lines of Section 1.2 in Part I of this volume, with a view to calculating R_0 and the probability of a major outbreak, then we soon encounter difficulties because of the household structure. An individual infected through a household infection and an individual infected through a global infection have different 'neighbourhoods' of susceptibles whom they might infect. Specifically, the person infected globally will have the remainder of their household susceptible, but for the individual infected through the household at least one other individual in their household (their infector) has already been infected and is thus not susceptible. Whilst it is possible to formulate and analyze an approximating branching process that reflects this structure, it is rather involved (see Section 3.3.3 below).

A crucial observation in what follows is that although within-household (i.e. local) contacts may have non-negligible probability of being with a non-susceptible individual, in the early stages of the epidemic (when the number of infections is small compared to m) global contacts will be with a susceptible individual with probability close to 1. We therefore think of the epidemic as evolving in stages, first considering the spread within a newly-infected household and then considering the global contacts made by those infected in the local epidemic. This leads to a Galton–Watson branching process approximation where the 'particles' correspond to infectious households, from which we can calculate a threshold parameter (which can be interpreted in terms of household to household spread) and then the probability of a major outbreak. (Cf. the real-time branching process approximation in Section 1.2 of Part I of this volume.) We say that a major outbreak occurs if, in the limit as $m \to \infty$, infinitely many households are infected. Since the mean household size is bounded, this is equivalent to infinitely many individuals being infected.

To specify this branching process of infected households we need to determine its offspring distribution. To that end, let R be a random variable giving the number of global contacts emanating from those infected in a within-household epidemic initiated by a single global contact. (In the early stages, all such global contacts will, with probability close to 1, be with individuals in previously uninfected households, and by construction their behaviour is independent of the previously infected households, so this is the appropriate random variable to act as the offspring distribution of our branching process.) We first calculate the threshold parameter $R_* = \mathbb{E}[R]$ which determines whether or not a large outbreak is possible and then the probability generating function $f_R(s) = \mathbb{E}[s^R]$, from which we can determine the probability of a large outbreak.

Consider an individual infected globally in the early stages of the epidemic. It is in a household that is otherwise uninfected (with probability close to 1) and that household is of size n with probability $\tilde{\alpha}_n$, since the newly infected individual is chosen uniformly from all individuals and the number of individuals in households of size n is proportional to $n\alpha_n$. Write $\mu_n(\lambda_L)$ for the mean size, including the initial infective, of the within-household epidemic that ensues. Then, since each infective makes global contacts at rate λ_G during an infectious period of mean $\mu_I = \mathbb{E}[I]$ and each such contact is with a different individual in a previously uninfected household, the mean number of global infectious contacts that emanate from this typical household is

$$R_* = \lambda_G \mu_I \sum_{n=1}^{n_{\max}} \tilde{\alpha}_n \mu_n(\lambda_L), \tag{2.2.1}$$

the sum being the (unconditional) mean size of a within-household outbreak. The conditional mean size $\mu_n(\lambda_L)$ can be calculated using Corollary 1.6.3; though unless n is very small this is only practical to evaluate numerically, not analytically. (We also note here that we may have $R_* = \infty$ if $\lim_{m\to\infty} \sum_{n=1}^{\infty} n^2 m_n^{(m)} / N^{(m)} = \infty$, i.e. if the limiting second moment of the household sizes is infinite.)

To compute the probability generating function f_R of the random variable R we start with the same conditioning on the size of the household that the globally infected individual is in: with probability $\tilde{\alpha}_n$ that size is n. Now, since each infective in the local epidemic makes global contacts at rate λ_G throughout its infectious period, the total number of such global contacts follows a Poisson distribution with random mean $\lambda_G A_n$, where A_n is the severity of the within-household epidemic. It then follows that

$$\mathbb{E}[s^{R_n}] = \mathbb{E}[\mathbb{E}[s^{R_n} \mid A_n]] = \mathbb{E}[\mathrm{e}^{-\lambda_G A_n(1-s)}] = \phi_{n-1,1}(1, \lambda_G(1-s))$$

(for all $s \in [0,1]$), where the Laplace transform $\phi_{n-1,1}(1,\theta)$ of the severity A_n may be calculated using Theorem 1.7.2. The law of total expectation thus implies that

$$f_R(s) = \sum_{n=1}^{n_{\max}} \tilde{\alpha}_n \mathbb{E}[s^{R_n}] = \sum_{n=1}^{n_{\max}} \tilde{\alpha}_n \phi_{n-1,1}(1, \lambda_G(1-s)); \tag{2.2.2}$$

and standard branching process theory implies that the chance of a large outbreak in the large population limit is $p_{\text{maj}} = 1 - \sigma$, where σ is the smallest non-negative solution of $f_R(s) = s$ (see Appendix A.1.1 in Part I of this volume).

Ball et al. [14] extend these ideas to derive expressions for the probability of a major outbreak with more general initial conditions, and to find some properties of the number of individuals and households infected in a minor outbreak (in a similar vein to Section 1.3 in Part I of this volume).

2.3 Final Outcome of a Major Outbreak

We now turn to the final outcome of a major outbreak; beginning with calculating z, the expected proportion of the population infected by a major outbreak. Under the assumption that there are few initial infectives, this can be viewed as the probability that a given initial susceptible, who is in a household that is not initially infectious, is ultimately infected by the large outbreak. Recall from Section 1.8 the model $\tilde{E}_{n,a}(\lambda, I, \pi)$ for an epidemic amongst a homogeneously mixing population with the additional feature that each initially susceptible individual is infected from outside the population, independently and with probability $1 - \pi$. We use this to help calculate z by considering an initially completely susceptible household, determining which individuals are infected from outside the household by global contacts at some point during a major outbreak, and then letting those infectives initiate a within-household epidemic.

Suppose that A is the total severity (i.e. the total length of the infectious periods of all infected individuals) of a major outbreak. Then for large m we have that A is approximately $Nz\mu_I$, since each of the Nz infected individuals is infectious for an average of μ_I time units. Each initially susceptible individual therefore experiences global infection a Poisson distributed number of times with mean $Nz\mu_I \cdot \lambda_G N^{-1}$, and thus avoids global infection with probability

$$\pi = \exp(-\lambda_G z \mu_I). \tag{2.3.1}$$

To express z in terms of π we follow the argument outlined at the end of the previous paragraph. A randomly chosen initial susceptible in the population belongs to a household of size n with probability $\tilde{\alpha}_n$ and conditional on this it will be ultimately infected with probability $\tilde{\mu}_{n,0}(\lambda_L, \pi)/n$. Here $\tilde{\mu}_{n,0}(\lambda_L, \pi)$ is the mean final size of the epidemic $\tilde{E}_{n,0}(\lambda_L, I, \pi)$, which may be computed using Corollary 1.8.2 (again this is only practical numerically unless n is very small). We therefore have that

$$z = \sum_{n=1}^{n_{\max}} \tilde{\alpha}_n \tilde{\mu}_{n,0}(\lambda_L, \pi)/n. \tag{2.3.2}$$

Equations (2.3.1) and (2.3.2) implicitly characterise the expected relative final size of a large outbreak, in a manner that resembles the equation $1 - z = \mathrm{e}^{-R_0 z}$ in the homogeneously mixing framework. (Indeed this latter equation can be recovered from (2.3.1) and (2.3.2) by considering the special case where all households are of size 1.) Analogously to the homogeneously mixing case, the equations (2.3.1) and (2.3.2) always have a trivial solution $z = 0$ (and $\pi = 1$), and there is a unique further solution $z \in (0,1)$ (with $\pi \in (0,1)$) if and only if $R_* > 1$. (Cf. Section 3.4.1 below.)

Having found z and therefore π, we can easily determine the *within-household final size distribution*, i.e. the distribution of the number of individuals ultimately infected within each household. In a household of size n this is simply the final size distribution of $\tilde{E}_{n,0}(\lambda_L, I, \pi)$, which can be computed (usually only numerically) via Corollary 1.8.3.

It is also possible to establish a Gaussian approximation to the number of initially susceptible individuals that are ultimately infected in the event of a large outbreak (as in Section 3.3 in Part I of this volume). Though an interesting and valuable part of the analysis of the households model, the arguments required to justify it are rather technical and thus do not fit with the spirit of this chapter. This central limit theorem is covered in Section 3.4.2 below in the case where all households are of the same size; see also Section 4 of Ball et al. [14] and Section 3.3 in Part I of this volume.

2.4 Vaccination

One of the motivations for studying the households model is that in real-life situations involving human diseases, vaccination strategies can be based on household structure. In this section we introduce a mathematical framework for determining how we should allocate a limited supply of vaccine; for example might we be better to vaccinate everyone in half of all households or half of the individuals in all households? We work exclusively in the framework where vaccinations are prophylactic; that is they are administered in advance of any outbreak. Reactive (as opposed to proactive) measures, for example contact tracing or ring vaccination, are of course interesting and worthwhile to study (see for example Becker et al. [26] and Ball et al. [10]). They are however more complex to analyse because their implementation, and thus their effect, is influenced by the real-time progression of the epidemic, which our method of analysis does not consider.

2.4.1 Modelling Vaccination

There are two distinct (although related) aspects of vaccination that we need to specify in order to capture the effect of vaccination in our mathematical model. These are the *allocation* and the *action* of the vaccine; which describe respectively (i) who gets vaccinated and (ii) what happens to vaccinated individuals in terms of susceptibility and infectivity. Broadly speaking, the practical approach that we take is to consider the vaccine action model as fixed (though an appropriate model will of course vary for different vaccines and/or diseases, and determining or inferring an appropriate model for a given situation is an interesting question in its own right) and then determine the allocation strategy that is in some sense optimal. This may involve, for example, determining a vaccine allocation which will minimise the amount of vaccine required subject to the requirement of rendering the epidemic model sub-critical; or minimising some outcome measure (like R_* or z) subject to a constraint on the amount of available vaccine. For this reason our focus is primarily on determining optimal vaccine allocation strategies, with the vaccine action model assumed fixed.

We use the vaccine action (or vaccine response) model proposed by Becker and Starczak [28] (see also Halloran et al. [38]), where the response of vaccinated individuals to the vaccine is described by independent realisations of the generic random vector (A,B). Here A is the relative susceptibility and B the relative infectivity of the vaccinated individual; both of these being relative to an unvaccinated individual. We include this in the epidemic model by multiplying the rates at which that individual receives infectious contacts by A and, should it become infectious, multiplying rates at which it makes infectious contacts by B. We usually think of (A,B) as taking values in $[0,1]^2$ so that vaccination reduces susceptibility and infectiousness, but the interpretation and analysis is equally valid if (A,B) takes values in $[0,\infty)^2$.

For mathematical tractability we usually require that (A,B) can take only a finite number of values, and we now describe some common vaccine action models that appear in the literature. The vaccine is called *all-or-nothing* if $\mathbb{P}(A=0, B=0) = \varepsilon = 1 - \mathbb{P}(A=1, B=1)$ for some $\varepsilon \in [0,1]$; i.e. the vaccine confers either total protection or no protection at all, independently across different vaccinees. The vaccine is called *non-random* if $\mathbb{P}(A=a, B=b) = 1$ for some $(a,b) \in [0,\infty)^2$; here every vaccinated individual has the same response to the vaccine. A non-random vaccine is called *leaky* if $b=1$, so the vaccine affects susceptibility but not infectivity. The simplest vaccine action model is the *perfect* vaccine, where $\mathbb{P}(A=0, B=0) = 1$, so every vaccinated individual is completely protected from infection. (Here $\mathbb{P}(A=0) = 1$ is the crucial part for most purposes, but careful interpretation may required if modelling assumptions make it possible for such a vaccinated individual to be chosen as an initial infective and $B > 0$.)

The vaccine allocation model describes how vaccinees are chosen from the population. Following Becker and Starczak [27], we specify this through the quantities $(x_{nv}, n = 1,2,\ldots,n_{\max}, v = 0,1,\ldots,n)$, where x_{nv} is the proportion of households of size n in which v individuals are vaccinated. (These quantities must be non-negative and satisfy $\sum_{v=0}^{n} x_{nv} = 1$ for all n.) By conditioning on the household size of an individual chosen uniformly at random from the population and then on the number of vaccinated individuals in that household we find that the vaccine *coverage*, defined as the proportion of the population that is vaccinated, is given by

$$c = \sum_{n=1}^{n_{\max}} \tilde{\alpha}_n \sum_{v=0}^{n} x_{nv} \frac{v}{n}. \tag{2.4.1}$$

In the remainder of this section we first investigate the effect of a given vaccine allocation strategy on the epidemic and then consider optimising these vaccine allocation parameters (x_{nv}) for fixed c.

2.4.2 Threshold Parameter

We can construct households-based branching process approximations for the early stages of the epidemic in the same spirit as for the basic model without vaccination. The ideas are exactly the same but the calculations can be rather more involved, depending on the details of the vaccine action and allocation. In this section we just focus on calculating the post-vaccination threshold parameter, which we call R_v. As a post-vaccination version of R_*, its derivation follows essentially the same method. Note, however, that one needs to be careful with the precise description of a generation, particularly with regard to whether an individual/particle in the branching process corresponds to a newly infected household or a newly contacted household (who if they are vaccinated might not actually get infected); the former interpretation is perhaps more intuitively natural but here we prefer the latter since it results in slightly simpler calculations.

With this in mind, let R_v be the expected number of global contacts made by those infected in the within-household epidemic initiated by an individual contacted globally, in the early stages of the outbreak. Conditioning on the size of the household and then the number of vaccinated individuals in the household that the newly infected individual is in, we find that

$$R_v = \sum_{n=1}^{n_{\max}} \tilde{\alpha}_n \sum_{v=0}^{n} x_{nv}\, \mu_{nv}, \tag{2.4.2}$$

where μ_{nv} is the mean number of global infections emanating from a single-household epidemic initiated by an individual chosen uniformly at random being contacted globally, in a household in state (n,v) (by which we mean a household with n individuals, of whom v are vaccinated). Bearing in mind previous results in this section, all that remains is to calculate the quantities μ_{nv} (for $n = 1,2,\ldots,n_{\max}$, $v = 1,2,\ldots,n$), which depend on the vaccine action model being considered. We now calculate these quantities for some specific vaccine action models.

2.4.2.1 All-or-nothing Vaccine Action

Under this model each vaccinated individual becomes completely immune (and thus plays no part in the epidemic, exactly as an individual in the recovered state) with probability ε; with the complementary probability $1-\varepsilon$ the vaccine fails and has no effect (so for the purposes of the epidemic they are indistinguishable from an unvaccinated individual). We therefore need only explicitly keep track of those individuals for whom the vaccine fails. A household in state (n,v) has $n-v$ individuals who are susceptible by virtue of not being vaccinated and up to v further susceptibles who were vaccinated but for whom the vaccine failed. Thus, for $k \in \{n-v, n-v+1,\ldots,n\}$, there are k susceptibles in the household precisely when $n-k$ of the v vaccines are successful, which happens with probability $\binom{v}{n-k}\varepsilon^{n-k}(1-\varepsilon)^{v-n+k}$. In such a household the globally contacted individual is susceptible, and thus initiates a within-household epidemic, with probability k/n; and if this is the case then the mean number of global contacts that result from the local epidemic is $\mu_k(\lambda_L)\lambda_G\mu_I$. We therefore have that

$$\mu_{nv} = \sum_{k=n-v}^{n} \binom{v}{n-k} \varepsilon^{n-k}(1-\varepsilon)^{v-n+k} \frac{k}{n} \mu_k(\lambda_L)\lambda_G\mu_I, \tag{2.4.3}$$

where the $\mu_k(\lambda_L)$ terms can be calculated using Corollary 1.6.3 in Section 1.6. Note that for a perfect vaccine we have $\varepsilon = 1$, so only the $k = n - v$ term in this sum is non-zero.

2.4.2.2 Non-random Vaccine Action

Now we suppose that all individuals respond identically to the vaccine, with the positive constants a and b characterising their relative susceptibility and infectivity, respectively. (Actually a and b are non-negative, but taking them to be strictly positive eliminates some degeneracies which are straightforward but a bit cumbersome to deal with.) Describing the local spread of the epidemic within a household now requires a 2-type SIR epidemic, with the types corresponding to vaccinated and unvaccinated individuals. We write Λ^L for the matrix of local infection rates

$$\Lambda^L = \begin{pmatrix} \lambda^L_{UU} & \lambda^L_{UV} \\ \lambda^L_{VU} & \lambda^L_{VV} \end{pmatrix} = \begin{pmatrix} \lambda_L & a\lambda_L \\ b\lambda_L & ab\lambda_L \end{pmatrix},$$

where, for $A, A' \in \{U, V\}$ representing the Unvaccinated and Vaccinated types respectively, $\lambda^L_{AA'}$ is the rate at which a type-A individual makes contact with a given type-A' individual in the same household. For a household with n_i individuals of type i we write $\mathbf{n} = (n_U, n_V)$ and let $\boldsymbol{\mu}_{\mathbf{n},i}(\Lambda^L) = (\mu_{\mathbf{n},i,j}(\Lambda^L),\ j = U, V)$ be a vector where the j-th entry is the mean number of type-j individuals that are ultimately infected (including the initial case if applicable) in the local epidemic in a household of $\mathbf{n}$ individuals of the two types, with one of the type-i individuals being the initial infective.

Now consider a household in state (n, v) that is contacted globally. If the contact is with a vaccinated (respectively, unvaccinated) individual then with probability a (respectively, 1) it becomes infected and thus initiates a local epidemic. Should this local epidemic occur then any individual infected by it makes on average $\lambda_G\mu_I$ or $b\lambda_G\mu_I$ global contacts during their infectious period, according as they are unvaccinated or vaccinated. Writing $\mathbf{n}^{(n,v)} = (n - v, v)$ and suppressing the Λ^L dependence of $\mu_{\mathbf{n},i,j}(\Lambda^L)$ for brevity, we therefore have that

$$\mu_{nv} = \left[\frac{n-v}{n}(\mu_{\mathbf{n}^{(n,v)},U,U} + b\mu_{\mathbf{n}^{(n,v)},U,V}) + \frac{v}{n} a(\mu_{\mathbf{n}^{(n,v)},V,U} + b\mu_{\mathbf{n}^{(n,v)},V,V})\right] \lambda_G\mu_I. \tag{2.4.4}$$

The quantities $\boldsymbol{\mu}_{\mathbf{n},i}(\Lambda^L)$ can be calculated using Proposition 1.9.1 in Section 1.9; which is a multitype analogue of Corollary 1.6.3 in Section 1.6.

2.4.2.3 General Discrete Vaccine Action

As mentioned in Section 2.4.1, we can handle vaccine action models where the random vector (A,B) describing vaccine response takes finitely many values. If it takes k values then each household contains (up to) $k+1$ types of individual; and conditional on the number of vaccinated individuals the numbers of each type follow a multinomial distribution. One can then calculate μ_{nv} using Proposition 1.9.1 in Section 1.9. (Note that the non-random case above fits into this framework with $k=1$.)

2.4.3 Vaccination Schemes

We can use equation (2.4.2) to compute the effect of specific vaccination strategies on the threshold parameter R_v. In particular we can determine whether or not some proposed vaccination strategy will control a supercritical epidemic, in the sense of reducing R_v below one so that major outbreaks are not possible. Two (mathematically) relatively simple allocation strategies involve (i) vaccinating all individuals in randomly chosen households and (ii) vaccinating randomly chosen individuals. We first briefly consider these before moving on to optimal schemes. Note that because of the often highly nonlinear dependence of μ_{nv} on v, we do not expect explicit formulae for R_v to be available except in some very simple cases. Numerical evaluation and exploration of the models is therefore an important tool; see for example Ball and Lyne [13]. We see later though that there is enough structure to be able to make some analytical progress in determining optimal vaccination schemes.

Since our analysis of these models is household based, analysis of the *random households* strategy is relatively straightforward, since every household is either completely unvaccinated or completely vaccinated. Vaccinating a proportion c of all households in the population gives (for all n) $x_{n0}=1-c$, $x_{nn}=c$ and $x_{nv}=0$ for $v=1,2,\ldots,n-1$. Substitution into equation (2.4.1) confirms that the overall coverage is indeed c, and the formula (2.4.2) for R_v simplifies considerably because many of the summands are zero. Indeed, for a perfect vaccine it is readily seen that $R_v=(1-c)R_*$, so when $R_*>1$ the critical vaccination coverage is $1-R_*^{-1}$; cf. equation (1.4.1) in Part I of this volume.

The *random individuals* strategy is slightly more complex, since now there are more than two possible 'vaccination structures' within a household. Assuming that we vaccinate a proportion c of individuals chosen uniformly at random from the population, the number of vaccinated individuals in a household of a given size follows a binomial distribution, so $x_{nv}=\binom{n}{v}c^v(1-c)^{n-v}$. Substitution into equation (2.4.1) again confirms that the coverage is c (as expected: any other result would indicate a serious problem with our model and/or calculations).

Now we consider optimal vaccination schemes, which arise naturally in the realistic contexts of (i) minimising the amount of vaccination required to 'control' the epidemic in the sense of eliminating the possibility of major outbreaks, or (ii) optimising (interpreted as minimising R_v) the allocation of a limited amount of available vaccine. Mathematically these amount to choosing the vaccine allocation parameters (x_{nv}) (for $n = 1,2,\ldots, v = 0,1,\ldots,n$) to either (i) minimise c subject to the constraint $R_v \leq 1$; or (ii) minimise R_v subject to a constraint on c. Since R_v and c are both linear functions of the decision variables x_{nv} (see equations (2.4.2) and (2.4.1)) and the constraints on the x_{nv} (described in the last paragraph of Section 2.4.1) are all linear, these are both linear programming problems.

In the linear programming framework it is also possible to compute worst-case scenarios, for example to determine the 'worst' vaccine allocation for a given coverage. Whilst not of direct practical interest this does allow comparison of proposed or actual vaccine allocation policies with the best-possible and worst-possible cases; which is helpful for establishing context when interpreting numerical results from such modelling calculations.

We now outline an analytical approach which allows us to characterise the optimal (and worst possible) vaccine allocation in the households model. It may be of interest in its own right if household-based transmission is a key driver of infection for some specific disease; but it is also indicative of the kind of analysis we might strive for when analysing vaccine allocation in more complex structured models.

The key tool, introduced by Ball and Lyne [13], is to re-write the formula in equation (2.4.2) for R_v as

$$R_v = \sum_{n=1}^{n_{\max}} \sum_{v=0}^{n} h_{nv} M_{nv},$$

were $h_{nv} = m_n x_{nv}$ is the number of households of size n that have v occupants vaccinated and $M_{nv} = n\mu_{nv}/N$. This representation implies that M_{nv} can be viewed as the contribution to R_v of each household in state (n,v). Building on this we can define (for $n = 1,2,\ldots,n_{\max}$ and $v = 0,1,\ldots,n-1$) the *gain* $G_{nv} = M_{nv} - M_{n,v+1} (\geq 0)$, which is the reduction in R_v that is achieved by vaccinating one further individual in a household currently in state (n,v). The *gain matrix* $G = (G_{nv}, n = 1,2,\ldots,n_{\max}, v = 0,1,\ldots,n-1)$ thus captures the impact (on this threshold parameter) of vaccinating different numbers of individuals in households of all possible states. When dealing with specific examples we usually work with the re-scaled gain matrix G' with entries $G'_{nv} = NG_{nv} = n(\mu_{nv} - \mu_{n,v+1})$; partly since these values are usually of a more practical order of magnitude and partly because G'_{nv} does not depend on the population size (and therefore may retain some meaning in the context of the infinite population size limiting framework that we are working in).

Interpretation of the gain matrix to reveal optimal vaccination schemes is straightforward if G_{nv} is decreasing in v for every fixed n, representing a diminishing return on vaccination for successive vaccinations in each household. For determining the optimal strategy the *ordering* of the entries of the gain matrix is the crucial feature: it determines which individuals should be prioritised for vaccination. Consider for example the gain matrix given in Table 2.4.1, for a model with households only of sizes 1, 2 and 3. In this example the largest entry is $G'_{3,0}$, so the first priority is to vaccinate a single individual in every household of size 3. This is followed by vaccinating a second individual in those households of size 3 and then vaccinating one individual in households of size 2. Finally we vaccinate the final unvaccinated individual in households of each size, starting with the largest.

Table 2.4.1 An example of a gain matrix with diminishing returns. Entries of the table are the scaled gains G'_{nv} and superscripts indicate the ordering of the entries (decreasing). Model parameters are $(\alpha_n, n = 1,2,3) = (1,2,3)/6$, $I \sim \exp(1)$, $\lambda_L = 3$, $\lambda_G = 1$ and the vaccine action is all or nothing with success probability $\varepsilon = 0.7$.

n	$v = 0$	1	2
1	0.69^6		
2	1.73^3	1.01^5	
3	3.11^1	2.14^2	1.35^4

We note here that the diminishing returns structure of the gain matrix (i.e. G_{nv} being decreasing in v for every n) that we observe above is a natural situation and indeed it necessarily obtains in the present modelling framework so long as $\mathbb{E}[A] < 1$ and $\mathbb{E}[B] < 1$. However, examples where G_{nv} is not decreasing in v do naturally arise in generalisations of the households model; for example if there is additional cost associated with vaccinating the first individual in each household (Ball and Lyne [12, Section 3.5]), if multiple types of individuals are present in the model (Ball et al. [8, Section 3]), or if the homogeneously mixing framework for global contacts is replaced by a network model (Ball and Sirl [20, Section 3.4]). In these situations of non-diminishing returns, the construction of optimal schemes is still possible but requires rather more care.

An important special case is that of a perfect vaccine, where all vaccinated individuals are completely immune to infection. In this situation G_{nv} depends on n and v only through $n - v$, the number of susceptible individuals in the household. One can show that if $n\mu_n(\lambda_L)$ is convex (as a function of n) then this function is decreasing in $n - v$; and in this case an *equalising* strategy, where one tries to equalise (as far as possible) the number of susceptible/unvaccinated individuals in the households, is optimal (Ball et al. [14, Section 5.2.1]). When the equalising strategy is not optimal there are plausible parameter sets where it is near-optimal, but also plausible parameter values where it is far from being so (see, for example, Keeling and Ross [44] and the non-random case in Exercise 2.6.3).

2.5 Other Measures of Epidemic Impact

The post-vaccination household-to-household reproduction number R_v is not necessarily a reliable indicator of overall epidemic impact. Whilst R_v quantifies an important aspect of the early proliferation of infection, infected households, it only indirectly takes into account how many individuals become infected in each household. Furthermore, it directly relates to the generation-based proliferation of infection in the early stages of an outbreak, not any other more direct measure of epidemic impact. (See also the discussion of the first paragraph of Section 3.3.3 below, which discusses several potential shortcomings of a reproduction number like R_*, and Keeling and Ross [44].)

It is possible to calculate modified versions of the probability generating function given by equation (2.2.2) and/or the balance equations (2.3.1) and (2.3.2); in much the same way as we modified the calculation of R_* to find R_v. Then we can calculate, at least numerically, the probability and size of a major outbreak. One might then aim to optimise these quantities instead of R_v. The resulting implicit equations, however, do not readily lend themselves to analytical results concerning the behaviour of their solutions. Nevertheless, the analysis performed above exemplifies the kind of exploration of these structured population models that can provide insight into vaccination strategies that one might hope to deploy, or at least to approximate, in a real-world epidemic planning situation where reliable information is available about the structure relating to inhomogeneous mixing of individuals in the population.

2.6 Exercises

A useful approach to these exercises, and indeed to much work in this area, is to complement analytical results with numerical methods. Here numerical methods include developing simulation code for the underlying stochastic models and numerical routines for calculating threshold parameters, properties of a large or small outbreak, etc. In addition to facilitating exploration of the behaviour of the model, these two numerical methods allow fairly reliable error checking: for example, if empirical estimates of the size of large outbreaks from simulations seem to converge to the approximate size one expects from asymptotic calculations (for a variety of different parameter values) then one can be fairly confident in the asymptotic analysis, the numerical implementation of it and the simulation code!

Exercise 2.6.1. Consider a simple version of the households model, with household size distribution $\alpha_1 = \frac{2}{3}$, $\alpha_2 = \frac{1}{3}$ (and $\alpha_i = 0$ for $i = 3, 4, 5, \ldots$) and a fixed infectious period of length 1.

For this model, calculate

(a) The value of the threshold parameter R_*.
(b) The Laplace transform of the severity of a single-household epidemic with specified household size, and thus the probability generating function of the offspring distribution for the branching process approximation of the early stages of the proliferation of infected households and an equation satisfied by $\sigma = 1 - \mathbb{P}(\text{major outbreak})$.
(c) The system of equations satisfied by the proportion of the population infected by a large outbreak, z, and the probability that each individual escapes global infection, π.
(d) The scaled gain matrix $G' = (G'_{nv})$ that results when a perfect vaccine is introduced into this model with infection rates $\lambda_G = 1.2$ and $\lambda_L = 3$; and hence a description of the optimal vaccine allocation policy.
(e) Determine an optimal vaccine allocation scheme if there is enough vaccine to cover 0.6 of the population. What is the effect of such a vaccination scheme on the epidemic?

Note that all necessary properties of within-household epidemics can be calculated using results from Chapter 1. However, with such small household sizes it is possible (and fairly straightforward) to derive them directly from their definitions and interpretations.

Exercise 2.6.2 (The highly locally infectious case).

Consider a special case of the households model where half of the households are of size 2 and the other half are of size 3; so $(\alpha_n, n = 1,2,\dots)$ satisfies $\alpha_2 = \alpha_3 = \frac{1}{2}$ and $\alpha_n = 0$ for all $n \neq 2,3$. Also suppose that $I \sim \mathrm{Exp}(\gamma)$, so that $\phi_I(\theta) = \mathbb{E}[\mathrm{e}^{-\theta I}] = \gamma/(\gamma+\theta)$. Assume that λ_G is fixed, but that the disease is *highly locally infectious.* This means that we consider the limit $\lambda_L \to \infty$. (This is a version of the model considered by Becker and Deitz [25].)

(a) State and justify the distribution (that is, the probability mass function) of $Z^{(n)}$, the final size (amongst the whole household; i.e. including any initial susceptibles who become infected *and* the initial infective) of an epidemic in a household of size n. Hint: think about $Z^{(n)}$ directly/intuitively, not in terms of Gontcharoff polynomials or other formulas.
(b) Hence (i) state the value of $\mu_n(\infty) = \lim_{\lambda_L \to \infty} \mu_n(\lambda_L)$ and (ii) find a formula for the threshold parameter R_* (it should depend on λ_G and γ only).
(c) Determine $m_n(\theta) = \lim_{\lambda_L \to \infty} \phi_{n-1,1}(1,\theta)$, the Laplace transform of the severity A_n of a single-household outbreak in a household of size n with $n-1$ initial susceptibles and 1 initial infective. Hint: look at the definition of severity and your answer to part (a).
(d) Hence find (i) a formula for $f_R(s)$, the probability generating function of the offspring distribution for the branching process approximation of the early stages of the proliferation of infected households, and (ii) an equation satisfied by $\sigma = 1 - \mathbb{P}(\text{major outbreak})$.
(e) For what values of (λ_G, γ) do we have this model including local infection supercritical, but the simpler model with global contacts only (which ignores within-household contacts) subcritical?

Exercise 2.6.3 (Vaccination in the highly locally infectious case). Consider introducing vaccination in the model of Exercise 2.6.2. Separately for each of the following vaccine action models, (i) determine a formula for the entries of the rescaled the gain matrix G', then (ii) taking $\lambda_G = 2$ and $\gamma = 1$, find G' numerically and interpret these results in terms of which 'types' of households should be the priority for vaccination.

(a) A perfect vaccine.
(b) An all-or-nothing vaccine with success probability $\frac{1}{2}$.
(c) A non-random vaccine with $a = b = 1/\sqrt{2}$.

(The latter two vaccine action models are comparable in the sense that they have the same value of the vaccine efficacy $1 - \mathbb{E}[AB]$, which is one possible high-level measure of vaccine effectiveness; see Becker et al. [24].)

(d) Show that with a leaky vaccine the optimal vaccine allocation concentrates vaccination in the largest households.

Exercise 2.6.4 (Self-isolation of the initial case in a household). Consider the following variant of the households model (which is quite similar to the "all-or-none case" discussed by Ball et al. [14, Section 5.2.1]) and similar in terms of mean behaviour to the approximation defined by Becker and Starczak [27, Equation (2)]). Suppose that with probability $\delta \in [0,1]$ the initial case in a household self-identifies their illness and completely isolates themself, so that they do not infect anyone else (locally or globally); otherwise (i.e. with probability $1-\delta$) the epidemic proceeds as usual.

(a) Determine a formula for a threshold parameter $R_* = \mathbb{E}[R]$ for this model, where R is defined as in Section 2.2.
(b) Determine a formula for f_R, analogous to (2.2.2). Use this to show that the chance of a major outbreak is bounded above by the corresponding probability when $\delta = 0$.

Chapter 3
A General Two-Level Mixing Model

In the households model analysed in Chapter 2, infectives make two types of infectious contacts: *local* contacts with individuals in their household and *global* contacts with individuals chosen uniformly at random from the whole population. This is an example of an epidemic in a population with two levels of mixing. We now define and analyse a general model for epidemics among populations that mix in this way. In Section 3.1, we define a general framework for such models and give a variety of examples that arise as special cases. In Section 3.2, we define the concepts of *local infectious clump* and *local susceptibility set*, which are crucial in analysing the early stages and final outcome of an epidemic in Sections 3.3 and 3.4, respectively. Finally, in Section 3.5, we illustrate the general theory by applying it to the above-mentioned special cases.

The chapter is long and can be read at different levels depending on the interest of the reader. A quick overview of the main results can be obtained by reading the model definition and special cases in Section 3.1, the definitions of local infectious clumps and susceptibility sets in Section 3.2 and the heuristic accounts of how they are used to analyse the early stages of an epidemic and the final outcome of a global epidemic (i.e. one that takes off) in Sections 3.3.2 and 3.4.1, respectively. The heuristic arguments are made rigorous in Sections 3.3.6 (early stages) and 3.4.2 (final outcome), respectively. These sections may be omitted by a reader who is not interested in detailed proofs, though the latter also contains a central limit theorem for the outcome of a global epidemic. We recommend that the reader reads at least the above (apart from the rigorous proofs) before turning to the analysis of the special cases in Section 3.5.

The early stages of an epidemic are analysed using an approximating branching process of local infectious clumps, which is a natural extension of the households model branching process of infected households, studied in Section 2.2, to the more general two-level mixing setting. As with the households model, the offspring mean of that branching process yields a threshold parameter R_* for the epidemic model. Suitable elaboration of that branching process leads to the definition of a basic reproduction number R_0 for the epidemic. The threshold parameter R_* is not an individual-based reproduction number, so typically $R_* \neq R_0$, though R_0 is also a threshold parameter and R_* takes the critical value one if and only if $R_0 = 1$. The

T. Britton, E. Pardoux (eds.), *Stochastic Epidemic Models with Inference*,
Lecture Notes in Mathematics 2255, https://doi.org/10.1007/978-3-030-30900-8_7

basic reproduction number R_0 is defined in Section 3.3.3 and its relation to the critical vaccination coverage for uniform vaccination with a perfect vaccine is studied in Section 3.3.4. A key finding is that the usual formula $1 - R_0^{-1}$ (cf. equation (1.4.1) on page 18 in Part I of this volume) yields only a lower bound for the critical vaccination coverage. Altering the time clock of the elaborated branching process enables the early exponential growth rate for an epidemic that takes off to be calculated; see Section 3.3.5. Readers interested in R_0, vaccination and early exponential growth rate for specific models should read these sections before studying the special cases in Section 3.5.

The presentation in Sections 3.3 and 3.4 is deliberately generic, with the aim of describing key concepts in a model-independent fashion. Thus Section 3.5 consists mainly of showing how the generic results are used to determine and calculate properties of epidemics in the various special cases. This is relatively straightforward for the standard SIR, households and great circle models but requires some further results for the households-workplaces and network with casual contacts models; see Exercise 3.5.7 and Lemma 3.5.19, respectively, the proofs of which may be omitted.

3.1 Definition and Examples

Consider a population $\mathcal{N} = \{1,2,\ldots,N\}$ of N individuals. Let $I_1, I_2, \ldots, I_N$ be i.i.d. copies of a non-negative random variable I, having an arbitrary but specified distribution; I_i is the length of individual i's infectious period if i becomes infected. For $i \in \mathcal{N}$, if individual i becomes infected then throughout its infectious period it makes *local* infectious contacts with individual j ($j \in \mathcal{N} \setminus \{i\}$) at the points of a Poisson process having rate λ_{ij}^L and *global* infectious contacts, with individuals chosen uniformly and independently from $\mathcal{N}$, at the points of a Poisson process having rate λ_G. If a contacted individual is susceptible then it is immediately able to infect other individuals. If a contacted individual is infective or recovered then nothing happens. Thus the model does not include an exposed period but incorporating an exposed period does not alter the distribution of the final outcome of the epidemic (cf. Remark 1.2.2 on page 127). An infective recovers at the end of its infectious period and is then immune to further infection. The epidemic is initiated by a number of individuals becoming infective at time $t = 0$, with the other individuals all being susceptible, and ends when there is no infective present if the population. Explicit assumptions about which individuals are initially infective are made as and when they are required. All infectious period random variables, all Poisson processes governing infective contacts and all uniform samplings for global contacts are mutually independent. We denote this model by E^N.

Note that the model is formulated so that it is possible for an individual to globally contact itself. This may appear odd but such contacts have no effect and their inclusion simplifies the analysis of the model. The key point is that the individual to individual global infection rate is λ_G/N. We analyse the limiting behaviour of the model as the population size $N \to \infty$. Observe that the distribution of the number of global contacts made by a typical infective is independent of N. The limiting results hold also if the global contact rate depends on N, say it is $\lambda_G^{(N)}$, and $\lambda_G^{(N)} \to \lambda_G$ as $N \to \infty$, though some require that the rate of convergence of $\lambda_G^{(N)}$ to λ_G is sufficiently fast. We do not consider that generalisation here and assume that λ_G is independent of N, which is sufficient for all practical purposes.

The local infection rates λ_{ij}^L $(i, j \in \mathcal{N}, i \neq j)$ reflect the structure of the population as the following special cases illustrate.

3.1.1 Standard SIR Model

If there is no local infection (i.e. $\lambda_{ij}^L = 0$ for all $i \neq j$) then the epidemic E^N is homogeneously mixing. The model E^N then reduces to the standard SIR epidemic model in Section 1.1 with $\lambda = \lambda_G/N$.

3.1.2 Households Model

Suppose that the population is partitioned into m households of size n, so $N = mn$, and that

$$\lambda_{ij}^L = \begin{cases} \lambda_H & \text{if } i \text{ and } j \text{ belong to the same household,} \\ 0 & \text{otherwise.} \end{cases}$$

Then E^N is the households model analysed in Section 2, but now with the restriction that the households all have the same size n. We are interested in the asymptotic situation where $m \to \infty$ with the household size n held fixed. We treat here just the case of equal household sizes, as it fits more easily into the general framework for E_N. The analysis can be extended to the case of unequal-sized households, as seen in Section 2.

3.1.3 Households-workplaces Model

Suppose that the population is partitioned into m_H households of size n_H and also into m_W workplaces of size n_W, so $m_H n_H = m_W n_W = N$. Thus each individual in the population belongs to precisely one household and precisely one workplace. Suppose also that

$$\lambda_{ij}^L = \begin{cases} \lambda_H & \text{if } i \text{ and } j \text{ belong to the same household,} \\ \lambda_W & \text{if } i \text{ and } j \text{ belong to the same workplace,} \\ \lambda_H + \lambda_W & \text{if } i \text{ and } j \text{ belong to the same household and the same workplace} \\ 0 & \text{otherwise.} \end{cases}$$

Hence infective individuals make two types of local contacts: household contacts, with individuals in their own household, and workplace contacts, with individuals in their own workplace. The model has its origins in Andersson [3, Section 6] (cf. Andersson [2]) and was analysed in Ball and Neal [15], where it is called the *overlapping groups* model; see also Pellis et al. [55, 54] and Ball et al. [19]. Of course the mixing groups need not be actual households and workplaces. They could for example be households and school classes. The model can be extended to include unequal-sized households and/or workplaces (note, for example, that allowing workplaces of size 1 means not everyone belongs to a workplace), and also to more that two local mixing groups.

We are interested in the asymptotic regime where the population size $N \to \infty$ with both the household size n_H and the workplace size n_W held fixed. In order to facilitate explicit asymptotic analysis, it is necessary to make strong assumptions about the configuration of households and workplaces as $N \to \infty$; specifically that the density of simple cycles of local contacts that are not either within the same household or within the same workplace tends to 0 as $N \to \infty$ (see Section 3.5.3 below). In particular this implies that the probability that two members of a given household have the same workplace tends to zero as $N \to \infty$.

3.1.4 Great Circle Model

In this model the N individuals are assumed to be equally spaced around a circle and local contacts are nearest-neighbour, so

$$\lambda_{ij}^{L} = \begin{cases} \lambda_L & \text{if } i-j = \pm 1 \text{ mod } N, \\ 0 & \text{otherwise.} \end{cases}$$

The model was motivated originally by the spread of infection between pigs in a line of stalls (M.C.M. de Jong, personal communication). It was introduced in Ball et al. [14] and analysed further in Ball and Neal [15]. The model is closely related to the 'small-world' model introduced by Watts and Strogatz [65], which has received much attention in the physics literature. The great circle model was extended by Ball and Neal [16] to include non-nearest-neighbour local contacts, though here we restrict attention to the nearest-neighbour case.

3.1.5 Network Model with Casual Contacts

As seen in Part III in this volume, in the past two decades there has been considerable interest in the analysis of models for epidemics on random graphs. The usual paradigm is that individuals in a population are nodes in an undirected random graph, $\mathscr{G}$ say, and are able to transmit infection only to their neighbours in $\mathscr{G}$. However, this does not allow for contacts outside a person's circle of social contacts, for example with people on a train or at a supermarket, and such casual contacts can have a significant impact on the spread of a disease. We include casual contacts by assuming that a given infective makes them at rate λ_G and that they are with individuals chosen independently and uniformly from the population. The model fits the general two-level-mixing framework with

$$\lambda_{ij}^L = \begin{cases} \lambda_L & \text{if } i \text{ and } j \text{ are neighbours in } \mathscr{G}, \\ 0 & \text{otherwise.} \end{cases} \tag{3.1.1}$$

Note that the households model is obtained by letting $\mathscr{G}$ be the union of m disjoint fully-connected cliques of size n and setting $\lambda_L = \lambda_H$. Also, the great circle model is obtained when $\mathscr{G}$ is a simple cycle of length N. We consider the case when $\mathscr{G}$ is a realisation of the configuration model; see Definition 1.2.5 on page 246 in Part III of this volume. The possibility of incorporating casual contacts into network models of epidemics is mentioned in the concluding comments of Diekmann et al. [31]. Kiss et al. [45] analyse an approximate deterministic model, which also includes degree-correlation. The model considered here was first analysed rigorously in Ball and Neal [17].

3.2 Local Infectious Clumps and Susceptibility Sets

Key tools in our asymptotic analysis of the epidemic E^N as $N \to \infty$ are local infectious clumps and local susceptibility sets, which we now define. Recall the random directed graph $\mathscr{G}_E$ defined for the standard SIR epidemic model in Section 1.2 on page 126. One can define a similar graph for the general two-level-mixing model E^N, in which the directed edges are also typed according to whether they correspond to a local or global contact. Thus now let $\mathscr{G}_E$ be a random directed graph with vertex set $\mathscr{N}$ in which for each $(i,j) \in \mathscr{N}^2$ there is a directed *local* edge from i to j if and only if i, if infected, contacts j locally and a directed *global* edge from i to j if and only if i, if infected, contacts j globally. (Note that there may be both a local and a global directed edge from i to j.)

Let $\mathscr{G}_L$ be the random directed graph obtained from $\mathscr{G}_E$ by deleting all global directed edges. For $(i,j) \in \mathscr{N}^2$, write $i \overset{\text{L}}{\rightsquigarrow} j$ if and only if there is a chain of directed edges in $\mathscr{G}_L$ from i to j, with the convention that $i \overset{\text{L}}{\rightsquigarrow} i$. For $i \in \mathscr{N}$, let

$$\mathscr{C}_i = \{j \in \mathscr{N} : i \overset{\text{L}}{\rightsquigarrow} j\}, \quad C_i = |\mathscr{C}_i| \quad \text{and} \quad A_i = \sum_{j \in \mathscr{C}_i} I_j. \tag{3.2.1}$$

Thus $\mathscr{C}_i$ is the set of individuals that are infected in the (local) epidemic in which there is only local contact and initially individual i is infective and all other individuals are susceptible; C_i and A_i are respectively the total size (including the initial infective) and severity of that local epidemic. We refer to $\mathscr{C}_i$ as i's *local infectious clump*.

For $i \in \mathcal{N}$, let

$$\mathcal{S}_i = \{j \in \mathcal{N} : j \overset{\mathrm{L}}{\rightsquigarrow} i\} \quad \text{and} \quad S_i = |\mathcal{S}_i|. \tag{3.2.2}$$

Thus, in the epidemic corresponding to the random graph directed $\mathcal{G}_E$, if any member of $\mathcal{S}_i$ becomes infected by a global contact then individual i will necessarily become infected by a chain of local contacts, possibly by a chain having length 0. We refer to $\mathcal{S}_i$ as i's *local susceptibility set*. With slight abuse of notation, we use $\mathcal{S}_i$ instead of $\mathcal{S}_{\{i\}}$.

Observe that in all of the special cases in Section 3.1, C_i $(i \in \mathcal{N})$ are identically distributed, as are A_i $(i \in \mathcal{N})$ and S_i $(i \in \mathcal{N})$; see Remark 3.5.18 on page 207 concerning the network model with casual contacts. Further, in the households model, the distributions of (C_i, A_i) and S_i are both independent of N (provided the household size n and the within-household infection rate λ_H do not depend N). This is not the case for the other special cases, so in general we write C_i, A_i and S_i as C_i^N, A_i^N and S_i^N, respectively, to show explicitly their dependence on N.

In the asymptotic analysis that follows we make the following assumptions concerning local infectious clumps and local susceptibility sets; $\xrightarrow{D}$ denotes convergence in distribution.

(A.1) For each N, the random vectors (C_i^N, A_i^N) $(i \in \mathcal{N})$ are identically distributed, according to (C^N, A^N) say. Further, there exists a random vector (C, A) such that
$$(C^N, A^N) \xrightarrow{D} (C, A) \quad \text{as} \quad N \to \infty. \tag{3.2.3}$$

(A.2) For each N, the random variables S_i^N $(i \in \mathcal{N})$ are identically distributed, according to S^N say. Further, there exists a random variable S such that
$$S^N \xrightarrow{D} S \quad \text{as} \quad N \to \infty. \tag{3.2.4}$$

It is immediate that these assumptions hold for the special cases of the standard SIR and households models, and easily seen that they hold for the households-workplaces model (subject to suitable assumptions concerning the configuration of households and workplaces), the great circle and the network model with casual contacts; see Section 3.5 below and also Remark 3.5.18 on page 207 concerning the network model with casual contacts.

Note that when $\mathbb{P}(I < \infty) = 1$, the random variables C, A and S are each finite (almost surely) in the great circle model but, depending on the parameters, they may have non-zero probability of being infinite in the households-workplaces model and the network model with casual contacts.

3.3 Early Stages of an Epidemic

3.3.1 Introduction

We consider the early stages of the epidemic E^N with few initial infectives and show that it can be approximated by a branching process, denoted by $\mathscr{B}$, of local infectious clumps. Heuristic arguments are given in Section 3.3.2, which use the branching process $\mathscr{B}$ to derive a threshold parameter R_*, which determines, in the limit as $N \to \infty$, whether a global outbreak (i.e. one infecting at least $\log N$ individuals) is possible and if so the probability of such an outbreak. The basic reproduction number R_0 for the epidemic E^N is defined in Section 3.3.3. Vaccination prior to an epidemic is considered in Section 3.3.4, where it is shown that if $R_* > 1$ and individuals are selected independently with probability v for vaccination with a perfect vaccine then the critical vaccination coverage v_c satisfies

$$1 - R_0^{-1} \leq v_c \leq 1 - R_*^{-1};$$

see Theorem 3.3.3. Note that the inequality $1 - R_0^{-1} \leq v_c$ can be strict, so the usual formula for the critical vaccination coverage (equation (1.4.1) on page 18 in Part I of this volume) may yield an underestimate. The early exponential growth rate of a global outbreak is studied in Section 3.3.5. Formal proofs that, as $N \to \infty$, the total size of E^N converges in distribution to the total number of 'individuals' (as opposed to clumps) in the branching process $\mathscr{B}$ and the probability that the total size of E^N is at least $\log N$ converges to the survival probability of $\mathscr{B}$ are given in Section 3.3.6.

3.3.2 Heuristics

The set of individuals that become infected during the epidemic E^N can be constructed using the random directed graph $\mathscr{G}_E$ as follows. To simplify the notation we do not index quantities by N. In the graph $\mathscr{G}_E$, write $i \xrightarrow{\mathrm{L}} j$ if there is a directed local edge from i to j, and $i \xrightarrow{\mathrm{G}} j$ if there a directed global edge from i to j. For simplicity, suppose that there is one initial infective which, without loss of generality, we assume is individual 1.

For $k = 1, 2, \ldots$, define sets $\mathscr{D}_k$ and $\mathscr{G}_k$ as follows. Let

$$\mathscr{D}_1 = \mathscr{G}_1 = \mathscr{C}_1, \tag{3.3.1}$$

and, for $k = 2, 3, \ldots$, let

$$\mathscr{K}_{k-1} = \{i \in \mathscr{N} \setminus \mathscr{G}_{k-1} : j \xrightarrow{\mathrm{G}} i \text{ for some } j \in \mathscr{D}_{k-1}\}, \tag{3.3.2}$$

$$\mathscr{D}_k = \left(\bigcup_{i \in \mathscr{K}_{k-1}} \mathscr{C}_i \right) \cap \mathscr{G}_{k-1}^c, \tag{3.3.3}$$

$$\mathscr{G}_k = \mathscr{G}_{k-1} \cup \mathscr{D}_k, \tag{3.3.4}$$

where ^{c} denotes set complement.

In words, the above iteration is as follows. It starts by forming the local infectious clump of individual 1. Members of that clump are necessarily infected by the epidemic E^N. Then, setting $k = 2$ in (3.3.2)–(3.3.4), it determines which individuals not in that clump are contacted globally by a member of that clump, to give $\mathscr{K}_1$. All individuals in the local infectious clumps of members of $\mathscr{K}_1$ are necessarily infected by the epidemic E^N; so $\mathscr{D}_2$ is the set of individuals in those clumps which are not in $\mathscr{C}_1$ (the latter have already been infected in the construction of the epidemic) and $\mathscr{G}_2$ is the set of all individuals infected so far in the construction. The construction then proceeds in the obvious fashion. It is determined which individuals are contacted globally by members $\mathscr{D}_2$ and then which individuals are in the local infectious clumps of such globally contacted individuals, and so on. This iteration terminates after a finite number of steps since N is finite. Let $k^* = \min\{k : \mathscr{G}_k = \mathscr{G}_{k-1}\}$. Then $\mathscr{G}_{k^*}$ is the set of all individuals that are infected during the epidemic E^N.

Now suppose that N is large and consider first the case when $\mathbb{P}(C < \infty) = 1$. Then, since global contacts are with individuals chosen uniformly at random from the population $\mathscr{N}$, in the early stages of the iteration given by (3.3.1)–(3.3.4), it is unlikely that the local infectious clump of a globally contacted individual will intersect with a local infectious clump used previously in the iteration. It follows that the process of local infectious clumps can be approximated by a Galton–Watson branching process (see Appendix A.1.1 of Part I in this volume), $\mathscr{B}^N$ say, in which individuals are (local infectious) clumps and the number of offspring of a typical individual is the number of global contacts that emanate from the corresponding clump.

Let R^N denote the offspring random variable of the branching process $\mathscr{B}^N$. Then, conditional upon A^N, R^N has an independent Poisson distribution with mean $\lambda_G A^N$, since individuals make global contacts at the points of independent Poisson processes, each having rate λ_G, throughout their infectious periods. We denote this distribution by $\mathrm{Poi}(\lambda_G A^N)$. Thus, if $X \sim \mathrm{Poi}(\lambda_G A^N)$, then $\mathbb{P}(X = k) = \mathbb{E}[(\lambda_G A^N)^k \exp(-\lambda_G A^N)/k!]$ $(k = 0, 1, \ldots)$ and we say that X has a mixed-Poisson distribution with mean $\lambda_G A^N$. Now $A^N \xrightarrow{D} A$ as $N \to \infty$, so $\mathscr{B}^N$ converges in distribution to a branching process, $\mathscr{B}$ say, as $N \to \infty$, where $\mathscr{B}$ has offspring random variable $R \sim \mathrm{Poi}(\lambda_G A)$. Thus, for large N, we can approximate the early stages of the epidemic E^N (on a clump basis – see Section 3.3.3) by the branching process $\mathscr{B}$.

For the present, we say that a *global outbreak* occurs if in the limit as $N \to \infty$ the epidemic infects infinitely many individuals (i.e. contains infinitely many clumps, as $\mathbb{P}(C < \infty) = 1$). Thus a global outbreak occurs if and only if the branching process $\mathscr{B}$ does not go extinct. This definition of a global outbreak is not fully satisfactory, as it requires $N \to \infty$ and in any practical setting N is finite. We show in Section 3.3.6 below that the current definition is asymptotically equivalent to defining a global outbreak as one which infects at least $\log N$ individuals. Moreover, $\log N$ can be replaced by εN, where $\varepsilon > 0$ depends on the parameters of the epidemic E^N.

Let $R_* = \mathbb{E}[R]$ and $f_R(s) = \mathbb{E}[s^R]$ $(0 \le s \le 1)$ be respectively the mean and probability-generating function of R. Now by the dominated convergence theorem, for $0 \le s \le 1$,

$$\begin{aligned} f_R(s) &= \lim_{N\to\infty} \mathbb{E}[s^{R^N}] \\ &= \lim_{N\to\infty} \mathbb{E}[\mathbb{E}[s^{R^N}|A^N]] \\ &= \lim_{N\to\infty} \mathbb{E}[\mathrm{e}^{-\lambda_G(1-s)A^N}] \qquad \left[\text{as } R^N|A^N \sim \mathrm{Poi}(\lambda_G A^N)\right] \\ &= \phi_A(\lambda_G(1-s)) \qquad \left[\text{since } A^N \xrightarrow{D} A \text{ as } N\to\infty\right], \end{aligned}$$

where $\phi_A(\theta) = \mathbb{E}[\exp(-\theta A)]$ $(\theta \ge 0)$ is the Laplace transform of A.

To determine R_*, observe using the third equation in (3.2.1) that

$$\mathbb{E}[A_1^N] = \mathbb{E}\left[\sum_{i\in\mathscr{N}} I_i 1_{\{i\in\mathscr{C}_1^N\}}\right] = \sum_{i\in\mathscr{N}} \mathbb{E}\left[I_i 1_{\{i\in\mathscr{C}_1^N\}}\right].$$

Now the event $\{i \in \mathscr{C}_1^N\}$ is independent of i's infectious period I_i, so

$$\mathbb{E}\left[I_i 1_{\{i\in\mathscr{C}_1^N\}}\right] = \mu_I \mathbb{P}(i \in \mathscr{C}_1^N),$$

where $\mu_I = \mathbb{E}[I]$, whence

$$\mathbb{E}[A_1^N] = \mu_I \sum_{i\in\mathscr{N}} \mathbb{P}(i \in \mathscr{C}_1^N) = \mu_I \mu_C^N,$$

where $\mu_C^N = \mathbb{E}[C^N]$. Recall that $R^N \sim \mathrm{Poi}(\lambda_G A^N)$. Thus, conditioning on A^N,

$$\mathbb{E}[R^N] = E[E[R^N|A^N]] = E[\lambda_G A^N] = \lambda_G \mu_I \mu_C^N.$$

We suppose further that C^N is stochastically increasing in N, i.e. $C^{N+1} \overset{\text{st}}{\ge} C^N$ for $N = 1, 2, \ldots$. (The random variable X is stochastically greater than the random variable Y, written $X \overset{\text{st}}{\ge} Y$, if

$$\mathbb{P}(X > a) \ge \mathbb{P}(Y > a) \quad \text{for all } a \in \mathbb{R};$$

see, for example, Ross [59, page 251].) This is shown easily for the special cases described in Section 3.1. Then the monotone convergence theorem implies that $\mu_C^N \uparrow \mu_C = \mathbb{E}[C]$ as $N \to \infty$; note that μ_C may be infinity. Hence,

$$R_* = \lambda_G \mu_I \mu_C. \tag{3.3.5}$$

By standard branching process theory (for example, Jagers [42, Theorem 2.3.1]; see Proposition A.1.1 on page 98 in Part I of this volume) a global outbreak occurs with strictly positive probability if and only if $R_* > 1$ and the probability that a global outbreak occurs is $1 - p_{\text{ext}}$, where p_{ext} is the smallest solution of $f_R(s) = s$ in $[0, 1]$.

The above arguments extend in the natural way to the case when $\mathbb{P}(C < \infty) < 1$. In that case a global outbreak is possible in the model with only local infection (i.e. with $\lambda_G = 0$). The process of infected clumps is still approximated by the branching process $\mathscr{B}$ but now the offspring random variable R of $\mathscr{B}$ has a strictly positive mass at infinity.

3.3.3 The Basic Reproduction Number R_0

The quantity R_* is sometimes called the clump-to-clump reproduction number, or simply the clump reproduction number. It is a threshold parameter for the epidemic E^N in that it determines whether a global epidemic can occur in the limit as $N \to \infty$. However, it does have some limitations, which are discussed by Pellis et al. [55] in the context of the households-workplaces model. First, R_* can be infinite; see, for example, the analyses of the households-workplaces model and the network model with casual contacts in Sections 3.5.3 and 3.5.5 below. In that case it is completely uninformative about how much effort (for example, by vaccination) is required to bring the epidemic below threshold. Secondly, when very large and even infinite clumps are possible, the time taken for a clump to form (when considering the epidemic in real time) can be very long and indeed comparable with the duration of the whole epidemic. Thirdly, R_* cannot generally be related to a critical vaccination coverage when a fraction of the population, chosen uniformly at random, is vaccinated with a perfect vaccine (i.e. one that necessarily renders the recipient immune to infection) prior to an epidemic. A fourth limitation of R_*, not discussed in Pellis et al. [55], is that it can be misleading when comparing different models as it is a clump-to-clump reproduction number and two models may have rather different distributions of clump size. For an example, see Figure 7 in Ball et al. [21], which is concerned with a network model that also incorporates household structure. The household structure induces clustering in the network, which normally slows down disease transmission; indeed, in this example, both the probability and size of a major epidemic decrease with clustering but R_* initially increases as clustering is introduced into the model.

The basic reproduction number R_0 is probably the most important quantity in epidemic theory. It determines whether or not an epidemic with few initial infectives in a large population can become established and lead to a large epidemic and, for a wide range of models, if $R_0 > 1$ then the critical vaccination coverage (with a vaccine that guarantees immunity) to prevent a large epidemic is given by $1 - R_0^{-1}$ (see equation (1.4.1) on page 18 in Part I of this volume). For many models, R_0 can be defined informally as 'the expected number of secondary cases produced by a typical infected individual during its entire infectious period, in a population consisting otherwise of susceptibles only'; see, for example, Heesterbeek and Dietz [40] and Heesterbeek [39]. However, for structured population models like those in this chapter it is far from clear how to define a typical infected individual. For example, in the households model, the initial infective in a household has more susceptibles in their household to which to transmit infection than subsequent infectives in that household. The above informal definition also needs modifying slightly for many epidemic models on networks (see, for example, Section 2.2 of Part III in this volume), since the initial infective is usually atypical, as its degree distribution is different from those of subsequent infectives. Consequently it is appropriate to consider a typical non-initial infective (in the early stages of an epidemic), for whom the population does not otherwise consist of susceptibles alone as that individual's infector is not susceptible. Several individual-based reproduction numbers have been proposed for the households model (see Ball et al. [19, Section 2] and the references therein). A definition for R_0 for epidemic models with households and other social structures was introduced by Pellis et al. [54]. We introduce and motivate this definition; show how this definition of R_0 and its calculation extend to the two-level mixing model of this chapter; and discuss both the comparison of R_0 with R_* and, in Section 3.3.4 below, its relationship to the above critical vaccination coverage.

A key component of this definition of R_0 is the generation of an infective individual. Consider the directed random graph representation $\mathscr{G}_E$ of the epidemic E^N (see page 127). As above, suppose that there is one initial infective, who is individual 1. The initial infective belongs to generation 0. For any other individual infected by the epidemic, i say, its generation is given by the length of (number of edges in) the shortest chain of directed edges (allowing for both global and local edges) from 1 to i in $\mathscr{G}_E$. Thus generation 0 consists of just individual 1, generation 1 consists of those individuals with whom the initial infective has at least one infectious contact (either local or global), generation 2 consists of those individuals that are contacted by at least one generation-1 infective but not by the initial infective, and so on. For $k=0,1,\ldots$, let $Y_k^{(N)}$ be the number of generation-k infectives in E^N.

Consider the standard SIR epidemic model so, in the setting of E^N, the clumps all have size 1. The branching process $\mathscr{B}$ is a branching process of infective individuals and its offspring mean $R_* = \lambda_G \mu_I$ coincides with R_0. By standard branching process, for $k=0,1,\ldots$, the mean size of the kth generation of $\mathscr{B}$ is R_0^k and, for large N, this approximates the mean number of generation-k infectives in the epidemic E^N. More precisely, using the coupling argument of Ball and Donnelly [9] and the dominated convergence theorem,

$$\lim_{N\to\infty} \mathbb{E}\left[Y_k^{(N)}\right] = R_0^k \qquad (k=0,1,\ldots).$$

Thus, for the standard SIR epidemic model, R_0 is the geometric rate of growth of the approximating branching process $\mathscr{B}$. Note that R_0 is also given by

$$R_0 = \lim_{k\to\infty}\lim_{N\to\infty}\left(\mathbb{E}\left[Y_k^{(N)}\right]\right)^{\frac{1}{k}}. \tag{3.3.6}$$

The outer limit in (3.3.6) is superfluous for the standard SIR epidemic model, since the sequence is independent of k, but the definition (3.3.6) of R_0 extends to more complicated models, such as multitype SIR epidemics where R_0 given by (3.3.6) agrees with that given by the usual definition as the maximum eigenvalue of the mean next-generation matrix. In particular, Pellis et al. [54] use (3.3.6) to define R_0 for models with small mixing groups such as households. The definition (3.3.6) also extends to the general two-level-mixing model E^N, assuming that the assumptions leading to the approximating branching process $\mathscr{B}$ are satisfied and that the probability law of the generation structure of a typical clump $\mathscr{C}_i^N$ is independent of i and converges suitably as $N \to \infty$.

To calculate R_0 for the epidemic E^N, recall that individuals in $\mathscr{B}$ correspond to infectious clumps in E^N and suppose that the time of the birth of an infectious clump is given by the generation of the initial case in that clump, so a typical individual in $\mathscr{B}$ reproduces only at ages $1, 2, \ldots$. (To ease the presentation we treat the limiting branching process $\mathscr{B}$ directly, rather than considering $\mathscr{B}_N$ and letting $N \to \infty$, and leave the technicalities required to make the argument fully rigorous to the interested reader.) Consider the local infectious clump $\mathscr{C}_i$ of a typical individual i. Individual i is said to have clump generation 0. Individuals contacted locally by i are said to have clump generation 1, and so on. Thus the clump generation of an individual $j \in \mathscr{C}_i$ is the length of the shortest chain of directed edges from i to j in the random graph $\mathscr{G}_L$ defined in Section 3.2.

Consider a typical individual in $\mathscr{B}$, i.e. a typical local infectious clump, $\mathscr{C}_i$ say. Then, with time given by generation, the global contacts made by the ancestor i of the clump occur when the clump has age 1 and, for $j \in \mathscr{C}_i$, the global contacts made by individual j occur when the clump has age $g_C(j)+1$, where $g_C(j)$ is the clump generation of individual j. For $k = 0, 1, \ldots$, let μ_k^C be the mean number of individuals in generation k of $\mathscr{C}_i$. Thus $\mu_0^C = 1$ and $\mu_C = \sum_{k=0}^{\infty} \mu_k^C$. Then, in $\mathscr{B}$, for $k = 1, 2, \ldots$, the mean number of offspring produced by an individual at age k is $\nu_k = \lambda_G \mu_I \mu_{k-1}^C$. It follows that the asymptotic (Malthusian) geometric growth rate of $\mathscr{B}$ is given by the unique positive solution of the discrete-time Lotka–Euler equation

$$\sum_{k=1}^{\infty} \frac{\nu_k}{\lambda^k} = 1; \tag{3.3.7}$$

see, for example, Haccou et al. [37, Section 3.3.1] adapted to the discrete-time setting. Thus, using (3.3.7), R_0 satisfies $g_0(R_0) = 0$, where

$$g_0(\lambda) = 1 - \lambda_G \mu_I \sum_{k=0}^{\infty} \frac{\mu_k^C}{\lambda^{k+1}} \qquad (\lambda \in (0,\infty)). \tag{3.3.8}$$

Now g_0 is strictly increasing on $(0,\infty)$ and $\lim_{\lambda \downarrow 0} g_0(\lambda) = -\infty$, so g_0 has either one or zero roots in $(0,\infty)$. In the former case then R_0 is given by that root, otherwise $R_0 = \infty$. The basic reproduction R_0 is finite for most models. If $R_0 = \infty$ then a clump must grow faster than geometrically on a generation basis. This happens in the network model with casual contacts if the degree distribution has infinite variance, see Section 3.5.5.4 below.

3.3.4 Uniform Vaccination

We now consider vaccination prior to the arrival of an epidemic; cf. Section 1.4 of Part I in this volume. Suppose that $R_* > 1$ and individuals in the population are vaccinated with a perfect vaccine independently, each with probability v. (A perfect vaccine is one which necessarily renders its recipient immune to infection.) Thus the (expected) vaccination coverage is v. Let $R_*(v)$ be the post-vaccination clump reproduction number and let v_c solve $R_*(v_c) = 1$, so v_c is the corresponding critical vaccination coverage. The notation v (and v_c) is consistent with that used in Section 1.4 of Part I in this volume. It differs from the notation in Section 2.4.1, where vaccine coverage is denoted by c and v denotes the number of individuals vaccinated in a household. The perfect vaccine-associated reproduction number R_V is defined by

$$R_V = \frac{1}{1-v_c}; \tag{3.3.9}$$

cf. Goldstein et al. [34], where it was introduced in the setting of the households model. Note from (3.3.9) that

$$v_c = 1 - \frac{1}{R_V}.$$

Thus, R_V is defined so that the formula for the critical vaccination coverage v_c parallels that for a homogeneously mixing population; cf. equation (1.4.1) on page 18 in Part I of this volume.

Remark 3.3.1. Note that choosing individuals uniformly at random for vaccination may not be optimal in the general two-level-mixing model, as demonstrated for the households model in Section 2.4.3. Indeed for most two-level-mixing models it is suboptimal.

Remark 3.3.2. Note that if $v_c = 1$, i.e. it is impossible to reduce the threshold parameter R_* to 1 by vaccination unless essentially the whole population is vaccinated, then $R_V = \infty$. This is the case for both the SIR epidemic on a configuration model random graph (see Section 2.6 of Part III in this volume) and the network model with casual contacts (see Section 3.5.5.4 below), when the degree distribution has infinite variance.

The following theorem compares R_*, R_0 and R_V; cf. Ball et al. [19, Theorems 1 and 3], which make similar comparisons for the households and households-workplaces models, respectively, and include other reproduction numbers not considered here. Following Ball et al. [19], we call an epidemic *growing* if $R_* > 1$ and *declining* if $R_* < 1$. Note that $R_V = 1$ if $R_* = 1$ and R_V is not defined for a declining epidemic. We adopt the convention that $\infty \geq \infty$.

Theorem 3.3.3.

(a) $R_* = 1 \iff R_0 = 1 \implies R_V = 1$.
(b) In a growing epidemic,

$$R_* \geq R_V \geq R_0 > 1,$$

and in a declining epidemic

$$R_* \leq R_0 < 1.$$

The inequalities $R_* \geq R_V$ *and* $R_* \leq R_0$ *are strict if* $\mathbb{P}(C > 1) > 0$.

Proof. First note that

$$g_0(1) = 1 - \lambda_G \mu_I \sum_{k=0}^{\infty} \mu_k^C = 1 - \lambda_G \mu_I \mu_C = 1 - R_*, \tag{3.3.10}$$

and part (a) follows, since $R_0 = 1$ if and only if $g_0(1) = 0$. In a growing epidemic, (3.3.10) implies that $g_0(1) < 0$, so $R_0 > 1$ as $g_0(R_0) = 0$ and g_0 is increasing on $(0, \infty)$. Similarly, in a declining epidemic, (3.3.10) implies that $g_0(1) > 0$, whence $R_0 < 1$.

Suppose that $R_* < 1$. Then,

$$\begin{aligned} g_0(R_*) &= 1 - \lambda_G \mu_I \sum_{k=0}^{\infty} \frac{\mu_k^C}{R_*^{k+1}} \\ &\leq 1 - \lambda_G \mu_I \sum_{k=0}^{\infty} \frac{\mu_k^C}{R_*} \\ &= 1 - \frac{\lambda_G \mu_I \mu_C}{R_*} \\ &= 0, \end{aligned} \tag{3.3.11}$$

so $R_0 \geq R_*$ as $g_0(R_0) = 0$ and g_0 is increasing on $(0, \infty)$. Further, the inequality (3.3.11) is strict if $\mathbb{P}(C > 1) > 0$, since then $\sum_{k=1}^{\infty} \mu_k^C > 0$, so in that case $R_0 > R_*$.

Turning to the inequalities involving R_V, clearly $R_* \geq R_V$ if $R_* = \infty$, so suppose that $R_* \in (1, \infty)$ and individuals in the population are vaccinated independently with probability v, where $v > 0$. The early stages of the epidemic can then be approximated by a branching process, $\mathscr{B}(v)$ say, defined analogously to $\mathscr{B}$ except the probability that a global contact is with an unvaccinated individual, and hence leads to a new clump, is $1 - v$. Also, if $\mathscr{C}(v)$ denotes a typical post-vaccination local infectious clump and $C(v) = |\mathscr{C}(v)|$, then $C \overset{\text{st}}{\geq} C(v)$, since a realisation of $\mathscr{C}(v)$ can be obtained from one of $\mathscr{C}$ by vaccinating members of $\mathscr{C}$, apart from the initial case, independently with probability v. The clump $\mathscr{C}(v)$ then consists of the initial case, i_0 say, in $\mathscr{C}$ together with all other unvaccinated $j \in \mathscr{C}$ with the property that there exists a chain of directed edges from i_0 to j in the underlying graph $\mathscr{G}_L$ used to construct $\mathscr{C}$ that involves only unvaccinated individuals. Hence, $\mu_{C(v)} \leq \mu_C$, where $\mu_{C(v)} = \mathbb{E}[C(v)]$. Let $R_*(v)$ denote the post-vaccination clump reproduction number, i.e. the mean of the offspring distribution of $\mathscr{B}(v)$. Then

$$\begin{aligned} R_*(v) &= (1 - v)\lambda_G \mu_I \mu_{C(v)} && (3.3.12) \\ &\leq (1 - v)\lambda_G \mu_I \mu_C && (3.3.13) \\ &= (1 - v)R_*. \end{aligned}$$

Hence, using (3.3.9) and (3.3.13),

$$1 = R_*(v_c) \leq \frac{R_*}{R_V},$$

whence $R_V \leq R_*$. The inequality (3.3.13) is strict if $\mathbb{P}(C > 1) > 0$, since then there is strictly positive probability that at least one member of $\mathscr{C}$ is vaccinated, so in that case $R_V < R_*$.

To show that $R_V \geq R_0$ in a growing epidemic, suppose first that $R_0 \in (1,\infty)$ and, as before, that individuals in the population are vaccinated independently with probability v, where $v > 0$, and let $\mathscr{C}(v)$ denote a typical post-vaccination local infectious clump. For $k = 0,1,\ldots$, let $\mu_k^C(v)$ be the mean number individuals in clump generation k of $\mathscr{C}(v)$. An infective in the clump $\mathscr{C}(v)$ makes successful global contacts (i.e. that lead to a new infective) at rate $\lambda_G(1-v)$, since a fraction v of global contacts are with vaccinated individuals. Thus, in $\mathscr{B}(v)$, the mean number of offspring produced by an individual at age k is $\nu_k(v) = \lambda_G(1-v)\mu_I\mu_{k-1}^C(v)$, so (cf. (3.3.7) and (3.3.8)) the post-vaccination basic reproduction number, $R_0(v)$ say, is given by the unique root in $(0,\infty)$ of $g_{0,v}$, where

$$g_{0,v}(\lambda) = 1 - \lambda_G(1-v)\mu_I \sum_{k=0}^{\infty} \frac{\mu_k^C(v)}{\lambda^{k+1}} \qquad (\lambda \in (0,\infty)).$$

As in the proof of $R_V \leq R_*$, construct a realisation of $\mathscr{C}(v)$ by first constructing a realisation of $\mathscr{C}$ and then vaccinating members of that clump, apart from the initial case, independently with probability v. Recall that i_0 is the initial case in $\mathscr{C}$, and hence also in $\mathscr{C}(v)$. For $k = 1,2,\ldots$, individual $j \in \mathscr{C} \setminus \{i_0\}$ has clump generation k in $\mathscr{C}$ if and only if there exists at least one chain of length k from i_0 to j in (the graph $\mathscr{G}_L$ underlying) $\mathscr{C}$, and there is no shorter chain from i_0 to j. Suppose j has clump generation k in $\mathscr{C}$. Then there is a path of length k from i_0 to j in $\mathscr{C}$ and individual j also has clump generation k in $\mathscr{C}(v)$ if both j and that path is retained in $\mathscr{C}(v)$, the probability of which is $(1-v)^k$ as all k members of that path, excluding i_0, must not be vaccinated. Hence,

$$\mu_k^C(v) \geq (1-v)^k \mu_k^C \qquad (k = 0,1,\ldots). \tag{3.3.14}$$

(The inequality (3.3.14) holds trivially when $k = 0$, since $\mu_0^C(v) = \mu_0^C = 1$.)

Let $v_* = 1 - R_0^{-1}$. Then,

$$\begin{aligned}
g_{0,v_*}(1) &= 1 - \lambda_G(1-v_*)\mu_I \sum_{k=0}^{\infty} \mu_k^C(v_*) \\
&\leq 1 - \lambda_G\mu_I \sum_{k=0}^{\infty} (1-v_*)^{k+1}\mu_k^C \qquad \text{[using (3.3.14)]} \\
&= 1 - \lambda_G\mu_I \sum_{k=0}^{\infty} \frac{\mu_k^C}{R_0^{k+1}} \\
&= g_0(R_0) \\
&= 0,
\end{aligned}$$

using the definition of R_0. Hence, $R_0(v_*) \geq 1$, since $g_{0,v_*}(R_0(v_*)) = 0$ and g_{0,v_*} is strictly increasing on $(0,\infty)$. Therefore, the critical vaccination coverage v_c is at least v_*, so

$$1 - \frac{1}{R_V} \geq 1 - \frac{1}{R_0} \iff R_V \geq R_0.$$

Finally, suppose that $R_0 = \infty$, so $g_0(\lambda) < 0$ for all $\lambda \in (0,\infty)$. Now, for any $v \in (0,1)$, (3.3.14) implies that

$$\begin{aligned} g_{0,v}(\lambda) &\leq 1 - \lambda_G \mu_I \sum_{k=0}^{\infty} (1-v)^{k+1} \frac{\mu_k^C}{\lambda^{k+1}} \\ &= g_0(\lambda/(1-v)) \\ &< 0, \end{aligned}$$

so $R_0(v) > 1$, whence $v_c \geq v$. It follows that $v_c = 1$ and hence that $R_V = \infty$, so $R_V \geq R_0$. □

Remark 3.3.4 (Condition for $R_V = R_0$). Observe from the above proof that, unless they are both infinite, $R_V = R_0$ if and only if there is equality in (3.3.14), i.e. if and only if

$$\mu_k^C(v) = (1-v)^k \mu_k^C \qquad (v \in (0,1), k = 0,1,\ldots), \tag{3.3.15}$$

otherwise $R_V > R_0$. Further a necessary and sufficient condition for (3.3.15) to hold is that, for $k = 1,2,\ldots$, the probability of there being more than one (self-avoiding) path of length k from i_0 to an individual j in $\mathscr{C}$ is zero. Note that (3.3.15) is satisfied in the great circle model (cf. Exercise 3.5.14) and also in the network model with casual contacts if the network is constructed via the configuration model, so for both of those models the critical vaccination coverage v_c is given by the usual formula $1 - R_0^{-1}$. However, it is not satisfied in the households and the households-workplaces models, unless all households and also all workplaces in the latter model have size at most 3. Thus for these models vaccinating a fraction $1 - R_0^{-1}$ of the population uniformly at random is insufficient to be sure of preventing a global outbreak.

Remark 3.3.5 (Bounds for R_V and v_c). Theorem 3.3.3 shows that $1 - R_0^{-1}$ and $1 - R_*^{-1}$ are respectively lower and upper bounds for the critical vaccination coverage v_c. Sharper upper bounds than $1 - R_*^{-1}$ for v_c for the households and households-workplaces models are given in Ball et al. [19].

3.3.5 Exponential Growth Rate

Recall the branching process $\mathscr{B}$ of local infectious clumps, which approximates the early stages of the epidemic E^N. Let $\mathscr{B}_R$ be the corresponding branching process run in real time. In the graph $\mathscr{G}_L$ defined in Section 3.2, attach to each directed edge $i \to j$ a weight W_{ij} giving the time elapsing after i's infection before i makes local contact with j; cf. Remark 1.2.1 on page 127. The weighted graph, together with the infectious periods $I_1, I_2, \ldots, I_N$, is sufficient to reconstruct the development of the local infectious clump $\mathscr{C}_1^N$ in real time.

Suppose that the clump $\mathscr{C}_1^N$ is initiated by individual 1 becoming infected at time $t = 0$. For $t \geq 0$, let $Y_1^N(t)$ be the number of infectives in $\mathscr{C}_1^N$ at time t. As usual, we assume that, for $t \geq 0$, there exists a random variable $Y_1(t)$ such that $Y_1^N(t) \xrightarrow{D} Y_1(t)$

and $\mu_Y^N(t) \to \mu_Y(t)$ as $N \to \infty$, where $\mu_Y^N(t) = \mathbb{E}[Y_1^N(t)]$ and $\mu_Y(t) = \mathbb{E}[Y_1(t)]$. The process $\mathscr{B}_R$ is a general (or Crump-Mode-Jagers) branching process. For $t \geq 0$, a typical individual (i.e. clump) in $\mathscr{B}_R$ having age t, reproduces at mean rate $\lambda_G \mu_Y(t)$, so the Malthusian parameter, r say, of $\mathscr{B}_R$ is given by the unique solution in $(-\infty, \infty)$ of

$$\int_0^\infty \lambda_G \mathrm{e}^{-rt} \mu_Y(t)\, \mathrm{d}t = 1. \tag{3.3.16}$$

The asymptotic theory of counts associated with supercritical general branching processes (see Haccou et al. [37, Chapter 6]) implies that, if $R_* > 1$ and $\mathscr{B}_R$ does not go extinct, the total number of infective individuals (as opposed to clumps) in $\mathscr{B}_R$ asymptotically grows exponentially at rate r. Thus, in the limit as $N \to \infty$, the early exponential growth rate of the epidemic E_N in the event of a global outbreak is given by r.

Note that

$$\int_0^\infty \mu_Y(t)\, \mathrm{d}t = \mathbb{E}[A] = \mu_I \mu_C,$$

so $w_G(t) = (\mu_I \mu_C)^{-1} \mu_Y(t)$ $(t \geq 0)$ may be interpreted as the probability density function of a random variable, W_G say. Let $\phi_{W_G}(\theta) = \mathbb{E}[\mathrm{e}^{-\theta W_G}]$ $(\theta \in (-\infty, \infty))$ be the Laplace transform of W_G. (For a function $f : [0, \infty) \to [0, \infty)$, we denote its Laplace transform by ϕ_f and for ease of notation we give the domain of ϕ_f as $(-\infty, \infty)$, though usually the domain is (θ_f, ∞), where θ_f depends on f, as the integral is infinite for $\theta \leq \theta_f$.) Recall that $R_* = \lambda_G \mu_I \mu_C$. It follows from (3.3.16) that

$$R_* = \frac{1}{\phi_{W_G}(r)}. \tag{3.3.17}$$

The practical usefulness of (3.3.17) is discussed in Section 3.5.1 below.

3.3.6 Formal Results and Proofs

In this section, we prove that the total size of the epidemic E^N converges in distribution to the total number of 'individuals' (as opposed to clumps) in the branching process $\mathscr{B}$ as $N \to \infty$ (Theorem 3.3.6) and also a result (Theorem 3.3.7) which includes as a special case that, as $N \to \infty$, the probability that the total size of E^N is at least $\log N$ tends to the survival probability of the branching process $\mathscr{B}$.

Consider the epidemic E^N. For $i \in \mathscr{N}$, let $\mathscr{C}_i^N$ denote the local infectious clump of individual i, $C_i^N = |\mathscr{C}_i^N|$ and

$$R_i^N = \sum_{j \in \mathscr{C}_i^N} \tilde{R}_j^N, \tag{3.3.18}$$

where $\tilde{R}_j^N$ is the number of attempted global contacts that emanate from individual j in E^N. Thus $R_i^N \sim \mathrm{Poi}(\lambda_G A_i^N)$, where $A_i^N = \sum_{j \in \mathscr{C}_i^N} I_j$ is the severity of the clump $\mathscr{C}_i^N$. In addition to assumption (A.1) on 164, we make the following assumptions concerning local infectious clumps.

(A.3) For each N, the random vectors (C_i^N, R_i^N) $(i \in \mathcal{N})$ are identically distributed, according to (C^N, R^N) say. Further, there exists a random vector (C, R) such that $(C^N, R^N) \xrightarrow{D} (C, R)$ as $N \to \infty$. As in Section 3.3.2, we allow the possibility that $\mathbb{P}(C < \infty) < 1$, in which case $\mathbb{P}(R < \infty) < 1$.

(A.4) For each N and $i = 2, 3, \dots, N$, a realisation of $\mathcal{C}_i^N$ can be obtained from one of $\mathcal{C}_1^N$.

(A.5) For each N, $k = 2, 3, \dots, N$ and any given set $F \subseteq \mathcal{N}$ with $|F| = k$, if J is uniformly distributed on $\mathcal{N}$ independently of $\mathcal{C}_i^N$ $(i \in \mathcal{N})$ then

$$\mathbb{P}(F \cap \mathcal{C}_J^N \neq \emptyset | C_J^N) \leq \frac{kC_J^N}{N}. \tag{3.3.19}$$

It is immediate that Assumption (A.3) holds for the special cases of the standard SIR model and the households model. We indicate how to prove that it holds for the other special cases described in Section 3.1 when we analyse them in Section 3.5 below. It is easily shown that Assumptions (A.4) and (A.5) hold for the special cases described in Section 3.1. For example, in the great circle model we may let $\mathcal{C}_i^N = \{i - 1 + j \bmod N : j \in \mathcal{C}_1^N\}$ and in that case the elements of $\mathcal{C}_J^N$ are each distributed as J (though not independently) and (3.3.19) follows easily. Note that the above assumptions do not preclude the case $\lambda_{ij}^L = \lambda_L > 0$ for all $i \neq j$, i.e. local mixing is also homogeneous, but in that case $\mathbb{P}(C < \infty) = \mathbb{P}(R < \infty) = 0$.

For ease of exposition we assume that there is one initial infective in E^N, who is chosen uniformly from $\mathcal{N}$. Let $(\mathcal{C}_i^N, R_i^N)$ $(i = 0, 1, \dots)$ be i.i.d. copies of $(\mathcal{C}_1^N, R_1^N)$ and $C_i^N = |\mathcal{C}_i^N|$ $(i = 0, 1, \dots)$. Then (C_i^N, R_i^N) $(i = 0, 1, \dots)$ can be used to construct a realisation of the branching process $\mathcal{B}^N$ defined in Section 3.3.2 below, in which clumps are labelled sequentially as they are born. Let Z_C^N denote the total number of clumps in $\mathcal{B}^N$, including the initial clump, and

$$Z_I^N = \sum_{i=0}^{Z_C^N - 1} C_i^N$$

denote the total number of 'individuals' in $\mathcal{B}^N$. Define Z_C and Z_I similarly for the branching process $\mathcal{B}$.

The *same* realisation $(\mathcal{C}_i^N, R_i^N)$ $(i = 0, 1, \dots)$ of random variables can also be used to construct a realisation of the set of individuals infected by the epidemic E^N as follows. Let $J_0^N, J_1^N, \dots$ be i.i.d. random variables, each distributed as J above, that are also independent of $(\mathcal{C}_i^N, R_i^N)$ $(i = 0, 1, \dots)$. The initial infective in E^N is individual J_0^N. The epidemic is constructed on a generation basis analogous to that given by (3.3.1)-(3.3.4) on page 165. The epidemic follows the branching process $\mathcal{B}^N$, with the individual in E^N corresponding to the ancestor of the kth clump in $\mathcal{B}^N$ being given by J_k^N, until a clump that has a non-empty intersection with a clump used previously in E^N is born. The construction of the epidemic then needs modifying but the details of such modification are not necessary for our arguments.

Let Z^N be the total number of individuals infected in E^N, including the initial infective. For $k = 0, 1, \dots$, let $\widehat{\mathcal{C}}_k^N$ be the set of individuals in $\mathcal{N}$ that belong to the clump in E^N that corresponds to the kth clump in $\mathcal{B}^N$. Let

$$M^N = \min\left\{k \geq 1 : \widehat{\mathscr{C}_k^N} \cap \bigcup_{i=0}^{k-1} \widehat{\mathscr{C}_i^N} \neq \emptyset\right\} + 1$$

be the number of clumps required until the construction of E^N needs modifying. The key observation is that

$$Z_C^N < M^N \implies Z^N = Z_I^N. \tag{3.3.20}$$

Theorem 3.3.6. *Suppose that Assumptions (A.3), (A.4) and (A.5) hold. Then*

$$Z^N \xrightarrow{D} Z_I \qquad \text{as } N \to \infty. \tag{3.3.21}$$

Proof. For $k = 1, 2, \ldots,$

$$\begin{aligned}\mathbb{P}(Z^N \leq k) &= \mathbb{P}(Z^N \leq k, M^N > k) + \mathbb{P}(Z^N \leq k, M^N \leq k) \\ &= \mathbb{P}(Z_I^N \leq k, M^N > k) + \mathbb{P}(Z^N \leq k, M^N \leq k),\end{aligned} \tag{3.3.22}$$

using (3.3.20). Also,

$$\mathbb{P}(Z_I^N \leq k) = \mathbb{P}(Z_I^N \leq k, M^N > k) + \mathbb{P}(Z_I^N \leq k, M^N \leq k). \tag{3.3.23}$$

Equations (3.3.22) and (3.3.23) imply

$$|\mathbb{P}(Z^N \leq k) - \mathbb{P}(Z_I^N \leq k)| \leq \mathbb{P}(M^N \leq k). \tag{3.3.24}$$

If the clump sizes are bounded, i.e. there exists an integer $K > 0$ such that $\mathbb{P}(C^N \leq K) = 1$ for all N, then, for $k = 1, 2, \ldots,$

$$\begin{aligned}\mathbb{P}(M^N \leq k) &= \mathbb{P}\left(\bigcup_{i=0}^{k-2} \bigcup_{j=i+1}^{k-1} \widehat{\mathscr{C}_i^N} \cap \widehat{\mathscr{C}_j^N}\right) \\ &\leq \sum_{i=0}^{k-2} \sum_{j=1}^{k-1} \mathbb{P}\left(\widehat{\mathscr{C}_i^N} \cap \widehat{\mathscr{C}_j^N}\right) \\ &\leq \binom{k}{2} \frac{K^2}{N},\end{aligned}$$

using (3.3.19). Thus, $\mathbb{P}(M^N \leq k) \to 0$ as $N \to \infty$ and, using (3.3.24),

$$\lim_{N\to\infty} \mathbb{P}(Z^N \leq k) = \lim_{N\to\infty} \mathbb{P}(Z_I^N \leq k) = \mathbb{P}(Z_I \leq k) \qquad (k = 1, 2, \ldots),$$

since $(C^N, R^N) \xrightarrow{D} (C, R)$ as $N \to \infty$, proving (3.3.21) when the clump sizes are bounded.

Turning to the general case, for $k = 1, 2, \ldots,$ equation (3.3.22) implies

$$\mathbb{P}(Z^N \leq k) \geq \mathbb{P}(Z_I^N \leq k)\mathbb{P}(M^N > k | Z_I^N \leq k).$$

Now $Z_I^N \leq k$ implies $Z_C^N \leq k$, as all clumps contain at least one individual, so using (3.3.19),

$$\mathbb{P}(M^N \leq k | Z_I^N \leq k) \leq (k-1)\frac{k^2}{N} \to 0 \qquad \text{as } N \to \infty,$$

whence $\mathbb{P}(M^N > k | Z_I^N \leq k) \to 1$ as $M \to \infty$. Thus,

$$\liminf_{N\to\infty} \mathbb{P}(Z^N \leq k) \geq \liminf_{N\to\infty} \mathbb{P}(Z_I^N \leq k) = \mathbb{P}(Z_I \leq k). \tag{3.3.25}$$

To show that $\limsup_{N\to\infty} \mathbb{P}(Z^N \leq k) \leq \mathbb{P}(Z_I \leq k)$, and hence complete the proof of Theorem 3.3.6, we consider, for each integer $K > 0$, modifications of the epidemic E^N and the branching processes $\mathscr{B}^N$ and $\mathscr{B}$ in which the clump sizes are capped at K. From (3.3.18) we may write R_N in an obvious notation as

$$R^N = \sum_{j=1}^{C^N} \tilde{R}_j^N.$$

Let

$$(C^N(K), R^N(K)) \stackrel{\mathrm{D}}{=} \begin{cases} (C^N, R^N) & \text{if } C^N \leq K, \\ (K, \sum_{j=1}^K \tilde{R}_j^N) & \text{if } C^N > K, \end{cases}$$

where $\stackrel{\mathrm{D}}{=}$ denotes equal in distribution. Let $E^N(K)$ denote the epidemic constructed analogously to E^N but using $(C^N(K), R^N(K))$ instead of (C^N, R^N), and define $\mathscr{B}^N(K)$ and $\mathscr{B}(K)$, similarly. We use a similar notation for quantities associated with these processes, for example, $Z^N(K)$ is the total number of individuals infected in $E^N(K)$.

Fix integers $k, K > 0$. Clearly, $Z^N \stackrel{\mathrm{st}}{\geq} Z^N(K)$, so

$$\mathbb{P}(Z^N \leq k) \leq \mathbb{P}(Z^N(K) \leq k),$$

whence

$$\begin{aligned} \limsup_{N\to\infty} \mathbb{P}(Z^N \leq k) &\leq \limsup_{N\to\infty} \mathbb{P}(Z^N(K) \leq k) \\ &= \mathbb{P}(Z_I(K) \leq k), \end{aligned} \tag{3.3.26}$$

as the clump sizes are bounded. Now $R(K) \xrightarrow{D} R$ as $K \to \infty$, so

$$\mathbb{P}(Z_I(K) \leq k) \to \mathbb{P}(Z_I \leq k) \qquad \text{as } K \to \infty,$$

and letting $K \to \infty$ in (3.3.26) yields

$$\limsup_{N\to\infty} \mathbb{P}(Z^N \leq k) \leq \mathbb{P}(Z_I \leq k),$$

which combined with (3.3.25) yields

$$\lim_{N\to\infty} \mathbb{P}(Z^N \le k) = \mathbb{P}(Z_I \le k) \qquad (k = 1,2,\dots),$$

proving (3.3.21). □

Recall from Section 3.3.2 that R_* and p_{ext} are respectively the offspring mean and extinction probability of the branching process $\mathscr{B}$. Thus it follows from Theorem 3.3.6 that if $R_* \le 1$ then, with probability tending to one as $N \to \infty$, the epidemic E^N infects only a very small fraction of the population. If $R_* > 1$ then the epidemic E^N infects a very small fraction of the population with probability tending to p_{ext} as $N \to \infty$. We now consider, for large N, the behaviour of E_N when the branching process $\mathscr{B}$ does not go extinct.

Theorem 3.3.7. *Suppose that Assumptions (A.3), (A.4) and (A.5) hold. Let (g_N) be any sequence of nonnegative real numbers satisfying $g_N \to \infty$ and $N^{-1}g_N \to 0$ as $N \to \infty$. Then*

$$\lim_{N\to\infty} \mathbb{P}(Z^N \ge g_N) = 1 - p_{\text{ext}}.$$

Proof. We prove the theorem by first obtaining, for fixed $\varepsilon \in (0,1)$, bounds on $\liminf_{N\to\infty} \mathbb{P}(Z^N \ge N\varepsilon)$ and $\limsup_{N\to\infty} \mathbb{P}(Z^N \ge N\varepsilon)$.

For any $k > 0$,

$$\limsup_{N\to\infty} \mathbb{P}(Z^N \ge N\varepsilon) \le \limsup_{N\to\infty} \mathbb{P}(Z^N \ge k) = \mathbb{P}(Z_I \ge k),$$

using Theorem 3.3.6. Letting $k \to \infty$ yields

$$\limsup_{N\to\infty} \mathbb{P}(Z^N \ge N\varepsilon) \le 1 - p_{\text{ext}}. \tag{3.3.27}$$

To get a lower bound for $\mathbb{P}(Z^N \ge N\varepsilon)$ we use a device that originates in Whittle [66]. Consider a typical clump, $(\mathscr{C}_i^N, R_i^N)$ say, used in the constructions of $\mathscr{B}^N$ and E^N. While the total number of infectives in E^N remains below $N\varepsilon$, it follows from (3.3.19) that the probability this clump intersects a clump previously used in E^N is at most εC_i^N. Thus, until the total number of infectives reaches $N\varepsilon$, the epidemic E^N is stochastically greater than a branching process, $\hat{\mathscr{B}}^N(\varepsilon)$ say, derived from $\mathscr{B}^N$, by independently deleting clumps (and all of their descendants in $\mathscr{B}^N$), with probability $\min(1, \varepsilon C^N)$ if the clump has size C^N. In particular,

$$\mathbb{P}(Z^N \ge N\varepsilon) \ge \mathbb{P}(\hat{Z}_I^N(\varepsilon) \ge N\varepsilon),$$

where $\hat{Z}_I^N(\varepsilon)$ is the total number of 'individuals' in $\hat{\mathscr{B}}^N(\varepsilon)$.

For integer $K > 0$, let $\mathscr{B}^N(\varepsilon, K)$ be obtained from $\hat{\mathscr{B}}^N(\varepsilon)$ in the same way that $\mathscr{B}^N(K)$ is obtained from $\mathscr{B}^N$, i.e. by truncating the clump sizes at K, and define $\mathscr{B}(\varepsilon, K)$ in the obvious fashion. Let $p_{\text{ext}}^N(\varepsilon, K)$ and $p_{\text{ext}}(\varepsilon, K)$ be the extinction probability of $\mathscr{B}^N(\varepsilon, K)$ and $\mathscr{B}(\varepsilon, K)$, respectively. Let $R^N(\varepsilon, K)$ and $R(\varepsilon, K)$ denote the offspring random variables of $\mathscr{B}^N(\varepsilon, K)$ and $\mathscr{B}(\varepsilon, K)$, respectively. Then $R^N(\varepsilon, K) \xrightarrow{D} R(\varepsilon, K)$ as $N \to \infty$, so $\lim_{N\to\infty} p_{\text{ext}}^N(\varepsilon, K) = p_{\text{ext}}(\varepsilon, K)$ (cf. Britton et al. [29, Lemma 4.1]). Now

$$\begin{aligned}\mathbb{P}(Z^N \geq N\varepsilon) &\geq \mathbb{P}(Z^N(K) \geq N\varepsilon)\\ &\geq \mathbb{P}(\hat{Z}_I^N(\varepsilon,K) \geq N\varepsilon)\\ &\geq 1 - p_{\text{ext}}^N(\varepsilon,K),\end{aligned} \tag{3.3.28}$$

so

$$\begin{aligned}\liminf_{N\to\infty} \mathbb{P}(Z^N \geq N\varepsilon) &\geq \liminf_{N\to\infty}[1 - p_{\text{ext}}^N(\varepsilon,K)]\\ &= 1 - p_{\text{ext}}(\varepsilon,K).\end{aligned} \tag{3.3.29}$$

Let (g_N) satisfy the conditions of the theorem. Then arguing as in the derivation of (3.3.27) yields

$$\limsup_{N\to\infty} \mathbb{P}(Z^N \geq g_N) \leq 1 - p_{\text{ext}}. \tag{3.3.30}$$

Also, for any $\varepsilon \in (0,1)$ and any $K > 0$,

$$\liminf_{N\to\infty} \mathbb{P}(Z^N \geq g_N) \geq \liminf_{N\to\infty} \mathbb{P}(Z^N \geq N\varepsilon) \geq 1 - p_{\text{ext}}(\varepsilon,K), \tag{3.3.31}$$

using (3.3.29). Note that $p_{\text{ext}}(\varepsilon,K) \downarrow p_{\text{ext}}(K)$ as $\varepsilon \downarrow 0$, since $R(\varepsilon,K) \xrightarrow{D} R(K)$, and $p_{\text{ext}}(K) \downarrow p_{\text{ext}}$ as $K \uparrow \infty$, since $R(K) \xrightarrow{D} R$. Thus, (ε,K) can be chosen so that $p_{\text{ext}}(\varepsilon,K)$ is arbitrarily close to p_{ext}, and it follows from (3.3.31) that

$$\liminf_{N\to\infty} \mathbb{P}(Z^N \geq g_N) \geq 1 - p_{\text{ext}}. \tag{3.3.32}$$

The theorem follows immediately from (3.3.30) and (3.3.32). □

Remark 3.3.8 (Definition of global outbreak). Theorem 3.3.7 implies immediately that $\lim_{N\to\infty} \mathbb{P}(Z^N \geq \log N) = 1 - p_{\text{ext}}$, so as indicated in Section 3.3.2 we can use $Z^N \geq \log N$ to define a global outbreak. Suppose that $R_* > 1$ and (g_N) satisfies $g_N \geq \log N$ for all N and $\lim_{N\to\infty} N^{-1} g_N = 0$. Then Theorem 3.3.7 implies that

$$\lim_{N\to\infty} \mathbb{P}(Z^N \geq g_N | Z^N \geq \log N) = 1,$$

so we could equivalently use such g_N to define a global outbreak.

Further, if $R_* > 1$ then $p_{\text{ext}} < 1$, so (ε,K) can be chosen so that $p_{\text{ext}}(\varepsilon,K) < 1$. Consider the epidemic E^N but having $\lfloor \log\log N \rfloor$ initial infectives, where for $x \in \mathbb{R}$, $\lfloor x \rfloor$ is the greatest integer $\leq x$. Then using the lower bounding branching process $\mathscr{B}^N(\varepsilon,K)$ and arguing as in the derivation of (3.3.28) yields

$$\liminf_{N\to\infty} \mathbb{P}(Z^N \geq \varepsilon N) \geq \liminf_{N\to\infty} \left\{1 - \left[p_{\text{ext}}^N(\varepsilon,K)\right]^{\lfloor \log\log N \rfloor}\right\} = 1. \tag{3.3.33}$$

This suggests that

$$\lim_{N\to\infty} \mathbb{P}(Z^N \geq \varepsilon N | Z^N \geq \log N) = 1, \tag{3.3.34}$$

so a global outbreak infects a strictly positive fraction of the population in the limit as $N \to \infty$.

The gap in the argument is that we have not proved anything about the number of infectives in E^N when the total number of infectives (which includes those who are no longer infectious) reaches $\log N$. We provide a proof of (3.3.34) for a closely related model in Section 3.4.2 below. Note that ε in (3.3.34) depends on the parameters of the epidemic model E^N.

3.4 Final Outcome of a Global Outbreak

We consider now the final outcome of a global outbreak in the limit as the population size $N \to \infty$. In Section 3.4.1, heuristic arguments are used to determine the fraction of the population that is infected by a global outbreak and also the distribution of the number ultimately infected in a fixed subset of initial susceptibles, such as an initially fully-susceptible household in the households model. In Section 3.4.2, a framework is described for proving these results and an associated central limit theorem.

3.4.1 Heuristics

Suppose that N is large, there are few initial infectives and a global outbreak occurs. Let z_N be the expected proportion of the population that is infected by the epidemic E^N and π_N be the probability that a given initial susceptible, i say, is not contacted globally during the course of E^N. (Note that i may still be infected in E^N by a local contact.) Let A^N be the sum of the infectious periods of all individuals infected during the epidemic E^N, i.e. the severity of E^N. Now a given infective, i_* say, makes global contacts at the points of a Poisson process having rate λ_G and such contacts are with individuals chosen independently and uniformly from the whole population $\mathscr{N}$. Thus i_* contacts i globally at the points of a Poisson process having rate $N^{-1}\lambda_G$. Further, distinct infectives behave independently, so, given A^N, individual i is not contacted globally if and only if there is no point of a Poisson process having rate $N^{-1}\lambda_G$ in an interval of length A^N. Hence,

$$\mathbb{P}(\text{individual } i \text{ not contacted globally during } E^N|A^N) = \exp(-N^{-1}\lambda_G A^N).$$

The number of individuals infected in the epidemic E^N is approximately Nz_N, and each infective is infectious on average for a time μ_I, so A^N is approximately $Nz_N\mu_I$. Thus,

$$\begin{aligned}\pi_N &= \mathbb{E}\left[\mathbb{P}(\text{individual } i \text{ not contacted globally during } E^N|A^N)\right] \\ &= \mathbb{E}\left[\exp(-N^{-1}\lambda_G A^N)\right] \\ &\approx \exp(-N^{-1}\lambda_G N z_N \mu_I) \\ &= \exp(-\lambda_G \mu_I z_N). \end{aligned} \tag{3.4.1}$$

Note that individual i is not infected by the epidemic E^N if and only if no member of individual i's local susceptibility set $\mathscr{S}_i$ is contacted globally during the epidemic and no member of $\mathscr{S}_i$ is an initial infective. For large N, individuals avoid global infection approximately independently, each with probability π_N, so if G_N is the event that all members of $\mathscr{S}_i$ avoid global infection then, conditioning on the size S^N of $\mathscr{S}_i$,

$$\begin{aligned}\mathbb{P}(G_N) &= \mathbb{E}\left[\mathbb{P}(G_N|S^N)\right] \\ &= \mathbb{E}\left[\pi_N^{S^N}\right] \\ &= f_{S^N}(\pi_N),\end{aligned} \tag{3.4.2}$$

where $f_{S^N}(s) = \mathbb{E}\left[(s)^{S^N}\right]$ $(0 \le s \le 1)$ is the probability-generating function of S_N.

Recall that we assume that $S^N \xrightarrow{D} S$ as $N \to \infty$, so $\lim_{N\to\infty} f_{S^N}(s) = f_S(s)$ $(0 \le s \le 1)$, where $f_S(s)$ $(0 \le s \le 1)$ is the probability-generating function of S. If $S < \infty$, then the probability that i's susceptibility set $\mathscr{S}_i$ contains an initial infective tends to 0 as $N \to \infty$. Also, if $S = \infty$, then the probability that all members of $\mathscr{S}_i$ avoid global infection tends to 0 as $N \to \infty$. Thus letting $N \to \infty$ in (3.4.1) and (3.4.2) yields

$$\lim_{N\to\infty} \mathbb{P}(i \text{ is not infected by a global outbreak}) = f_S(\pi), \tag{3.4.3}$$

where

$$\pi = \exp(-\lambda_G \mu_I z) \tag{3.4.4}$$

and z is the expected fraction of the population infected by a global outbreak. Further, if the fraction of the population that is initially infected tends to 0 as $N \to \infty$, then z is given by the (limiting) probability that a typical initial susceptible is infected by a global outbreak, so substituting (3.4.4) into (3.4.3) yields that z satisfies

$$1 - z = f_S(\mathrm{e}^{-\lambda_G \mu_I z}). \tag{3.4.5}$$

To investigate the solutions of (3.4.5), consider a Galton–Watson branching process with offspring random variable, $\tilde{R}$ say, that has a mixed-Poisson distribution with mean $\lambda_G \mu_I S$, i.e. $\tilde{R} \sim \mathrm{Poi}(\lambda_G \mu_I S)$. Then, for $s \in [0,1]$,

$$\begin{aligned}f_{\tilde{R}}(s) &= \mathbb{E}\left[s^{\tilde{R}}\right] \\ &= \mathbb{E}\left[\mathbb{E}\left[s^{\tilde{R}}|S\right]\right] \\ &= \mathbb{E}\left[\mathrm{e}^{-\lambda_G \mu_I S(1-s)}\right] \qquad \left[\text{as } \tilde{R}|S \sim \mathrm{Poi}(\lambda_G \mu_I S)\right] \\ &= f_S(\mathrm{e}^{-\lambda_G \mu_I (1-s)}),\end{aligned}$$

so, from (3.4.5), $s = 1 - z$ satisfies the equation governing the extinction probability of this branching process: viz. $f_{\tilde{R}}(s) = s$. Let

$$\mu_{\tilde{R}} = \mathbb{E}[\tilde{R}] = \lambda_G \mu_I \mu_S. \tag{3.4.6}$$

By standard branching process theory (Proposition A.1.1 on page 98 in Part I of this volume), the equation $f_{\tilde{R}}(s) = s$ has exactly one root in $[0,1)$ if $\mu_{\tilde{R}} > 1$ and none if $\mu_{\tilde{R}} \leq 1$. Thus the equation (3.4.5) governing z has exactly one root in $(0,1]$, giving the limiting mean fraction of the population infected by a global outbreak as $N \to \infty$ (assuming few initial infectives), if $\mu_{\tilde{R}} > 1$ and none if $\mu_{\tilde{R}} \leq 1$.

We show now that $\mu_{\tilde{R}} = R_*$. Note from (3.2.1) and (3.2.2) on page 163 that, for $i \in \mathscr{N}$,

$$C_i^N = \sum_{j \in \mathscr{N}} 1_{\{i \overset{\mathrm{L}}{\rightsquigarrow} j\}} \qquad \text{and} \qquad S_i^N = \sum_{j \in \mathscr{N}} 1_{\{j \overset{\mathrm{L}}{\rightsquigarrow} i\}},$$

so

$$\mathbb{E}[C_i^N] = \sum_{j \in \mathscr{N}} \mathbb{P}(i \overset{\mathrm{L}}{\rightsquigarrow} j) \qquad \text{and} \qquad \mathbb{E}[S_i^N] = \sum_{j \in \mathscr{N}} \mathbb{P}(j \overset{\mathrm{L}}{\rightsquigarrow} i).$$

Now C_i^N $(i \in \mathscr{N})$ are identically distributed, as are S_i^N $(i \in \mathscr{N})$, so

$$\begin{aligned}
\mathbb{E}[C_1^N] &= \frac{1}{N} \sum_{i \in \mathscr{N}} \mathbb{E}[C_i^N] \\
&= \frac{1}{N} \sum_{i \in \mathscr{N}} \sum_{j \in \mathscr{N}} \mathbb{P}(i \overset{\mathrm{L}}{\rightsquigarrow} j) \\
&= \frac{1}{N} \sum_{j \in \mathscr{N}} \sum_{i \in \mathscr{N}} \mathbb{P}(i \overset{\mathrm{L}}{\rightsquigarrow} j) \\
&= \frac{1}{N} \sum_{j \in \mathscr{N}} \mathbb{E}[S_j^N] \\
&= \mathbb{E}[S_1^N],
\end{aligned}$$

and letting $N \to \infty$ yields $\mu_C = \mu_S$. Thus, using (3.3.5) on page 167 and (3.4.6),

$$\mu_{\tilde{R}} = \lambda_G \mu_I \mu_S = \lambda_G \mu_I \mu_S = R_*. \tag{3.4.7}$$

Summarising, if $R_* \leq 1$, the only solution of the equation (3.4.5) in $[0,1]$ is $z = 0$, corresponding to there being no large epidemic, which is consistent with the approximating branching process $\mathscr{B}$ going extinct almost surely. If $R_* > 1$, then the equation (3.4.5) has two solutions in $[0,1]$, $z = 0$ and $z = \hat{z}$ say, and we still need to determine which of these solutions gives the fraction of the population infected by a global outbreak. We explore this more rigorously in Section 3.4.2 below, where we show that if $\bar{Z}^N$ is the fraction of the population infected during the epidemic E^N then $\bar{Z}^N \xrightarrow{D} \bar{Z}$ as $N \to \infty$, where the limiting random variable $\bar{Z}$ takes only the values 0 and $\hat{z}$, corresponding to a non-global and a global outbreak, respectively. We also derive a central limit theorem for the the size of a global outbreak.

The above heuristic argument can be extended to the finer structure of the final outcome of a global outbreak. Let H denote a set of initial susceptibles that is held fixed as $N \to \infty$. Thus, for example, H could be a typical initially fully-susceptible household in the households (or the households-workplaces) model or, for fixed $k \geq 2$, a typical chain of k initially susceptible individuals in the great circle model. Let

$$X_H = \{i \in H : i \text{ is ultimately uninfected by the epidemic } E^N\}.$$

We calculate the distribution of the set X_H in the limit as $N \to \infty$.

For $F \subseteq H$, let

$$\mathscr{S}_F = \{j \in \mathscr{N} : j \overset{\text{L}}{\rightsquigarrow} i \text{ for some } i \in F\}, \tag{3.4.8}$$

denote the local susceptibility set of F, with the convention that $\mathscr{S}_\emptyset = \emptyset$. Let

$$S_F = |\mathscr{S}_F| \qquad \text{and} \qquad f_{S_F}(s) = \mathbb{E}[s^{S_F}] \;\; (0 \le s \le 1). \tag{3.4.9}$$

All members of F avoid infection by the epidemic E^N if and only if all members of $\mathscr{S}_F$ avoid global infection, so

$$\mathbb{P}(X_H \supseteq F) = f_{S_F}(\mathrm{e}^{-\lambda_G \mu_I \hat{z}}) \qquad (F \subseteq H), \tag{3.4.10}$$

since, in the limit as $N \to \infty$, each member of $\mathscr{S}_F$ avoids global infection independently and with probability $\mathrm{e}^{-\lambda_G \mu_I \hat{z}}$ (see (3.4.4) with z replaced by $\hat{z}$). Thus, using the Möbius inversion formula (1.3.2) on page 128,

$$\mathbb{P}(X_H = F) = \sum_{F \subseteq G \subseteq H} (-1)^{|G|-|F|} f_{S_G}(\mathrm{e}^{-\lambda_G \mu_I \hat{z}}) \qquad (F \subseteq H). \tag{3.4.11}$$

3.4.2 'Rigorous' Argument and Central Limit Theorem

In this section, we describe a framework for proving rigorously a law of large numbers and a central limit theorem for the final outcome of a global outbreak. This involves adapting the embedding technique of Scalia-Tomba [60, 61], see Section 3.3 of Part I in this volume, to the present general two-level mixing model. We describe the general argument. In a few places, which we point out, further details are required to make the arguments fully rigorous. These details are model dependent, so they are different for different special cases. The starting point is the following alternative construction of the model E^N, which uses a Sellke-type construction (see Sellke [62] and Section 3.2 of Part I of this volume) for global contacts.

As in Section 3.1 on page 160, label the individuals in the population $1, 2, \ldots, N$, and let $I_1, I_2, \ldots, I_N$ be i.i.d. copies of I, where I_i is the infectious period of individual i if it becomes infected. Local spread of infection is modelled as in Section 3.1, leading to a directed graph of local contacts $\mathscr{G}_L^N$ and for $i \in \mathscr{N}$, local susceptibility sets $\mathscr{S}_i^N$ $(i \in \mathscr{N})$ (see Section 3.2), where now we show explicitly the dependence of $\mathscr{G}_L$ and $\mathscr{S}$ on the population size N. We assume that Assumption (A.2) on page 164 is satisfied, i.e. that $S^N \xrightarrow{D} S$ as $N \to \infty$. Global spread of infection is modelled as follows. Let $L_1, L_2, \ldots, L_N$ be i.i.d. exponential random variables, having rate λ_G and hence mean λ_G^{-1}. At any given time, t say, each susceptible accumulates exposure to global infection at rate $N^{-1}Y(t)$, where $Y(t)$ is the total number of infectives at time t. For $i \in \mathscr{N}$, individual i is infected globally when its total exposure to global infection reaches L_i, provided that it is still susceptible at that time. It is easily seen, using the lack-of-memory property of both the Poisson process and the exponential distribution, together with the thinning property of the Poisson process, that this yields an epidemic process which satisfies the same probability law as E^N.

Construct a related epidemic model as follows. Suppose that initially all N individuals are susceptible and then each individual is exposed to t units of global infection. Now use $L_1, L_2, \ldots, L_N$ to determine which individuals, if any, are infected globally so, for $i \in \mathscr{N}$, individual i is infected globally if and only if $L_i \leq t$. Then use the random directed graph $\mathscr{G}_L^N$ to determine which individuals are subsequently infected locally. Denote this epidemic by $\tilde{E}^N(t)$. Note that in the construction of $\tilde{E}^N(t)$ the individuals do not make global contacts. Note also that individual $i \in \mathscr{N}$ is infected in $\tilde{E}^N(t)$ if and only if i's local susceptibility set $\mathscr{S}_i^N$ contains at least one individual that is contacted globally.

For $i = 1, 2, \ldots, N$, let

$$\chi_i^N(t) = 1_{\{i \text{ infected in } \tilde{E}^N(t)\}} = \begin{cases} 1 \text{ if} & \min_{j \in \mathscr{S}_i^N} L_j \leq t, \\ 0 \text{ otherwise.} \end{cases}$$

Further, let

$$R^N(t) = \sum_{i=1}^N \chi_i^N(t) \qquad \text{and} \qquad A^N(t) = \sum_{j=1}^N I_j \chi_j^N(t)$$

be respectively the size and severity of $\tilde{E}^N(t)$.

Now return to the epidemic E^N and suppose that E^N is initiated by exposing the population to T_0^N units of global infection, so each individual is exposed to $\bar{T}_0^N = N^{-1} T_0^N$ units of global infection. These T_0^N units of global infection will infect some individuals globally and trigger local infections. The total amount of global infection created by the individuals contacted globally and the ensuing local infectious clumps is given by $A^N(\bar{T}_0^N)$, so the population has now been exposed to a total of $T_0^N + A^N(\bar{T}_0^N)$ units of infection. The process is continued in the obvious fashion, viz.

$$\begin{aligned} \bar{T}_1^N &= \bar{T}_0^N + N^{-1} A^N(\bar{T}_0^N) \\ \bar{T}_2^N &= \bar{T}_0^N + N^{-1} A^N(\bar{T}_1^N) \\ &\vdots \\ \bar{T}_\infty^N &= \bar{T}_{k^*}^N, \end{aligned}$$

where $k^* = \min\{j : \bar{T}_{j+1}^N = \bar{T}_j^N\}$. Note that the process must stop after a finite number of iterations as the population is finite. Note also that

$$\bar{T}_\infty^N = \min\{t > 0 : t = \bar{T}_0^N + N^{-1} A^N(t)\}. \tag{3.4.12}$$

(An illustration of the above iteration and the stopping time $\bar{T}_\infty^N$ is given in Figure 3.4.1.) Further the size of the epidemic E^N is given by

$$R^N(\bar{T}_\infty^N) = \sum_{i=1}^{N} \chi_i^N(\bar{T}_\infty^N) \tag{3.4.13}$$

and the severity of E^N is given by

$$T_0^N + \sum_{j=1}^{N} \chi_j^N(\bar{T}_\infty^N) I_j = T_0^N + A^N(\bar{T}_\infty^N). \tag{3.4.14}$$

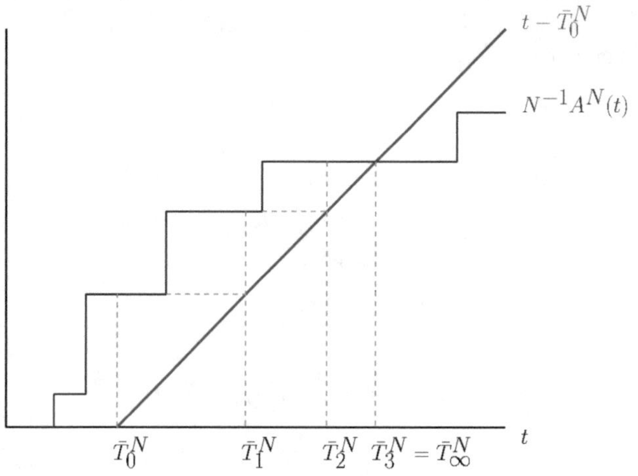

Fig. 3.4.1 Example of the iteration $\bar{T}_k^N$ $(k = 0, 1, \ldots)$ and the associated stopping time $\bar{T}_\infty^N$, which satisfies (3.4.12).

For $i = 1, 2, \ldots, N$,

$$\begin{aligned}
\mathbb{E}[\chi_i^N(t)]] &= \mathbb{P}\left(\min_{j \in \mathscr{S}_i^N} L_j \le t\right) \\
&= 1 - \mathbb{P}(L_j > t \text{ for all } j \in \mathscr{S}_i^n) \\
&= 1 - \mathbb{E}\left[\mathrm{e}^{-\lambda_G t S_i^N}\right] \\
&= 1 - f_{S^N}(\mathrm{e}^{-\lambda_G t}) \\
&\to 1 - f_S(\mathrm{e}^{-\lambda_G t}) \qquad \text{as } N \to \infty,
\end{aligned}$$

since $S^N \xrightarrow{D} S$ as $N \to \infty$. Also, since I_i and $\mathscr{S}_i^N$ are independent,

$$\begin{aligned}
\mathbb{E}[I_i \chi_i^N(t)]] &= \mu_I \mathbb{E}[\chi_i^N(t)]] \\
&\to \mu_I(1 - f_S(\mathrm{e}^{-\lambda_G t})) \qquad \text{as } N \to \infty.
\end{aligned}$$

By an appropriate weak law of large numbers, for all $t \ge 0$,

$$N^{-1}R^N(t) \xrightarrow{p} r(t) \quad \text{and} \quad N^{-1}A^N(t) \xrightarrow{p} a(t) \quad \text{as} \quad N \to \infty, \tag{3.4.15}$$

where

$$r(t) = \lim_{N\to\infty} \mathrm{E}[\chi_1^N(t)] = 1 - f_S(\mathrm{e}^{-\lambda_G t}) \quad \text{and} \quad a(t) = \lim_{N\to\infty} \mathrm{E}[\chi_1^N(t) I_1] = \mu_I r(t). \tag{3.4.16}$$

This of course needs justifying. It is straightforward to prove (3.4.15) for the households model, since both $R^N(t)$ and $A^N(t)$ can be expressed as a sum of contributions from the different households, which are independent and identically distributed, so (3.4.15) follows immediately from the weak law of large numbers; indeed (3.4.15) holds with $\xrightarrow{p}$ replaced by almost sure convergence. More generally, using Chebyshev's inequality, sufficient conditions for the first and second results in (3.4.15) are $N^{-2}\mathrm{Var}(R^N(t)) \to 0$ and $N^{-2}\mathrm{Var}(A^N(t)) \to 0$ as $N \to \infty$, respectively.

By construction the random functions $R^N(t)$ and $A^N(t)$ are non-decreasing with t, as are $r(t)$ and $a(t)$. Using this, it is straightforward to extend (3.4.15) to

$$\sup_{0\le t<\infty} |N^{-1}R^N(t) - r(t)| \xrightarrow{p} 0 \quad \text{and} \quad \sup_{0\le t<\infty} |N^{-1}A^N(t) - a(t)| \xrightarrow{p} 0, \tag{3.4.17}$$

as we now show.

Fix $\varepsilon > 0$ and choose $0 = t_0 < t_1 < t_2 < \cdots < t_p = \infty$ such that

$$0 < r(t_i) - r(t_{i-1}) \le \frac{\varepsilon}{2}, \qquad i = 1, 2, \ldots, p,$$

this being possible since $r(t)$ is non-decreasing, $r(0) = 0$ and $r(\infty) = 1$. Then, observing that (3.4.15) holds also when $t = \infty$,

$$\lim_{N\to\infty} \mathbb{P}\left(\bigcap_{i=0}^{p} \left\{ |N^{-1}R^N(t_i) - r(t_i)| \le \frac{\varepsilon}{2} \right\}\right) = 1. \tag{3.4.18}$$

For $i = 0, 1, \ldots, p-1$, since $R^N(t)$ and $r(t)$ are non-decreasing in t,

$$N^{-1}R^N(t_i) - r(t_i) - \frac{\varepsilon}{2} \le N^{-1}R^N(t) - r(t) \le N^{-1}R^N(t_{i+1}) - r(t_{i+1}) + \frac{\varepsilon}{2},$$

for all $t \in [t_i, t_{i+1})$, which together with (3.4.18), yields

$$\lim_{N\to\infty} \mathbb{P}\left(\sup_{0\le t<\infty} |N^{-1}R^N(t) - r(t)| \le \varepsilon \right) = 1.$$

The first result in (3.4.17) then follows as $\varepsilon > 0$ is arbitrary. The second result is proved similarly. (Note that the above proof of (3.4.17) is nothing but a proof of the second Dini theorem, adapted to convergence in probability. The same theorem for almost sure convergence is used in the proof of Proposition 2.2.6 of Part I in this volume.)

Observe from (3.4.12) that $\bar{T}_\infty^N$ satisfies

$$\bar{T}_\infty^N = \bar{T}_0^N + N^{-1}A^N(\bar{T}_\infty^N). \tag{3.4.19}$$

Suppose $\bar{T}_0^N \xrightarrow{p} \mu$ as $N \to \infty$, where $\mu \geq 0$ is constant. The situation of a trace of initial infection, considered in Section 3.4.1, yields $\mu = 0$. We consider first the simpler case of $\mu > 0$.

Consider the equation

$$t = a(t) + \mu. \tag{3.4.20}$$

Now $a(0) = 0$, $a(\infty) = \mu_I$ and, for $t \in [0, \infty)$,

$$a''(t) = -\mu_I \lambda_G^2 \mathrm{e}^{-\lambda_G t} \left[f_S'(\mathrm{e}^{-\lambda_G t}) + \mathrm{e}^{-\lambda_G t} f_S''(\mathrm{e}^{-\lambda_G t}) \right] < 0,$$

where $'$ and $''$ denote first and second derivative, respectively. Thus, $a(t)$ is concave on $(0, \infty)$ and the equation (3.4.20) has a unique solution, τ say, in $[0, \infty)$. Moreover, $a'(\tau) < 1$, so (3.4.17) implies that

$$\bar{T}_\infty^N \xrightarrow{p} \tau \qquad \text{and} \qquad \bar{Z}^N \xrightarrow{p} z \qquad \text{as } N \to \infty, \tag{3.4.21}$$

where $\bar{Z}^N = N^{-1} R^N(\bar{T}_\infty^N)$ is the fraction of the population that is infected by the epidemic and $z = \mu_I^{-1}\tau$. Note that (3.4.16) and (3.4.20) imply that

$$z = \mu_I^{-1}\mu + 1 - f_S(\mathrm{e}^{-\lambda_G \mu_I z}),$$

which reduces to (3.4.5) when $\mu = 0$.

We can also obtain a central limit theorem for Z_N. Suppose that

$$\frac{1}{\sqrt{N}} \left\{ \begin{pmatrix} R^N(t) - Nr(t) \\ A^N(t) - Na(t) \end{pmatrix} : t \geq 0 \right\} \xrightarrow{w} \left\{ \begin{pmatrix} X_R(t) \\ X_A(t) \end{pmatrix} : t \geq 0 \right\} \quad \text{as} \quad N \to \infty, \tag{3.4.22}$$

where $\left\{ \begin{pmatrix} X_R(t) \\ X_A(t) \end{pmatrix} : t \geq 0 \right\}$ is a zero-mean Gaussian process and $\xrightarrow{w}$ denotes weak convergence in an appropriate space. This again needs justifying and details, which can be lengthy, are application dependent; see Ball et al. [14] and Ball and Lyne [11] for the households model, Ball and Neal [16] for the great circle model and Neal [51, Chapter 4] for the households-workplaces model. Note that (3.4.22) implies the weak law of large numbers at (3.4.15).

Recalling that $\bar{T}_\infty^N \xrightarrow{p} \tau$ as $N \to \infty$, it follows from (3.4.22), using Slutsky's lemma and the continuous mapping theorem, that

$$\frac{1}{\sqrt{N}} \begin{pmatrix} R^N(\bar{T}_\infty^N) - Nr(\bar{T}_\infty^N) \\ A^N(\bar{T}_\infty^N) - Na(\bar{T}_\infty^N) \end{pmatrix} \xrightarrow{D} \begin{pmatrix} X_R(\tau) \\ X_A(\tau) \end{pmatrix} \quad \text{as} \quad N \to \infty, \tag{3.4.23}$$

where

$$\begin{pmatrix} X_R(\tau) \\ X_A(\tau) \end{pmatrix} \sim \mathrm{N}(\mathbf{0}, \Sigma(\tau)) \quad \text{and} \quad \Sigma(\tau) = \begin{bmatrix} \sigma_R^2(\tau) & \sigma_{RA}(\tau) \\ \sigma_{RA}(\tau) & \sigma_A^2(\tau) \end{bmatrix}$$

with

$$\sigma_R^2(\tau) = \lim_{N \to \infty} N^{-1} \mathrm{Var}(R^N(\tau)),$$

$$\sigma_{RA}(\tau) = \lim_{N \to \infty} N^{-1} \mathrm{cov}(R^N(\tau), A^N(\tau)),$$

$$\sigma_A^2(\tau) = \lim_{N \to \infty} N^{-1} \mathrm{Var}(A^N(\tau)).$$

By the mean value theorem,

$$\begin{aligned}\frac{1}{\sqrt{N}}\left(R^N(\bar{T}_\infty^N) - Nr(\tau)\right) &= \frac{1}{\sqrt{N}}\left(R^N(\bar{T}_\infty^N) - Nr(\bar{T}_\infty^N)\right) + \sqrt{N}\left(r(\bar{T}_\infty^N) - r(\tau)\right) \\ &= \frac{1}{\sqrt{N}}\left(R^N(\bar{T}_\infty^N) - Nr(\bar{T}_\infty^N)\right) + \sqrt{N} r'(\xi_N)\left(\bar{T}_\infty^N - \tau\right),\end{aligned}$$

for some ξ_N between τ and $\bar{T}_\infty^N$.

Now (3.4.19) and (3.4.20) imply

$$\bar{T}_\infty^N - \tau = \bar{T}_0^N + N^{-1} A^N(\bar{T}_\infty^N) - a(\tau),$$

and $\bar{T}_\infty^N \xrightarrow{p} \tau$ (see (3.4.21)) implies that $\xi_N \xrightarrow{p} \tau$ as $N \to \infty$, so

$$\begin{aligned}\frac{1}{\sqrt{N}}\left(R^N(\bar{T}_\infty^N) - Nr(\tau)\right) &= \frac{1}{\sqrt{N}}\left(R^N(\bar{T}_\infty^N) - Nr(\bar{T}_\infty^N)\right) \\ &+ r'(\tau)\left[\sqrt{N}(\bar{T}_0^N - \mu) + \frac{1}{\sqrt{N}}\left(A^N(\bar{T}_\infty^N) - Na(\tau)\right)\right] + o_{\mathrm{p}}(1), \quad (3.4.24)\end{aligned}$$

where a sequence of random variables (X^N) is $o_{\mathrm{p}}(1)$ if $X^N \xrightarrow{p} 0$ as $N \to \infty$. Similarly,

$$\begin{aligned}\frac{1}{\sqrt{N}}\left(A^N(\bar{T}_\infty^N) - Na(\tau)\right) &= \frac{1}{\sqrt{N}}\left(A^N(\bar{T}_\infty^N) - Na(\bar{T}_\infty^N)\right) \\ &+ a'(\tau)\left[\sqrt{N}(\bar{T}_0^N - \mu) + \frac{1}{\sqrt{N}}\left(A^N(\bar{T}_\infty^N) - Na(\tau)\right)\right] + o_{\mathrm{p}}(1). \quad (3.4.25)\end{aligned}$$

Suppose that $\sqrt{N}(\bar{T}_0^N - \mu) \xrightarrow{p} 0$ as $N \to \infty$. Then, (3.4.23)-(3.4.25) imply

$$H \frac{1}{\sqrt{N}} \begin{pmatrix} R^N(\bar{T}_\infty^N) - Nr(\tau) \\ A^N(\bar{T}_\infty^N) - Na(\tau) \end{pmatrix} \xrightarrow{D} \begin{pmatrix} X_R(\tau) \\ X_A(\tau) \end{pmatrix} \quad \text{as} \quad N \to \infty,$$

where

$$H = \begin{bmatrix} 1 & -r'(\tau) \\ 0 & 1 - a'(\tau) \end{bmatrix} = \begin{bmatrix} 1 & -r'(\tau) \\ 0 & 1 - \mu_I r'(\tau) \end{bmatrix},$$

using (3.4.16), so

$$\frac{1}{\sqrt{N}} \begin{pmatrix} R^N(\bar{T}_\infty^N) - Nr(\tau) \\ A^N(\bar{T}_\infty^N) - Na(\tau) \end{pmatrix} \xrightarrow{D} \mathrm{N}\left(\mathbf{0}, H^{-1}\Sigma(\tau)(H^{-1})^\top\right) \quad \text{as} \quad N \to \infty.$$

Let $Z^N = R^N(\bar{T}_\infty^N)$ and $A^N = A^N(\bar{T}_\infty^N)$ so, recalling (3.4.13) and (3.4.14), the size and severity of E^N are Z^N and $A^N + T_0^N$, respectively. Then calculating $H^{-1}\Sigma(\tau)(H^{-1})^\top$ yields the following theorem.

Theorem 3.4.1. *Suppose that Assumption (A.2) (see page 164) and* (3.4.22) *hold, and* $\sqrt{N}(\bar{T}_0^N - \mu) \xrightarrow{p} 0$ *as* $N \to \infty$*, where* $\mu > 0$*. Then*

$$\frac{1}{\sqrt{N}} \begin{pmatrix} Z^N - Nr(\tau) \\ A^N - Na(\tau) \end{pmatrix} \xrightarrow{D} \mathrm{N}(\mathbf{0}, \Sigma),$$

where

$$\Sigma = \begin{bmatrix} \sigma_R^2 & \sigma_{RA} \\ \sigma_{RA} & \sigma_A^2 \end{bmatrix} \tag{3.4.26}$$

with

$$\begin{aligned}
\sigma_R^2 &= \frac{1}{(1-\mu_I r'(\tau))^2} \left[(1-\mu_I r'(\tau))^2 \sigma_{\tilde{R}}^2(\tau) + 2r'(\tau)(1-\mu_I r'(\tau))\sigma_{\tilde{R}\tilde{A}}(\tau) + r'(\tau)^2 \sigma_{\tilde{A}}^2(\tau) \right], \\
\sigma_{RA} &= \frac{1}{(1-\mu_I r'(\tau))^2} \left[(1-\mu_I r'(\tau))\sigma_{\tilde{R}\tilde{A}}(\tau) + r'(\tau)\sigma_{\tilde{A}}^2(\tau) \right], \\
\sigma_A^2 &= \frac{1}{(1-\mu_I r'(\tau))^2} \sigma_{\tilde{A}}^2(\tau).
\end{aligned}$$

The next corollary follows immediately from Theorem 3.4.1 on noting that when I is almost surely constant, $\sigma_{\tilde{R}\tilde{A}}(\tau) = \mu_I \sigma_{\tilde{R}}^2(\tau)$ and $\sigma_{\tilde{A}}^2(\tau) = \mu_I^2 \sigma_{\tilde{R}}^2(\tau)$.

Corollary 3.4.2. *Suppose that* $\mathbb{P}(I = \mu_I) = 1$*. Then, under the conditions of Theorem 3.4.1,*

$$\frac{1}{\sqrt{N}} (Z^N - Nr(\tau)) \xrightarrow{D} \mathrm{N}\left(0, \frac{1}{(1-\mu_I r'(\tau))^2} \sigma_{\tilde{R}}^2(\tau)\right) \qquad \textit{as } N \to \infty.$$

Suppose now that $\mu = 0$. The equation (3.4.20) becomes

$$t = a(t). \tag{3.4.27}$$

Clearly $t = 0$ is a solution of (3.4.27). Using (3.4.7), (3.4.16) and the concavity of $a(t)$, there is a (unique) solution, $\hat{\tau}$ say, in $(0, \infty)$ if and only if $R_* > 1$. Suppose that $R_* > 1$. Then (3.4.17) implies that, as $N \to \infty$,

$$\min\{\bar{T}_\infty^N, |\bar{T}_\infty^N - \hat{\tau}|\} \xrightarrow{p} 0 \qquad \text{and} \qquad \min\{\bar{Z}^N, |\bar{Z}^N - \hat{z}|\} \xrightarrow{p} 0, \tag{3.4.28}$$

where $\hat{z}$ is the unique solution of (3.4.5) in $(0, 1]$. Hence, with probability tending to 1 as $N \to \infty$, the fraction of the population infected by the epidemic, $\bar{Z}^N$, is close to either 0 or $\hat{z}$.

Suppose that $R_* > 1$, $\bar{T}_0^N \xrightarrow{p} 0$ as $N \to \infty$ but $\lim_{N\to\infty} \mathbb{P}(T_0^N \geq K) = 1$ for all $K > 0$. Then an analogous argument to the derivation of (3.3.33) in Section 3.3.6 shows that there exists an $\varepsilon > 0$ such that $\lim_{N\to\infty} \mathbb{P}(\bar{Z}_\infty^N > \varepsilon) = 1$. It then follows from (3.4.28) that (3.4.21) holds, with (τ, z) replaced by $(\hat{\tau}, \hat{z})$, as do Theorem 3.4.1 and Corollary 3.4.2 (both with $\mu = 0$).

Theorem 3.4.1 and its above extension with $\mu = 0$ are for a version of the epidemic E^N, in which the entire population is initially susceptible and the epidemic is initiated by exposing each individual in the population to $\bar{T}_0^N$ units of global infection. This is different from the assumption made when using branching processes to approximate the early stages of an epidemic in Section 3.3, where it is assumed that the epidemic is initiated by an individual chosen uniformly at random from the population becoming infected. When $R_* > 1$, we would like to develop a central limit theorem analogous to Theorem 3.4.1, for epidemics that are initiated by a single infective and result in a global outbreak. For the special case of the standard SIR epidemic this can be achieved by assuming that initially there are N susceptibles, labelled $1, 2, \dots, N$ and setting $T_0^N = I_0$, where I_0 is the infectious period of the initial infective. In the households model, we can similarly add an extra household, which contains the initial infective, and let T_0^N be the severity of the corresponding local infectious clump (single-household epidemic). In the latter there is a slight complication because it is possible for the initially infected household to be reinfected later in the epidemic, unless the single-household epidemic infects all individuals in that household. However, it is easily shown that possibility does not effect the limiting distribution in Theorem 3.4.1, since the extra severity owing to such reinfection is stochastically bounded above by $\check{T}^N = I_1 + I_2 + \cdots + I_n$, so $N^{-1/2}\check{T}^N \xrightarrow{p} 0$ as $N \to \infty$. (Recall that the household size is n.)

In view of the above, suppose finally that $R_* > 1$ and there exists a non-negative random variable T_0 such that $T_0^N \xrightarrow{D} T_0$ as $N \to \infty$. Then $R^N(T_0) \xrightarrow{D} \text{Poi}(\lambda_G T_0)$ as $N \to \infty$ and arguing as in Section 3.3.6 shows that Theorem 3.3.7 holds, with p_{ext} replaced by $\tilde{p}_{\text{ext}} = \mathbb{E}\left[\mathrm{e}^{-\lambda_G T_0(1-p_{\text{ext}})}\right]$. (In the limit as $N \to \infty$ the epidemic E^N is initiated by $\text{Poi}(\lambda_G T_0)$ infectives, so can be approximated by the branching process $\mathscr{B}$ having $\text{Poi}(\lambda_G T_0)$ initial ancestors. It is easily verified, and left as an exercise, that $\tilde{p}_{\text{ext}} = p_{\text{ext}}$ in the two special cases discussed in previous paragraph.) Thus, in particular,

$$\lim_{N\to\infty} \mathbb{P}(Z^N \geq \log N) = 1 - \tilde{p}_{\text{ext}}. \tag{3.4.29}$$

Also,

$$\limsup_{N\to\infty} \mathbb{P}(\bar{Z}^N > \hat{z}/2) \leq 1 - \tilde{p}_{\text{ext}}. \tag{3.4.30}$$

In an obvious notation, arguing as in the derivation of (3.3.28) shows that, for $\varepsilon \in (0,1)$,

$$\liminf_{N\to\infty} \mathbb{P}(\bar{Z}^N > \varepsilon) \geq 1 - \tilde{p}_{\text{ext}}(\varepsilon, K),$$

which together with (3.4.28) implies that

$$\liminf_{N\to\infty} \mathbb{P}(\bar{Z}^N > \hat{z}/2) \geq 1 - \tilde{p}_{\text{ext}}(\varepsilon, K). \tag{3.4.31}$$

Now (ε, K) can be chosen so that $p_{\text{ext}}(\varepsilon, K)$ is arbitrarily close to p_{ext}, and hence so that $\tilde{p}_{\text{ext}}(\varepsilon, K)$ is arbitrarily close to $\tilde{p}_{\text{ext}}$. Therefore, (3.4.30) and (3.4.31) imply that

$$\lim_{N\to\infty} \mathbb{P}(\bar{Z}^N > \hat{z}/2) = 1 - \tilde{p}_{\text{ext}},$$

which, together with (3.4.28), yields the following theorem. (Assumptions (A.2) to (A.5) are stated on page 176.)

Theorem 3.4.3. *Suppose that Assumptions (A.2) to (A.5) and* (3.4.15) *hold, and that* $T_0^N \xrightarrow{D} T_0$ *as* $N \to \infty$. *Then*

$$\bar{Z}^N \xrightarrow{D} \bar{Z} \qquad \text{as } N \to \infty,$$

where

$$\mathbb{P}(\bar{Z} = 0) = \tilde{p}_{\text{ext}} = 1 - \mathbb{P}(\bar{Z} = \hat{z}).$$

Theorem 3.4.3 and (3.4.29) yield the following law of large numbers for global outbreaks.

Corollary 3.4.4. *Suppose that* $R_* > 1$ *and* $T_0^N \xrightarrow{D} T_0$ *as* $N \to \infty$. *Then, under the conditions of Theorem 3.4.3,*

$$\bar{Z}^N | Z^N \geq \log N \xrightarrow{p} \hat{z} \qquad \text{as } N \to \infty.$$

Note that, under the conditions of Corollary 3.4.4, $\bar{T}_\infty^N | Z^N \geq \log N \xrightarrow{p} \hat{\tau}$ as $N \to \infty$. It is tempting to conclude that the argument leading to Theorem 3.4.1 yields the following theorem.

Theorem 3.4.5. *Suppose that* $R_* > 1$, *Assumptions (A.2) to (A.5) and* (3.4.22) *hold and* $T_0^N \xrightarrow{D} T_0$ *as* $N \to \infty$. *Then,*

$$\frac{1}{\sqrt{N}} \left[\begin{pmatrix} Z^N - Nr(\hat{\tau}) \\ A^N - Na(\hat{\tau}) \end{pmatrix} \right] | \; Z^N \geq \log N \xrightarrow{D} \mathrm{N}(\mathbf{0}, \hat{\Sigma}) \qquad \text{as } N \to \infty,$$

where $\hat{\Sigma}$ *is given by* (3.4.26) *with* $\tau = \hat{\tau}$.

The result is generally true but the above argument fails because the distribution of the sample paths of $\{(R^N(t), A^N(t)) : t \geq 0\}$ conditional upon $Z^N \geq \log N$ is different from the unconditional distribution. One way to obtain a valid proof for some models, which also works for other initial conditions, is to use a branching process approximation to the epidemic until there are $\log N$ infectives and then apply the above-mentioned version of Theorem 3.4.1 (with $\mu = 0$) to the remaining susceptible population. The details are messy and are not considered here. Theorem 3.4.5 has an equivalent corollary to Corollary 3.4.2 when the infectious period random variable I is almost surely constant.

3.5 Applications to Special Cases

We now apply the general theory developed in Sections 3.2–3.4 to the special cases in Section 3.1 on pages 161 to 163. Further details on the application to the reproduction number R_*, and the probability and size of a global outbreak, may be found for the households, households-workplaces and great circle model in Ball and Neal [15] and for the network model with casual contacts in Ball and Neal [17].

Further details on the calculation of the basic reproduction number R_0 and the exponential growth rate r for the households and households-workplaces models are given in Ball et al. [19].

3.5.1 Standard SIR Model

As noted previously, setting $\lambda_{ij}^L = 0$ for all $i \neq j$ yields the standard SIR epidemic model of Section 1.1 with $\lambda = \lambda_G/N$, which has the same final size distribution as the corresponding SEIR model incorporating a latent period. Thus results about the asymptotic distribution of the final size of a homogeneously mixing SEIR epidemic presented in Section 3.3 of Part I in this volume arise as special cases of the theorems in Section 3.3 and 3.4. The local infectious clumps all have size 1 so, using (3.3.5) on page 167, $R_* = \lambda\mu_I$. Further, $\mu_0^C = 1$ and $\mu_k^C = 0$ $(k = 1, 2, \ldots)$, and it follows from (3.3.8) that $R_0 = \lambda\mu_I$, so $R_0 = R_*$.

Exercise 3.5.1. Derive the central limit theorem (Theorem 3.3.2 of Part I in this volume) using Theorem 3.4.5.

Turning to the exponential growth rate (see Section 3.3.5 on page 174), note that $Y_1(t) = 1_{\{I_1 > t\}}$. It follows that $\mu_Y(t) = \mathbb{P}(I > t)$ and $w_G(t) = \mu_I^{-1}\mathbb{P}(I > t)$ $(t \geq 0)$, whence

$$\phi_{W_G}(\theta) = (\mu_I\theta)^{-1}(1 - \phi_I(\theta))$$

and, since $R_0 = R_*$, (3.3.17) gives

$$R_0 = \frac{\mu_I r}{1 - \phi_I(r)}. \tag{3.5.1}$$

The practical usefulness of (3.5.1) is that if estimates of the exponential growth rate r and the distribution of I are available from data on an emerging epidemic, then (3.5.1) yields an estimate of R_0 and hence of the critical vaccination coverage v_c; see Nowak et al. [53], Lloyd [48], Wallinga and Lipsitch [64] and Roberts and Heesterbeek [58], which consider homogeneously mixing models with more general infectivity curves (see Section 1.1.2 of Part I in this volume). However, it should be borne in mind that $\phi_{W_G}(\theta)$ can be difficult to estimate unbiasedly owing to the emerging nature of the data (Britton and Scalia-Tomba [30]). For example, early in an epidemic completed infectious periods are likely to be atypically short.

One can also use (3.5.1) to estimate R_0 for more complicated models, though of course such an estimate has no theoretical grounding without further work. However, for many common departures from homogeneous mixing, such as those owing to household and network structures, (3.5.1) typically yields overestimates of both R_0 and v_c (Trapman et al. [63] and Section 2.6 of Part III in this volume).

Exercise 3.5.2. Determine the exponential growth rate r for the Markovian SEIR model, defined in Section 1.1.2 of Part I in this volume, with $I \sim \text{Exp}(\gamma)$ and $L \sim \text{Exp}(\nu)$. (For $\gamma > 0$, $\text{Exp}(\gamma)$ denotes an exponential random variable with probability density function $f(t) = \gamma e^{-\gamma t}$ $(t \geq 0)$ and hence mean γ^{-1}.)

3.5.2 Households Model

Recall from Section 3.1.2 on page 161 that we consider the special case of the households model in which all the households have size n. The more general case of unequal-sized households is analysed extensively in Chapter 2, so here we focus mainly on the basic reproduction number R_0 and the exponential growth rate r, which are not considered in Section 3.1.2, and the final outcome of a global outbreak, where the results obtained by specialising the general two-level mixing theory yield different (though of course equivalent) expressions to those obtained in Section 3.1.2. In the following $q_i = \phi_I(i\lambda_H)$ $(i=0,1,\dots)$.

3.5.2.1 Threshold Parameter R_*

First note that the size C of a typical local infectious clump is distributed as the total size (including the initial infective) of the standard SIR epidemic $E_{n-1,1}(\lambda_H, I)$ so, using (3.3.5) on page 167 and Corollary 1.6.3 on page 135,

$$R_* = \lambda_G \mu_I \left[n - \sum_{i=1}^{n-1} (n-1)_{[i]} q_i^{n-i} G_{i-1}(1 \mid V) \right],$$

where V is given by $v_i = q_{i+1}$ $(i=0,1,\dots)$.

3.5.2.2 Basic Reproduction Number R_0

To calculate R_0 we need the clump generation means μ_k^C $(k=0,1,\dots)$. In the households model, the clumps are single-household epidemics, so we call clump generations, household generations, and denote the mean number of individuals in household generation k by μ_k^H $(k=0,1,\dots,n-1)$. (The maximum household generation is $n-1$ as the households all have size n.)

For small household size n, we can calculate the μ_k^Hs by considering all possible chains of infection as in Section 3.1 of Part I of this volume.

Exercise 3.5.3. Suppose I is constant, so $\mathbb{P}(I = \mu_I) = 1$, and $n = 3$.

(a) Show that $\mu_0^H = 1, \mu_1^H = 2p_H$ and $\mu_2^H = 2p_H^2(1-p_H)$, where $p_H = 1 - \mathrm{e}^{-\lambda_H \mu_I}$.
(b) Determine μ_0^H, μ_1^H and μ_2^H when I is not constant.
(c) Repeat parts (a) and (b) when $n = 4$, calculating all non-zero μ_k^H.

For larger household sizes, such enumeration becomes tedious and we present a method that is amenable to numerical calculation. Consider the standard SIR epidemic model $E_{n,a}(\lambda_H, I)$, defined in Section 1.1 and recall the probabilities $P_{n,a}(k)$ $(k=0,1,\dots n)$ defined in Exercise 1.3.2 on page 129. For $k=0,1,\dots,n$, let $Y_{n,a,k}$ be the number of infectives in household generation k and let $\mu_{n,a,k} = \mathbb{E}[Y_{n,a,k}]$, so

$$\mathbb{P}(Y_{n,a,1} = i) = P_{n,a}(n-i) \qquad (i=0,1,\dots,n).$$

Then, for $n,a = 1,2,\dots$ and $k = 1,2,\dots,n$,

$$\begin{aligned}\mu_{n,a,k} &= \mathbb{E}[\mathbb{E}[Y_{n,a,k}|Y_{n,a,1}]]\\ &= \sum_{i=1}^{n-k+1} \mathbb{E}[Y_{n,a,k}|Y_{n,a,1}=i]\mathbb{P}(Y_{n,a,1}=i)\\ &= \sum_{i=1}^{n-k+1} P_{n,a}(n-i)\mu_{n-i,i,k-1},\end{aligned}$$

which, together with $\mu_{n,a,0} = a$ and $\mu_{0,a,k} = 0$ ($n,a = 1,2,\dots$ and $k = 1,2,\dots,n$), can be solved recursively for the $\mu_{n,a,k}$. Note that $\mu_k^H = \mu_{n-1,1,k}$ ($k = 0,1,\dots,n-1$). See Appendix A in Pellis et al. [54] for further discussion, including another method of computing the μ_k^Hs.

3.5.2.3 Exponential Growth Rate r

The difficulty in calculating r for the households model is the absence in general of a closed-form expression of $\mu_Y(t)$, the mean number of infectives at time t in the single-household epidemic $E_{n,1}(\lambda_H, I)$. Various approximations to r are discussed in Ball et al. [19, Section 2.8] (see also Fraser [33]). If I is exponentially distributed, $E_{n,1}(\lambda_H, I)$ is described by a continuous-time Markov chain, and the Laplace transform $\mathscr{L}_{\mu_Y}(\theta)$ of $\mu_Y(t)$ can be computed as follows (see Pellis et al. [56, Section 4.2]).

Suppose $I \sim \text{Exp}(\gamma)$. For $t \geq 0$, let $X(t)$ and $Y(t)$ be respectively the numbers of susceptibles and infectives at time t in $E_{n,1}(\lambda_H, I)$. Then $\{(X(t),Y(t))\} = \{(X(t),Y(t)) : t \geq 0\}$ is a continuous-time Markov chain with $(X(0),Y(0)) = (n-1,1)$ and state space

$$E = \{(i,j) : i = 0,1,\dots,n-1, j = 0,1,\dots,n-i\}$$

having size $n_E = n(n+3)/2$. For $(i,j) \neq (i',j')$, the transition rates of $\{(X(t),Y(t))\}$ are

$$q_{(i,j),(i',j')} = \begin{cases} \lambda_H ij & \text{if } (i',j') = (i-1,j+1),\\ \gamma j & \text{if } (i',j') = (i,j-1),\\ 0 & \text{otherwise;}\end{cases}$$

the first transition corresponds to an infection and the second to a recovery. For $(i,j) \in E$, let

$$q_{(i,j),(i,j)} = -\sum_{(i',j')\neq(i,j)} q_{(i,j),(i',j')}.$$

Give the states of E the labels $1,2,\dots,n_E$. For $(i,j) \in E$, let $h(i,j)$ denote the label of state (i,j). Choose the labels so that $h(n-1,1) = 1$ and $h(i,0) = n_E - i$ ($i = 0,1,\dots,n-1$). Thus the initial state is given the label 1 and the terminal states (i.e. those with no infective) are given the labels $n_A+1, n_A+2,\dots,n_A+n$, where $n_A = n_E - n = n(n+1)/2$ is the number of active states (i.e. those with at least one infective). For $k = 1,2,\dots,n_E$, let $(x(k),y(k)) = h^{-1}(k)$, so $x(k)$ and $y(k)$ are respectively the numbers of susceptibles and infectives in the state having label k. Let $\tilde{Q} = [\tilde{q}_{kl}]$ be the $n_E \times n_E$ matrix with elements given by $\tilde{q}_{kl} = q_{(x(k),y(k)),(x(l),y(l))}$. Thus $\tilde{Q}$ is the transition-rate matrix of $\{h(X(t),Y(t)) : t \geq 0\}$ and, for $t \geq 0$,

$$\mathbb{P}[(X(t),Y(t)) = (i,j)] = \left[\mathrm{e}^{\tilde{Q}t}\right]_{1,h(i,j)} \qquad ((i,j) \in E),$$

where $\mathrm{e}^{\tilde{Q}t} = \sum_{k=0}^{\infty} t^k \tilde{Q}^k / k!$ is the usual matrix exponential. Further, if E_A denotes set of active states in E and $\tilde{Q}_{AA}$ is the $n_A \times n_A$ submatrix of $\tilde{Q}$ corresponding to E_A, then

$$\mathbb{P}[(X(t),Y(t)) = (i,j)] = \left[\mathrm{e}^{\tilde{Q}_{AA}t}\right]_{1,h(i,j)} \qquad ((i,j) \in E_A).$$

Let $\mathbf{u}_0 = (1,0,0,\ldots,0)$ have dimension n_A and $\mathbf{v}_Y = (y(1),y(2),\ldots,y(n_A))^\top$. Then

$$\mu_Y(t) = \mathbb{E}[Y(t)] = \mathbf{u}_0 \mathrm{e}^{\tilde{Q}_{AA}t} \mathbf{v}_Y,$$

whence

$$\mathscr{L}_{\mu_Y}(\theta) = \mathbf{u}_0 [\theta I_{n_A} - \tilde{Q}_{AA}]^{-1} \mathbf{v}_Y, \tag{3.5.2}$$

where I_{n_A} is the $n_A \times n_A$ identity matrix. Equation (3.5.2) enables $\mathscr{L}_{\mu_Y}(\theta)$ and hence r to be computed numerically.

By enlarging suitably the state space E, the above argument can be extended to the case when I has a gamma distribution with an integer shape parameter, and more generally to when I has a phase type distribution (see Asmussen [5, pages 71–78]). However, the state space E can become prohibitively large for numerical calculation. When the household size n is very small, $\mathscr{L}_{\mu_Y}(\theta)$ can be found by enumerating all possible real-time chains of infection, as in the following exercise.

Exercise 3.5.4. Suppose that $n = 2$.

(a) Suppose that I has an arbitrary but specified distribution. Show that, when it is finite,

$$\mathscr{L}_{\mu_Y}(\theta) = \psi_I(\theta)\,[1 + \lambda_H \psi_I(\lambda_H + \theta)], \tag{3.5.3}$$

where $\psi_I(\theta) = \theta^{-1}[1 - \phi_I(\theta)]$.
Hint: the contribution of the initial infective to $\mathscr{L}_{\mu_Y}(\theta)$ is $\psi_I(\theta)$.

(b) Determine r when $I \sim \mathrm{Exp}(\gamma)$.

3.5.2.4 Final Outcome of Global Outbreak

Turning to the final outcome, let H denote the set of individuals in a household and $F \subseteq H$ having size $|F| = j$, where $j = 0,1,\ldots,n$. (If $j = 0$ then $F = \emptyset$.) Recall the definitions of $\mathscr{S}_F$ and S_F from (3.4.8) and (3.4.9). The distribution of S_F depends only on F through j, so write $\mathbb{P}_{jn}(S_F = k)$ for the probability that $S_F = k$, where $k = j, j+1,\ldots,n$. Now $\mathbb{P}_{0n}(S_F = 0) = 1$, as $\mathscr{S}_\emptyset = \emptyset$ by convention, and application of Lemma 1.5.2 on page 132 yields that, for $j = 1,2,\ldots,n$,

$$\mathbb{P}_{jn}(S_F = k) = (n-j)_{[k-j]} q_k^{n-k} G_{k-j}(1 \mid E^j U) \qquad (k = j, j+1,\ldots,n), \tag{3.5.4}$$

where U is given by $u_k = q_k$ $(k = 0, 1, \ldots)$ and $E^j U$ is the sequence $u_j, u_{J+1}, \ldots$.

Recall also that $f_{S_F}(s) = \mathbb{E}[s^{S_F}]$ $(0 \leq s \leq 1)$, so write $f_{S_F}(s)$ as $f_{jn}(s)$. Then $f_{0n}(s) = 1$ and, for $j = 1, 2, \ldots, n$,

$$f_{jn}(s) = \sum_{k=j}^{n} (n-j)_{[k-j]} s^k q_k^{n-k} G_{k-j}(1 \mid E^j U). \tag{3.5.5}$$

Suppose that $R_* > 1$. Noting that S is distributed as S_F when $j = 1$, it follows using (3.4.5) that, as $N \to \infty$, the fraction of the population that is infected by a global outbreak, $\hat{z}$, is given by the unique solution in $(0, 1]$ of

$$1 - z = f_{1n}(\mathrm{e}^{-\lambda_G \mu_I z}). \tag{3.5.6}$$

Exercise 3.5.5. Show that equation (3.5.6) for $\hat{z}$ is the same as equation (2.3.2) in Section 2.3 (assuming a common household size).

Now let H be a household that initially contained only susceptibles and let X_H be the set of susceptibles in that household at the end of a global outbreak. Then X_H is a set obtained from a symmetric sampling procedure (see Section 1.3) on H, so $\mathbb{P}(|X_H| = k) = \binom{n}{k}\mathbb{P}(X_H = G)$, where G is any given size-k subset of H, and it follows from (3.4.11) on page 184 that

$$\mathbb{P}(|X_H| = k) = \binom{n}{k} \sum_{j=k}^{n} (-1)^{j-k} \binom{n-k}{j-k} f_{jn}(\mathrm{e}^{-\lambda_G \mu_I \hat{z}}) \qquad (k = 0, 1, \ldots, n). \tag{3.5.7}$$

Exercise 3.5.6. Show that (3.5.7) yields the same distribution for the number infected in a typical household in the event of a global outbreak as that derived in Section 2.3, i.e. that $|X_H| \stackrel{\mathrm{D}}{=} \tilde{S}$, where $\tilde{S}$ is the final number of susceptibles in the epidemic $\tilde{E}_{n,0}(\lambda_H, I, \hat{\pi})$, defined in Section 1.8, and $\hat{\pi} = \mathrm{e}^{-\lambda_G \mu_I \hat{z}}$.

3.5.3 Households-workplaces Model

For reasons explained later, the distribution of the size C of a typical local infectious clump is difficult to obtain unless the infectious period I is constant, so we focus first on the size S of a typical local susceptibility set. When I is constant, C and S have the same distribution as we now explain (cf. Remark 1.5.3 on page 133).

If I is constant, say $\mathbb{P}(I = \mu_I) = 1$ for some $\mu_I > 0$, the random directed graph $\mathscr{G}_L$, defined in Section 3.2 on page 163, can be replaced by an undirected random graph, $\hat{\mathscr{G}}_L$ say, in which for any unordered pair (i, j) of distinct vertices in $\mathscr{N}$ the edge between i and j is present independently with probability $p_L(i, j)$, where

$$p_L(i,j) = \begin{cases} 1 - \mathrm{e}^{-\lambda_H \mu_I} & \text{if } i \text{ and } j \text{ belong to the same household,} \\ 1 - \mathrm{e}^{-\lambda_W \mu_I} & \text{if } i \text{ and } j \text{ belong to the same workplace,} \\ 0 & \text{otherwise.} \end{cases}$$

For $i \in \mathcal{N}$, the random graph $\hat{\mathcal{G}}_L$ can be used to construct the local infectious clump $\mathcal{C}_i$ of individual i, in an analogous fashion to that used to construct the final outcome of the Reed–Frost epidemic in Remark 1.2.3 on page 128. The random graph $\hat{\mathcal{G}}_L$ can also be used to construct the local susceptibility set $\mathcal{S}_i$ of individual i. For $j \neq i$, individual $j \in \mathcal{S}_i$ if and only if their is a path of edges from i to j in $\hat{\mathcal{G}}_L$. Note that $\mathcal{C}_i = \mathcal{S}_i$ by construction, so C and S above are identically distributed.

3.5.3.1 Size of Local Susceptibility Set

For $i \in \mathcal{N}$, let H_i and W_i denote the sets of individuals in i's household and workplace, respectively, and define i's household and workplace local susceptibility sets by $\mathcal{S}_i^H = \{j \in H_i : j \overset{\mathrm{L}}{\rightsquigarrow} i\}$ and $\mathcal{S}_j^W = \{j \in W_i : j \overset{\mathrm{L}}{\rightsquigarrow} i\}$. For $i \in \mathcal{N}$, the local susceptibility set $\mathcal{S}_i$ of individual i can be constructed on a generation basis as follows. Let

$$\mathcal{P}_0 = \mathcal{S}_i^H,$$

and, for $k = 1, 2, \dots$, let

$$\mathcal{P}_k = \begin{cases} \left(\bigcup_{j \in \mathcal{P}_{k-1}} \mathcal{S}_j^W\right) \setminus \left(\bigcup_{l=0}^{k-1} \mathcal{P}_l\right) & \text{if } k \text{ is odd,} \\ \left(\bigcup_{j \in \mathcal{P}_{k-1}} \mathcal{S}_j^H\right) \setminus \left(\bigcup_{l=0}^{k-1} \mathcal{P}_l\right) & \text{if } k \text{ is even.} \end{cases}$$

Let $k^* = \min(k : \mathcal{P}_k = \emptyset)$ and note that $k^* < \infty$ since $\mathcal{N}$ is finite. Then

$$\mathcal{S}_i = \bigcup_{k=0}^{k^*-1} \mathcal{P}_k.$$

In words, the local susceptibility set $\mathcal{S}_i$ is constructed by first forming the household susceptibility set of individual i, to give generation 0, then forming the workplace susceptibility set of each generation-0 individual to form generation-1, then forming the household susceptibility set of each generation-1 individual to form generation-2, and so on, where at each generation an individual is not included if it has already been used in the construction of $\mathcal{S}_i$.

The above construction of $\mathcal{S}_i$ can be approximated by a two-type branching process $\hat{\mathcal{B}}$, which assumes that, for $k = 0, 1, \dots$, if k is even then the households of the individuals in $\mathcal{P}_k$ are disjoint and also have empty intersection with the households of individuals used in previous generations of the construction, and similarly if k is odd but with households replaced by workplaces. In the branching process $\hat{\mathcal{B}}$, individuals in generation k all have type H if k is even and all have type W if k is odd, so individuals beget only individuals of the opposite type. The initial ancestors (i.e. generation 0) in $\hat{\mathcal{B}}$ comprise all individuals in individual i's household susceptibility set $\mathcal{S}_i^H$. The offspring of a typical generation-0 individual, $j \in \mathcal{S}_i^H$ say, are all individuals in j's workplace susceptibility set excluding j, i.e. $\mathcal{S}_j^W \setminus \{j\}$, and so on. Let S^H and S^W denote the size of a typical household and workplace susceptibility set, respectively. Then, in $\hat{\mathcal{B}}$, the number of initial ancestors, $\hat{Y}_0$ say, is distributed as S^H, the number of offspring of a typical type-H individual is distributed as $S^W - 1$, and the number of offspring of a typical type-W individual is distributed as $S^H - 1$. The distribution of S_H is given by setting $j = 1, n = n_H$ and $q_i = \phi_I(i\lambda_H)$ $(i = 0, 1, \dots)$ in (3.5.4). The distribution of S^W is given similarly, with (n_H, λ_H) replaced by (n_W, λ_W).

For $k = 0, 1, \dots$, let $\hat{Y}_k$ be the size of generation k in $\hat{\mathscr{B}}$, and let $\hat{Z} = \sum_{k=0}^{\infty} \hat{Y}_k$ be the total size of $\hat{\mathscr{B}}$ including the initial ancestors. We assume that $S^N \xrightarrow{D} \hat{Z}$ as $N \to \infty$ (see Exercise 3.5.7 below), so, as detailed in the next two subsections, we may set $S = \hat{Z}$ in the results in Section 3.4.1. This implicitly imposes strong conditions on the configuration of households and workplaces in the population, as indicated at the end of Section 3.1.3, which are unrealistic in many practical settings. One situation when $S^N \xrightarrow{D} \hat{Z}$ as $N \to \infty$ is when the partitioning of the population $\mathscr{N}$ into households is independent of the partitioning into workplaces, as follows.

Recall that the individuals in $\mathscr{N}$ are labelled $1, 2, \dots, N$, Label the m_H households $1, 2, \dots, m_H$ and, for $i = 1, 2, \dots, N$, assign individual i to household $\lceil i/n_H \rceil$. (For $x \in \mathbb{R}$, $\lceil x \rceil$ is the smallest integer $\geq x$.) Thus individuals $1, 2, \dots, n_H$ are assigned to household 1, individuals $n_H + 1, n_H + 2, \dots, 2n_H$ are assigned to household 2, and so on. Now let $(\sigma(1), \sigma(2), \dots, \sigma(N))$ be a (uniform) random permutation of $(1, 2, \dots, N)$. Label the m_W workplaces $1, 2, \dots, m_W$. Then for $i = 1, 2, \dots, N$, individual i is assigned to workplace $\lceil \sigma(i)/n_W \rceil$.

Exercise 3.5.7. Show that $S^N \xrightarrow{D} \hat{Z}$ as $N \to \infty$ under the above allocation of individuals to households and workplaces, so Assumption (A.2) on page 164 holds. Hint: consider the above construction of $\mathscr{S}_i$ and for fixed $k = 1, 2, \dots$, obtain an upper bound for the probability that $\mathscr{P}_k$ contains two individuals that belong to the same household and the same workplace.

3.5.3.2 Threshold Parameter R_*

Let $\mu_H = \mathbb{E}[S^H]$ and $\mu_W = \mathbb{E}[S^W]$. Then $\mathbb{E}[\hat{Y}_0] = \mu_H$ and, conditioning on $\hat{Y}_0$,

$$\mathbb{E}[\hat{Y}_1] = \mathbb{E}[\mathbb{E}[\hat{Y}_1 | \hat{Y}_0]] = \mathbb{E}[(\mu_W - 1)\hat{Y}_0] = (\mu_W - 1)\mu_H,$$

where in the second equality we have used that, given $\hat{Y}_0$, $\hat{Y}_1$ is the sum of $\hat{Y}_0$ i.i.d. copies of $S^W - 1$. Continuing in a similar fashion, it is easily shown by induction that, for $k = 0, 1, \dots$,

$$\mathbb{E}[\hat{Y}_k] = \begin{cases} \mu_H[(\mu_H - 1)(\mu_W - 1)]^l & \text{if } k = 2l, \\ \mu_H(\mu_W - 1)[(\mu_H - 1)(\mu_W - 1)]^{l-1} & \text{if } k = 2l + 1. \end{cases}$$

Now $\mathbb{E}[S] = \mathbb{E}[\hat{Z}] = \sum_{k=0}^{\infty} \mathbb{E}[\hat{Y}_k]$ so, using (3.4.7) on page 183,

$$R_* = \begin{cases} \frac{\lambda_G \mu_I \mu_H \mu_W}{\mu_H + \mu_W - \mu_H \mu_W} & \text{if } (\mu_H - 1)(\mu_W - 1) < 1, \\ \infty & \text{otherwise.} \end{cases}$$

Expressions for μ_H and μ_W in terms of Gontcharoff polynomials are obtained easily using (3.5.4).

3.5.3.3 Final Outcome of Global Outbreak

To determine the fraction of the population infected by a global outbreak, we need the probability-generating function of $S = \hat{Z}$. Let $f_H(s) = \mathbb{E}[s^{S_H}]$ $(0 \le s \le 1)$ be the probability-generating function of S_H. Let $f_{ZH}(s) = \mathbb{E}[s^{\hat{Z}_H}]$ $(0 \le s \le 1)$, where $\hat{Z}_H$ is the total size of the branching process which has the same offspring distributions as $\hat{\mathscr{B}}_H$ but starts with a single individual whose type is H. Define the probability-generating functions f_W and f_{ZW} similarly. Then, conditioning on $\hat{Y}_1$ yields that

$$f_{ZH}(s) = f_W(f_{ZW}(s)) \qquad \text{and} \qquad f_{ZW}(s) = f_H(f_{ZH}(s)),$$

whence

$$f_{ZW}(s) = f_H(f_W(f_{ZW}(s))) \qquad (0 \le s \le 1). \tag{3.5.8}$$

The equation (3.5.8) has a unique solution (cf. Jagers [42, page 39]). Conditioning on $\hat{Y}_0$ then yields

$$f_S(s) = f_H(f_{ZH}(s)) = f_{ZW}(s),$$

which can also be obtained directly. The fraction $\hat{z}$ of the population that is infected by a global outbreak can now be obtained using (3.4.5) on page 182.

The distribution of the final size, Z_H say, within a typical, initially fully-susceptible household in the event of a global outbreak can be obtained using (3.4.11) on page 184.

Exercise 3.5.8. Show that if $\lambda_H, n_H, \hat{z}$ and the distribution of I are fixed, then any choice of $(n_W, \lambda_W, \lambda_G)$ consistent with $\hat{z}$ yields the same distribution of Z_H.

3.5.3.4 Size of Local Infectious Clump

The size C of a typical local infectious clump can be approximated by a two-type process, $\check{\mathscr{B}}$ say, that is similar to $\hat{\mathscr{B}}$ but with household and workplace local susceptibility sets replaced by household and workplace local infectious clumps (i.e. single-household and single-workplace epidemics). A similar argument to Exercise 3.5.7 shows that Assumptions (A.1) and (A.3) (see pages 164 and 176) hold. However, unless the infectious period I is constant, $\check{\mathscr{B}}$ is not a branching process since the infectious periods of infectives in a single-household epidemic, which are the initial cases in the ensuing single-workplace epidemics, are not independent of the size of the single-household epidemic. This dependence does not affect calculation of the means required for R_*, or R_0 below, but it does make calculation of the probability of a global outbreak difficult. If individuals in $\check{\mathscr{B}}$ are also typed by the length of the initial infective in the single-household (or workplace) epidemic then $\check{\mathscr{B}}$ becomes a branching process with a larger (infinite if the support of I is infinite) type space;

cf. Ball et al. [22]. The difficulty disappears if I is constant; the processes $\hat{\mathscr{B}}$ and $\check{\mathscr{B}}$ are then identically distributed.

3.5.3.5 Basic Reproduction Number R_0

As in Ball et al. [19, Section 4.2], the basic reproduction number R_0 for the households-workplaces model can be obtained by considering the following three-type branching process, $\bar{\mathscr{B}}$ say, which approximates the process of infectives on a generation basis. The three types of individuals in $\bar{\mathscr{B}}$ are: *double-primary* cases (type 1), who are infected by a global contact; *household-primary* cases (type 2), who are infected by a within-workplace contact; and *workplace-primary* cases (type 3), who are infected by a within-household contact. Recall from Section 3.5.2 the household mean generation sizes μ_k^H $(k=0,1,\dots,n_H-1)$ and define the workplace mean generation sizes μ_k^W $(k=0,1,\dots,n_W-1)$ similarly.

In $\bar{\mathscr{B}}$, the mother of a double-primary (type-1) individual, is the person who infected it in the epidemic; the mother of a household-primary (type-2) individual is the initial case in the corresponding within-workplace epidemic; and the mother of a workplace-primary (type-3) individual is the initial case in the corresponding within-household epidemic. As indicated above, time in the branching process $\bar{\mathscr{B}}$ corresponds to generation in the epidemic E^N. All individuals in $\bar{\mathscr{B}}$ produce a mean number $\mu_G=\lambda_G\mu_I$ of type-1 individuals (corresponding to global contacts in E^N) at age 1. In addition, a type-2 individual triggers a within-household epidemic in its household, so it produces a mean number μ_k^H of type-3 individuals at age k, where $k=1,2,\dots,n_H-1$. Similarly, a type-3 individual produces a mean number μ_k^W of type-2 individuals at age k, where $k=1,2,\dots,n_W-1$. Finally, a type-1 individual triggers both a within-household and a within-workplace epidemic, so it produces a mean number of μ_k^W of type-2 individuals at age k, where $k=1,2,\dots,n_W-1$, and a mean number μ_k^H of type-3 individuals at age k, where $k=1,2,\dots,n_H-1$. The basic reproduction number R_0 is given by the asymptotic geometric growth rate of the branching process $\bar{\mathscr{B}}$.

For $i,j=1,2,3$ and $k=1,2,\dots$, let $v_{i,j}(k)$ be the mean number of type-j individuals produced by a type-i individual at age k, and let

$$v_{ij}(\lambda)=\sum_{k=1}^{\infty}\frac{v_{i,j}(k)}{\lambda^k} \qquad (\lambda\in(0,\infty)).$$

Let $V(\lambda)$ be the 3×3 matrix with elements $v_{ij}(\lambda)$ and let $v_*(\lambda)$ be the dominant eigenvalue of $V(\lambda)$. Then, using multitype general branching process theory (for example, Haccou et al. [37, Section 3.3.2] and Jagers [43]), R_0 is given by the unique solution in $(0,\infty)$ of $v_*(\lambda)=1$.

The matrix $V(\lambda)$ is given by

$$V(\lambda)=\begin{bmatrix} v_G(\lambda) & v_W(\lambda) & v_H(\lambda) \\ v_G(\lambda) & 0 & v_H(\lambda) \\ v_G(\lambda) & v_W(\lambda) & 0 \end{bmatrix},$$

where

$$\nu_G(\lambda) = \frac{\mu_G}{\lambda} \qquad \nu_H(\lambda) = \sum_{k=1}^{n_H-1} \frac{\mu_k^H}{\lambda^k} \qquad \text{and} \qquad \nu_W(\lambda) = \sum_{k=1}^{n_W-1} \frac{\mu_k^W}{\lambda^k}.$$

Exercise 3.5.9. Show that the characteristic polynomial of $V(\lambda)$ is

$$x^3 - \nu_G(\lambda)x^2 - [\nu_G(\lambda)\nu_H(\lambda) + \nu_G(\lambda)\nu_W(\lambda) + \nu_H(\lambda)\nu_W(\lambda)]x - \nu_G(\lambda)\nu_H(\lambda)\nu_W(\lambda),$$

and hence that $\nu_*(\lambda) = 1$ if and only if

$$\nu_G(\lambda)(\nu_H(\lambda)+1)(\nu_W(\lambda)+1) + \nu_H(\lambda)\nu_W(\lambda) - 1 = 0. \tag{3.5.9}$$

It follows from (3.5.9) that R_0 is given by the unique solution in $(0,\infty)$ of $g_0^{HW}(\lambda) = 0$, where

$$g_0^{HW}(\lambda) = 1 - \sum_{k=0}^{n_H+n_W-2} \frac{c_k}{\lambda^{k+1}}, \tag{3.5.10}$$

with $c_0 = \mu_G$ and, for $k = 1,2,\ldots,n_H+n_W-2$,

$$c_k = \mu_G \sum_{i=\max(0,k-n_W+1)}^{\min(k,n_H-1)} \mu_i^H \mu_{k-i}^W + \sum_{i=\max(1,k-n_W+2)}^{\min(k,n_H-1)} \mu_i^H \mu_{k+1-i}^W, \tag{3.5.11}$$

where the second sum in (3.5.11) is zero if $k = n_H + n_W - 2$. The equation (3.5.10) governing R_0 was first obtained by Pellis et al. [54] using a different derivation.

3.5.3.6 Exponential Growth Rate r

The Malthusian parameter of the branching process $\mathscr{B}_R$ (see Section 3.3.5 on page 174) is given by that of the three-type branching process, $\bar{\mathscr{B}}_R$ say, corresponding to $\bar{\mathscr{B}}$ but run in real time. For $i,j = 1,2,3$ and $t \geq 0$, let $\lambda_{ij}(t)$ be the mean rate that a type-i individual has a type-j child at age t. Let $\Lambda(t)$ be the 3×3 matrix with elements $\lambda_{ij}(t)$. Then,

$$\Lambda(t) = \begin{bmatrix} \lambda_G \mathbb{P}(I>t) & \nu_W(t) & \nu_H(t) \\ \lambda_G \mathbb{P}(I>t) & 0 & \nu_H(t) \\ \lambda_G \mathbb{P}(I>t) & \nu_W(t) & 0 \end{bmatrix},$$

where $\nu_H(t)$ is the mean rate that new infections occur at time t in the epidemic $E_{n_H-1,1}(\lambda_H, I)$ and $\nu_W(t)$ is defined similarly. For $\theta \in (-\infty,\infty)$, let $\mathscr{L}_\Lambda(\theta) = \int_0^\infty \mathrm{e}^{-\theta t}\Lambda(t)\,\mathrm{d}t$, where the integration is elementwise. The exponential growth rate r is given by the unique $r \in (-\infty,\infty)$ such that the dominant eigenvalue of $\mathscr{L}_\Lambda(r)$ is one.

Note that $\int_0^\infty \mathrm{e}^{-\theta t}\mathbb{P}(I>t)\,\mathrm{d}t = \psi_I(\theta)$, where $\psi_I(\theta)$ is defined in Exercise 3.5.4 on page 196. The matrix $\mathscr{L}_\Lambda(r)$ has the same structure of non-zero elements as $V(\lambda)$, so the argument of Exercise 3.5.9 shows that r is given by the unique solution in $(-\infty,\infty)$ of the equation

$$\lambda_G \psi_I(r)(\mathscr{L}_{v_H}(r)+1)(\mathscr{L}_{v_W}(r)+1)+\mathscr{L}_{v_H}(r)\mathscr{L}_{v_W}(r)=1.$$

The difficulty in calculating r is the absence of closed-form expressions for $\mathscr{L}_{v_H}(r)$ and $\mathscr{L}_{v_W}(r)$. Note that $\mathscr{L}_{v_W}(r)$ can be obtained from $\mathscr{L}_{v_H}(r)$ by substituting (n_W,λ_W) for (n_H,λ_H). Various approximations to $\mathscr{L}_{v_H}(r)$ are discussed in Ball et al. [19, Section 4.7] (see also Pellis et al. [56]). If I is exponentially distributed then $\mathscr{L}_{v_H}(r)$ can be computed numerically as follows (see Pellis et al. [56, Section 4.3]).

We use the same notation as in Section 3.5.2 and let $n=n_H$. Note that if $(X(t),Y(t))=(i,j)$ a new infection occurs at rate $\lambda_H ij$. Let

$$\mathbf{v}_{XY}=(x(1)y(1),x(2)y(2),\ldots,x(n_A)y(n_A))^\top.$$

Then,

$$v_H(t)=\lambda_H \mathbf{u}_0 \mathrm{e}^{\tilde{Q}_{AA}t}\mathbf{v}_{XY},$$

whence

$$\mathscr{L}_{v_H}(r)=\lambda_H \mathbf{u}_0[rI_{n_A}-\tilde{Q}_{AA}]^{-1}\mathbf{v}_{XY},$$

thus enabling $\mathscr{L}_{v_H}(r)$ to be computed.

3.5.4 Great Circle Model

3.5.4.1 Threshold Parameter R_* and Probability of a Global Outbreak

Consider first the early stages of an epidemic. The local infectious clump of a typical individual, i say, assuming an infinite population can be partitioned as

$$\mathscr{C}_i=\mathscr{C}_L\cup\{i\}\cup\mathscr{C}_R, \tag{3.5.12}$$

where $\mathscr{C}_L$ and $\mathscr{C}_R$ are the sets of individuals in $\mathscr{C}_i$ that are to the left and right of $\{i\}$, respectively. Thus, $C=1+C_L+C_R$, where $C_L=|\mathscr{C}_L|$ and $C_R=|\mathscr{C}_R|$ and we have written C for C_i. In the population $\mathscr{N}$,

$$C^N \stackrel{\mathrm{D}}{=} \min(C,N), \tag{3.5.13}$$

from which it is seen easily that $C^N \xrightarrow{D} C$ and $\mu_C^N \to \mu_C$ as $N\to\infty$. Note that C_L and C_R are identically distributed but they are not independent unless the infectious period I is constant.

Let $p_L=1-\phi_I(\lambda_L)$ be the probability that a given individual infects locally a given neighbour. Then,

$$\mathbb{P}(i+k\in\mathscr{C}_i)=p_L^k \qquad (k=1,2,\ldots), \tag{3.5.14}$$

since infectives behave independently. Hence,

$$E[C_R] = \sum_{k=1}^{\infty} p_L^k = \frac{p_L}{1-p_L},$$

so, $\mu_C = 1 + 2p_L/(1-p_L)$ and, using (3.3.5) on page 167,

$$R_* = \lambda_G \mu_I \left(\frac{1+p_L}{1-p_L}\right).$$

Turning to the probability of a global outbreak, note that A admits the decomposition

$$A = I + A_L + A_R, \tag{3.5.15}$$

where I $(= I_i)$ is the infectious period of individual i, $A_L = \sum_{j \in \mathscr{C}_L} I_j$ is the severity of the left clump $\mathscr{C}_L$ and A_R is defined similarly for the right clump $\mathscr{C}_R$. Note that $A_L | A_L > 0$ and $A_R | A_R > 0$ are independent but, unless I is constant, A_L and A_R are dependent.

Exercise 3.5.10. Show that

$$\mathbb{E}[\mathrm{e}^{-\theta A_R} | A_R > 0] = \frac{\phi_I(\lambda_L + \theta)}{1 - \phi_I(\theta) + \phi_I(\lambda_L + \theta)} \qquad (\theta \geq 0) \tag{3.5.16}$$

and hence, by conditioning on I, that

$$\phi_A(\theta) = \frac{\phi_I(\theta + 2\lambda_L)(1-\phi_I(\theta))^2 + \phi_I(\lambda_L+\theta)^2(2-\phi_I(\theta))}{(1-\phi_I(\theta)+\phi_I(\lambda_L+\theta))^2} \qquad (\theta \geq 0). \tag{3.5.17}$$

Recall from the end of Section 3.3.2 on page 167 that the probability of a global outbreak is given by the $1 - p_{\mathrm{ext}}$, where p_{ext} is the smallest solution of $f_R(s) = s$ in $[0,1]$ with $f_R(s) = \phi_A(\lambda_G(1-s))$. Thus (3.5.17) enables the probability of a global outbreak to be calculated.

Remark 3.5.11 (Proof of Assumptions (A1) and (A3)). Note that since $\mathbb{P}(C < \infty) = 1$, it is easily shown using (3.5.13) that Assumptions (A.1) on page 164 and (A.3) on page 176 are satisfied.

3.5.4.2 Basic Reproduction Number R_0 and Vaccination

The early stages of the great circle epidemic can also be analysed using a two-type approximating branching process, $\tilde{\mathscr{B}}$ say, of infected *individuals*, in which infectives are typed G or L according to whether they are infected by a global or a local contact. The initial infective is of type G. A type-G [type-L] infective has two [one] susceptible local neighbours so in $\tilde{\mathscr{B}}$, conditional upon its infectious period I, it produces $\mathrm{Poi}(\lambda_G I)$ type-G offspring and $\mathrm{Bin}(2, 1-\mathrm{e}^{-\lambda_G I})$ [$\mathrm{Bin}(1, 1-\mathrm{e}^{-\lambda_G I})$] type-$L$ offspring. Thus the mean offspring matrix of $\tilde{\mathscr{B}}$ is

$$\tilde{M} = \begin{bmatrix} m_{GG} & m_{GL} \\ m_{LG} & m_{LL} \end{bmatrix} = \begin{bmatrix} \mu_I \lambda_G & 2p_L \\ \mu_I \lambda_G & p_L \end{bmatrix}, \tag{3.5.18}$$

where, for example, m_{GL} is the mean number of type-L offspring of a typical type-G individual. By standard branching process theory, for example, Haccou et al. [37, Section 5.5], the branching process $\tilde{\mathscr{B}}$ has a non-zero probability of not going extinct if and only if the dominant eigenvalue of $\tilde{M}$ is strictly greater than one. Let R_0 be the dominant eigenvalue of $\tilde{M}$ and note that this coincides with the classical definition of R_0 as, in the epidemic setting, $\tilde{M}$ is an individual-to-individual mean offspring matrix. A simple calculation shows that

$$R_0 = \frac{1}{2}\left[\lambda_G\mu_I + p_L + \sqrt{(\lambda_G\mu_I)^2 + 6\lambda_G\mu_I p_L + p_L^2}\right]. \tag{3.5.19}$$

Exercise 3.5.12. Determine the clump generation means μ_k^C $(k = 0, 1, \ldots)$ for the great circle model and show that the positive solution of (3.3.8) (see page 170) is indeed given by (3.5.19).

Remark 3.5.13. Note that the above typing cannot be used to analyse the households model, unless the household size $n = 2$, since in that model the distribution of the number of local (within-household) infections made by a type-L individual depends on how many susceptibles are remaining in that household and is not independent for different individuals in the same household.

Exercise 3.5.14 (Uniform vaccination in the great circle model). Suppose that $R_* > 1$ and individuals are vaccinated with a perfect vaccine independently, each with probability v. Compute the post-vaccination clump reproduction number $R_*(v)$, defined in Section 3.3.4 on page 170. Hence determine the critical vaccination coverage v_c and verify that it is given by $1 - R_0^{-1}$.

Exercise 3.5.15 (Optimal vaccination in the great circle model). Suppose that $R_* > 1$ (or equivalently that $R_0 > 1$, see Theorem 3.3.3 on page 171) and a fraction v of individuals are vaccinated with a perfect vaccine. Note that the corresponding post-vaccination clump reproduction number, $\tilde{R}_*(v)$ say, is determined by the distribution of the length, L_S, of runs of susceptibles between vaccinated individuals. (If two vaccinated individuals are adjacent the corresponding $L_S = 0$.) Show that, for given $v \in (0,1)$, the reproduction number $\tilde{R}_*(v)$ is minimised by making the distribution of L_S as constant as possible subject to the constraint imposed by v, i.e. that the support of L_S is concentrated on a single integer, if $vN \in \mathbb{Z}$, and on a pair of consecutive integers, otherwise. Thus the equalising strategy is optimal for the great circle model (Ball et al. [14]).

Hint: consider the finite N problem, as in Section 2.4.3, so analogous to (3.3.12),

$$\tilde{R}_*(v) = \mu_G(1-v)\mathbb{E}[\tilde{C}(v)],$$

where $\tilde{C}(v) = |\tilde{\mathscr{C}}(v)|$ and $\tilde{\mathscr{C}}(v)$ is the post-vaccination local infectious clump of an individual, i_0 say, chosen uniformly at random from the unvaccinated individuals in the population $\mathscr{N}$. Suppose that post-vaccination the population contains a run of k susceptibles and a run of $k+l$ susceptibles, for some $k \geq 0$ and $l \geq 2$. Consider the effect on $\tilde{R}_*(v)$ of replacing these runs by one of length $k+1$ and one of length $k+l-1$.

3.5.4.3 Exponential Growth Rate r

The exponential growth rate r can be calculated by a similar method to that used in Section 3.5.3.6 for the households-workplaces model, i.e. by determining the Malthusian parameter of the two-type branching process, $\tilde{\mathscr{B}}_R$ say, corresponding to the branching process $\tilde{\mathscr{B}}$ but run in real time. For $t \geq 0$, let $\lambda_{GG}(t)$ be the mean rate that a type-G individual has a type-G child at age t in $\tilde{\mathscr{B}}_R$ and define $\lambda_{GL}(t)$, $\lambda_{LG}(t)$ and $\lambda_{LL}(t)$ similarly.

Note that $\lambda_{GG}(t) = \lambda_{LG}(t) = \lambda_G \mathbb{P}(I > t)$, so $\mathscr{L}_{\lambda_{GG}}(\theta) = \lambda_G \psi_I(\theta)$. Consider a type-$L$ individual, i say. It has one susceptible neighbour, j $(= i \pm 1)$ say, who it infects (locally) at age t if and only if (i) it contacts j at age t (which occurs at rate λ_L), (ii) it is still infectious at age t (which happens with probability $\mathbb{P}(I > t)$) and (iii) it has not previously contacted j (which happens with probability $\mathrm{e}^{-\lambda_L t}$). These three events are independent, so $\lambda_{LL}(t) = \lambda_L \mathbb{P}(I > t)\mathrm{e}^{-\lambda_L t}$ and $\mathscr{L}_{\lambda_{LL}}(\theta) = \lambda_L \psi_I(\theta + \lambda_L)$. A type-$G$ individual has two susceptible neighbours, so $\mathscr{L}_{\lambda_{GL}}(\theta) = 2\lambda_L \psi_I(\theta + \lambda_L)$.

Let $\mathscr{L}_\Lambda(\theta) = \int_0^\infty \mathrm{e}^{-\theta t} \Lambda(t)\,\mathrm{d}t$, where

$$\Lambda(t) = \begin{bmatrix} \lambda_{GG}(t) & \lambda_{GL}(t) \\ \lambda_{LG}(t) & \lambda_{LL}(t) \end{bmatrix}.$$

Then

$$\mathscr{L}_\Lambda(\theta) = \begin{bmatrix} \lambda_G \psi_I(\theta) & 2\lambda_L \psi_I(\theta + \lambda_L) \\ \lambda_G \psi_I(\theta) & \lambda_L \psi_I(\theta + \lambda_L) \end{bmatrix} \tag{3.5.20}$$

and r is given by the unique $r \in (-\infty, \infty)$ such that the dominant eigenvalue of $\mathscr{L}_\Lambda(r)$ is one.

Exercise 3.5.16 (Great circle model exponential growth rate r). Show that r is given by the unique real solution of

$$\lambda_G \psi_I(r) + \lambda_L \psi_I(r + \lambda_L) + \lambda_G \lambda_L \psi_I(r) \psi_I(r + \lambda_L) = 1.$$

3.5.4.4 Final Outcome of Global Outbreak

The local susceptibility set $\mathscr{S}_i$ of a typical individual i, assuming an infinite population, can be partitioned analogously to $\mathscr{C}_i$ at (3.5.12), leading to, in an obvious notation, $S = 1 + S_L + S_R$. Note that S_L and S_R are independent, and

$$\mathbb{P}(S_L = k) = \mathbb{P}(S_R = k) = p_L^k (1 - p_L) \qquad (k = 0, 1, \dots),$$

whence

$$f_S(s) = s\left(\frac{1 - p_L}{1 - p_L s}\right)^2 \qquad (s \in (-p_L^{-1}, p_L^{-1}).$$

It then follows using (3.4.5) that $\hat{z}$, the fraction of the population infected by a global outbreak, is given by the unique solution in $(0, 1]$ of

$$1 - z = e^{-\lambda_G \mu_I z} \left(\frac{1 - p_L}{1 - p_L e^{-\lambda_G \mu_I z}} \right)^2. \qquad (3.5.21)$$

At a more detailed level, note that at the end of an epidemic the great circle consists of alternating runs of susceptible and recovered individuals, which form an alternating renewal process (see, for example, Grimmett and Stirzaker [36, page 403]) in the limit as $N \to \infty$. Let T_S and T_R denote the lengths of typical runs of susceptibles and recovered individuals, respectively, in this alternating renewal process.

Exercise 3.5.17.

(a) Show that

$$\mathbb{P}(T_S = k) = \hat{\pi}^{k-1}(1 - \hat{\pi}) \qquad (k = 1, 2 \dots), \qquad (3.5.22)$$

where $\hat{\pi} = e^{-\lambda_G \mu_I \hat{z}}$. Thus, given $\hat{\pi}$, the distribution of T_S is independent of the local infection rate λ_L, which may seem surprising at first sight.

(b) Show that

$$\mathbb{E}[T_R] = \frac{1 - p_L^2 \hat{\pi}}{\hat{\pi}(1 - p_L)^2}. \qquad (3.5.23)$$

3.5.5 Network Model with Casual Contacts

3.5.5.1 Configuration Model Random Graph

We assume that a configuration model random graph is defined on the population $\mathcal{N}$, as follows. Let $D_1, D_2, \dots, D_N$ be i.i.d. copies of a random variable D, which describes the degree of a typical individual. (These random variables are independent of the infectious periods and Poisson process used to define the epidemic E^N.) For $i = 1, 2, \dots, N$, attach D_i half-edges to individual i. Then pair up the $D_1 + D_2 + \cdots + D_N$ half-edges uniformly at random to form the edges in the random graph, which we refer to as the network. If $D_1 + D_2 + \cdots + D_N$ is odd, there is a left-over half-edge, which is ignored; this has no effect on the asymptotic properties of the epidemic model as $N \to \infty$. The network may have some imperfections, specifically self-loops and multiple edges, but they are sparse as $N \to \infty$, provided $\sigma_D^2 = \text{Var}(D) < \infty$ (Durrett [32, Theorem 3.1.2]). The above construction gives the Newman–Strogatz–Watts (Newman et al. [52]) version of the configuration model. In the Molloy–Reed version (Molloy and Reed [50]) the degrees of individuals are prescribed deterministically. As indicated in Section 3.1.5, we assume that any given infectives makes local contacts with its neighbours in the network, at rate λ_L per neighbour (see (3.1.1)). Let $p_k = \mathbb{P}(D = k)$ $(k = 0, 1, \dots)$ and $\mu_D = \mathbb{E}[D]$, which we assume to be finite.

Remark 3.5.18. The model described above does not fit exactly the framework defined in Section 3.1 on page 160, since the local infection rates λ_{ij}^L $(i, j \in \mathcal{N}, i \neq j)$ depend on the realisation of the configuration model network. We consider the analysis of a single epidemic defined on a single realisation of the configuration model.

Local infectious clumps and local susceptibility sets can then be defined as in Section 3.2 on page 163. Note, for example, that the random variable C_i^N describing the size of individual i's local infectious clump is not conditioned on i's degree since the random variables $D_1, D_2, \dots, D_N$ are i.i.d.

3.5.5.2 Size of Local Infectious Clump

The local infectious clump $\mathscr{C}_i$ of individual $i \in \mathscr{N}$ is a realisation of the outcome of an SIR epidemic on the configuration model random graph $\mathscr{G}$ defined on $\mathscr{N}$ as above (cf. Chapter 3 of Part III in this volume), with individual i as the initial infective. The early stages of the clump $\mathscr{C}_1$ can be approximated on a generation basis by the (forward) branching process, $\mathscr{B}_F$ say, defined as follows. The branching process $\mathscr{B}_F$ has one initial ancestor, who corresponds to individual 1 in E^N. This individual has D_1 neighbours in the network, so the number of individuals it infects locally is distributed as $\text{Bin}(D, 1 - e^{\lambda_L I})$. (If D and I are independent random variables, then $\text{Bin}(D, 1 - e^{\lambda_L I})$ denotes a mixed-Binomial random variable obtained by first sampling D and I independently and then, conditional on (D, I), sampling independently from the binomial distribution having D trials and success probability $1 - e^{\lambda_L I}$.) Note that, since the half-edges are paired up uniformly at random, for $k = 1, 2, \dots$, a given half-edge is k times as likely to be paired with a half-edge attached to a given individual having degree k than with one attached to a given individual having degree 1. It follows that, in the limit as $N \to \infty$, the degree $\tilde{D}$ of a typical neighbour of a typical individual has the size-biased distribution given by $\mathbb{P}(\tilde{D} = k) = \tilde{p}_k = \mu_D^{-1} k p_k$ $(k = 1, 2, \dots)$. Thus, apart from individual 1, the number of susceptible neighbours of a typical infective in the early stages of the clump $\mathscr{C}_1$ is distributed as $\tilde{D} - 1$, since one of the neighbours of that individual (i.e. its infector) is not susceptible. Hence, the number of individuals infected locally by such an individual is distributed as $\text{Bin}(\tilde{D} - 1, 1 - e^{\lambda_L I})$. Thus the offspring distribution of the branching process $\mathscr{B}_F$ is $\text{Bin}(D, 1 - e^{\lambda_L I})$ in the initial generation and $\text{Bin}(\tilde{D} - 1, 1 - e^{\lambda_L I})$ in all subsequent generations. Let Z_F denote the total size of $\mathscr{B}_F$, including the initial ancestor, and recall that C^N is the size of a typical local infectious clump in E^N.

Lemma 3.5.19.

$$C^N \xrightarrow{D} Z_F \qquad \text{as } N \to \infty.$$

Proof. We construct realisations of C^N $(N = 1, 2, \dots)$ and Z_F on the same probability space and show that $C^N \xrightarrow{a.s.} Z_F$ as $N \to \infty$, where $\xrightarrow{a.s.}$ denotes almost sure convergence. The lemma then follows as almost sure convergence implies convergence in distribution.

To that end, let $(\Omega, \mathscr{F}, \mathbb{P})$ be a probability space on which are defined the following independent sets of random variables.

(i) $D_1, D_2, \dots$, i.i.d. copies of D.
(ii) $U_0, U_1, \dots$, i.i.d., each uniformly distributed on $(0, 1)$.
(iii) $R_{i,j}$ $(i, j = 0, 1, \dots)$, independent with $R_{i,j} \sim \text{Bin}(i, 1 - e^{\lambda_L I})$.

Let $c_k = \sum_{l=0}^{k} p_l$ $(k = 0, 1, \dots)$ and $\tilde{c}_k = \sum_{l=1}^{k} \tilde{p}_l$ $(k = 1, 2, \dots)$. For $x \in (0, 1)$, let $d(x) = \min(k : c_k \leq x)$ and $\tilde{d}(x) = \min(k : \tilde{c}_k \leq x)$.

A realisation of the branching process $\mathscr{B}_F$ is defined on $(\Omega, \mathscr{F}, \mathbb{P})$ as follows. The initial individual has degree $d_0 = d(U_0)$ and $R_{d_0,0}$ offspring. For $k = 1, 2, \ldots$, the kth individual born in $\mathscr{B}_F$ has degree $d_k = \tilde{d}(U_k)$ and $R_{d_k-1,l+1}$ offspring, where l is the number of individuals used previously in the construction of $\mathscr{B}_F$ which have degree d_k, excluding the initial ancestor.

For $N = 1, 2, \ldots$, define a branching process $\mathscr{B}_F^N$ on $(\Omega, \mathscr{F}, \mathbb{P})$ as follows. Let

$$p_k^N = N^{-1} \sum_{i=1}^{N} 1_{\{D_i = k\}} \quad (k = 0, 1, \ldots),$$

$$\mu_D^N = N^{-1} \sum_{i=1}^{N} D_i \text{ and}$$

$$\tilde{p}_k^N = (N\mu_D^N)^{-1} \sum_{i=1}^{N} k 1_{\{D_i = k\}} \quad (k = 1, 2, \ldots).$$

Let $c_k^N = \sum_{l=0}^{k} p_l^N$ $(k = 0, 1, \ldots)$ and $\tilde{c}_k^N = \sum_{l=1}^{k} \tilde{p}_l^N$ $(k = 1, 2, \ldots)$. For $x \in (0, 1)$, let $d^N(x) = \min(k : c_k^N \leq x)$ and $\tilde{d}^N(x) = \min(k : \tilde{c}_k^N \leq x)$. The branching process $\mathscr{B}_F^N$ is defined analogously to $\mathscr{B}_F$, using the functions $d^N(x)$ and $\tilde{d}^N(x)$ instead of $d(x)$ and $\tilde{d}(x)$, respectively. (If $\mu_D^N = 0$, the $\tilde{p}_k^N$s, and hence also $\tilde{d}^N(x)$, are not well-defined but in that case $\mathscr{B}_F^N$ dies out immediately.)

For $N = 1, 2, \ldots$, define on $(\Omega, \mathscr{F}, \mathbb{P})$ a realisation of a typical local infectious clump, $\mathscr{C}^N$ say, in E^N as follows. The N individuals in $\mathscr{N}$ have degrees given by $D_1, D_2, \ldots, D_N$. Without loss of generality, label the individuals $1, 2, \ldots, N$ in increasing order of degree. Label the $N\mu_D^N$ half-edges $1, 2, \ldots, N\mu_D^N$, starting with the half-edges attached to individual 1, then the half-edges attached to individual 2, and so on. The initial member of the clump, i_0 say, is individual $\lceil NU_0 \rceil$. Note that this individual has degree $d_0^N = d^N(U_0)$, i.e. the same as the initial ancestor in $\mathscr{B}_F^N$. It makes local contacts down $R_{d_0^N,0}$ of its d_0^N half-edges. For $k = 1, 2, \ldots$, the kth half-edge down which a contact is made is paired with half-edge $\lceil N\mu_D^N U_k \rceil$. Note that this latter half-edge is attached to an individual, i_* say, having degree $d_k^N = \tilde{d}^N(U_k)$, i.e. the same as the corresponding individual in $\mathscr{B}_F^N$. Suppose that i_* has not been used previously in the construction of $\mathscr{C}^N$. Then i_* joins $\mathscr{C}^N$ and makes local contacts down $R_{j,l+1}$ of those half-edges, where l is the number of individuals with j unpaired half-edges used previously in the construction of $\mathscr{C}^N$, excluding the initial the initial member i_0. The construction continues in the obvious fashion but needs modifying when an attempt is made to pair a half-edge with one attached to a previously-used individual. The details of that modification are not important for proving the lemma. The key observation is that the sizes of $\mathscr{B}_F^N$ and $\mathscr{C}^N$ are necessarily equal if no such modification is required.

Let $\tilde{c}_0 = 0$ and define the piecewise-linear function $f : [0, 1) \to [0, 1)$ by

$$f(x) = \tilde{c}_i + \left(\frac{\tilde{c}_{i+1} - \tilde{c}_i}{c_{i+1} - c_i} \right) \qquad (x \in [c_i, c_{i+1}); i = 0, 1, \ldots).$$

(This function is well-defined as $[c_i, c_{i+1})$ is empty if $c_i = c_{i+1}$.) For $N = 1, 2, \ldots$, define $f^N : [0, 1) \to [0, 1)$ analogously, using $(c_i^N, \tilde{c}_i^N)$ $(i = 0, 1, \ldots)$, with $\tilde{c}_0^N = 0$.

Note that in the construction of $\mathscr{C}^N$, the lowest-numbered half-edge attached to the initial member i_0 is $\lceil N\mu_D^N f^N(U_0)\rceil$.

By the strong law of large numbers, $p_k^N \xrightarrow{a.s.} p_k$ $(k=0,1,\dots)$ and $\mu_D^N \xrightarrow{a.s.} \mu_D$ as $N\to\infty$, so there exists an $F_0\in\mathscr{F}$, with $\mathbb{P}(F_0)=1$, such that $\lim_{N\to\infty} p_k^N(\omega)=p_k$ $(k=0,1,\dots)$ and $\lim_{N\to\infty}\mu_D^N(\omega)=\mu_D$ for all $\omega\in F_0$. Let

$$F_{11}=\left\{\omega\in\Omega:\bigcup_{i=0}^{\infty}\{U_0=c_i\}\right\}\quad\text{and}\quad F_{12}=\left\{\omega\in\Omega:\bigcup_{i=0}^{\infty}\bigcup_{k=1}^{\infty}\{U_k=\tilde{c}_i\}\right\}.$$

Then $\mathbb{P}(F_{11})=\mathbb{P}(F_{12})=0$, as both F_{11} and F_{12} are countable unions of events having probability zero. Thus $\mathbb{P}(F_1)=1$, where $F_1=F_{11}^c\cap F_{12}^c$. Let

$$F_{21}=\left\{\omega\in\Omega:\bigcup_{i=1}^{\infty}\{f(U_0)=U_i\}\right\}\quad\text{and}\quad F_{12}=\left\{\omega\in\Omega:\bigcup_{i=1}^{\infty}\bigcup_{j=i+1}^{\infty}\{U_i=U_j\}\right\}.$$

Then $\mathbb{P}(F_{21})=\mathbb{P}(F_{22})=0$, as F_{21} and F_{22} are also countable unions of events having probability zero, since $F(U_0),U_1,U_2,\dots$ are independent continuous random variables. Hence, $\mathbb{P}(F_2)=1$, where $F_2=F_{21}^c\cap F_{22}^c$. Let $F=F_0\cap F_1\cap F_2$, so $\mathbb{P}(F)=1$.

Fix $\omega\in F$ and let $k=Z_F(\omega)$. Suppose that $k<\infty$. Now $\omega\in F_0$ implies that $\lim_{N\to\infty}c_k^N(\omega)=c_k$ and $\lim_{N\to\infty}\tilde{c}_k^N(\omega)=\tilde{c}_k$. It follows that $d_l^N(\omega)=d_l(\omega)$ $(l=0,1,\dots,k)$ for all sufficiently large N, say $N\ge N_1(\omega)$, since $\omega\in F_1$. Thus, $Z_F^N(\omega)=k$ for $N\ge N_1(\omega)$, where Z_F^N is the total size of $\mathscr{B}_F^N$.

Let $d_{\max}=\max(d_1,d_2,\dots,d_k)$ be the maximum degree of the k individuals in $\mathscr{B}$. In the construction of $\mathscr{C}^N$ (the local infectious clump of an individual chosen uniformly at random from $\mathscr{N}$), for $1\le i<j\le k$, the half-edges $\lceil N\mu_D^N U_i\rceil$ and $\lceil N\mu_D^N U_j\rceil$ are attached to the same individual only if

$$|N\mu_D^N(\omega)U_i(\omega)-N\mu_D^N(\omega)U_j(\omega)|\le d_{\max}(\omega)\implies|U_i(\omega)-U_j(\omega)|\le\frac{d_{\max}(\omega)}{N\mu_D^N(\omega)}.$$

Now $\frac{d_{\max}(\omega)}{N\mu_D^N(\omega)}\to 0$ as $N\to\infty$, since $\mu_D^N\to\mu_D>0$. Thus, since $\omega\in F_2$, there exists an $N_2(\omega)$ such that, for all $N\ge N_2(\omega)$, the individuals attached to the half-edges $\lceil N\mu_D^N U_i\rceil$ $(i=1,2,\dots,k-1)$ in the construction of $\mathscr{C}^N$ are all distinct.

Note that $\lim_{N\to\infty}f^N(x,\omega)=f(x)$, for $x\in[\tilde{c}_0,1)\setminus\{\tilde{c}_1,\tilde{c}_2,\dots\}$, since $\omega\in F_0$. A similar argument to the above shows that there exists an $N_3(\omega)$ such that for all $N\ge N_3(\omega)$, the individuals attached to the half-edges $\lceil N\mu_D^N U_i\rceil$ $(i=1,2,\dots,k-1)$ in the construction of $\mathscr{C}^N$ are all distinct from $i_0=\lceil NU_0\rceil$. It follows that $C^N(\omega)=Z_F^N(\omega)=k$ for all $N\ge\max(N_1(\omega),N_2(\omega),N_3(\omega))$.

Suppose instead that $Z_F(\omega)=\infty$. Then, for any $K\in\mathbb{N}$, we can use the above argument to show that $C^N(\omega)\ge K$ for all sufficiently large N, so $C^N(\omega)\to\infty$ as $N\to\infty$. Thus, $C^N(\omega)\to Z_F(\omega)$ as $N\to\infty$, for all $\omega\in F$, which completes the proof of the lemma as $\mathbb{P}(F)=1$. □

Remark 3.5.20 (Proof of Assumptions (A1) and (A3)). The proof of Lemma 3.5.19 can be extended in an obvious fashion to show that Assumptions (A.1) on page 164 and (A.3) on page 176 are satisfied.

3.5.5.3 Threshold Parameter R_*

Let m_{GL} and m_{LL} denote respectively the offspring means of the initial individual and all subsequent individuals in $\mathscr{B}_F$. Then $m_{GL} = \mu_D p_L$ and $m_{LL} = \mu_{\tilde{D}-1} p_L$, where $p_L = 1 - \phi_I(\lambda_L)$ and

$$\mu_{\tilde{D}-1} = \mathbb{E}[\tilde{D}-1] = \mu_D + \frac{\sigma_D^2}{\mu_D} - 1.$$

For $k = 1, 2, \ldots$, the mean size of the kth generation in $\mathscr{B}_F$ is $m_{GL} m_{LL}^{k-1}$, so

$$\mu_C = \mathbb{E}[Z_F] = 1 + \sum_{k=1}^{\infty} m_{GL} m_{LL}^{k-1} = \begin{cases} 1 + \frac{m_{GL}}{1-m_{LL}} & \text{if } m_{LL} < 1, \\ \infty & \text{otherwise,} \end{cases}$$

so, using (3.3.5),

$$R_* = \begin{cases} \lambda_G \mu_I \left(1 + \frac{m_{GL}}{1-m_{LL}}\right) & \text{if } m_{LL} < 1, \\ \infty & \text{otherwise.} \end{cases} \tag{3.5.24}$$

It is possible to derive an expression for $\phi_A(\theta)$ $(\theta \geq 0)$, and hence enable the probability of a global outbreak to be calculated (see Ball and Neal [17, Section 3.3]). However, it does not take a pleasant form, unless I is constant, and we do not consider it here.

3.5.5.4 Basic Reproduction Number R_0 and Exponential Growth Rate r

As with the great circle model, the early stages of E^N can be approximated by a two-type branching process $\tilde{\mathscr{B}}$ of infected individuals, in which infectives are typed G or L according to whether they were infected by a global or a local contact.

Exercise 3.5.21 (Basic reproduction number R_0). Determine the mean offspring matrix of $\tilde{\mathscr{B}}$. Hence, or otherwise, show that

$$R_0 = \frac{1}{2}\left[\lambda_G \mu_I + m_{LL} + \sqrt{(\lambda_G \mu_I - m_{LL})^2 + 4\lambda_G \mu_I m_{GL}}\right]. \tag{3.5.25}$$

Note that $R_0 = \infty$ if $\sigma_D^2 = \infty$.

Exercise 3.5.22 (Exponential growth rate r).

(a) Using the real-time version of $\tilde{\mathscr{B}}$, show that the exponential growth rate r is given by the largest real solution of

$$\lambda_G \psi_I(r) + \lambda_L \mu_{\tilde{D}-1} \psi_I(r+\lambda_L) + \lambda_G \lambda_L (\mu_D - \mu_{\tilde{D}-1}) \psi_I(r) \psi_I(r+\lambda_L) = 1.$$

(b) Determine r when $I \sim \text{Exp}(\gamma)$.

3.5.5.5 Size of Local Susceptibility Set

Turning to the final outcome of a global outbreak, the local susceptibility set $\mathscr{S}_1$ of individual 1 can be approximated on a generation basis by a (backward) branching process, $\mathscr{B}_B$, in much the same way as $\mathscr{C}_1$ is approximated by $\mathscr{B}_F$. Individual 1 has D_1 neighbours, each of which, if they were infected, would infect individual 1 independently with probability p_L. Thus, in $\mathscr{B}_B$, the offspring distribution of the initial ancestor is, in an obvious notation, $\text{Bin}(D, p_L)$ and, by a similar argument, the offspring distribution of any subsequent individual is $\text{Bin}(\tilde{D}-1, p_L)$. Let Z_B denote the total size of $\mathscr{B}_B$, including the initial ancestor. A similar argument to the proof of Lemma 3.5.19 shows that

$$S^N \xrightarrow{D} Z_B \qquad \text{as } N \to \infty,$$

so assumption (A.2) on page 164 is satisfied and we may set $S = Z_B$ in the results in Section 3.4.1.

3.5.5.6 Final Outcome of Global Outbreak

The branching process $\mathscr{B}_B$ is simpler to analyse than $\mathscr{B}_F$ (unless the infectious period is constant, in which case $\mathscr{B}_F \stackrel{\text{D}}{=} \mathscr{B}_B$), as its offspring distribution depends on the distribution of I only through p_L. We now derive the probability-generating function of Z_B, and hence of S. Let Y be the number of offspring of the initial ancestor in $\mathscr{B}_B$. Then,

$$Z_B = 1 + \sum_{i=1}^{Y} \tilde{Z}_B(i), \tag{3.5.26}$$

where $\tilde{Z}_B(1), \tilde{Z}_B(2), \dots$ are i.i.d. copies of a random variable $\tilde{Z}_B$ giving the total size of the branching process started by a typical child of the initial ancestor in $\mathscr{B}_B$. (Note that $\tilde{Z}_B(1), \tilde{Z}_B(2), \dots$ are independent of Y.) A similar decomposition yields

$$\tilde{Z}_B = 1 + \sum_{i=1}^{\tilde{Y}} \tilde{Z}'_B(i), \tag{3.5.27}$$

where $\tilde{Z}'_B(1), \tilde{Z}'_B(2), \dots$ are i.i.d. copies of $\tilde{Z}_B$ that are independent of $\tilde{Y}$.

For $0 \le s \le 1$, let $g(s) = \mathbb{E}[s^D]$, as in Section 1.2 of Part III in this volume, $f_Y(s) = \mathbb{E}[s^Y]$, $f_{\tilde{Y}}(s) = \mathbb{E}[s^{\tilde{Y}}]$, $\psi(s) = \mathbb{E}[s^{Z_B}]$ and $\tilde{\psi}(s) = \mathbb{E}[s^{\tilde{Z}_B}]$. Then,

$$f_Y(s) = \mathbb{E}[E[s^Y|D]] = \mathbb{E}[(1-p_L+p_L s)^D] = g(1-p_L+p_L s) \qquad (0 \le s \le 1);$$

the second equality follows as $Y \sim \text{Bin}(D, p_L)$. Similarly,

$$f_{\tilde{Y}}(s) = \mathbb{E}[(1-p_L+p_L s)^{\tilde{D}-1}] = \mu_D^{-1} g'(1-p_L+p_L s) \qquad (0 \le s \le 1).$$

Further, using (3.5.26),

$$\begin{aligned}\psi(s) &= \mathbb{E}[s^{1+\sum_{i=1}^{Y}\tilde{Z}_B(i)}] \\ &= \mathbb{E}[\mathbb{E}[s^{1+\sum_{i=1}^{Y}\tilde{Z}_B(i)}|Y]] \\ &= s\mathbb{E}[(\tilde{\psi}(s))^Y] \\ &= sg(1-p_L+p_L\tilde{\psi}(s)) \end{aligned} \tag{3.5.28}$$

and similarly, using (3.5.27),

$$\tilde{\psi}(s) = \frac{s}{\mu_D}g'(1-p_L+p_L\tilde{\psi}(s)). \tag{3.5.29}$$

Equation (3.5.29) uniquely determines $\tilde{\psi}(s)$ $(0 \leq s \leq 1)$ (see Jagers [42, page 39]) so, when $R_* > 1$, it follows using (3.4.5) on page 182 that $\hat{z}$, the fraction of the population infected by a global outbreak, is given by the unique solution in $(0,1]$ of

$$1-z = \psi(\mathrm{e}^{-\lambda_G \mu_I z}), \tag{3.5.30}$$

where $\psi(\cdot)$ is given by (3.5.28) and (3.5.29).

Exercise 3.5.23. For most choices of degree distribution D, equation (3.5.29) does not admit a closed-form solution. An exception is when D has a logarithmic distribution, i.e.

$$\mathbb{P}(D=k) = -\frac{1}{\log(1-p)}\frac{p^k}{k} \qquad (k=1,2,\ldots),$$

where $p \in (0,1)$ is a fixed parameter. For this degree distribution, determine R_* and an equation governing $\hat{z}$.

Solutions

Problems of Chapter 1

1.3.2 Note that $\mathscr{S}_1^{\rm sus}$ is a symmetric sampling procedure on $\mathscr{S}_0^{\rm sus}$. For $k = 1,2,\ldots,n$, let $A_k \subseteq \mathscr{S}_0^{\rm sus}$ with $|A_k| = k$. Using notation from Section 1.2, the probability that all members of A_k are not contacted by the infective with label 0 is

$$\begin{aligned}\mathbb{P}\left(\bigcap_{i\in A_k}\{W_{0i} > I_0\}\right) &= \mathbb{E}\left[\mathbb{P}\left(\bigcap_{i\in A_k}\{W_{0i} > I_0\}|I_0\right)\right]\\ &= \mathbb{E}\left[\mathrm{e}^{-k\lambda I_0}\right]\\ &= q_k,\end{aligned}$$

so $\mathbb{P}(\mathscr{S}_1^{\rm sus} \supseteq A_k) = q_k^a$, as distinct infectives behave independently. Thus, by Lemma 1.3.1, $\mathbb{E}[S_{1,[k]}] = q_k^a$ $(k = 1,2,\ldots,n)$ and (1.3.4) follows. (When $k = 0$, (1.3.4) becomes $\sum_{i=0}^{n} P_{n,a}(k) = 1$.) Part (b) follows immediately using (1.3.3).

Problems of Chapter 2

2.6.1 Firstly, we can find that $\mu_H = \sum_i i\alpha_i = \frac{4}{3}$, so $\tilde{\alpha}_1 = \tilde{\alpha}_2 = \frac{1}{2}$. Also $\mathbb{P}(I = 1) = 1$ implies that $\phi_I(\theta) = \mathbb{E}[\mathrm{e}^{-\theta I}] = \mathrm{e}^{-\theta}$. We also use the fact that in the households of size 2 the initial case in a household infects the other individual with probability $1 - q_1 = 1 - \phi_I(\lambda_L) = 1 - \mathrm{e}^{-\lambda_L}$.

(a) From equation (2.2.1) and the calculations above, we have $R_* = \lambda_G[\frac{1}{2}\mu_1(\lambda_L) + \frac{1}{2}\mu_2(\lambda_L)]$. Since there are no possible secondary cases in a household of size 1 we have $\mu_1(\lambda_L) = 1$; and since the initially susceptible individual gets infected with probability $\mathrm{e}^{-\lambda_L}$, we have $\mu_2(\lambda_L) = \mathrm{e}^{-\lambda_L} + 2(1 - \mathrm{e}^{-\lambda_L}) = 2 - \mathrm{e}^{-\lambda_L}$. We therefore find that $R_* = \lambda_G\frac{1}{2}[3 - \mathrm{e}^{-\lambda_L}]$.

(b) First we find $m_n(\theta) = \phi_{n-1,1}(1,\theta)$, the Laplace transform of the total severity. It is immediate that $m_1(\theta) = \mathrm{e}^{-\theta}$, and by conditioning on the size of the outbreak we find that $m_2(\theta) = \mathrm{e}^{-\lambda_L}\mathrm{e}^{-\theta} + (1-\mathrm{e}^{-\lambda_L})\mathrm{e}^{-2\theta}$. We therefore have $\mathbb{P}(\text{major outbreak}) = 1-\sigma$, where σ is the smallest solution in $[0,1]$ of $s = f_R(s)$ and (using equation (2.2.2))

$$\begin{aligned} f_R(s) &= \frac{1}{2}m_1(\lambda_G(1-s)) + \frac{1}{2}m_2(\lambda_G(1-s)) \\ &= \frac{1}{2}(1+\mathrm{e}^{-\lambda_L})\mathrm{e}^{-\lambda_G(1-s)} + \frac{1}{2}(1-\mathrm{e}^{-\lambda_L})\mathrm{e}^{-2\lambda_G(1-s)}. \end{aligned}$$

(c) To use equations (2.3.1) and (2.3.2), we first need to calculate $\tilde{\mu}_{1,0}(\lambda_L,\pi)$ and $\tilde{\mu}_{2,0}(\lambda_L,\pi)$. It is immediate that $\tilde{\mu}_{1,0}(\lambda_L,\pi) = 0\cdot\pi + 1\cdot(1-\pi) = 1-\pi$, since the size of the local outbreak is zero or one according as the individual under consideration avoids or does not avoid outside infection. A household of size 2 will have size 0 precisely when both individuals avoid outside infection; it will have size 1 when one is infected from outside and the other avoids infection both from outside and inside the household. From this we deduce that

$$\begin{aligned} \tilde{\mu}_{2,0}(\lambda_L,\pi) &= 0\cdot\pi^2 + 1\cdot 2\pi(1-\pi)\mathrm{e}^{-\lambda_L} + 2\cdot[1-\pi^2-\pi(1-\pi)\mathrm{e}^{-\lambda_L})] \\ &= 2(1-\pi)(1+\pi(1-\mathrm{e}^{-\lambda_L})). \end{aligned}$$

It then follows that

$$\begin{aligned} z &= \frac{1}{2}\tilde{\mu}_{1,0}(\lambda_L,\pi) + \frac{1}{2}\tilde{\mu}_{2,0}(\lambda_L,\pi) \\ &= (1-\pi)[\frac{3}{2} + \pi(1-\mathrm{e}^{-\lambda_L})], \end{aligned}$$

where $\pi = \mathrm{e}^{-\lambda_G z}$.

(d) Using equation (2.4.3) we find that $\mu_{nv} = \lambda_G \cdot \mu_I \cdot \mu_{n-v}(\lambda_L)$, and using the formulae for $\mu_k(\lambda_L)$ from part (a) and the given parameter values yields $\mu_{10} = 1.2$, $\mu_{20} = 2.34$ and $\mu_{21} = 0.6$ (to 2 decimal places). This gives the following scaled gain matrix (again to two decimal places).

n	$v=0$	1
1	1.2	
2	3.48	1.2

We therefore see that the highest priority is to vaccinate one of the individuals in households of size 2. These households are then effectively of size 1 (since the vaccinated individual is completely unaffected by the epidemic), so vaccinating a second individual in a household of size 2 has the same effect on R_v as vaccinating a single individual in its own household.

(e) Following the ordering from (d) above, we vaccinate one individual in households of size 2 first: since $\tilde{\alpha}_2 = \frac{1}{2}$, half of the population are in such households, so vaccinating one in each such household gives coverage of $\frac{1}{4}$. Then there is enough vaccine left to vaccinate a further $\frac{3}{5} - \frac{1}{4} = \frac{7}{20}$ of the population. Since $G'_{10} = G'_{21}$ it is equally effective (in terms of R_*) to allocate this vaccine to any combination of the half of the population that are in single-resident households and the quarter that are unvaccinated in 2-resident households. For simplicity

of calculation, allocate it to the singletons: we can vaccinate $0.35/\tilde{\alpha}_1 = 0.7$ of them. Thus we have $(x_{10}, x_{11}) = (0.3, 0.7)$ and $(x_{20}, x_{21}, x_{22}) = (0, 1, 0)$.
For this (or any other specified) vaccine allocation regime (x_{nv}, $n = 1, 2$, $v = 0, \ldots, n$), equation (2.4.2) can be used to find the resulting value of R_* (using the values for μ_{nv} from (d) above). The resulting value of R_v is 0.48, so the epidemic is certainly under control in the sense that major outbreaks are not possible. (Compare with the original R_* value, without vaccination, of approximately 1.77 which implies that major outbreaks are possible.)

2.6.2

(a) Since the infection is highly locally infectious, the initial infective in the household instantly infects all susceptibles in the household. Thus the whole household will become infected (with probability 1) and we have

$$\mathbb{P}(Z^{(n)} = z) = \begin{cases} 0 & z = 1, 2, \ldots, n-1, \\ 1 & z = n. \end{cases}$$

(b) (i) Following directly from part (a) we have $\mu_n(\infty) = \mathbb{E}[Z^{(n)}] = n$.
(ii) We also have $\mu_H = \sum_n n\alpha_n = 2 \cdot \frac{1}{2} + 3 \cdot \frac{1}{2} = \frac{5}{2}$, so using $\tilde{\alpha}_n = n\alpha_n/\mu_H$ we find that $\tilde{\alpha}_2 = 2 \cdot \frac{1}{2}/\frac{5}{2} = \frac{2}{5}$ and $\tilde{\alpha}_3 = 3 \cdot \frac{1}{2}/\frac{5}{2} = \frac{3}{5}$. (This makes sense: with equal numbers of households of size 2 and 3 there will be two fifths of individuals in households of size 2 and three fifths in households of size 3.) Therefore

$$R_* = \sum_n \tilde{\alpha}_n n \lambda_G \frac{1}{\gamma} = (\frac{2}{5} \cdot 2 + \frac{3}{5} \cdot 3) \times \frac{\lambda_G}{\gamma} = \frac{13}{5} \frac{\lambda_G}{\gamma}.$$

(c) The severity A_n is the sum of the infectious periods of all individuals infected, including the initial infective. Since everyone in the household gets infected, this is the sum of n independent $\text{Exp}(\gamma)$ random variables; that is $A_n = \sum_{j=1}^n 1_{\{\text{individual } j \text{ is infected}\}} I_j = \sum_{j=1}^n I_j$. Since the variables I_j are independent and have common Laplace transform $\phi_I(\theta) = \mathbb{E}[e^{-\theta I}] = \gamma/(\gamma+\theta)$, we have

$$m_n(\theta) = \mathbb{E}[e^{-\theta \sum_{j=1}^n I_j}] = \prod_{j=1}^n \phi_I(\theta) = \left(\frac{\gamma}{\gamma+\theta}\right)^n.$$

(d) (i) Using the formula (2.2.2),

$$\begin{aligned} f_R(s) &= \sum_n \tilde{\alpha}_n m_n(\lambda_G(1-s)) \\ &= \frac{2}{5}\left(\frac{\gamma}{\gamma+\lambda_G(1-s)}\right)^2 + \frac{3}{5}\left(\frac{\gamma}{\gamma+\lambda_G(1-s)}\right)^3. \end{aligned}$$

(ii) Then $\sigma = 1 - \mathbb{P}(\text{major outbreak})$ is a fixed point of this function, that is it satisfies $f_R(\sigma) = \sigma$.

(e) We seek values of (λ_G, γ) which satisfy $R_0 = \lambda_G/\gamma < 1$ (standard SIR model subcritical) but $R_* = \frac{13}{5}\lambda_G/\gamma > 1$ (households model supercritical). Values of (λ_G, γ) satisfying both of these criteria are $\{(\lambda_G, \gamma) : \lambda_G/\gamma \in (\frac{5}{13}, 1)\}$.

2.6.3 In all cases the key is calculating μ_{nv} for all relevant values of n and v (i.e. $v = 0, 1, \ldots, n$ for each $n = 2, 3$); then it is straightforward (though maybe a bit tedious) to compute $G'_{nv} = n(\mu_{nv} - \mu_{n,v+1})$. If household sizes larger than 3 or 4 are to be used then it is advisable to do the numerical calculations using a computer package.

(a) With a perfect vaccine, a within-household outbreak in a household in state (n, v) will have size 0 with probability v/n and will have size $n-v$ with probability $(n-v)/n$. Thus $\mu_{nv} = (n-v)^2/n \cdot \lambda_G \mu_I$ and then $G'_{nv} = (2(n-v)-1)\lambda_G \mu_I$. (One can also derive the formula for μ_{nv} from equation (2.4.3), taking $\varepsilon = 1$.) Using the given parameter values this yields the following scaled gain matrix G'.

n	$v=0$	1	2
2	6	2	
3	10	6	2

From this we see that vaccinating a single individual in households of size 3 is the highest priority. Such households are then effectively households of size 2, so vaccinating a second individual in a household of size 3 has the same effect (on R_v) as vaccinating one individual in a household of size 2 (i.e. $G'_{31} = G'_{20}$), and doing either of these is the next priority. Similar reasoning applies to vaccinating the last susceptible in each household.

(b) With an all-or-nothing vaccine we could calculate μ_{nv} using equation (2.4.3), but again direct reasoning is simpler. If the contacted individual is unvaccinated (which happens with probability $(n-v)/n$) then the mean size of the local epidemic is $n - v + v(1-\varepsilon)$ and if it is vaccinated (which occurs with probability v/n) then the mean size is $(1-\varepsilon)(1+n-v+(v-1)(1-\varepsilon))$. We then find that

$$\mu_{nv} = \frac{\lambda_G \mu_I}{n}\left(n^2 - (2n-1)\varepsilon v + \varepsilon^2 v(v-1)\right),$$

from which it follows that $G'_{nv} = \varepsilon[2(n-\varepsilon v)-1]$.
The given numerical parameter values thus yield the following scaled gain matrix.

n	$v=0$	1	2
2	3	2	
3	5	4	3

In this situation the first priority is to vaccinate a first individual in households of size 3, followed by a second individual in those households. Then vaccinating the last individual in 3-households and the first individual in 2-households have equal priority (though perhaps in practice with limited vaccine we might prioritise vaccinating in the 3-households since we will already be visiting them to vaccinate the first two individuals there); and if we still have vaccine available then the lowest priority individuals are the remaining lone unvaccinated individuals in households of size 2.

(c) Again we rely on the fact that within-household epidemic completely infects the household (as the local infection rate is very large) to simplify the calculations.

It is clear that $\mu_{\mathbf{n}^{(n,v)},A,V} = v$ and $\mu_{\mathbf{n}^{(n,v)},A,U} = n - v$ for both $A = U, V$. (This can also be derived from Proposition 1.9.1.) Making these substitutions into equation (2.4.4) and simplifying yields $\mu_{nv} = \lambda_G \mu_I (n - (1-a)v)(n - (1-b)v)/n$, from which it follows that $G'_{nv} = \lambda_G \mu_I [(2-a-b)n - (1-a)(1-b)(2v+1)]$. The scaled gain matrix that results from the parameter values $a = b = 1/\sqrt{2}$ is as follows (to 2 decimal places).

n	$v=0$	1	2
2	2.17	1.83	
3	3.34	3	2.66

Here we see that the optimal course of action is to first vaccinate one individual in each household of size 3, then a second and third individual in those households. Only after households of size 3 are completely vaccinated do we vaccinate a first then a second individual in households of size 2. Note that this is *not* an equalising strategy.

(d) With a leaky vaccine we are in the framework of (c) above, but with $b = 1$. The formula for G'_{nv} from (c) simplifies to $G'_{nv} = \lambda_G \mu_I (1-a)n$. This is independent of v and also (so long as $a \in (0,1)$) decreasing in n; thus the optimal vaccine allocation scheme involves vaccinating all individuals in the largest households, then in the next largest households, and so on. If there is insufficient vaccine to cover everyone in households of a given size, then there is no preference (in terms of R_v) of how to allocate the vaccine.

2.6.4

(a) Consider a globally infected individual in a household of size n. With probability δ she self-isolates and infects no-one else, so the local epidemic causes no subsequent global infections. With the complementary probability the initial case does not self-isolate and the within-household epidemic proceeds as normal, with an average of $\mu_n(\lambda_L)$ individuals becoming infected in the household and each of them making an average of $\lambda_G \mu_I$ global contacts. Thus

$$R_* = \mathbb{E}[R] = \sum_{n=1}^{n_{\max}} \tilde{\alpha}_n [\delta \cdot 0 + (1-\delta)\mu_n(\lambda_L)\lambda_G \mu_I]$$
$$= (1-\delta) \sum_{n=1}^{n_{\max}} \tilde{\alpha}_n \mu_n(\lambda_L)\lambda_G \mu_I.$$

(b) Since self-isolation effectively means zero severity for the within-household epidemic (although the initial case is infected, the self-isolation means that she is guaranteed to not infect anyone else in the population), one can condition on whether or not the initial case self-isolates to find that

$$E[s^{R_n}] = \delta + (1-\delta)\phi_{n-1,1}(1, \lambda_G(1-s)),$$

so that

$$f_R^{\delta}(s) = \delta + (1-\delta) \sum_{n=1}^{n_{\max}} \tilde{\alpha}_n \phi_{n-1,1}(1, \lambda_G(1-s)).$$

Letting $\sigma_\delta = f_R^\delta(\sigma_\delta)$ be the probability of a minor outbreak, it follows that $f_R^\delta(\sigma_0) = \delta + (1-\delta)\sigma_0 \geq \sigma_0$ and thus that $\sigma_\delta = f_R^\delta(\sigma_\delta) \geq \sigma_0$ (draw a diagram of the probability generating functions to help see this last inequality). This implies that the major outbreak probabilities satisfy $1-\sigma_\delta \leq 1-\sigma_0$.

Problems of Chapter 3

3.5.1 Note that the local susceptibility set of an individual, i say, comprises just that individual, so $\chi_i^N(t) = 1_{\{L_i \leq t\}}$. Thus, using (3.4.16), $r(t) = \mathbb{P}(L_1 \leq t) = 1-\mathrm{e}^{-\lambda t}$ and $a(t) = \mu_I(1-\mathrm{e}^{-\lambda t})$, both for $t \geq 0$. Hence, using (3.4.27), $\hat{\tau}$ solves $\tau = \mu_I(1-\mathrm{e}^{-\lambda\tau})$. Recalling that $R_0 = \lambda\mu_I$, it follows that $\hat{z} = \mu_I^{-1}\hat{\tau}$ is the unique solution in $(0,1]$ of $z = 1-\mathrm{e}^{-\lambda R_0 z}$, so $\hat{z} = z^*$ where z^* is defined in Theorem 3.3.1 of Part I in this volume. Note that $r(\hat{\tau}) = 1-\hat{z}$.

Further, since $L_1, L_2, \ldots, L_N, I_1, I_2, \ldots, I_N$ are independent,

$$\sigma_R^2(\hat{\tau}) = \mathrm{Var}(\chi_1^N(\hat{\tau})) = \mathrm{e}^{-\lambda\hat{\tau}}(1-\mathrm{e}^{-\lambda\hat{\tau}}) = \hat{z}(1-\hat{z}), \tag{3.5.31}$$

$$\sigma_{RA}(\hat{\tau}) = \mathrm{cov}(\chi_1^N(\hat{\tau}), I_1\chi_1^N(\hat{\tau})) = \mu_I \mathrm{Var}(\chi_1^N(\hat{\tau})) = \mu_I\hat{z}(1-\hat{z}) \tag{3.5.32}$$

and

$$\begin{aligned}\sigma_R^2(\hat{\tau}) &= \mathrm{Var}(I_1\chi_1^N(\hat{\tau})) = (\sigma_I^2+\mu_I^2)(1-\mathrm{e}^{-\lambda\hat{\tau}}) - \mu_I^2(1-\mathrm{e}^{-\lambda\hat{\tau}})^2 \\ &= \mu_I^2\hat{z}(1-\hat{z}) + \sigma_I^2\hat{z}.\end{aligned} \tag{3.5.33}$$

Substituting (3.5.31)–(3.5.33) into σ_R^2, given by (3.4.26) with $\tau = \hat{\tau}$, and rearranging yields the asymptotic variance in Theorem 3.3.2 of Part I in this volume.

3.5.2 Consider the approximating branching process $\mathscr{B}_R$, defined on page 174 in Section 3.3.5, for the special case of the Markovian SEIR model. A typical individual has offspring at the points of a Poisson process having rate λ during the age interval $[L, L+I)$, where $L \sim \mathrm{Exp}(\nu)$ and $I \sim \mathrm{Exp}(\gamma)$ are independent, so in the notation of Section 3.3.5,

$$\begin{aligned}\mu_Y(t) &= \mathbb{P}(L \leq t < L+I) \\ &= [\mathbb{P}(L \leq t) - \mathbb{P}(L+I \leq t)] \qquad (t > 0).\end{aligned}$$

(A local infectious clump consists of a single infective, who is infective at infectious age t if and only if $t \in [L, L+I)$.) Thus, using (3.3.16) on page 175 with $\lambda_G = \lambda$, the exponential growth rate r is given by the unique solution in $(-\infty, \infty)$ of

$$\int_0^\infty \lambda\mathrm{e}^{-rt}[\mathbb{P}(L \leq t) - \mathbb{P}(L+I \leq t)]\,\mathrm{d}t = 1. \tag{3.5.34}$$

Now

$$\int_0^\infty \mathrm{e}^{-rt}\mathbb{P}(L \le t)\,\mathrm{d}t = \int_0^\infty \mathrm{e}^{-rt}(1-\mathrm{e}^{-\nu t})\,\mathrm{d}t = \frac{\nu}{(\nu+r)r} \qquad (r > -\nu)$$

and, using the formula for the Laplace transform of a convolution of two functions,

$$\begin{aligned}\int_0^\infty \mathrm{e}^{-rt}\mathbb{P}(L+I \le t)\,\mathrm{d}t &= \int_{t=0}^\infty \mathrm{e}^{-rt}\int_{u=0}^t \nu\mathrm{e}^{-\nu u}\mathbb{P}(I \le t-u)\,\mathrm{d}u\,\mathrm{d}t\\ &= \frac{\nu}{\nu+r}\frac{\gamma}{(\gamma+r)r} \qquad (r > -\min(\nu,\gamma)),\end{aligned}$$

so

$$\lambda\int_0^\infty \mathrm{e}^{-rt}\mathbb{P}(L \le t < L+I)\,\mathrm{d}t = \frac{\nu}{(\nu+r)(\gamma+r)} \qquad (r > -\min(\nu,\gamma)). \quad (3.5.35)$$

Substituting (3.5.35) into (3.5.34) and rearranging shows that r satisfies the quadratic equation

$$r^2 + (\gamma+\nu)r + (\gamma-\lambda)\nu = 0, \qquad (3.5.36)$$

whence

$$r = \frac{1}{2}\left[\sqrt{(\gamma-\nu)^2+4\lambda\nu} - (\gamma+\nu)\right].$$

(The other solution of (3.5.36) can be excluded as it is $\le -\min(\nu,\gamma)$.)

3.5.3 For the epidemic $E_{n-1,1}(\lambda_H, I)$, let $Y_{n,k}$ be the number of individuals in household generation k ($k = 0,1,\ldots,n-1$), so $\mu_k^H = \mathbb{E}[Y_{n,k}]$. Note that household generation 0 always consists of the initial infective, so $\mu_k^H = 1$ for all n.

(a) As the infectious period is constant, the initial infective infects the other two household members independently with probability p_H, so $Y_{3,1} \sim \mathrm{Bin}(2, p_H)$ and $\mu_1^H = 2p_H$. (A binomial distribution with n trials and success probability p is denoted by $\sim \mathrm{Bin}(n,p)$.) The only way an individual can be in household generation 2 is if the initial infective infects precisely one of the two initial susceptibles, who then infects the other initial susceptible (i.e., in the notation of Section 3.1 of Part I of this volume, the chain $1 \to 1 \to 1$ occurs), which happens with probability $2p_H(1-p_H)p_H$, so $\mu_2^H = 2p_H^2(1-p_H)$.

(b) If I is not constant then $Y_{3,1}|I \sim \mathrm{Bin}(2, 1-\mathrm{e}^{-\lambda_H I})$, so letting I_0 denote the length of the initial infective's infectious period,

$$\mu_1^H = \mathbb{E}[Y_{3,1}] = \mathbb{E}[\mathbb{E}[Y_{3,1}|I_0]] = \mathbb{E}[2(1-\mathrm{e}^{-\lambda_H I_0})] = 2(1-\phi_I(\lambda_H)).$$

The probability that the initial infective infects precisely one of the two initial susceptibles is

$$\mathbb{E}[2(1-\mathrm{e}^{-\lambda_H I_0})\mathrm{e}^{-\lambda_H I_0}] = 2\left(\phi_I(\lambda_H) - \phi_I(2\lambda_H)\right)$$

and, letting I_1 denote the length of the infected susceptible's infectious period, the probability it infects the other susceptible is $\mathbb{E}[1-\mathrm{e}^{-\lambda_H I_1}] = 1-\phi_I(\lambda_H)$, so since I_0 and I_1 are independent,

$$\mu_2^H = 2\left(\phi_I(\lambda_H) - \phi_I(2\lambda_H)\right)\left(1 - \phi_I(\lambda_H)\right).$$

(c) Suppose $n = 4$ and I is constant. Then $Y_{4,1} \sim \text{Bin}(3, p_H)$, so $\mu_1^H = 3p_H$. Note that

$$\begin{aligned}\mathbb{E}[Y_{4,2}] &= \mathbb{E}[\mathbb{E}[Y_{4,2}|Y_{4,1}]] \\ &= \mathbb{P}(Y_{4,1} = 1)\mathbb{E}[Y_{4,2}|Y_{4,1} = 1] + \mathbb{P}(Y_{4,1} = 2)\mathbb{E}[Y_{4,2}|Y_{4,1} = 2],\end{aligned} \tag{3.5.37}$$

since the possible values of $Y_{4,1}$ are $0, 1, 2, 3$ and $Y_{4,2} = 0$ if $Y_{4,1}$ is 0 or 3. Now $Y_{4,2}|Y_{4,1} = 1 \sim \text{Bin}(2, p_H)$, since at that stage there are two remaining susceptibles, so $\mathbb{E}[Y_{4,2}|Y_{4,1} = 1] = 2p_H$. If $Y_{4,1} = 2$ then there is one remaining susceptible, who avoids infection from the two generation-1 infectives with probability $(1 - p_H)^2$, so $\mathbb{E}[Y_{4,2}|Y_{4,1} = 2] = 1 - (1 - p_H)^2$. Thus, since $Y_{4,1} \sim \text{Bin}(3, p_H)$, (3.5.37) yields

$$\begin{aligned}\mu_2^H &= \left(3p_H(1 - p_H)^2\right)2p_H + \left(3p_H^2(1 - p_H)\right)\left(1 - (1 - p_H)^2\right) \\ &= 3p_H^2(1 - p_H)(2 - p_H^2).\end{aligned}$$

The only way an individual can be in household generation 3 is if the chain $1 \to 1 \to 1 \to 1$ occurs. Thus,

$$\mu_3^H = \left(3p_H(1 - p_H)^2\right)\left(2p_H(1 - p_H)\right)(p_H) = 6p_H^3(1 - p_H)^3.$$

If I is not constant, then $Y_{4,1}|I_0 \sim \text{Bin}(3, 1 - \mathrm{e}^{-\lambda_H I_0})$, where I_0 is the length of the initial infective's infectious period, so

$$\mu_1^H = \mathbb{E}[Y_{4,1}] = \mathbb{E}[\mathbb{E}[Y_{4,1}|I_0]] = \mathbb{E}[3(1 - \mathrm{e}^{-\lambda_H I_0})] = 3(1 - \phi_I(\lambda_H)). \tag{3.5.38}$$

To determine μ_2^H, note that

$$\mathbb{P}(Y_{4,1} = 1) = \mathbb{E}[3(1 - \mathrm{e}^{-\lambda_H I_0})\mathrm{e}^{-2\lambda_H I_0}] = 3\left(\phi_I(2\lambda_H) - \phi_I(3\lambda_H)\right)$$

and

$$\mathbb{P}(Y_{4,1} = 2) = \mathbb{E}[3(1 - \mathrm{e}^{-\lambda_H I_0})^2\mathrm{e}^{-\lambda_H I_0}] = 3\left(\phi_I(\lambda_H) - 2\phi_I(2\lambda_H) + \phi_I(3\lambda_H)\right).$$

Further, if $Y_{4,1} = 1$, let I_1 be the infectious period of the generation-1 infective. Then

$$\mathbb{E}[Y_{4,2}|Y_{4,1} = 1] = \mathbb{E}[\mathbb{E}[Y_{4,2}|Y_{4,1} = 1, I_1]] = \mathbb{E}[2(1 - \mathrm{e}^{-\lambda_H I_1})] = 2(1 - \phi_I(\lambda_H)).$$

Conditional on $Y_{4,1} = 2$, the remaining susceptible avoids infection from the two generation-1 infectives independently, each with probability $\phi(\lambda_H)$, so

$$\mathbb{E}[Y_{4,2}|Y_{4,1} = 2] = 1 - \phi_I(\lambda_H)^2.$$

Thus (3.5.37) now yields

$$\begin{aligned}\mu_2^H =& \left(3[\phi_I(2\lambda_H) - \phi_I(3\lambda_H)]\right)2(1 - \phi_I(\lambda_H)) \\ &+ 3[\phi_I(\lambda_H) - 2\phi_I(2\lambda_H) + \phi_I(3\lambda_H)]\left(1 - \phi_I(\lambda_H)^2\right).\end{aligned}$$

Finally, as the infectives in the chain $1 \to 1 \to 1 \to 1$ have independent infectious periods, arguing as in the derivation of (3.5.38) yields

$$\mu_3^H = 6\left(\phi_I(2\lambda_H) - \phi_I(3\lambda_H)\right)\left(\phi_I(\lambda_H) - \phi_I(2\lambda_H)\right)\left(1 - \phi_I(\lambda_H)\right).$$

3.5.4 (a) Label the two individuals in a household 0 and 1, where 0 is the initial infective. For $t \geq 0$,

$$Y(t) = \chi_0(t) + \chi_1(t), \tag{3.5.39}$$

where, for $i = 0, 1$,

$$\chi_i(t) = \begin{cases} 1 & \text{if } i \text{ is infective at time } t, \\ 0 & \text{otherwise}. \end{cases}$$

For simplicity we assume that the distribution of the infectious period I is absolutely continuous with density $f_I(t)$ $(t \geq 0)$. Denote the infectious periods of individuals 0 and 1 (if it is infected) by I_0 and I_1, respectively. Then,

$$\begin{aligned}
\int_0^\infty e^{-\theta t}\mathbb{E}[\chi_0(t)]\,dt &= \int_0^\infty e^{-\theta t}\mathbb{P}(I_0 > t)\,dt \\
&= \int_{t=0}^\infty e^{-\theta t}\int_{u=t}^\infty f_I(u)\,du\,dt \\
&= \int_{u=0}^\infty f_I(u)\int_{t=0}^u e^{-\theta t}\,dt\,du \\
&= \int_{u=0}^\infty f_I(u)\frac{1}{\theta}\left(1 - e^{-\theta u}\right)du \\
&= \frac{1}{\theta}\left[1 - \phi_I(\theta)\right] \\
&= \psi_I(\theta).
\end{aligned} \tag{3.5.40}$$

Let T_1 denote the time when individual 0 infects individual 1, where $T_1 = \infty$ if individual 0 fails to infect individual 1. For $t > 0$, $T_1 = t$ if and only if the first contact of individual 1 by individual 0 occurs at time t (which happens with density $\lambda_H e^{-\lambda_H t}$) and $I_0 > t$. Hence, T_1 has density $f_{T_1}(t) = \lambda_H e^{-\lambda_H t}\mathbb{P}(I_0 > t)$ $(t > 0)$, since the Poisson process which governs the times when individual 0 contacts individual 1, is independent of I_0. Further, $\chi_1(t) = 1$ if and only if $T_1 \leq t$ and $T_1 + I_1 > t$. Thus,

$$\mathbb{E}[\chi_1(t)] = \int_0^t f_{T_1}(u)\mathbb{P}(I_1 > t - u)\,du,$$

so, using the formula for the Laplace transform of a convolution of two functions,

$$\begin{aligned}
\int_0^\infty e^{-\theta t}\mathbb{E}[\chi_1(t)]\,dt &= \int_0^\infty e^{-\theta t}\lambda_H e^{-\lambda t}\mathbb{P}(I_0 > t)\,dt\,\psi_I(\theta) \\
&= \lambda_H\psi_I(\lambda_H + \theta)\psi_I(\theta).
\end{aligned} \tag{3.5.41}$$

Note that using a Stieltjes integral shows that (3.5.40) and (3.5.41) also hold when I is not absolutely continuous. The expression (3.5.3) for $\mathscr{L}_{\mu_Y}(\theta)$ now follows using (3.5.39).

(b) Suppose $I \sim \text{Exp}(\gamma)$. Then $f_I(t) = \gamma \mathrm{e}^{-\gamma t}$ $(t \geq 0)$, so $\phi_I(\theta) = \gamma/(\gamma+\theta)$ and $\psi_I(\theta) = 1/(\gamma+\theta)$ $(\theta > -\gamma)$. It follows from (3.3.16) on page 175 that r satisfies $\lambda_G \mathscr{L}_{\mu_Y}(r) = 1$. Thus, using part (a),

$$\frac{\lambda_G}{\gamma+r}\left[1+\frac{\lambda_H}{\gamma+\lambda_H+r}\right] = 1,$$

which on rearranging yields

$$r^2 + (2\gamma+\lambda_H-\lambda_G)r + (\gamma-\lambda_G)(\gamma+\lambda_H) - \lambda_H\lambda_G = 0, \tag{3.5.42}$$

so

$$r = \frac{1}{2}\left[\lambda_H - \lambda_G - 2\gamma + \sqrt{\lambda_H^2 + 6\lambda_H\lambda_G + \lambda_G^2}\right].$$

(The other solution of (3.5.36) is less than

$$\frac{1}{2}[\lambda_H - \lambda_G - 2\gamma - (\lambda_H + \lambda_G)] = -(\gamma+\lambda_G) < -\gamma,$$

so it can be excluded.)

3.5.5 Setting $j = 1$ in (3.5.5) yields

$$f_S(s) = \sum_{k=1}^{n} (n-1)_{[k-1]} s^k q_k^{n-k} G_{k-1}(1 \mid U'),$$

where U' $(= EU)$ is given by $u'_k = q_{k+1}$ $(k = 0, 1, \ldots)$. Let $\tilde{\mu}_n(\lambda_H, I, \pi)$ be the mean total size of $\tilde{E}_{n,0}(\lambda_H, I, \pi)$. Then Corollary 1.8.2 on page 139 yields

$$\tilde{\mu}_n(\lambda_H, I, \pi) = n - \sum_{i=1}^{n} n_{[i]} q_i^{n-i} \pi^i G_{i-1}(1 \mid U'),$$

so

$$\frac{\tilde{\mu}_n(\lambda_H, I, \pi)}{n} = 1 - \sum_{i=1}^{n} (n-1)_{[i-1]} q_i^{n-i} \pi^i G_{i-1}(1 \mid U').$$

Thus,

$$1 - f_S(\mathrm{e}^{-\lambda_G \mu_I z}) = \frac{\tilde{\mu}_n(\lambda_H, I, \mathrm{e}^{-\lambda_G \mu_I z})}{n}$$

and the two equations governing $\hat{z}$ are the same.

3.5.6 A simple way of showing that $|X_H| \stackrel{\mathrm{D}}{=} \tilde{S}$ is to show that the factorial moments of the two distributions are the same. It follows using Lemma 1.3.1 on page 129, (3.4.10) on page 184 and (3.5.5) that, for $j = 0, 1, \ldots, n$,

$$\begin{aligned}\mathbb{E}\left[|X_H|_{[j]}\right] &= n_{[j]} f_{jn}(\hat{\pi}) \\ &= n_{[j]} \sum_{k=j}^{n} (n-j)_{[k-j]} \hat{\pi}^k q_k^{n-k} G_{k-j}(1 \mid E^j U),\end{aligned} \tag{3.5.43}$$

where U is given by $u_k = q_k$ $(k = 0, 1, \dots)$. Setting $a = 0, \pi = \hat{\pi}$ and $x = 1$ in (1.8.3) on page 140 yields, for $j = 0, 1, \dots, n$, that

$$\mathbb{E}\left[\tilde{S}_{[j]}\right] = \sum_{k=j}^{n} n_{[k]} q_k^{n-k} \hat{\pi}^k G_k^{(j)}(1 \mid U). \tag{3.5.44}$$

Noting that $n_{[j]}(n-j)_{[k-j]} = n_{[k]}$ and $G_k^{(j)}(1 \mid U) = G_{k-j}(1 \mid E^j U)$ (using Property 1.4.5 on page 131), it follows from (3.5.43) and (3.5.44) that $\mathbb{E}\left[|X_H|_{[j]}\right] = \mathbb{E}\left[\tilde{S}_{[j]}\right]$ $(j = 0, 1, \dots, n)$, so $|X_H| \stackrel{D}{=} \tilde{S}$ as both $|X_H|$ and $\tilde{S}$ have support $\{0, 1, \dots, n\}$.

Alternatively, one can show directly that $\mathbb{P}(\tilde{S} = k)$ is given by (3.5.7). Let $f_{\tilde{S}}(x)$ denote the probability-generating function of $\tilde{S}$. Then setting $\theta = 0$ in Theorem 1.8.1 on page 138 yields

$$f_{\tilde{S}}(x) = \sum_{l=0}^{n} n_{[l]} q_l^{n-l} \hat{\pi}^l G_l(x \mid U) \qquad (x \in \mathbb{R}),$$

so, for $k = 0, 1, \dots, n$,

$$\mathbb{P}(\tilde{S} = k) = \frac{1}{k!} f_{\tilde{S}}^{(k)}(0) = \frac{1}{k!} \sum_{l=k}^{n} n_{[l]} q_l^{n-l} \hat{\pi}^l G_l^{(k)}(0 \mid U),$$

since $G_l(x \mid U)$ is a polynomial of degree l. Further, $G_l^{(k)}(x \mid U)$ is a polynomial of degree $l - k$, so its Taylor expansion about $x = 1$ yields

$$\begin{aligned}G_l^{(k)}(0 \mid U) &= \sum_{j=0}^{l-k} \frac{(-1)^j}{j!} G_l^{(k+j)}(1 \mid U) \\ &= \sum_{j=k}^{l} \frac{(-1)^j}{(j-k)!} G_{l-j}(1 \mid E^J U),\end{aligned}$$

where we have used Property 1.4.5 on page 131. Thus, for $k = 0, 1, \dots, n$,

$$\begin{aligned}\mathbb{P}(\tilde{S} = k) &= \frac{1}{k!} \sum_{l=k}^{n} n_{[l]} q_l^{n-l} \hat{\pi}^l \sum_{j=k}^{l} \frac{(-1)^j}{(j-k)!} G_{l-j}(1 \mid E^J U) \\ &= \binom{n}{k} \sum_{j=k}^{n} (-1)^j \binom{n-k}{j-k} \sum_{l=j}^{n} (n-j)_{[l-j]} q_l^{n-l} \hat{\pi}^l G_{l-j}(1 \mid E^J U) \\ &= \binom{n}{k} \sum_{j=k}^{n} (-1)^j \binom{n-k}{j-k} f_{jn}(\hat{\pi}),\end{aligned}$$

using (3.5.5).

3.5.7 Recall that, for $i \in \mathscr{N}$, the sets of individuals in i's household and workplace are denoted by H_i and W_i, respectively. Fix $i \in \mathscr{N}$ and consider the following iterative process, which is analogous to the construction of i's local susceptibility set $\mathscr{S}_i$ in Section 3.5.3.1 but assumes that at each stage all household (or workplace) members join a household (or workplace) local susceptibility set. Let

$$\hat{\mathscr{P}}_0 = H_i,$$

and, for $k = 1,2,\ldots$, let

$$\hat{\mathscr{P}}_k = \begin{cases} \left(\bigcup_{j\in\hat{\mathscr{P}}_{k-1}} W_j\right) \setminus \left(\bigcup_{l=0}^{k-1} \hat{\mathscr{P}}_l\right) & \text{if } k \text{ is odd,} \\ \left(\bigcup_{j\in\hat{\mathscr{P}}_{k-1}} H_j\right) \setminus \left(\bigcup_{l=0}^{k-1} \hat{\mathscr{P}}_l\right) & \text{if } k \text{ is even.} \end{cases}$$

Note that forming $\hat{\mathscr{P}}_1$ involves determining the workplaces of n_H individuals (i.e. of the n_H members of i's household), forming $\hat{\mathscr{P}}_2$ then involves determining the households of $n_H(n_W - 1)$ individuals (the members of i's household are already known), forming $\hat{\mathscr{P}}_3$ then involves determining the workplaces of $n_H(n_W - 1)(n_H - 1)$ individuals, and so on. Thus, for $k = 1,2,\ldots$, in forming $\hat{\mathscr{P}}_{2k}$ the total number of individuals whose workplace has been determined is

$$\begin{aligned} N_W(k) &= \sum_{l=0}^{k-1} n_H[(n_W - 1)(n_H - 1)]^l \\ &= n_H \left[\frac{[(n_W - 1)(n_H - 1)]^k - 1}{n_W n_H - n_W - n_H}\right] \end{aligned}$$

and the total number of individuals whose household has been determined is

$$\begin{aligned} N_H(k) &= \sum_{l=0}^{k-1} n_H(n_W - 1)[(n_W - 1)(n_H - 1)]^l \\ &= n_H(n_W - 1) \left[\frac{[(n_W - 1)(n_H - 1)]^k - 1}{n_W n_H - n_W - n_H}\right]. \end{aligned}$$

Let $M_W(k)$ be the event that at least two of the workplaces of the above $N_W(k)$ individuals are the same. For $i \neq j$,

$$\mathbb{P}(\sigma(i) \text{ and } \sigma(j) \text{ belong to the same workplace}) = \frac{n_W - 1}{N - 1},$$

so, for fixed k,

$$\mathbb{P}(M_W(k)) \leq \binom{N_W(k)}{2} \frac{n_W - 1}{N - 1} \to 0 \qquad \text{as } N \to \infty. \tag{3.5.45}$$

Let $M_H(k)$ be the event that at least two of the households of individual i and the above $N_H(k)$ individuals are the same. A similar argument shows that, for fixed k,

$$\mathbb{P}(M_H(k)) \le \binom{N_H(k)+1}{2}\frac{n_W-1}{N-1} \to 0 \qquad \text{as } N \to \infty. \tag{3.5.46}$$

Similar to the proof of Theorem 3.3.6 on page 177, the approximating branching process $\hat{\mathscr{B}}$ and the local susceptibility set $\mathscr{S}_i$ can be constructed on a common probability space so that, for $k = 1,2,\ldots$,

$$|\mathbb{P}(S^N \le k) - \mathbb{P}(\hat{Z} \le k)| \le \mathbb{P}(M_W(k) \cup M_H(k)),$$

cf. (3.3.24). Now (3.5.45) and (3.5.46) imply that $\mathbb{P}(M_W(k) \cup M_H(k)) \to 0$ as $N \to \infty$ ($k = 1,2,\ldots$), so $S^N \xrightarrow{D} \hat{Z}$ as $N \to \infty$.

3.5.8 Let H be an initially fully susceptible household. For $i \in H$, let $\bar{\mathscr{S}}_i^N$ be the local susceptibility set of i among $\mathscr{N} \setminus H$ and $\bar{S}_i^N = |\bar{\mathscr{S}}_i^N|$. Then $\bar{S}_i^N \xrightarrow{D} \hat{Z}_H$ as $N \to \infty$. In the event of a global outbreak, the members of H avoid external infection (i.e. from a global or a workplace contact) independently with probability $\bar{\pi} = f_{ZH}(\mathrm{e}^{-\lambda_G \mu_I \hat{z}})$. It follows that Z_H is distributed as the total size of the epidemic $\tilde{E}_{n_H,0}(\lambda_H, I, \bar{\pi})$ defined in Section 1.8 on page 138.

Let $\tilde{\mu}_{n_H}(\lambda_H, I, \bar{\pi})$ be the mean total size of $\tilde{E}_{n_H,0}(\lambda_H, I, \bar{\pi})$. Then, as in Section 2.3 (cf. (2.3.2) on page 147), $\hat{z}$ satisfies

$$\hat{z} = \frac{1}{n_H}\tilde{\mu}_{n_H}(\lambda_H, I, \bar{\pi}). \tag{3.5.47}$$

For fixed n_H, λ_H and distribution of I, the right-hand side of (3.5.47) is strictly decreasing in $\bar{\pi}$, so fixing $\hat{z}$ also fixes $\bar{\pi}$ and hence also the distribution of Z_H. Thus any choice of $(n_W, \lambda_W, \lambda_G)$ consistent with $\hat{z}$ yields the same distribution of Z_H.

3.5.9 The characteristic polynomial of the matrix $V(\lambda)$ is $f(x) = \det(xI - V(\lambda))$, where I is the 3×3 identity matrix. Expanding the determinant $\det(xI - V(\lambda))$ yields that $f(x)$ is given by the expression in the exercise. Let $A = v_G(\lambda), B = v_H(\lambda)$ and $C = v_W(\lambda)$. Then,

$$\begin{aligned} f(x) = 0 &\iff x^3 - Ax^2 - (AB+AC+BC)x - ABC = 0 \\ &\iff \frac{ABC}{x^3} + \frac{AB+AC+BC}{x^2} + \frac{A}{x} = 1. \end{aligned} \tag{3.5.48}$$

The left-hand side of (3.5.48) is decreasing in $x \in (0,\infty)$, tends to ∞ as $x \to 0-$ and to 0 as $x \to \infty$. Thus $f(x) = 0$ has a unique solution in $(0,\infty)$. The dominant eigenvalue $v_*(\lambda)$ of $V(\lambda)$ satisfies $f(v_*(\lambda)) = 0$. Moreover, by the Perron–Frobenius theorem (see, for example, Haccou et al. [37, page 293]), $v_*(\lambda) \in (0,\infty)$, so $v_*(\lambda) = 1$ if and only if $f(1) = 0$, i.e. if and only if

$$ABC + AB + AC + BC + A - 1 = 0 \iff A(B+1)(C+1) + BC - 1 = 0.$$

The equation (3.5.9) then follows.

3.5.10 Note that $(A_R | A_R > 0) \stackrel{\mathrm{D}}{=} A'$, where $A' = I + A_R$. Recall that I is the infectious period of individual i. Conditioning on I,

$$A' = \begin{cases} I & \text{if } i \text{ does not infect } i+1 \text{ locally}, \\ I + A'' & \text{otherwise}, \end{cases} \tag{3.5.49}$$

where A'' is an independent copy of A'. Let $\phi_{A'}(\theta) = \mathbb{E}[\mathrm{e}^{-\theta A'}]$ $(\theta \geq 0)$. Now

$$\mathbb{P}(i \text{ does not infect } i+1 \text{ locally}|I) = \mathrm{e}^{-\lambda_L I},$$

so, using (3.5.49),

$$\mathbb{E}[\mathrm{e}^{-\theta A'}|I] = \mathrm{e}^{-\lambda_L I}\mathrm{e}^{-\theta I} + (1-\mathrm{e}^{-\lambda_L I})\mathrm{e}^{-\theta I}\phi_{A'}(\theta).$$

Thus,

$$\begin{aligned} \phi_{A'}(\theta) &= \mathbb{E}[\mathbb{E}[\mathrm{e}^{-\theta A'}|I]] \\ &= \phi_I(\lambda_L + \theta) + [\phi_I(\theta) - \phi_I(\lambda_L + \theta)]\phi_{A'}(\theta), \end{aligned}$$

which on rearranging yields (3.5.16).

Given I, the events $\{A_R > 0\}$ and $\{A_L > 0\}$ occur independently, each with probability $1 - \mathrm{e}^{-\lambda_L I}$. Now $A = I + A_L + A_R$, so

$$\begin{aligned} \phi_A(\theta) &= \mathbb{E}\left[\mathbb{E}\left[\mathrm{e}^{-\theta(I+A_L+A_R)}|I\right]\right] \\ &= \mathbb{E}\left[\mathrm{e}^{-\theta I}\left\{\mathrm{e}^{-2\lambda_L I} + 2\mathrm{e}^{-\lambda_L I}(1-\mathrm{e}^{-\lambda_L I})\phi_{A'}(\theta) + (1-\mathrm{e}^{-\lambda_L I})^2(\phi_{A'}(\theta))^2\right\}\right] \\ &= \phi_I(\theta + 2\lambda_L) + 2[\phi_I(\theta+\lambda_L) - \phi_I(\theta+2\lambda_L)]\phi_{A'}(\theta) \\ &\quad + [\phi_I(\theta) - 2\phi_I(\theta+\lambda_L) + \phi_I(\theta+2\lambda_L)](\phi_{A'}(\theta))^2. \end{aligned} \tag{3.5.50}$$

Equation (3.5.17) follows by substituting (3.5.16) into (3.5.50).

3.5.12 The clump $\mathscr{C}_i$ has one index case, individual i, so $\mu_0^C = 1$. For $k = 1, 2 \ldots$, the only two possible clump generation-k individuals are individuals $i+k$ and $i-k$, who by (3.5.14) each belong to the clump with probability p_L^k. Thus $\mu_k^C = 2p_L^k$ $(k = 1, 2, \ldots)$.

Let $\mu_G = \lambda_G \mu_I$. Substituting the above μ_k^Cs into (3.3.8) on page 170 yields

$$\begin{aligned} g_0(\lambda) &= 1 - \mu_G \left[\frac{1}{\lambda} + 2\sum_{k=1}^{\infty} \frac{p_L^k}{\lambda^{k+1}}\right] \\ &= 1 - \frac{\mu_G(\lambda + p_L)}{\lambda(\lambda - p_L)} \qquad (\lambda \in (p_L, \infty)). \end{aligned} \tag{3.5.51}$$

It follows that $g_0(\lambda) = 0$ if and only if $f(\lambda) = 0$, where

$$f(\lambda) = \lambda^2 - (\mu_G + p_L)\lambda - \mu_G p_L = 0,$$

so R_0 is given by the positive solution of this quadratic. It is easily verified that $f(\lambda)$ is the characteristic polynomial of the matrix $\tilde{M}$ defined at (3.5.18), so R_0 is given by (3.5.19).

3.5.14 Let $\mathscr{C}_i(v)$ be the post-vaccination local infectious clump of individual i; see the proof of Theorem 3.3.3 in Section 3.3.4. Partition $\mathscr{C}_i(v) = \mathscr{C}_L(v) \cup \{i\} \cup \mathscr{C}_R(v)$ analogously to $\mathscr{C}_i$ at (3.5.12). For $k = 1, 2, \dots$,

$$i+k \in \mathscr{C}_R(v) \iff i+k \in \mathscr{C}_R \text{ and } i+1, i+2, \dots, i+k \text{ are unvaccinated.}$$

Thus, similarly to (3.5.14),

$$\mathbb{P}(i+k \in \mathscr{C}_R(v)) = p_L^k (1-v)^k \qquad (k = 1, 2, \dots),$$

whence $\mu_{C(v)} = 1 + 2p_L(1-v)/[1 - p_L(1-v)]$. Hence, using (3.3.12) on page 172,

$$R_*(v) = \mu_G(1-v)\left[\frac{1+(1-v)p_L}{1-(1-v)p_L}\right]. \tag{3.5.52}$$

Let $u = (1-v_c)^{-1}$, where v_c solves $R_*(v) = 1$. Then (3.5.52) implies that

$$\frac{\mu_G(u+p_L)}{u(u-p_L)} = 1,$$

so, recalling (3.5.51), $g_0(u) = 0$. Thus $u = R_0$, whence $v_c = 1 - R_0^{-1}$.

3.5.15 As suggested in the hint, we consider the finite N problem and let

$$\tilde{R}_*(v) = \mu_G(1-v)\mathbb{E}[\tilde{C}(v)],$$

where $\tilde{C}(v) = |\tilde{\mathscr{C}}(v)|$ and $\tilde{\mathscr{C}}(v)$ is the post-vaccination local infectious clump of an individual, i_0 say, chosen uniformly at random from the unvaccinated individuals in the population $\mathscr{N}$. Note that $\mu_G(1-v)$ is unaffected by the vaccine allocation, so the problem is to find the distribution of L_S which minimises $\mu_{\tilde{C}(v)} = \mathbb{E}[\tilde{C}(v)]$ subject to the constraint that a fraction v of the population is vaccinated. Partitioning $\tilde{\mathscr{C}}(v)$ analogously to $\mathscr{C}_i$ at (3.5.12) yields, in an obvious notation, that

$$\mu_{\tilde{C}(v)} = 1 + \mu_{\tilde{C}_L(v)} + \mu_{\tilde{C}_R(v)} = 1 + 2\mu_{\tilde{C}_R(v)}. \tag{3.5.53}$$

Suppose that the nearest vaccinated individual to i_0's right is at $i_0 + V_R + 1$. For $j = 1, 2, \dots, V_R$, the probability $i_0 + j$ belongs to $\tilde{\mathscr{C}}_R(v)$ is p_L^j, so

$$\mathbb{E}[\tilde{C}_R(v)|V_R] = \sum_{j=1}^{V_R} p_L^j = \frac{p_L(1-p_L^{V_R})}{1-p_L}.$$

Now consider a given run, U_k say, of k unvaccinated individuals between two vaccinated individuals. Given $i_0 \in U_k$, it is equally likely to be any of the k individuals in U_k, so

$$\mathbb{E}[\tilde{C}_R(v)|i_0 \in U_k] = \frac{1}{k}\sum_{j=0}^{k-1} \frac{p_L(1-p_L^j)}{1-p_L}$$
$$= \frac{p_L}{k(1-p_L)^2}(k-1-p_L+p_L^k).$$

Further, $\mathbb{P}(i_0 \in U_k) = ck$ for some constant c that is independent of k, so the contribution of U_k to $\mu_{\tilde{C}_R(v)}$ is

$$a(k) = \frac{cp_L}{(1-p_L)^2}(k-1-p_L+p_L^k).$$

Thus, by (3.5.53), the contribution of U_k to $\mu_{\tilde{C}(v)}$ is

$$b(k) = kc + 2a(k). \tag{3.5.54}$$

For $k \geq 1$ and $l \geq 2$, compare the combined contributions to $\mu_{\tilde{C}(v)}$ of (i) U_k and U_{k+l} and (ii) U_{k+1} and U_{k+l-1}, i.e.

$$b_1 = b(k) + b(k+l) \qquad \text{and} \qquad b_2 = b(k+1) + b(k+l-1).$$

Now

$$b_1 - b_2 = \frac{2cp_L}{(1-p_L)^2}(p_L^k + p_L^{k+l} - p_L^{k+1} - p_L^{k+l-1})$$
$$= \frac{2cp_L^{k+1}}{1-p_L}\left(1-p_L^{l-1}\right) > 0.$$

Thus, if the vaccinated population contains two runs of unvaccinated individuals whose lengths differ by at least 2, then $\tilde{R}_*(v)$ is made smaller by replacing them by two runs of more equal lengths but having the same total of lengths.

Also, for $k \geq 2$, compare the contributions to $\mu_{\tilde{C}_R(v)}$ of (iii) a run U_k preceded by two neighbouring vaccinated individuals and (iv) U_1 and U_{k-1}, i.e. $b_3 = b(k)$ and $b_4 = b(1) + b(k-1)$. Using (3.5.54) and noting that $a(1) = 0$,

$$b_3 - b_4 = 2[a(k) - a(k-1)] = \frac{2cp_L}{(1-p_L)^2}\left[1 - p_L^{k-1}(1-p_L)\right] > 0.$$

Thus, if the vaccinated population contains two consecutive vaccinated individuals next to a run of $k \geq 2$ unvaccinated individuals, then $\tilde{R}_*(v)$ is made smaller by replacing the $k+2$ individuals by a run of length 1 and a run of length $k-1$.

The above two observations concerning reduction of $\tilde{R}_*(v)$ imply that if v is held fixed then $\tilde{R}_*(v)$ is minimised by making the lengths of runs of unvaccinated individuals as equal as possible. See Ball et al. [14, Section 5.2.4] for an alternative, more sophisticated proof.

3.5.16 The characteristic polynomial of the matrix $\mathscr{L}_\Lambda(r)$ defined at (3.5.20) is

$$f(x) = x^2 - [\lambda_G \psi_I(r) + \lambda_L \psi_I(r+\lambda_L)] - \lambda_G \lambda_L \psi_I(r) \psi_I(r+\lambda_L).$$

Now $f(0) < 0$ and it is easily shown that $f(x) = 0$ has one positive and one negative solution, so $\mathscr{L}_\Lambda(r)$ has one positive and one negative eigenvalue. It follows that the dominant eigenvalue of $\mathscr{L}_\Lambda(r)$ is one if and only if $f(1) = 0$, i.e. if and only if

$$\lambda_G \psi_I(r) + \lambda_L \psi_I(r+\lambda_L) + \lambda_G \lambda_L \psi_I(r) \psi_I(r+\lambda_L) = 1. \tag{3.5.55}$$

Recall that $\psi_I(r) = \int_0^\infty \mathrm{e}^{-rt} \mathbb{P}(I > t)\,\mathrm{d}t$. Thus $\psi_I(r)$ is decreasing in r and there exists $r_0 \leq 0$ (may be $-\infty$) such that $\psi_I(r) \uparrow \infty$ as $r \downarrow r_0$. Further, $\lim_{r\to\infty} \psi_I(r) = 0$. It follows that the left-hand side of (3.5.55) is decreasing in r, converges to 0 as $r \uparrow \infty$ and to ∞ as $r \downarrow r_0$. Thus (3.5.55) has a unique solution in (r_0, ∞), which gives the exponential growth rate of the epidemic.

3.5.17 (a) We calculate $\mathbb{P}(T_S > k | T_S > k-1)$ $(k = 1,2,\dots)$. Without loss of generality suppose that a run of susceptible individuals starts at individual 1. Fix $k \in \mathbb{N}$, so $T_S > k-1$ if and only if individuals $1,2,\dots,k$ are all susceptible. Let $X = \min\{l > 0 :$ individual $k+l$ is contacted globally$\}$, so $\mathbb{P}(X = l) = \hat{\pi}^{l-1}(1-\hat{\pi})$ $(l = 1,2,\dots)$. Further, given $X = l$, the probability that this global contact does not lead to individuals k being infected locally is $1 - p_L^l$; the corresponding probability for individual $k+1$ is $1 - p_L^{l-1}$ Thus,

$$\mathbb{P}(X = l | T_S > k-1) = \frac{\hat{\pi}^{l-1}(1-\hat{\pi})(1-p_L^l)}{\sum_{i=1}^\infty \hat{\pi}^{i-1}(1-\hat{\pi})(1-p_L^i)} \qquad (l = 1,2,\dots)$$

and

$$\begin{aligned}\mathbb{P}(T_S > k | T_S > k-1) &= \sum_{l=2}^\infty \mathbb{P}(T_S > k | T_S > k-1, X = l)\mathbb{P}(X = l | T_S > k-1)\\ &= \frac{\sum_{l=2}^\infty \hat{\pi}^{l-1}(1-\hat{\pi})(1-p_L^{l-1})}{\sum_{i=1}^\infty \hat{\pi}^{i-1}(1-\hat{\pi})(1-p_L^i)}\\ &= \hat{\pi}.\end{aligned}$$

It follows that $\mathbb{P}(T_S > k) = \hat{\pi}^k$ $(k = 1,2,\dots)$, which yields (3.5.22).

(b) Since the runs of infectives form an alternating renewal process, the probability $\hat{z}$ that a typical initial susceptible is ultimately infected is given by $\frac{\mathbb{E}[T_R]}{\mathbb{E}[T_S]+\mathbb{E}[T_R]}$ (see, for example, Grimmett and Stirzaker [36, page 404]). Thus, noting that $\mathbb{E}[T_S] = (1-\hat{\pi})^{-1}$,

$$\mathbb{E}[T_R] = \frac{\hat{z}}{(1-\hat{\pi})(1-\hat{z})}. \tag{3.5.56}$$

Substituting $\hat{\pi} = \mathrm{e}^{-\lambda_G \mu_I \hat{z}}$ into (3.5.21) yields

$$1 - \hat{z} = \frac{\hat{\pi}(1-p_L)^2}{1 - p_L\hat{\pi})^2}. \tag{3.5.57}$$

The expression (3.5.23) for $\mathbb{E}[T_R]$ follows from (3.5.56) and (3.5.57).

3.5.21 As in Section 3.5.4.2, R_0 is given by the dominant eigenvalue of the mean offspring matrix $\tilde{M}$ of $\tilde{\mathscr{B}}$. As at (3.5.18) on page 204, $\tilde{M}$ takes the form

$$\tilde{M} = \begin{bmatrix} m_{GG} & m_{GL} \\ m_{LG} & m_{LL} \end{bmatrix}.$$

It is shown in Section 3.5.5.3 that $m_{GL} = \mu_D p_L$ and $m_{LL} = \mu_{\tilde{D}-1} p_L$. As at (3.5.18), $m_{GG} = m_{LG} = \lambda_G \mu_I$. A simple calculation shows that the dominant eigenvalue of $\tilde{M}$ is given by (3.5.25).

3.5.22 (a) Arguing as in the derivation of (3.5.20) on page 206 shows that the exponential growth rate of the network model with casual contacts is given by the unique $r \in (-\infty, \infty)$ such the dominant eigenvalue of $\mathscr{L}_\Lambda(r)$ is one, where

$$\mathscr{L}_\Lambda(r) = \begin{bmatrix} \lambda_G \psi_I(r) & 2\lambda_L \mu_D \psi_I(r+\lambda_L) \\ \lambda_G \psi_I(r) & \lambda_L \mu_{\tilde{D}-1} \psi_I(\theta+\lambda_L) \end{bmatrix}. \tag{3.5.58}$$

(The difference here between the current model and the great circle model is that in the branching process approximation, the mean number of neighbours a globally contacted individual may infect is μ_D, instead of 2, and the mean number of neighbours a locally contacted individual may infect is $\mu_{\tilde{D}-1}$, instead of 1.)

The characteristic polynomial of $\mathscr{L}_\Lambda(r)$ is

$$f(x) = x^2 - [\lambda_G \psi_I(r) + \lambda_L \mu_D \psi_I(r+\lambda_L)] + \lambda_G \lambda_L (\mu_{\tilde{D}-1} - \mu_D) \psi_I(r) \psi_I(r+\lambda_L). \tag{3.5.59}$$

It follows that one is an eigenvalue of $\mathscr{L}_\Lambda(r)$ if and only if

$$\lambda_G \psi_I(r) + \lambda_L \mu_{\tilde{D}-1} \psi_I(r+\lambda_L) + \lambda_G \lambda_L (\mu_D - \mu_{\tilde{D}-1}) \psi_I(r) \psi_I(r+\lambda_L) = 1. \tag{3.5.60}$$

If $\mu_{\tilde{D}-1} < \mu_D$, then $\mathscr{L}_\Lambda(r)$ has one positive and one negative eigenvalue and arguing as in the solution of Exercise 3.5.16 shows that (3.5.60) has a unique real solution, which gives the required exponential growth rate.

If $\mu_{\tilde{D}-1} = \mu_D$ (as happens if the degree distribution D is Poisson), then one of the eigenvalues of $\mathscr{L}_\Lambda(r)$ is zero and it is easily shown that again the required exponential growth rate r is given by the unique real solution of (3.5.16).

Finally, if $\mu_{\tilde{D}-1} > \mu_D$ then, for any r for which $\mathscr{L}_\Lambda(r)$ is finite, the eigenvalues of $\mathscr{L}_\Lambda(r)$ are both positive. The elements of $\mathscr{L}_\Lambda(r)$ each decrease with r and tend to 0 as $r \to \infty$, hence so does the dominant eigenvalue, $\lambda_{\max}(r)$ say. It follows that the value of r for which $\lambda_{\max}(r) = 1$ is given by the largest real solution of (3.5.60).

(b) When $I \sim \text{Exp}(\gamma)$, $\mathbb{P}(I > t) = \mathrm{e}^{-\gamma t}$ $(t \geq 0)$, so $\psi(\theta) = \int_0^\infty \mathrm{e}^{-\theta t} \mathbb{P}(I > t)\,\mathrm{d}t = \frac{1}{\gamma + r}$ $(\theta > -\gamma)$. Substituting $\psi(\theta) = \frac{1}{\gamma+\theta}$ into (3.5.60) and rearranging shows that r satisfies a quadratic equation, which is readily solved.

3.5.23 First note that

$$g(s) = -\frac{1}{\log(1-p)} \sum_{k=1}^{\infty} \frac{p^k s^k}{k} = \frac{\log(1-ps)}{\log(1-p)} \qquad (|s| < p^{-1}). \tag{3.5.61}$$

Hence,

$$\mu_D = g'(1) = -\frac{p}{(1-p)\log(1-p)}$$

and

$$\mu_D^{-1}g'(s) = \frac{1-p}{1-ps} \qquad (|s| < p^{-1}). \tag{3.5.62}$$

Noting that $\mathbb{E}[s^{\tilde{D}-1}] = \mu_D^{-1}g'(s)$, we have

$$\mu_{\tilde{D}-1} = \mu_D^{-1}g''(1) = \frac{p}{1-p}.$$

Thus, in the notation of Section 3.5.5.3, $m_{GL} = -\frac{pp_L}{(1-p)\log(1-p)}$ and $m_{LL} = \frac{pp_L}{1-p}$, so $m_{LL} < 1$ if an only if $p_L < p^{-1} - 1$. Substitution into (3.5.24) then yields

$$R_* = \begin{cases} \lambda_G \mu_I \left(1 - \frac{pp_L}{(1-p-pp_L)\log(1-p)}\right) & \text{if } p_L < p^{-1} - 1, \\ \infty & \text{otherwise.} \end{cases}$$

Turning to $\hat{z}$, it follows from (3.5.29) on page 213 and (3.5.62) that, for $s \in [0,1]$, $\tilde{\psi}(s)$ is the unique solution in $(0,1]$ of

$$\tilde{\psi}(s) = \frac{s(1-p)}{1-p+pp_L - pp_L\tilde{\psi}(s)}. \tag{3.5.63}$$

Thus,

$$pp_L(\tilde{\psi}(s))^2 - (1-p+pp_L)\tilde{\psi}(s) + s(1-p) = 0, \tag{3.5.64}$$

whence

$$\tilde{\psi}(s) = \frac{1-p+pp_L - \sqrt{(1-p+pp_L)^2 - 4s(1-p)pp_L}}{2pp_L}. \tag{3.5.65}$$

(The other solution, $\hat{\psi}(s)$ say, of (3.5.64) does not belong to $(0,1]$, since $\hat{\psi}(s)$ is decreasing in s for $s \in [0,1]$ and $\hat{\psi}(1) > \tilde{\psi}(1) = 1$.)

Further, (3.5.63) implies that

$$1 - p(1 - p_L + p_L\tilde{\psi}(s) = \frac{s(1-p)}{\tilde{\psi}(s)},$$

so substituting (3.5.61) into (3.5.28) on page 213 yields

$$\psi(s) = \frac{s}{\log(1-p)}\left[\log s + \log(1-p) - \log\tilde{\psi}(s)\right].$$

An equation governing $\hat{z}$ follows using (3.5.30) on page 213 and (3.5.65).

References for Part II

1. C.L. Addy, I.M. Longini and M. Haber, A generalized stochastic model for the analysis of infectious disease final size data, *Biometrics* **47**, 961–974, 1991.
2. H. Andersson, Epidemics in a population with social structures, *Math. Biosci.* **140**, 79–84, 1997.
3. H. Andersson, Epidemic models and social networks, *Math. Scientist.* **24**, 128–147, 1999.
4. H. Andersson and T. Britton, *Stochastic Epidemic Models and Their Statistical Analysis – Lecture Notes in Statistics*, **151**, Springer-Verlag, New York, 2000.
5. S. Asmussen, *Applied Probability and Queues*, Wiley, 1987.
6. F.G. Ball, A unified approach to the distribution of total size and total area under the trajectory of infectives in epidemic models, *Adv. Appl. Prob.* **18**, 289–310, 1986.
7. F.G. Ball, Susceptibility sets and the final outcome of collective Reed–Frost epidemics, *Methodology Computing Appl. Prob.* **21**, 401–421, 2019.
8. F.G. Ball, T. Britton and O.D. Lyne, Stochastic multitype epidemics in a community of households: estimation and form of optimal vaccination schemes, *Math. Biosci.* **191**, 19–40, 2004.
9. F.G. Ball and P. Donnelly, Strong approximations for epidemic models, *Stoch. Proc. Appl.* **55**, 1–21, 1995.
10. F.G. Ball, E.S. Knock and P.D. O'Neill, Control of emerging infectious diseases using responsive imperfect vaccination and isolation, *Math. Biosci.* **216**, 100–113, 2008.
11. F.G. Ball and O.D. Lyne, Stochastic multitype SIR epidemics among a population partitioned into households, *Adv. Appl. Prob.* **33**, 99–123, 2001.
12. F.G. Ball and O.D. Lyne, Optimal vaccination policies for stochastic epidemics among a population of households, *Math. Biosci.* **177&178**, 333–354, 2002.
13. F.G. Ball and O.D. Lyne, Optimal vaccination schemes for epidemics among a population of households, with application to variola minor in Brazil, *Stat. Methods Med. Res.* **15**, 481–497, 2006.
14. F.G. Ball, D. Mollison and G. Scalia-Tomba, Epidemics with two levels of mixing, *Ann. Appl. Probab.* **7**, 46–89, 1997.
15. F.G. Ball and P.J. Neal, A general model for stochastic SIR epidemics with two levels of mixing, *Math. Biosci.* **180**, 73–102, 2002.
16. F.G. Ball and P.J. Neal, The great circle epidemic model, *Stoch. Proc. Appl.* **107**, 233–268, 2003.
17. F.G. Ball and P.J. Neal, Network epidemic models with two levels of mixing, *Math. Biosci.* **212**, 69–87, 2008.
18. F.G. Ball and P.D. O'Neill, The distribution of general final state random variables for stochastic epidemic models, *J. Appl. Prob.* **36**, 473–491, 1999.
19. F.G. Ball, L. Pellis and P. Trapman, Reproduction numbers for epidemic models with households and other social structures II: Comparisons and implications for vaccination, *Math. Biosci.* **274**, 108–139, 2016.
20. F.G. Ball and D.J. Sirl, Evaluation of vaccination strategies for SIR epidemics on random networks incorporating household structure, *J. Math. Biol.* **76**, 483–530, 2018.

21. F.G. Ball, D. Sirl and P. Trapman, Analysis of a stochastic SIR epidemic on a random network incorporating household structure, *Math. Biosci.* **224**, 53–73, 2010.
22. F.G. Ball, D. Sirl and P. Trapman, Epidemics on random intersection graphs, *Ann. Appl. Probab.* **24**, 1081–1128, 2014.
23. R. Bartoszyński, On a certain model of an epidemic, *Applicationes Mathematicae* **13**, 139–151, 1972.
24. N.G. Becker, T. Britton and P.D. O'Neill, Estimating vaccine effects from studies of outbreaks in household pairs, *Statist. Med.* **25**, 1079–1093, 2006.
25. N.G. Becker and K. Deitz, The effect of household distribution on transmission and control of highly infectious diseases, *Math. Biosci.* **127**, 207–219, 1995.
26. N.G. Becker, K. Glass, Z. Li and G.K. Aldis, Controlling emerging infectious diseases like SARS, *Math. Biosci.* **193**, 205–221, 2005.
27. N.G. Becker and D.N. Starczak, Optimal vaccination strategies for a community of households, *Math. Biosci.* **139**, 117–132, 1997.
28. N.G. Becker and D.N. Starczak, The effect of random vaccine response on the vaccination coverage required to prevent epidemics, *Math. Biosci.* **154**, 117–135, 1998.
29. T. Britton, S. Janson, and A. Martin-Löf, Graphs with specified degree distributions, simple epidemics, and local vaccination strategies, *Adv. Appl. Prob.* **39**, 922–948, 2007.
30. T. Britton and G. Scalia-Tomba, Estimation in emerging epidemics: biases and remedies, *J. R. Soc. Interface* **16**, 20180670, 2019.
31. O. Diekmann, M.C.M. de Jong and J.A.J. Metz, A deterministic epidemic model taking account of repeated contacts between the same individuals, *J. Appl. Prob.* **35**, 448–462, 1998.
32. R. Durrett, *Random Graph Dynamics*, Cambridge, 2007.
33. C. Fraser, Estimating individual and household reproduction numbers in an emerging epidemic, *PLoS One* **2**, e758, 2007.
34. E. Goldstein, K. Paur, C. Fraser, E. Kenah, J. Wallinga and M. Lipsitch, Reproductive numbers, epidemic spread and control in a community of households, *Math. Biosci.* **221**, 11–25, 2009.
35. W. Gontcharoff, *Détermination des Fonctions Entières par Interpolation*, Hermann, Paris, 1937.
36. G. Grimmett and D. Stirzaker, *Probability and Random Processes*, Oxford, 1992.
37. P. Haccou, P. Jagers and V.A. Vatutin, *Branching Processes: Variation, Growth and Extinction of Populations*, Cambridge, 2005.
38. M.E. Halloran, M. Haber and I.M. Longini, Jr., Interpretation and estimation of vaccine efficacy under heterogeneity, *Am. J. Epidemiology* **136**, 328–343, 1992.
39. J.A.P. Heesterbeek, A brief history of R_0 and a recipe for its calculation, *Acta Biotheoretica* **50**, 189–204, 2002.
40. J.A.P. Heesterbeek and K. Dietz, The concept of R_0 in epidemic theory, *Statistica Neerlandica* **50**, 89–110, 1996.
41. T. House, J.V. Ross and D. Sirl, How big is an outbreak likely to be? Methods for epidemic final-size calculation, *Proc. R. Soc. Lond. A* **469**, 20120436, 2013.
42. P. Jagers, *Branching Processes with Biological Applications*, Wiley, 1975.
43. P. Jagers, General branching processes as Markov fields, *Stoch. Proc. Appl.* **32**, 183–212, 1989.
44. M. Keeling and J.V. Ross, Optimal prophylactic vaccination in segregated populations: When can we improve on the equalising strategy?, *Epidemics* **11**, 7–13, 2015.
45. I. Kiss, D. Green and R. Kao, The effect of contact heterogeniety and multiple routes of transmission on final epidemic size, *Math. Biosci.* **203**, 124–136, 2006.
46. C. Lefèvre and P. Picard, A non-standard family of polynomials and the final size distribution of Reed–Frost epidemic processes, *Adv. Appl. Prob.* **22**, 25–48, 1990.
47. C. Lefèvre and P. Picard, *Collective epidemic processes: A general modelling approach to the final outcome of SIR infectious diseases*, In *Epidemic Models: their Structure and Relation to Data*, D. Mollison (ed.), Cambridge Univerity Press, pp. 53–70, 1995.
48. A.L. Lloyd, Realistic distributions of infectious periods in epidemic models: Changing patterns of persistence and dynamics, *Theor. Pop. Biol.* **60**, 59–71, 2001.
49. A. Martin-Löf, Symmetric sampling procedures, general epidemic processes and their threshold limit theorems, *J. Appl. Prob.* **23**, 265–282, 1986.

50. M. Molloy and B. Reed, A critical point for random graphs with a given degree sequence, *Rand. Struct. Algor.* **6**, 161–180, 1995.
51. P.J. Neal, *Epidemics with two levels of mixing*, PhD Thesis, University of Nottingham, 2001.
52. M.E.J. Newman, S.H. Strogatz and D.J. Watts, Random graphs with arbitrary degree distributions and their applications, *Phys. Rev. E* **64**, 026118, 2001.
53. M.A. Nowak, A.L. Lloyd, G.M. Vasquez, T.A. Wiltrout, L.M. Wahl, N. Bischofberger, J. Williams, A. Kinter, A.S. Fauci, V.M. Hirsch and J.D. Lifson, Viral dynamics of primary viremia and antiretroviral therapy in simian immunodeficiency virus infection, *J. Virol.* **71**, 7518–7525, 1997.
54. L. Pellis, F. Ball and P. Trapman, Reproduction numbers for epidemic models with households and other social structures. I. Definition and calculation of R_0, *Math. Biosci.* **235**, 85–97, 2012.
55. L. Pellis, N. Ferguson and C. Fraser, Threshold parameters for a model of epidemic spread among households and workplaces, *J. R. Soc. Interface* **6**, 979–987, 2009.
56. L. Pellis, N. Ferguson, C. Fraser, Epidemic growth rate and household reproduction number in communities of households, schools and workplaces, *J. Math. Biol.* **63**, 691–734, 2011.
57. P. Picard and C. Lefèvre, A unified analysis of the final size and severity distribution in collective Reed–Frost epidemic processes, *Adv. Appl. Prob.* **22**, 269–294, 1990.
58. M.G. Roberts and J.A.P. Heesterbeek, Model-consistent estimation of the basic reproduction number from the incidence of an emerging infection, *J. Math. Biol.* **55**, 803–816, 2007.
59. S.M. Ross, *Stochastic Processes*, Wiley, 1983.
60. G. Scalia-Tomba, Asymptotic final-size distribution for some chain-binomial processes, *Adv. Appl. Prob.* **17**, 477–495, 1985.
61. G. Scalia-Tomba, *On the asymptotic final size distribution of epidemics in heterogeneous populations*, In *Stochastic Processes in Epidemic Theory*, J.-P. Gabriel, C. Lefèvre and P. Picard (eds.), *Lecture Notes in Biomath.* **86**, 189–196. Springer, Berlin, 1990.
62. T. Sellke, On the asymptotic distribution of the size of a stochastic epidemic, *J. Appl. Prob.* **20**, 390–394, 1983.
63. P. Trapman, F.G. Ball, J.-S. Dhersin, V.C. Tran, J. Wallinga and T. Britton, Inferring R_0 in emerging epidemics—the effect of common population structure is small, *J. R. Soc. Interface* **13**, 20160288, 2016.
64. J. Wallinga and M. Lipsitch, How generation intervals shape the relationship between growth rates and reproductive numbers, *Proc. R. Soc. Lond. B* **274**, 599–604, 2007.
65. D.J. Watts and S.H. Strogatz, Collective dynamics of 'small-world' networks, *Nature* **393**, 440–442, 1998.
66. P. Whittle, The outcome of a stochastic epidemic—A note on Bailey's paper, *Biometrika* **42**, 116–122, 1995.

Part III
Stochastic Epidemics in a Heterogeneous Community

Viet Chi Tran

Viet Chi Tran, Marne la Vallée
e-mail: chi.tran@u-pem.fr

Introduction

Recently, network concepts have received much attention in infectious disease modelling, essentially for modeling purposes, and the reader is also referred to earlier references of Durrett [49], Newman [88], House [61] or Kiss et al. [70]. In the compartmental models presented in Part I of this volume, any infected individual can contaminate any susceptible individuals. In many public health problems, heterogeneity issues have to be taken into account, in particular some diseases such as AIDS or HCV (Hepatitis C Virus) may spread only along a social network: the network of people having sexual intercourse or of injecting drug partners. The need to take into account the network along which an epidemic spreads has been underlined by numerous papers, starting for example from [43, 50], and more recently [18, 61].

After introducing random networks and describing how the spread of disease can be modelled on such structures, we explain how to approximate the dynamics by deterministic differential equations when the graphs are large. Mathematical models for epidemics on large networks are obtained by mean-field approximation (e.g. [49, 71, 91]) or through large population approximations (e.g. [13, 44, 58, 19, 65]). They generally stipulate simple structures for the network: small worlds (e.g. [71, 81]), configuration models (e.g. [69, 75, 93, 110, 111]), random intersection graphs and graphs with overlapping communities (e.g. [27, 16, 40])...

In the last section, real data from the AIDS epidemic in Cuba is studied (data from [35] and that can be found in supplementary materials of this book). We show how to conduct descriptive statistical procedures. By performing clustering and simplification of the graph, we decompose it into smaller clusters where the probabilistic models of the previous sections can be used.

Notation 0.0.1. In this part, we denote by $\mathbb{N}$ the set of strictly positive integers and by $\mathbb{Z}_+$ the set $\mathbb{N} \cup \{0\}$.
For any real bounded function f on $\mathbb{Z}_+$, let $\|f\|_\infty$ denote the supremum of f on $\mathbb{Z}_+$. For all such f and $y \in \mathbb{Z}_+$, we denote by $\tau_y f$ the function $x \mapsto f(x-y)$. For all $n \in \mathbb{Z}_+$, χ^n is the function $x \mapsto x^n$, and in particular, $\chi \equiv \chi^1$ is the identity function, and $\mathbf{1} \equiv \chi^0$ is the function constant equal to 1.

We denote by $\mathscr{M}_F(\mathbb{Z}_+)$ the set of finite measures on $\mathbb{Z}_+$, equipped with the topology of weak convergence. For all $\mu \in \mathscr{M}_F(\mathbb{Z}_+)$ and real bounded function f on $\mathbb{Z}_+$, we write

$$\langle \mu, f \rangle = \sum_{k \in \mathbb{Z}_+} f(k)\,\mu(k), \tag{0.0.66}$$

where we use the notation $\mu(k) = \mu(\{k\})$.
For $k \in \mathbb{Z}_+$, we write δ_k for the Dirac measure at k. In particular, for any test function f from $\mathbb{Z}_+$ to $\mathbb{R}$, $\langle \delta_k, f \rangle = f(k)$.
For a sequence $D_1, \ldots D_n \in \mathbb{Z}_+$, if $\mu = \sum_{k=1}^n \delta_{D_k}$, then

$$\langle \mu, f \rangle = \sum_{k=1}^{n} f(D_k),$$

implying in particular that $\langle \mu, 1 \rangle = n$ and $\langle \mu, \chi \rangle = \sum_{k=1}^n D_k$.

Chapter 1
Random Graphs

1.1 Definitions

Usually, social networks on which disease spread are very complex. It is thus convenient to model them by *random* networks. We start with some definitions, and then present some common families of random networks. There is a growing literature on random networks to which we refer the reader for further developments (e.g. [25, 109]).

Definition 1.1.1. A random graph $\mathscr{G} = (V, E)$ is a set of vertices V and a set of edges $E \subset V \times V$. If u, $v \in V$ are connected in the random graph, then $(u, v) \in E$.

The set of vertices of $\mathscr{G}$ is V, but when we will need to make precise that it is the set of vertices of $\mathscr{G}$, we will use the notation $V(\mathscr{G})$. The population size is $|V| = N$. In the sequel, we will label the vertices with integers, so that $V = \{1, \dots N\}$.

Definition 1.1.2. The adjacency matrix of the graph $\mathscr{G}$ is a matrix $G \in \mathscr{M}_{V \times V}(\mathbb{R})$ such that $\forall u, v \in V$,

$$G_{uv} = 1 \text{ if } (u, v) \in E,$$
$$G_{uv} = 0 \text{ if } (u, v) \notin E.$$

If the matrix is symmetric, the graph in undirected: to any edge from u to v corresponds an edge from v to u. Else, if $(u, v) \in E$ and $(v, u) \notin E$, the graph is oriented with only the directed edge from u to v belonging to E. We say that u is the *ego* and v the *alter* of the edge.
If we consider weighted graphs, we can generalize the entries of G to real non-negative numbers.

In this chapter, we will focus on undirected non-weighted graphs.

T. Britton, E. Pardoux (eds.), *Stochastic Epidemic Models with Inference*,
Lecture Notes in Mathematics 2255, https://doi.org/10.1007/978-3-030-30900-8_8

Definition 1.1.3. The degree of a vertex $u \in V$ in the graph $\mathscr{G}$ is

$$D_u = \sum_{v \in V} G_{uv}.$$

D_u hence corresponds to the number of neighbours of the vertex u, i.e. the number of the vertices of $\mathscr{G}$ that can be reached in one step starting from u.
If the graph is oriented, the above notion corresponds to the out-degree, and similarly we can define as in-degree the number of vertices of $\mathscr{G}$ that lead to u in one step:

$$D_u^{\text{in}} = \sum_{v \in V} G_{vu}.$$

For undirected graphs, the out and in-degrees coincide.

Definition 1.1.4. The degree distribution of a finite graph $\mathscr{G}$ is:

$$\frac{1}{N} \sum_{u \in V} \delta_{D_u} = \sum_{d \in \mathbb{Z}_+} \frac{\text{Card}\{u \in V : D_u = d\}}{N} \delta_d.$$

For $d \in \mathbb{Z}_+$, $\text{Card}\{u \in V : D_u = d\}/N$ is the proportion of vertices with degree d.

We see that the notion of degree distribution can be generalized to graphs with infinitely many vertices: the degree distribution is a probability measure on $\mathbb{Z}_+$, $\sum_{d \in \mathbb{Z}_+} p_d \delta_d$, where the weight p_d of the atom $d \in \mathbb{Z}_+$ is the proportion of vertices with degree d.

Let us consider the product of the matrix G with itself: $G^2 = G \times G$. Notice that

$$G^2_{uv} = \sum_{w \in V} G_{uw} G_{wv},$$

and thus, $G^2_{uv} > 0$ if there is a path consisting of two edges of G that links u and v. More precisely, G^2_{uv} counts the number of paths of length exactly 2 that link u and v. Generalizing this definition, and with the convention that $G^0 = \text{Id}$ the identity matrix of $\mathbb{R}^N$, we obtain that:

Definition 1.1.5. Two vertices u and v of the graph $\mathscr{G}$ are connected if there is a path in $\mathscr{G}$ going from u to v, i.e. if there exists some integer $n \geq 1$ such that $G^n_{uv} > 0$. We can then define the graph distance between u and v by:

$$d_G(u,v) = \inf\{n \geq 0,\ G^n_{uv} > 0\}. \tag{1.1.1}$$

By convention, $\inf \emptyset = +\infty$.
For $r \geq 0$, we define by $B_G(u,r)$ the ball of $\mathscr{G}$ with center u and radius r for the graph distance:

$$B_G(u,r) = \big\{v \in V : d_G(u,v) \leq r\big\}.$$

Several important descriptors of the graph depend on this graph distance. We remark for instance that $D_u = \text{Card}(B_G(u,1)) - 1$. Also, we can define a shortest path (for the graph distance) between two vertices u and v. The diameter of the graph is:

$$\mathrm{diam}(\mathscr{G}) = \sup\{d_G(u,v) : u,v \in V\}.$$

Definition 1.1.6. For a vertex u in a graph $\mathscr{G}$, we denote by $\mathscr{C}(u)$ the connected component of u, i.e. the set of vertices $v \in V$ that are connected to u:

$$\mathscr{C}(u) = \big\{v \in V : d_G(u,v) < +\infty\big\}.$$

1.2 Classical Examples of Random Graphs

Random graphs, especially those arising from applications, can have very complex distributions and topologies. There are some simple families of random graphs. We now present the complete graph, the Erdös–Rényi graphs, the stochastic block model, the configuration model and the household model.

Definition 1.2.1 (Complete graph). The complete graph K_N is the graph where all the pairs of vertices are linked by an edge, i.e. $E = V \times V$.

The complete graph is in fact a deterministic graph, and $\forall u,v \in V(K_N)$, $d_G(u,v) = 1$ if $u \neq v$.

Definition 1.2.2 (Erdös–Rényi random graph (ER)). Erdös–Rényi random graphs are undirected graphs where each pair of vertices $(u,v) \in V^2$ is linked by an edge with probability $p \in [0,1]$ independently from the other pairs.
The distribution $\mathrm{ER}(N,p)$ of Erdös–Rényi random graphs is completely defined by the family $(G_{uv};\ u,v \in V,\ u < v)$ of i.i.d. random variables with Bernoulli distribution $\mathrm{Ber}(p)$, $p \in [0,1]$.

Notice that for $p = 1$, the Erdös–Rényi graph corresponds to the complete graph K_N.

These graphs can be generalized if we introduce a partition of the population according to a discrete type, taking K values, say $\{1,\dots,K\}$: to each vertex $u \in V$ is associated a type $k_u \in \{1,\dots K\}$. This corresponds to cases where a community contains different types of individuals that display specific roles in contact behaviour. Types might be related to age-groups, social behaviour or occupation.

Definition 1.2.3 (Stochastic block model graph (SBM)). A stochastic block model graph is a undirected graph, where each vertex is given a type independently from the others, all with the same probability, and where each pair of vertices is linked independently of the other pairs with a probability depending on the types of the vertices. If there are K types, say $\{1,\dots K\}$, we will denote by $(\rho_i)_{i\in\{1,\dots K\}}$ the probability distribution of the types, and by π_{ij} the probability of linking a vertex of type i with a vertex of type j.

If there is just one type of vertex ($K = 1$), the SBM resumes to ER graphs. For $K = 2$ where vertices of the same type cannot be connected ($\pi_{11} = \pi_{22} = 0$), we obtain *bipartite* graphs. For instance, sexual networks in heterosexual populations are bipartite networks. The interested reader is referred to the review of Abbe [1].

Proposition 1.2.4. *The degree distribution of a vertex u in an* $\mathrm{ER}(N,p)$ *random graph with N vertices and connection probability p is a binomial distribution* $\mathrm{Bin}(N,p)$. *When the connection probability is λ/N, with $\lambda > 0$, then for any integer $d \geq 0$,*

$$\lim_{N\to+\infty} \mathbb{P}_N(D_u = d) = \frac{\lambda^d}{d!}e^{-\lambda},$$

showing that the probability distribution converges to a Poisson distribution with expectation λ.

The proof of this result is easy and let to the reader.

A detailed presentation and study of Erdös–Rényi graphs and their limits when $N \to +\infty$ can be found in [109] for example. In particular, the case where the connection probability is λ/N, is carefully discussed. The case $\lambda > 1$ is termed the supercritical case, while the case $\lambda < 1$ is the subcritical case.

Proposition 1.2.4 emphasizes the importance of graphs defined from their degree distributions. The next class of graphs has been introduced by Bollobas [25] and Molloy and Reed [79]. The reader is referred to Durrett [49] and van der Hofstad [109] for more details.

Definition 1.2.5 (Configuration model graph (CM)). Let $\mathbf{p} = (p_k,\ k \in \mathbb{Z}_+)$ be a probability distribution on $\mathbb{Z}_+$. The Bollobás–Molloy–Reed or Configuration model random graph with vertices V is constructed as follows. We associate with each vertex $u \in V$ an independent random variable X_u drawn from the distribution $\mathbf{p}$, that corresponds to the number of half edges attached to u. Conditionally on $\{\sum_{u\in V} X_u \text{ even}\}$, the Configuration model random graph is a multigraph (a graph with possibly self-loops and multiple edges) obtained by pairing the half-edges uniformly at random.

A possible algorithm for pairing the half edges (also called stubs) is the following:

- Associate with each half edge an independent uniform random variable on $[0,1]$ and sort the half-edges by decreasing values.
- Pair each odd stub with the following even stub. Note that if the number of stubs $\sum_{u\in V} X_u$ is odd, it is possible to add or remove one stub arbitrarily.

Note that this linkage procedure does not exclude self-loops or multiple edges. When the size of the graph $N \to +\infty$ with a fixed degree distribution, self-loops and multiple edges become less and less apparent in the global picture (see e.g. [49, Theorem 3.1.2]).

In [109], it is carefully studied how one can turn a multigraph into a simple graph (without self-loop nor multi-edge), either by erasing self-loops and merging multi-edges, or by conditioning on obtaining a simple graph. Note that in this respect, a Configuration model with a Binomial distribution $\mathscr{B}(N, p/N)$ looks like an Erdös–Rényi graph with multiple-edges and self-loops.

Because of this construction, we see that in such a network, given an edge of ego u, the alter v is chosen proportionally to his/her number of half-edges (i.e. his/her degree). Thus, the following degree distribution $\mathbf{q} = (q_k, k \in \mathbb{Z}_+)$ defined as the size-biased degree distribution of $\mathbf{p}$ will play a major role in the understanding of disease dynamics on CM graphs:

$$q_k = \frac{k p_k}{\sum_{\ell \in \mathbb{Z}_+} \ell p_\ell}. \tag{1.2.1}$$

Example 1.2.6. Particular graphs of this family include the regular graphs, where all the vertices have the same degree d (that is $p_d = 1$ and $\forall k \neq d, p_k = 0$) and the graphs whose degree distribution is a power law: for some $\alpha > 1$,

$$p_k \overset{k \to +\infty}{\sim} k^{-\alpha}.$$

A key quantity when dealing with configuration models is the generating function of its degree distribution, defined as:

$$g(z) = \sum_{k \geq 0} z^k p_k = \mathbb{E}_{\mathbf{p}}\big(z^D\big), \tag{1.2.2}$$

where the notation in the right-hand side recalls that the random variable D has distribution $\mathbf{p}$.
In case it exists, the moment of order q of the degree distribution can be written by means of the generating function:

$$\forall q \geq 0,\ \mathbb{E}_{\mathbf{p}}\big(D^q\big) = g^{(q)}(1).$$

Example 1.2.7. Let us recall the probability generating function of some usual parametric distributions:

(i) For a Poisson distribution with parameter α: $g(z) = e^{\alpha(z-1)}$.
(ii) For a Geometric distribution with parameter ρ: $g(z) = \frac{\rho z}{1 - z(1-\rho)}$.
(iii) For a Binomial with parameters (n, ρ): $g(z) = (z\rho + 1 - \rho)^n$.

Assumption 1.2.8. Let us assume that $\mathbf{p} = (p_k, k \in \mathbb{Z}_+)$ admits a second order moment:

$$m = g'(1) = \sum_{k \in \mathbb{Z}_+} k p_k, \qquad \sigma^2 = g''(1) + g'(1) - (g'(1))^2 = \sum_{k \in \mathbb{Z}_+} (k - m)^2 p_k.$$

Notice that under Assumptions 1.2.8, the size-biased degree distribution $\mathbf{q}$ defined in (1.2.1) admits a moment of order 1, which is referred to as the mean excess degree:

$$\kappa = \sum_{k\geq 0} \frac{k(k-1)p_k}{m} = \frac{\sigma^2}{m} + m - 1 = \frac{g''(1)}{g'(1)}. \tag{1.2.3}$$

The household models (see Part II of the present volume) can be built on the previous graph models. They were first analysed in detail in [12] and we also refer to Chapter 2 in Part II of this volume. They account for several levels of mixing, for instance local and global in case of 2 levels. In the latter case, the population is partitioned into clusters or households. A first possible approach is to consider a graph model on the entire population (for example a CM in [12, 13, 16]) on which the household structure is superposed independently. The links are considered stronger between individuals of the same household (for example they can transmit diseases at higher rates). Another possibility is to define the graph between individuals by taking into account the household structure, which results into clustering effects.

Definition 1.2.9 (Household models). A graph belong to the family of Household model if it is an SBM where the types are the households.

Each household can be viewed as a vertex in a graph describing the global connections, while the intra-group connections between individuals of the same group are described by a local graph model.
How clustering affects epidemics using household models has for example been studied by [9, 39].

Let us also mention other families of random graphs: for example, the exponential random graphs, which are defined by their Radon–Nikodym densities. We refer to [31] for developments.

Definition 1.2.10 (Exponential random graph model (ERGM)). A random graph belongs to the family of exponential random graphs if its distribution is of the following form. For a positive integer K, for a vector of parameters $\theta = (\theta_1, \ldots \theta_K) \in \mathbb{R}^K$ and for a vector of statistics $(T_1, \ldots T_K)$ of the graph, we have for any deterministic graph g:

$$\mathbb{P}_\theta\big(G = g\big) = \exp\Big(\sum_{k=1}^{K} \theta_k T_k(g) - c(\theta)\Big).$$

The renormalizing constant $c(\theta)$ is also called partition function in statistical mechanics.

Examples of statistics T_k are the number of edges, the degrees of vertices, the number of triangles or other patterns. In Rolls et al. [100], ERGMs are for example used to estimate parameters describing the social networks of people who inject drugs in Australia. This has inspired a similar study for the French case, see [41].

1.3 Sequences of Graphs

Let us consider a sequence of graphs $(\mathscr{G}_N)_{N\geq 1}$, such that for all $N \geq 1$, $\mathrm{Card}(V(\mathscr{G}_N)) = N$.

For a given graph $\mathscr{G}$ and for an integer $j \geq 1$, let us denote by $\mathscr{C}_{(j)}(\mathscr{G})$ the jth largest connected component of $\mathscr{G}$.

Definition 1.3.1 (Giant component). Consider a sequence of graphs $(\mathscr{G}_N)_{N\geq 1}$ such that for all $N \geq 1$, $\mathrm{Card}(V(\mathscr{G}_N)) = N$. If

$$\liminf_{N\to+\infty} \frac{\mathrm{Card}\big(V(\mathscr{C}_{(1)}(\mathscr{G}_N))\big)}{N} > 0,$$

then we say that the sequence $(\mathscr{G}_N)_{N\geq 1}$ is highly connected and that the graph $\mathscr{G}_N$ admits a giant component, $\mathscr{C}_{(1)}(\mathscr{G}_N)$.

For $\mathrm{ER}(N,p)$ in the supercritical regime (with $Np > 1$), there exists a giant component [109, Theorem 4.8]. So does it for the CM, as shown by Molloy and Reed [79, 80]. The condition for the existence with positive probability of a giant component in CM graphs is that the expectation of the size biased distribution minus 1, κ, is larger than 1:

$$\kappa := \sum_{k\in\mathbb{Z}_+} (k-1)\frac{kp_k}{\sum_{\ell\in\mathbb{Z}_+} \ell p_\ell} = \mathbb{E}_{\mathbf{q}}(D-1) > 1.$$

This is connected with results on the super-criticality of Galton–Watson trees (see [49, Section 3.2 p. 75] for example). Heuristically, a CM graph looks like a tree locally, and a vertex of degree k of the graph corresponds in the tree to a node with 1 parent and $k-1$ offspring. From the construction of the CM graphs given after Definition 1.2.5, the degrees of the vertices encountered along the CM graph are given by the size-biased distribution.

If $\mathrm{Card}\big(V(\mathscr{C}_{(2)}(\mathscr{G}_N))\big) = o(N)$, then the giant component $\mathscr{C}_{(1)}(\mathscr{G}_N)$ is said to be unique. In many models such as ER, it is shown that the second largest component is of order $\log N$ (see [109, Corollary 4.13]).

The notion of being 'highly connected', as introduced in Definition 1.3.1, can also be extended.

Definition 1.3.2 (Sequence of dense graphs). We say that the graph sequence $(\mathscr{G}_N)_{N\geq 1}$ is a sequence of dense graphs if:

$$\liminf_{N\to+\infty} \frac{\mathrm{Card}\big(E(\mathscr{G}_N)\big)}{N^2} > 0.$$

Of course, the next important notion is the notion of convergence of a sequence of graphs $(\mathscr{G}_N)_{N\geq 1}$. The topologies and notions of convergence depend on the order of the edge numbers. For graphs that are not dense, such as tree-like graphs, a large literature around the Hausdorff-Gromov topology has developed and we refer for instance to Addario-Berry et al. [2, 3]. When the graph is dense, the topology is inspired by ideas coming from the topologies of measure spaces (see Borgs et al. [26] or Lovasz and Szegedy [73]).

1.4 Definition of the SIR Model on a Random Graph

We now describe the spread of infectious diseases on graphs. We consider a population of size N whose individuals are the vertices of a random graph $\mathscr{G}_N$. As in compartmental models, the population is partitioned into three classes that can change in time: susceptible individuals who can contract the disease (individuals of type S), infectious individuals who transmit the disease (type I) and removed individuals who were previously infectious and can not transmit the disease any more (type R). The corresponding sets of vertices, at time t, are respectively denoted by S_t, I_t and R_t, and the corresponding sizes by S_t, I_t and R_t.

On the graph $\mathscr{G}_N$, the dynamics is as follows. To each I individual is associated an exponential random clock with rate γ to determine its removal. To each edge with an infectious ego and a susceptible alter, we associate a random exponential clock with rate λ. When it rings, the edge transmits the disease and the susceptible alter becomes infectious.

Example 1.4.1 (Compartmental models). When the graph $\mathscr{G}_N = K_N$ is the complete graph, we recover the compartmental model of Part I of this volume.

Example 1.4.2 (Household models). The above mechanisms can of course be generalized. For household models [13, 16], for example, the infection probability λ depends on whether ego and alter belong or not to the same household. See Part II of this volume.

Notice also that for modelling real data, several studies require to take into account the dynamics of the social network itself (e.g. [51, 111]). For sexual network, for instance, accounting for the changes of sexual partners (contacts) is important (e.g. [72, 82, 103]). Also, the epidemics itself can act on the structure of the network (see [68]), such as the changes of sexual behaviour due to the spread of the AIDS epidemic (e.g. [74]). These aspects are however not treated here.

Chapter 2
The Reproduction Number R_0

We consider the early stage of the epidemics. Let us consider a single first infective of degree d_1 in a population of large size N.

For this, we proceed as in Section 1.2 of Part I of this volume and couple the process $(I_t)_{t\geq 0}$ with a branching process. As for the mixing case, it is more precisely a stochastic domination. The coupling remains exact as long as no infected or removed individual is contaminated for the second time, in which case the branching process creates an extra individual, who is named 'ghost'.

Definition 2.0.1 **(R_0).** The basic reproduction number of the epidemic, denoted by R_0, is the mean offspring number of the branching process approximating the infectious population in early stages.
If we denote by $\beta(t)$ the birth rate at time $t > 0$ in this branching process, then:

$$R_0 = \int_0^{\infty} \beta(t)dt. \tag{2.0.1}$$

Notice that in the above definition, the measure $\beta(t)dt$ represents the intensity measure of the point process describing the occurrence of new infections due to a chosen infective (e.g. [64]).

A large literature is devoted to this indicator R_0 and extensions. Recall indeed that the nature and importance of the disease is usually classified according to whether $R_0 > 1$ or $R_0 \leq 1$.
When $R_0 > 1$, the branching process is super-critical and with positive probability its size is infinite, in which case we say that there is a major outbreak of the disease. The probability for this to happen can be computed [47, Eq. 3.10] and is less than 1. When the branching process does not get extinct, its size grows roughly proportional to $e^{\alpha t}$, where α is termed the (initial) epidemic growth rate (see [64]). In this case, the positive constant α depends on the parameters of the model through the equation

$$1 = \int_0^{\infty} e^{-\alpha t}\beta(t)dt. \tag{2.0.2}$$

T. Britton, E. Pardoux (eds.), *Stochastic Epidemic Models with Inference*,
Lecture Notes in Mathematics 2255, https://doi.org/10.1007/978-3-030-30900-8_9

When $R_0 \leq 1$, the branching process is critical or subcritical and its size is almost surely finite. Then, the total number of individuals who have been infected when the epidemic stops (at the time t when $I_t = 0$) is upper bounded by an almost surely finite random variable with distribution independent of the total population size N, and we talk of a small epidemic. We refer to [7, 107] for reviews.

2.1 Homogeneous Mixing

In the case where $\mathscr{G}_N = K_N$ is the complete graph, as stated in Part I of this volume, many results for epidemics in large homogeneous mixing populations can be obtained since the initial phase of the epidemic is well approximated by a branching process (see e.g. [11]).

Proposition 2.1.1 (R_0 for homogeneous mixing). *The reproduction number is given by:*

$$R_0 = \frac{\lambda}{\gamma}.$$

In the case where $\lambda > \gamma$, then $\alpha = \lambda - \gamma$ and

$$R_0 = \frac{\lambda}{\gamma} = 1 + \frac{\alpha}{\gamma}.$$

Notice that the second expression of R_0 does not depend on λ, which is sometimes complicated to estimate, especially at the beginning of an epidemic, but only on the removal rate γ, that is usually documented, and on the Malthusian parameter α, that can be estimated from the dynamics of the emerging epidemics.

Proof. The reproduction number R_0 for the homogeneous mixing case has already been studied in Part I of this volume, but let us give here another proof of the proposition using (2.0.1). In this case, $\beta(t) = \lambda e^{-\gamma t}$. This can be understood by observing that λ is the rate at which an infected individual makes contacts if he or she is still infectious, while $e^{-\gamma t}$ is the probability that the individual is still infectious t time units after he or she became infected. Then, (2.0.2) and (2.0.1) translate to

$$1 = \frac{\lambda}{\gamma + \alpha} \quad \text{and} \quad R_0 = \frac{\lambda}{\gamma} = 1 + \frac{\alpha}{\gamma}. \tag{2.1.1}$$

This completes the proof. □

2.2 Configuration Model

Assume that $\mathscr{G}_N$ is a configuration model graph whose degree distribution $\mathbf{p}$ admits a mean μ and a variance σ^2. Recall also the definition of the size-biased distribution $\mathbf{q}$ in (1.2.1), and of the mean excess degree κ in (1.2.3). The mean excess degree

κ, is in the context of SIR epidemics spreading on graphs, the mean number of susceptibles that are contaminated by a typical infective (other than his or her own infector).

Let us consider the following continuous time birth-death process $(X_t)_{t\geq 0}$. Individuals live during exponential independent times with expectation $1/\gamma$. To each individual is associated a maximal number of offspring $k-1$, where k (the 'degree' of the individual) is drawn in the size-biased distribution $\mathbf{q}$. We associate to such an individual $k-1$ independent exponential random variables with expectations $1/\lambda$. The ages at which the individual gives birth are the exponential random variables that are smaller than the lifetime of the individual. There is an intuitive coupling between $(X_t)_{t\geq 0}$ and $(I_t)_{t\geq 0}$ such as $X_t \geq I_t$ for every t, with the equality as long as no 'ghost' has appeared.
We can associate with the process $(X_t)_{t\geq 0}$ its discrete-time skeleton (time counting the generations) that is a Galton–Watson process $(Z_n)_{n\geq 0}$ ($Z_0 = 1$). Conditionally on the degree k and the fact that the chosen individual remains infectious for a duration y, the number of contacts contaminated by this individual follows a binomial distribution with parameters $k-1$ and $1-e^{-\lambda y}$. Summing over k and integrating with respect to y, we can write the probability that in this Galton–Watson process an individual of generation $n \geq 1$ has $\nu = \ell$ offspring:

$$\mathbb{P}(\nu = \ell) = \sum_{k=\ell+1}^{+\infty} \frac{kp_k}{m} \binom{k-1}{\ell} \Big(\frac{\lambda}{\lambda+\gamma}\Big)^{\ell} \Big(\frac{\gamma}{\lambda+\gamma}\Big)^{k-1-\ell}.$$

Proposition 2.2.1 (R_0 for CM). *Recall the definition of the mean excess degree κ in* (1.2.3)*. We have:*

$$R_0 = \frac{\kappa\lambda}{\lambda+\gamma}. \tag{2.2.1}$$

In the super-critical case, R_0 can also be rewritten as

$$R_0 = \frac{\gamma+\alpha}{\gamma+\alpha/\kappa} = 1 + \frac{\alpha}{\lambda+\gamma}.$$

Proof. With the description of the process $(Z_n)_{n\geq 1}$:

$$\begin{aligned} R_0 =& \sum_{k\geq 0} \frac{kp_k}{m} \int_0^{+\infty} (k-1)(1-e^{-\lambda y})\, \gamma e^{-\gamma y} dy \\ =& \sum_{k\geq 0} (k-1) \frac{kp_k}{\mu} \frac{\lambda}{\lambda+\gamma} \\ =& \Big(\frac{g''(1)}{g'(1)} - 1\Big) \frac{\lambda}{\lambda+\gamma} \\ =& \frac{\kappa\lambda}{\lambda+\gamma}. \end{aligned}$$

We obtain

$$\beta(t) = \kappa\lambda e^{-(\lambda+\gamma)t}.$$

This can be seen by noting that κ is the expected number of susceptible acquaintances a typical newly infected individual has in the early stages of the epidemic, while $e^{-\lambda t}$ is the probability that a given susceptible individual is not contacted by the infective over a period of t time units, and $e^{-\gamma t}$ is the probability that the infectious individual is still infectious t time units after he or she became infected. From (2.0.2), we obtain that

$$\alpha = \kappa\lambda - \lambda - \gamma,$$

from which we conclude the proof. □

Example 2.2.2. Let us compute R_0 for particular choices of degree distribution $\mathbf{p}$:
(i) For a Poisson distribution with parameter $a > 0$,

$$R_0 = \frac{a\lambda}{\lambda+\gamma}.$$

Thus, $R_0 > 1$ if and only if $a > 1 + \gamma/\lambda$.
(ii) For a Geometric distribution with parameter $a \in (0,1)$, $R_0 = \frac{\lambda}{\lambda+\gamma}\frac{2(1-a)}{a}$. Thus, $R_0 > 1$ if and only if $a < 2\lambda/(3\lambda+\gamma)$. □

We can now connect the considerations on the skeleton with the epidemic in continuous time.

Proposition 2.2.3. *Let us consider the continuous time birth-death process* $(X_t)_{t\geq 0}$.

(i) If $R_0 \leq 1$, *the process* $(X_t)_{t\geq 0}$ *dies out almost surely.*

(ii) If $R_0 > 1$, *the process* $(X_t)_{t\geq 0}$ *dies with a probability* $z \in (0,1)$ *that is the smallest solution of*

$$z = \frac{\gamma}{g'(1)} \int_{\mathbb{R}_+} g'\big(z + e^{-\lambda y}(1-z)\big) e^{-\gamma y} dy. \tag{2.2.2}$$

(iii) Let us define the times $\tau_0 = \inf\{t \geq 0 \mid X_t = 0\}$ *and* $\tau_{\varepsilon n} = \inf\{t \geq 0 \mid X_t \geq \varepsilon n\}$. *If* $R_0 > 1$, *then for all sequence* $(t_n)_{n\in\mathbb{Z}_+}$ *such that* $\lim_{n\to+\infty} t_n/\log(n) = +\infty$,

$$\lim_{n\to+\infty} \mathbb{P}(\tau_0 \leq t_n \wedge \tau_{\varepsilon n}) = z \tag{2.2.3}$$

$$\lim_{n\to+\infty} \mathbb{P}(\tau_{\varepsilon n} \leq t_n \wedge \tau_0) = 1 - z. \tag{2.2.4}$$

Proof. Points (i) and (ii) are consequences of Proposition 2.2.1 and the connections between the discrete time Galton–Watson tree and the continuous time birth-death process $(X_t)_{t\geq 0}$ that is coupled with $(I_t)_{t\geq 0}$ as long as no ghost has appeared.

The proof of (iii) is an adaptation of Lemma A.1 in Méléard and Tran [77] (see also [29, 106]). Heuristically, (iii) says that at the beginning of the epidemics, the population either gets extinct with probability z or, with probability $1-z$, reaches

the size εn before time t_n and before extinction. The time t_n should be thought of as of order $\log(n)$, since the supercritical process has an exponential growth when it does not go to extinction.
For the birth-death process $(X_t)_{t\geq 0}$ there is no accumulation of birth and death events and almost surely,

$$\lim_{n\to+\infty} t_n \wedge \tau_{\varepsilon n} = +\infty.$$

So, we have by dominated convergence that $\lim_{n\to+\infty}\mathbb{P}(\tau_0 \leq t_n \wedge \tau_{\varepsilon n}) = \mathbb{P}(\tau_0 < +\infty)$. This last probability is the extinction probability of the process $(X_t)_{t\geq 0}$ which solves (2.2.2). For the second limit, we have:

$$\mathbb{P}(\tau_{\varepsilon n} \leq t_n \leq \tau_0) = \mathbb{P}(\tau_{\varepsilon n} \leq t_n \text{ and } \tau_0 = +\infty) + \mathbb{P}(\tau_{\varepsilon n} \leq t_n \leq \tau_0 < +\infty). \quad (2.2.5)$$

The second term of (2.2.5) is upper bounded by $\mathbb{P}(t_n \leq \tau_0 < +\infty)$ which converges to 0 by dominated convergence when $n \to +\infty$. For the second term, we can prove that with martingale techniques (e.g. [64]) that:

$$\lim_{t\to+\infty} \frac{\log X_t}{t} = \alpha, \quad (2.2.6)$$

where α is the initial epidemic growth rate defined in (2.0.2) and that is positive when $R_0 > 1$.

Let us consider $n > 1/\varepsilon$, so that $\log(\varepsilon n) > 0$. Since $\lim_{n\to+\infty} \tau_{\varepsilon n} = +\infty$ almost surely, we have on $\{\tau_0 = +\infty\}$ that:

$$\lim_{n\to+\infty} \frac{\log(\varepsilon n)}{\tau_{\varepsilon n}} \geq \lim_{n\to+\infty} \frac{\log(X_{\tau_{\varepsilon n}-})}{\tau_{\varepsilon n}} = \alpha > 0.$$

We deduce that:

$$\begin{aligned}\lim_{n\to+\infty} \mathbb{P}(\tau_{\varepsilon n} \leq t_n,\ \tau_0 = +\infty) = & \lim_{n\to+\infty} \mathbb{P}\Big(\frac{\tau_{\varepsilon n}}{\log(\varepsilon n)} \leq \frac{t_n}{\log(\varepsilon n)},\ \tau_0 = +\infty\Big) \\ = & \mathbb{P}(\tau_0 = +\infty) = 1 - z,\end{aligned}$$

since by our choice of t_n, $\lim_{n\to+\infty} t_n/\log(\varepsilon n) = +\infty$. □

Using similar results and fine couplings with branching properties, Barbour and Reinert [19] approximate the epidemic curve from the initial stages to the extinction of the disease.

2.3 Stochastic Block Models

We assume that there are K types of individuals, labeled $\{1, 2, \cdots, K\}$ and that for $k = 1, \cdots, K$ a fraction η_k of the N individuals in the population is of type k. We assume that the infection rate from an ego of type i to an alter of type j is λ_{ij}/N.

Proposition 2.3.1 **(R_0 for SBM).** *Consider a SBM as in Definition 1.2.3. Denote by ρ be the largest eigenvalue of the matrix with elements $\lambda_{ij}\rho_j$. Then:*

$$R_0 = \frac{\rho}{\gamma} = 1 + \frac{\alpha}{\gamma}.$$

Proof. We can hence couple here the infection process with a multi-type branching process. The rate at which a given i individual gives birth to a j individual corresponds to the rate, in the epidemic process, at which an i individual infects j individuals at time t since infection: it is $a_{ij}(t) = \lambda_{ij}\rho_j e^{-\gamma t}$. Here, λ_{ij}/N is the rate at which the i individual contacts a given j individual, $N\rho_j$ is the number of j individuals and $e^{-\gamma t}$ is the probability that the i individual is still infectious t time units after being infected. For multi-type branching processes, it is well known (e.g. [10, 46, 47]) that the basic reproduction number $R_0 = \rho_M$ is the largest eigenvalue of the matrix M with elements $m_{ij} = \int_0^{+\infty} a_{ij}(t)dt$, and the epidemic growth rate α is such that $1 = \int_0^{\infty} e^{-\alpha t}\rho_{A(t)}dt$, where $\rho_{A(t)}$ is the largest eigenvalue of the matrix $A(t)$ with elements $a_{ij}(t)$. Note that $\rho_{A(t)} = \rho e^{-\gamma t}$. Therefore,

$$R_0 = \rho \int_0^{\infty} e^{-\gamma t}dt = \frac{\rho}{\gamma}$$

and

$$1 = \rho \int_0^{+\infty} e^{-(\alpha+\gamma)t}dt \quad \text{leading to} \quad \rho = \alpha + \gamma.$$

These equalities imply that

$$R_0 = 1 + \frac{\alpha}{\gamma},$$

which shows that the relation between R_0 and α for a multi-type Markov SIR epidemic is the same as for such an epidemic in a homogeneous mixing population (cf. equation (2.1.1)). □

2.4 Household Structure

It is possible to define several different measures for the reproduction numbers for household models [14, 15, 23, 57]. For this model it is hard to find explicit expressions for R_0. We refer to Part II of this volume, for discussion on the early stages of the an epidemic spreading on a household graph or on a two-level mixing graph.

2.5 Statistical Estimation of R_0 for SIR on Graphs

Since we often have observations on symptom onset dates of cases for a new, emerging epidemic, as was the case for the Ebola epidemic in West Africa, it is often possible to estimate α from observations. In addition, we often have observations on the typical duration between time of infection of a case and infection of its infector, which allow us to estimate, assuming a Markov SIR model, the average duration of the infectious period, $1/\gamma$ [112].

In [107], it is shown that estimates of R_0 obtained by assuming homogeneous mixing are always larger than the corresponding estimates if the contact structure follows the configuration network model. For virtually all standard models studied in the literature, assuming homogeneous mixing leads to conservative estimates.

2.6 Control Effort

Definition 2.6.1. The control effort v_c is defined as the proportion of infected individuals that we should prevent from spreading the disease and immunize to stop the outbreak (have $R_0 < 1$), the immunized people being chosen uniformly at random.

For the homogeneous mixing contact structure, the required control effort for epidemics on the network structures under consideration, is known to depend solely on R_0 through equation [28, p. 69]

Proposition 2.6.2. *On the complete graph K_N, we have that:*

$$v_c = 1 - \frac{1}{R_0} = \frac{\alpha}{\alpha+\gamma}. \tag{2.6.1}$$

Proof. Consider a given infectious non-immunized individual whose infectious period is of length $y > 0$. In case we immunize a fraction v_c of the infected individuals, the number of new infectious and non-immunized individuals contaminated by this individual is not a Poisson random variable with parameter λy, but a thinned Poisson random variable of parameter $\lambda(1-v_c)y$. The condition that the new $R_0 = \lambda(1-v_c)/\gamma$ is less than 1 provides the expression of v_c announced in the proposition. □

Notice that if we estimate the initial epidemic growth rate α and the mean duration of the infectious period $1/\gamma$ from the data, (2.6.1) allows us to propose a natural estimator of v_c.

For CM graphs, we can establish a similar formula for v_c that depends also on the mean excess degree κ:

Proposition 2.6.3 (**v_c for CM graphs**). *For a CM graph with degree distribution* $\mathbf{p}$ *and mean excess degree κ:*

$$v_c = \frac{\kappa-1}{\kappa}\frac{\alpha}{\alpha+\gamma}.$$

The results obtained for Markov SIR epidemics in the complete graph model, CM and SBM are summarized in Table 2.6.1. The results from household models are not in the table, since the expressions are hardly insightful. These results are taken from [107].

Model	Quantity of interest	Quantity of interest as function of λ, γ and κ	α, γ and κ	Ratio with complete graph
Complete graph	α	$\lambda-\gamma$	-	-
	R_0	$\frac{\lambda}{\gamma}$	$1+\frac{\alpha}{\gamma}$	-
	v_c	$\frac{\lambda-\gamma}{\lambda}$	$\frac{\alpha}{\alpha+\gamma}$	-
CM	α	$(\kappa-1)\lambda-\gamma$	-	-
	R_0	$\frac{\kappa\lambda}{\lambda+\gamma}$	$\frac{\gamma+\alpha}{\gamma+\alpha/\kappa}$	$1+\frac{\alpha}{\gamma\kappa}$
	v_c	$1-\frac{\lambda+\gamma}{\kappa\lambda}$	$\frac{\kappa-1}{\kappa}\frac{\alpha}{\alpha+\gamma}$	$1+\frac{1}{\kappa-1}$
SBM	α	$\gamma(\rho_M-1)$	-	-
	R_0	ρ_M	$1+\frac{\alpha}{\gamma}$	1
	v_c	$1-\frac{1}{\rho_M}$	$\frac{\alpha}{\alpha+\gamma}$	1

Table 2.6.1 *The epidemic growth rate α, the basic reproduction number R_0 and required control effort v_c for a Markov SIR epidemic model as function of model parameters in the complete graph K_N, in the CM and in the SBM. In the fourth column, the ratio has been made between the R_0 in the CM and SBM cases (numerators) and the R_0 obtained in mixing populations (complete graphs) given the estimations of α, γ and κ.*

Let us comment on these results. First, we find that the estimator of R_0 obtained assuming homogeneous mixing (complete graph) overestimates by a factor $1+\frac{1}{\kappa-1}$ the R_0 in configuration models. This factor is always strictly greater than 1, since the mean excess degree κ is strictly greater than 1. Thus, v_c obtained by assuming homogeneous mixing is always larger than that of the configuration model. Consequently, if the actual infectious contact structure is made up of a CM and a perfect vaccine is available, we need to vaccinate a smaller proportion of the population than predicted assuming homogeneous mixing.

The overestimation of R_0 is small whenever R_0 is not much larger than 1 or when κ is large. The same conclusion applies to the required control effort v_c. The observation that the R_0 and v_c for the homogeneous mixing model exceed the corresponding values for the network model extends to the full epidemic model allowing for an arbitrarily distributed latent period followed by an arbitrarily distributed independent infectious period, during which the infectivity profile (the rate of close contacts) may vary over time but depends only on the time since the start of the infectious period. Figure 2.6.1(a) shows that for SIR epidemics with Gamma distributed infectious periods, the factor by which the homogeneous mixing estimator overestimates the actual R_0 increases with increasing epidemic growth rate α, and suggests that this factor increases with increasing standard deviation of the infectious period. Figure 2.6.1(b) shows that the factors by which the homogeneous mixing estimator overestimates the actual v_c, decreases with increasing α and increases with increasing standard deviation of the infectious period. When the standard deviation of the infectious period is low, which is a realistic assumption for most emerging infectious diseases (see e.g. [38]), and R_0 is not much larger than 1, then ignoring the contact structure in the network model and using the simpler estimators for the homogeneous mixing results in a slight overestimation of R_0 and v_c.

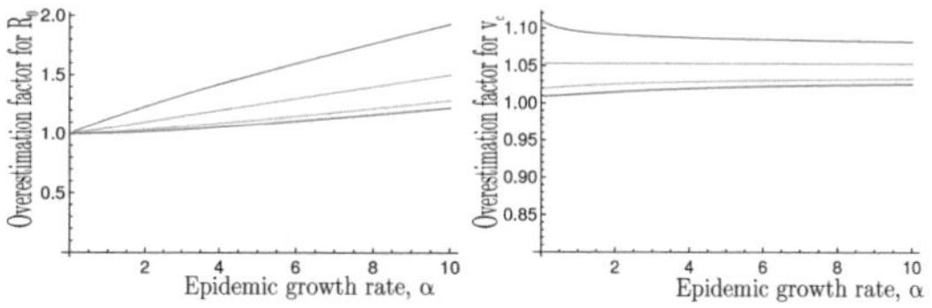

Fig. 2.6.1 *The factor by which estimators based on homogeneous mixing will overestimate (a) the basic reproduction number R_0 and (b) the required control effort v_c for the network case. Here the epidemic growth rate α is measured in multiples of the mean infectious period $1/\gamma$. The mean excess degree $\kappa = 20$. The infectious periods are assumed to follow a gamma distribution with mean 1 and standard deviation $\sigma = 1.5$, $\sigma = 1$, $\sigma = 1/2$ and $\sigma = 0$, as displayed from top to bottom. Note that the estimate of R_0 based on homogeneous mixing is $1+\alpha$. Furthermore, note that $\sigma = 1$, corresponds to the special case of an exponentially distributed infectious period, while if $\sigma = 0$, the duration of the infectious period is not random.*

When considering epidemics spreading on SBM graphs (see [107, Supplementary materials]), we can derive that estimators for R_0 and (if control measures are independent of the types of individuals) v_c are exactly the same as for homogeneous mixing in a broad class of SEIR epidemic models. This class includes the full epidemic model allowing for arbitrarily distributed latent and infectious periods and models in which the rates of contacts between different types keep the same proportion all of the time, although the rates themselves may vary over time (cf. [48]). We illustrate our findings on multitype structures through simulations of SEIR epidemics in an age stratified population with known contact structure as described in [113]. We use values of the average infectious period $1/\gamma$ and the average latent period $1/\delta$ close to the estimates for the 2014 Ebola epidemic in West Africa [115]. Two estimators for R_0 are computed. The first of these estimators is based on the average number of infections among the people who were infected early in the epidemic. This procedure leads to a very good estimate of R_0 if the spread of the disease is observed completely. The second estimator for R_0 is based on $\hat{\alpha}$, an estimate of the epidemic growth rate α, and known expected infectious period $1/\gamma$ and expected latent period $1/\delta$. This estimator of R_0 is $(1+\hat{\alpha}/\delta)(1+\hat{\alpha}/\gamma)$. We calculate estimates of R_0 using these two estimators for 250 simulation runs. As predicted by the theory, the simulation results show that for each run the estimates are close to the actual value (Figure 2.6.2(a)), without a systematic bias (Figure 2.6.2(b)).

Let us now consider an epidemic spreading on a household structure. It is also argued that the required control effort satisfies $v_c \geq 1 - 1/R_0$ for this model, which implies that if we know R_0 and we base our control effort on this knowledge, we might fail to stop an outbreak. However, we usually do not have direct estimates for R_0 and even though it is not true in general that using R_0 leads to conservative estimates for v_c [17], numerical computations suggest that the approximation of v_c using α and the homogeneous mixing assumption is often conservative.

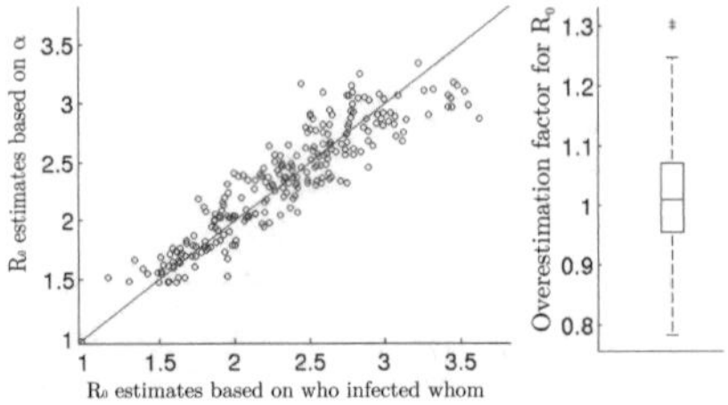

Fig. 2.6.2 *The estimated basic reproduction number, R_0, for a Markov SEIR model in a multi-type population as described in [113], based on the real infection process (who infected whom) plotted against the computed R_0, assuming homogeneous mixing, based on the estimated epidemic growth rate, α, and given expected infectious period (5 days) and expected latent period (10 days). The infectivity is chosen at random, such that the theoretical R_0 is uniform between 1.5 and 3. The estimate of α is based on the times when individuals become infectious. In the right plot, a boxplot of the ratios is given.*

To illustrate this last point, we consider in Figure 2.6.3 a household structure with within and global infectivities. The within household infection rate is λ_H. In the simulations, we show estimates for R_0 and v_c over a range of values for the relative contribution of the within-household spread. For each epidemic growth rate α, the estimated values remain below the value obtained for homogeneous mixing (neglecting the partition into households).

We use two types of epidemics: in (a) and (b) the Markov SIR epidemic is used, while in (c) the so-called Reed–Frost model is used, which can be interpreted as an epidemic in which infectious individuals have a long latent period of non-random length, after which they are infectious for a very short period of time. We note that for the Reed–Frost model the relationship between α and R_0 does not depend on the household structure (cf. [17]) and therefore, for this model, only the dependence of v_c on the relative contribution of the within household spread is shown in Figure 2.6.3.

The household size distribution is taken from a 2003 health survey in Nigeria [45]. For Markov SIR epidemics, as the within-household infection rate λ_H is varied, the global infection rate is varied in such a way that the computed epidemic growth rate α is kept fixed. For this model, α is calculated using the matrix method described in Section 4.1 of [94].

For the Reed–Frost epidemic model, the probability that an infectious individual infects a given susceptible household member during its infectious period, p_H is varied, while the corresponding probability for individuals in the general population varies with p_H so that α is kept constant. For this model, R_0 coincides with the initial geometric rate of growth of infection, so $\alpha = \log(R_0)$. From Figure 2.6.3, we see that estimates of v_c assuming homogeneous mixing are reliable for Reed–Frost type epidemics, although as opposed to all other analysed models and structures, the estimates are not conservative. We see also that for the Markov SIR epidemic, estimating R_0 and v_c based on the homogeneously mixing assumption might lead to conservative estimates which are up to 40% higher than the real R_0 and v_c.

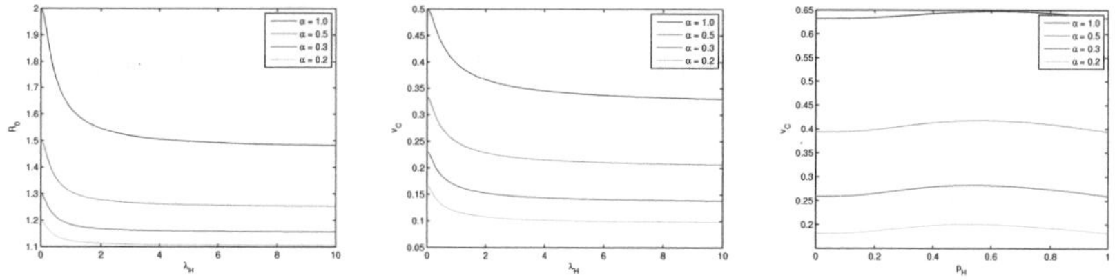

Fig. 2.6.3 *Estimation of key epidemiological variables in a population structured by households (see Part II of this volume). The basic reproduction number R_0 for Markov SIR epidemics (a), critical vaccination coverage v_c for Markov SIR epidemics (b) and v_c for Reed–Frost epidemics (c), as a function of the relative influence of within household transmission, in a population partitioned into households. The household size distribution is given by $m_1 = 0.117, m_2 = 0.120, m_3 = 0.141, m_4 = 0.132, m_5 = 0.121, m_6 = 0.108, m_7 = 0.084, m_8 = 0.051, m_9 = 0.126$, for $i = 1, 2, \cdots, 9$, m_i is the fraction of the households with size i. The global infectivity is chosen so that the epidemic growth rate α is kept constant while the within household transmission varies. Homogeneous mixing corresponds to $\lambda_H = p_H = 0$.*

Chapter 3
SIR Epidemics on Configuration Model Graphs

We now turn to establishing limit theorems for approximating the dynamics of the disease in large populations, when $N \to +\infty$, similarly to Chapter 2 in Part I of this book. We focus here on the case where $\mathscr{G}_N$ is a Configuration model graph, and we will let $N \to +\infty$. Several strategies have been developed for epidemics spreading on such random graphs (see e.g. Newman [86, 88], Durrett [49], Barthélemy et al. [20], Kiss et al. [70]).

Contrarily to the classical mixing compartmental SIR epidemic models (e.g. [67, 21] see also Part I of this book for a presentation), heterogeneity in the number of contacts makes it difficult to describe the dynamical behaviour of the epidemic. An important literature, starting from Andersson [7], deals with moment closure, mean field approximations (e.g. [91, 20, 49, 70]) or large population approximations (e.g. [13], see also Eq. (3) of [6] in discrete time). In 2008, Ball and Neal [13] proposed to describe the dynamics with an infinite system of ordinary differential equations, by obtaining an equation for each subpopulation of individuals with same degree k, $k \in \mathbb{Z}_+$. The same year, Volz [110] proposed a large population approximation with only 5 ordinary differential equations and without moment closure, which was a major advance for prediction and tractability. The key concept behind his work was to focus not only on node-based quantities, but rather of edge-based ones (see also [78]). Rigorous proofs have then been proposed by [44, 19, 65]).

Recall that we have denoted the sets of S, I and R vertices at time t by S_t, I_t and R_t (see Section 1.4). The sizes of these sub-populations are S_t, I_t and R_t. We will say that an edge linking an infectious ego and susceptible alter is of type $\mathrm{I}-\mathrm{S}$ (accordingly $\mathrm{R}-\mathrm{S}$, $\mathrm{I}-\mathrm{I}$ or $\mathrm{I}-\mathrm{R}$).

3.1 Moment Closure in Large Populations

For the presentation in this section, we follow the work of [7]. Let us introduce some notation. For $u \in V$, denote

T. Britton, E. Pardoux (eds.), *Stochastic Epidemic Models with Inference*,
Lecture Notes in Mathematics 2255, https://doi.org/10.1007/978-3-030-30900-8_10

$$S_u(t) = \mathbf{1}_{u\in \mathrm{S}_t} \qquad \text{and} \qquad I_u(t) = \mathbf{1}_{u\in \mathrm{I}_t}.$$

Then, $S_t = \sum_{u\in V} S_u(t)$ and $I_t = \sum_{u\in V} I_u(t)$. Because the size N of the graph $\mathscr{G}_N$ converges to infinity, we will be lead to study the proportions of susceptible, infectious and removed individuals, that are denoted by:

$$S_t^N = \frac{S_t}{N}, \qquad I_t^N = \frac{I_t}{N}, \qquad R_t^N = \frac{R_t}{N}. \tag{3.1.1}$$

Notice that $S_t^N + I_t^N + R_t^N = 1$ since our population is closed. Hence, knowing the evolution of $S_.^N$ and $I_.^N$ is sufficient for describing the size and evolution of the outbreak.
For A, B, C being S or I, we denote by

$$[a] = \lim_{N\to+\infty} \frac{1}{N} \sum_{u\in V} A_u = a, \qquad [ab] = \lim_{N\to+\infty} \frac{1}{N} \sum_{u,v\in V} A_u G_{uv} B_v,$$

$$[abc] = \lim_{N\to+\infty} \frac{1}{N} \sum_{u,v,w\in V} A_u G_{uv} B_v G_{vw} C_w,$$

where we recall that G is the adjacency matrix of the graph (see Definition 1.1.2).

In the sequel, we will work under the following assumption.

Assumption 3.1.1. We assume that $\lim_{N\to+\infty}(S_0^N, I_0^N) = (s_0, i_0) \in (\mathbb{R}_+ \setminus \{0\})^2$ and that for all N, $R_0^N = 0$.

The idea is that in the large population limit, the initial fraction of infectious individuals should be positive to allow the observation of an outbreak. That is why we assume that it is of order $i_0 N$ with $i_0 > 0$ but possibly small with respect to 1.

Let us present a system of limiting deterministic equations. The limit theorems allowing to obtain the following equations from the finite stochastic system are not shown here. In fact, we will later detail how Volz' equations are obtained.

Andersson [7] proposes the following ODEs for the sizes of the S and I classes.

$$\frac{ds_t}{dt} = -\lambda [s_t i_t], \qquad \frac{di_t}{dt} = \lambda [s_t i_t] - \gamma i_t. \tag{3.1.2}$$

Let us comment on these equations. In a closed population, susceptible individuals disappear when they are contaminated, i.e. when an edge with susceptible ego and infectious alter transmits the disease. Thus, the rate at which the number of susceptible individuals decreases due to infection (which equals to the rate at which the number of infectious individuals increases) should be proportional to the proportion of edges with susceptible ego and infectious alter, $[s_t i_t]$. The rate at which infectious individuals disappear is $-\gamma i_t$ as in the compartmental case, since removals are node-related events and not edge-related events like infections.

Equations 3.1.2 are not closed, and this leads Andersson to propose the following assumption.

Assumption 3.1.2. Let A, B, C be S or I. If $\{u,w\} \notin E$, we assume that

$$\mathbb{P}(A_u = 1 \mid B_v C_w = 1) = \mathbb{P}(A_u = 1 \mid B_v = 1) = \frac{\mathbb{P}(A_u = 1,\, B_v = 1)}{\mathbb{P}(B_v = 1)}.$$

Let us comment on this assumption. As the Bayes formula says that:

$$\mathbb{P}(A_u B_v C_w = 1) = \mathbb{P}(A_u = 1 \mid B_v C_w = 1)\mathbb{P}(B_v C_w = 1),$$

Assumption (3.1.2) implies that

$$\mathbb{P}(A_u C_w = 1 \mid B_v = 1) = \mathbb{P}(A_u = 1 \mid B_v = 1)\mathbb{P}(C_w = 1 \mid B_v = 1).$$

Thus, Assumption 3.1.2 amounts to assuming that conditionally on having a B friend, having an A and a C friends are independent events, and is heuristically true when

$$[abc] \approx \frac{[ab][bc]}{[b]}.$$

This assumption fails when we are in graphs with strong correlations between edges so that 'the friend of my friend is also my friend'.

Let us define the selection pressure by

$$\widetilde{i}_t = \frac{[s_t i_t]}{s_t}. \tag{3.1.3}$$

It is the mean number of edges toward I_t for individuals in S_t. This quantity allows Andersson [7] to close the system of ODEs (3.1.2) under Assumption 3.1.2.

Theorem 3.1.3. *Under Assumption 3.1.2, the epidemic on the network can be described by the following equations:*

$$\frac{ds_t}{dt} = -\lambda s_t \widetilde{i}_t, \tag{3.1.4}$$

$$\frac{di_t}{dt} = \lambda s_t \widetilde{i}_t - \gamma i_t \tag{3.1.5}$$

$$\frac{d\widetilde{i}_t}{dt} = (C\lambda s_t - \lambda - \gamma)\widetilde{i}_t. \tag{3.1.6}$$

Proof. The equations proposed in Theorem 3.1.3 are derived in several steps. Recall Equations (3.1.2). To close them, it is needed to describe how the quantities of edges $[s_t s_t]$ and $[s_t i_t]$ evolve. An edge $\text{S}-\text{S}$ disappears when one of its vertices is infected. For each motif $\text{S}-\text{S}-\text{I}$, the edge $\text{S}-\text{I}$ transmits the disease independently with rate λ. Thus, the rate of disappearance of $\text{S}-\text{S}$ edges is proportional to the $\lambda[s_t s_t i_t]$. Similarly, $\text{S}-\text{I}$ edges appear when edges $\text{S}-\text{S}$ become $\text{S}-\text{I}$, and disappear when becoming $\text{I}-\text{I}$ (which happens when the susceptible vertex is infected by its infectious alter, or by another infectious contact) or when becoming S – R (when the infectious individual is removed). Then:

$$\frac{d[s_t s_t]}{dt} = -2\lambda [s_t s_t i_t],$$
$$\frac{d[s_t i_t]}{dt} = \lambda\big([s_t s_t i_t] - [i_t s_t i_t] - [s_t i_t]\big) - \gamma[s_t i_t]. \tag{3.1.7}$$

These equations are still not closed, as they depend on the numbers of motifs S – S – I and I – S – I renormalized by N. The equations that we might write for these quantities depend on motifs with four vertices etc. To close the equations, we use Assumption 3.1.2. Then, the equations (3.1.7) become:

$$\frac{d[s_t s_t]}{dt} = -2\lambda \frac{[s_t s_t][s_t i_t]}{s_t},$$
$$\frac{d[s_t i_t]}{dt} = \lambda\Big(\frac{[s_t s_t][s_t i_t]}{s_t} - \frac{[s_t i_t]^2}{s_t} - [s_t i_t]\Big) - \gamma[s_t i_t].$$

Notice that

$$\frac{d(s_t^2)}{dt} = 2s_t \frac{ds_t}{dt} = -2\lambda s_t [s_t i_t] = -2\lambda \frac{[s_t i_t]}{s_t} s_t^2.$$

Thus, (s_t^2) and $[s_t s_t]$ satisfy the same ODE and we deduce that there exists a $C > 0$ such that $[s_t s_t] = C s_t^2$.

Using the definition of the selection pressure $\widetilde{i}_t$,

$$\begin{aligned}\frac{d\widetilde{i}_t}{dt} =& \frac{d[s_t i_t]}{dt}\frac{1}{s_t} - \frac{[s_t i_t]}{s_t^2}\frac{ds_t}{dt}\\ =& \frac{1}{s_t}\Big(\lambda\big(C s_t^2 \times \widetilde{i}_t s_t \times \frac{1}{s_t} - \widetilde{i}_t^2 s_t^2 \times \frac{1}{s_t} - \widetilde{i}_t s_t\big) - \gamma \widetilde{i}_t s_t\Big) + \frac{\widetilde{i}_t s_t}{s_t^2} \times \lambda \widetilde{i}_t s_t\\ =& (C\lambda s_t - \lambda - \gamma)\widetilde{i}_t.\end{aligned}$$

The system can then be reformulated as the announced system with three ODEs in s_t, i_t and $\widetilde{i}_t$. □

When the infection rate is low and the number of S – S edges is very high, we recover the Kermack–McKendrick ODEs describing the dynamics of an epidemic in a homogeneous case:

Proposition 3.1.4. *If $C \to +\infty$ and $\lambda \to 0$ with $\lambda' = C\lambda$ constant, we recover in the limit the Kermack–McKendrick system of ODE:*

$$\frac{ds_t}{dt} = -\lambda' s_t i_t$$
$$\frac{di_t}{dt} = \lambda' s_t i_t - \gamma i_t.$$

Proof. If $C \to +\infty$ and $\lambda \to 0$ with $\lambda' = C\lambda$ constant, then 'in the limit':

$$\frac{d\widetilde{i}_t}{dt} = \lambda' \, s_t\widetilde{i}_t - \gamma\widetilde{i}_t.$$

Consider $f(t) = \widetilde{i}_t - Ci_t$. This quantity satisfies

$$\frac{df}{dt}(t) = -\gamma f_t.$$

Applying Gronwall's inequality, this yields that $\widetilde{i}_t = Ci_t$. We recover as announced, the Kermack–McKendrick ODEs with infection rate λ'. □

From Equation (3.1.6), we can for example predict the total size of the epidemics, i.e. the number of removed individuals when the infective population vanishes and the epidemics stops.

Proposition 3.1.5. *Based on the equations* (3.1.6)*, we can compute the final size of the epidemics:*

$$z := s_0 - s_\infty = s_0 \, \big(1 - \exp\big(-\frac{\lambda}{\lambda+\gamma}(Cz + \widetilde{i}_0)\big)\big).$$

Proof. Because $t \mapsto s_t$ is a continuous non-negative decreasing function, it converges to a limit s_∞ when $t \to +\infty$. From (3.1.6):

$$\frac{d\widetilde{i}_t}{dt} = -\lambda s_t \widetilde{i}_t\big(-C + \frac{1}{s_t} + \frac{\gamma}{\lambda s_t}\big) = \frac{ds_t}{dt}\big(-C + \frac{1+\frac{\gamma}{\lambda}}{s_t}\big)$$

from which we obtain by integration:

$$\widetilde{i}_t - \widetilde{i}_0 = -C(s_t - s_0) + \big(1 + \frac{\gamma}{\lambda}\big)\log\frac{s_t}{s_0}.$$

Since $\widetilde{i}_\infty = 0$:

$$-\widetilde{i}_0 + C(s_\infty - s_0) = \big(1 + \frac{\gamma}{\lambda}\big)\log\frac{s_\infty}{s_0}.$$

Computing $z := s_0 - s_\infty$, we recover the announced result. □

For further and recent developments on moment closures, we refer the reader to e.g. [92] or [70].

3.2 Volz and Miller Approach

In 2008, Volz [110] proposed a system of only 5 ODEs to describe the spread of an epidemic on a random CM graph. Volz approximation is based on an edge-centered point of view, in an 'infinite' CM graph setting, without any assumption of moment closure. We present Volz equations and then explain how to recover them with Miller's approach [78]. The derivation of these equations as limit of epidemics spreading on finite graphs is detailed following the approach of Decreusefond et al. [44].

The spread of diseases on random graphs involves two sources of randomness: one for the random graph, the other for describing the way the epidemic propagates on this random environment. An idea coming from statistical mechanics is to build the random graph progressively as the epidemic spreads over it, instead of first constructing the random graph, conditioning on it and studying the epidemic on the frozen environment. We detail the process that we will consider in the rest of the section.
Assume that only the edges joining the I and R individuals are observed. This means that the cluster of infectious and removed individuals is built, while the network of susceptible individuals is still not defined. We further assume that the degree of each individual is known. To each I individual is associated an exponential random clock with rate γ to determine its removal. To each open edge (directed to S), we associate a random exponential clock with rate λ. When it rings, an infection occurs. The infectious ego chooses the edge of a susceptible alter at random. Hence the latter individual is chosen proportionally to her/his degree, in the size biased distribution, as explained in (1.2.1). When this susceptible individual becomes infected, she/he is connected and uncovers the edges to neighbours that were already in the subgraph: we determine whether her/his remaining edges are linked with I, R-type individuals (already in the observed cluster) or to S, in which case the edges remains 'open' (the alter is not chosen yet).

Let us consider the limit when the size of the graph converges to infinity, and let us denote as before by s_t and i_t the proportion of susceptible and infectious individuals in the population at time t. A key quantity in the approach of Volz [110] and Miller [78] is the probability $\theta(t)$ that an directed edge picked uniformly at random at t has not transmitted the disease. Let $u \in V$ be a vertex of degree k. The vertex u is still susceptible at time t if none of its k edges has transmitted the disease. By the construction of the stochastic process, where the random graph is built simultaneously to the spread of the disease on it, any infectious individual that transmits the disease pairs one of her/his half-edge with a half-edge of a susceptible individual chosen uniformly at random. Thus, the probability that none of the k edges of a susceptible has transmitted the disease up to time t is $\theta^k(t)$. Hence,

$$s_t = \sum_{k=0}^{+\infty} \theta(t)^k p_k = g(\theta(t)), \tag{3.2.1}$$

where g is the generating function of the probability distribution $(p_k)_{k\geq 0}$ (see (1.2.2)). Notice that in Equation (3.2.1), the proportion s_t of susceptibles is assumed to coincide with the expectation of the proportion of the number of susceptible individuals at t. We recall that a rigorous derivation of Volz' equations is given in Section 3.3.7 below.

3.2.1 Dynamics of $\theta(t)$

To deduce an equation for s_t from (3.2.1), an equation for $\theta(t)$ is needed.

Proposition 3.2.1. *We have that:*

$$\frac{d\theta}{dt} = -\lambda\theta(t) + \gamma(1-\theta(t)) + \lambda\frac{g'(\theta(t))}{g'(1)}.$$

Proof. Denote by $h(t)$ the probability that the alter is still susceptible at time t. Define $\phi(t)$ as the probability that a random edge has not transmitted the disease and that its alter is infectious. Notice that

$$\frac{d\theta}{dt} = -\lambda\phi(t). \tag{3.2.2}$$

Given an edge satisfying the definition of $\phi(t)$ (an edge that has not transmitted the disease yet and whose alter is infectious), the probability that the alter is of degree k is given by (1.2.1) and given its degree, the probability that it is still susceptible at time t is $\theta^{k-1}(t)$, because the considered edge did not transmit the disease before t. Then:

$$h(t) = \sum_{k=0}^{+\infty}\frac{kp_k}{m}\theta^{k-1}(t) = \frac{g'(\theta(t))}{g'(1)},$$

from which we deduce that

$$\frac{dh}{dt} = \frac{g''(\theta(t))}{g'(1)}\frac{d\theta}{dt} = -\lambda\phi(t)\frac{g''(\theta(t))}{g'(1)}.$$

An equation for the evolution of $\phi(t)$ can be written by noticing that:

- An edge stops satisfying the definition of ϕ if it transmits the disease or if the alter is removed.
- An edge starts satisfying the definition of ϕ if its alter becomes infectious.

Thus

$$\begin{aligned}\frac{d\phi}{dt} &= -(\lambda+\gamma)\phi(t) - \frac{dh}{dt}\\ &= -(\lambda+\gamma)\phi(t) + \lambda\phi(t)\frac{g''(\theta(t))}{g'(1)}\\ &= \frac{\lambda+\gamma}{\lambda}\frac{d\theta}{dt} - \frac{g''(\theta(t))}{g'(1)}\frac{d\theta}{dt},\end{aligned} \tag{3.2.3}$$

which gives for a constant C:

$$\phi(t) = \frac{\lambda+\gamma}{\lambda}\theta(t) - \frac{g'(\theta(t))}{g'(1)} + C.$$

Using that $\phi(0) = 0$ and $\theta(0) = 1$, we deduce that $C = -\gamma/\lambda$ and hence

$$\phi(t) = \theta(t) - \frac{\gamma}{\lambda}(1-\theta(t)) - \frac{g'(\theta(t))}{g'(1)}. \tag{3.2.4}$$

We deduce the announced result from (3.2.2) and (3.2.4). □

3.2.2 Miller's Equations

We can now deduce the equations for the proportions s_t, i_t and r_t of susceptible, infectious and recovered individuals proposed by Miller [78].

Proposition 3.2.2 (Miller's equations [78]). *We have:*

$$\begin{aligned}
s_t &= g(\theta(t))\\
\frac{dr_t}{dt} &= \gamma i_t\\
\frac{di_t}{dt} &= -g'(\theta(t))\Big(-\lambda\theta(t)+\gamma(1-\theta(t))+\lambda\frac{g'(\theta(t))}{g'(1)}\Big) - \gamma i_t.\\
\frac{d\theta}{dt} &= -\lambda\theta(t)+\gamma(1-\theta(t))+\lambda\frac{g'(\theta(t))}{g'(1)}.
\end{aligned}$$

Proof. By (3.2.1), we have that $s_t = g(\theta(t))$. From the node-centered removal dynamics of infectious nodes, we have that $\frac{dr_t}{dt} = \gamma i_t$. Using $i_t = 1 - s_t - r_t$ and Proposition 3.2.1, we obtain the two last equations. □

We can now recover the equations proposed by Volz [110] by introducing the proportion of edges $\mathrm{I}-\mathrm{S}$ that have not transmitted the disease yet

$$p_I(t) = \frac{\phi(t)}{\theta(t)} \tag{3.2.5}$$

and the proportion of edges $\mathrm{S}-\mathrm{S}$ that have not transmitted the disease

$$p_S(t) = \frac{g'(\theta(t))}{\theta(t)g'(1)}. \tag{3.2.6}$$

From Miller's equations, we obtain by straightforward computation:

Proposition 3.2.3 (Volz' equations [110]). *We have:*

$$\begin{aligned}
\theta(t) &= \exp\Big(-\lambda\int_0^t p_I(s)\,ds\Big), \qquad s_t = g(\theta(t)),\\
\frac{di_t}{dt} &= \lambda p_I(t)\theta(t)g'(\theta(t)) - \gamma i_t\\
\frac{dp_I}{dt} &= \lambda\, p_I(t)p_S(t)\theta(t)\frac{g''(\theta(t))}{g'(\theta(t))} - \lambda\, p_I(t)(1-p_I(t)) - \gamma p_T(t).\\
\frac{dp_S}{dt} &= \lambda p_I(t)p_S(t)\Big(1-\theta(t)\frac{g''(\theta(t))}{g'(\theta(t))}\Big).
\end{aligned}$$

Let us compare Volz' equations with the Kermack–McKendrick equations:

$$\frac{ds}{dt} = -\lambda\, s_t i_t, \qquad \frac{di}{dt} = \lambda\, s_t i_t - \gamma i_t.$$

In Volz' equations, denoting by $\bar{N}_t^{\mathrm{S}} = p_I(t)\theta(t)g'(\theta(t))$ the 'quantity' of edges from I to S:

$$\begin{aligned}\frac{ds_t}{dt} &= g'(\theta(t))\frac{d\theta}{dt} = -\lambda g'(\theta(t))\theta(t)p_I(t) = -\lambda \bar{N}_t^{\mathrm{S}} p_I(t) = -\lambda \bar{N}_t^{\mathrm{IS}} \\ \frac{di_t}{dt} &= \lambda \times \bar{N}_t^{\mathrm{IS}} - \gamma i_t.\end{aligned}$$

These equations account for the fact that not all the I and S vertices are connected, which modifies the infection pressure compared with the mixing models (Part I of this volume).

3.3 Measure-valued Processes

Decreusefond et al. [44] proved the convergence that was left open by Volz [110]. The proof that we now present underlines the key objects that lie at the core of the phenomenon: because degree distributions are central in CMs, these objets are not surprisingly measures representing some particular degree distributions. Three degree distributions are sufficient to describe the epidemic dynamics which evolve in the space of measures on the set of nonnegative integers, and of which Volz' equations are a by-product.
A rigorous individual-based description of the epidemic on a random graph is provided. Starting with a node-centered description, we show that the individual dimension is lost in the large graph limit. Our construction heavily relies on the choice of a CM for the graph underlying the epidemic, which was also made in [110].

3.3.1 Stochastic Model for a Finite Graph with N Vertices

Recall the notation of Section 1.4. The idea of Volz is to use network-centric quantities (such as the number of edges from I to S) rather than node-centric quantities. For a vertex $u \in \mathrm{S}$, D_u corresponds to the degree of u. For $u \in \mathrm{I}$ (respectively R), $D_u(\mathrm{S})$ represents the number of edges with u as infectious (resp. removed) ego and susceptible alter. The numbers of edges with susceptible ego (resp. of edges of types $\mathrm{I}-\mathrm{S}$ and $\mathrm{R}-\mathrm{S}$) are denoted by N_t^{S} (resp. N_t^{IS} and N_t^{RS}). All these quantities are in fact encoded into three degree distributions, that we now introduce and on which we will work to establish Volz' equations. Notice that with the notations of Section 3.1, $\frac{1}{N}N_t^{\mathrm{IS}} = [SI]_t$ and $\frac{1}{N}N_t^{\mathrm{RS}} = [SR]_t$. However, we drop this notation with brackets for simplification of later formula and because we will not need motifs other than edges.

Definition 3.3.1. We consider here the following three degree distributions of $\mathcal{M}_F(\mathbb{Z}_+)$, given for $t \geq 0$ as:

$$\mu_t^{\mathrm{S}} = \sum_{u \in \mathrm{S}_t} \delta_{D_u}, \quad \mu_t^{\mathrm{IS}} = \sum_{u \in \mathrm{I}_t} \delta_{D_u(\mathrm{S}_t)}, \quad \mu_t^{\mathrm{RS}} = \sum_{u \in \mathrm{R}_t} \delta_{D_u(\mathrm{S}_t)}, \tag{3.3.1}$$

where we recall that δ_D is the Dirac mass at $D \in \mathbb{Z}_+$ (see Notation 0.0.1).

Notice that the measures μ_t^{S}/S_t, μ_t^{IS}/I_t and μ_t^{RS}/R_t are probability measures that correspond to usual (probability) degree distributions. The degree distribution μ_t^{S} of susceptible individuals is needed to describe the degrees of the new infected individuals. The measure μ_t^{IS} provides information on the number of edges from I_t to S_t, through which the disease can propagate. Similarly, the measure μ_t^{RS} is used to describe the evolution of the set of edges linking S_t to R_t.
Using Notation 0.0.1, we can see that

$$I_t = \langle \mu_t^{\mathrm{IS}}, 1 \rangle, \qquad N_t^{\mathrm{IS}} = \langle \mu_t^{\mathrm{IS}}, \chi \rangle = \sum_{u \in \mathrm{I}_t} D_u(\mathrm{S}_t),$$

and accordingly for N_t^{S}, N^{RS}, S_t and R_t.

Definition 3.3.2 (Labelling the nodes). For an integer-valued measure $\mu \in \mathcal{M}_F(\mathbb{Z}_+)$, we can rank its atoms by increasing degrees and label them with this order. A way of deducing this labelling from μ by using its cumulative distribution function is proposed in [44]. We omit it here for the sake of simplicity.

Example 3.3.3. Consider for instance the measure $\mu = 2\delta_1 + 3\delta_5 + \delta_7$. If μ is a degree distribution, this means that 2 individuals have degree 1, 3 individuals have degree 5 and 1 individual has degree 7. Ranking the atoms by increasing degrees, we can label them from 1 to 6 such that $D_1 = D_2 = 1$, $D_3 = D_4 = D_5 = 5$, $D_6 = 7$.□

3.3.2 Dynamics and Measure-valued SDEs

Suppose that at initial time, we are given a set of S and I nodes together with their degrees. The graph of relationships between the I individuals is in fact irrelevant for studying the propagation of the disease. The minimal information consists in the sizes of the classes S, I, R and the number of edges to the class S for every infectious or removed node. Each node of class S comes with a given number of half-edges of undetermined types ; each node of class I (resp. R) comes with a number of $\mathrm{I}-\mathrm{S}$ (resp. $\mathrm{R}-\mathrm{S}$) edges. The numbers of $\mathrm{I}-\mathrm{R}$, $\mathrm{I}-\mathrm{I}$ and $\mathrm{R}-\mathrm{R}$ edges need not to be retained. The three descriptors in (3.3.1) are hence sufficient to describe the evolution of the SIR epidemic.

Recall the graph construction of Section 3.2 explaining how to handle simultaneously the two sources of randomness of the problem. The random network of social relationships is explored while the disease spreads on it: only the clusters of I and R individuals are observed and constructed, with $\mathrm{I}-\mathrm{S}$ and $\mathrm{R}-\mathrm{S}$ edges having their S alter still unaffected. Susceptible individuals remain unattached until they become infected, in which case their connections to the cluster of I's and R's are revealed. We assume that the degree distribution of S_0 and the size N of the total population are known.

We now explain the dynamics, that is summarized in Figure 3.3.1. Recall that to each half-edge of type $I-S$, an independent exponential clock with parameter λ is associated, and to each I vertex, an independent exponential clock with parameter γ is associated. The first of all these clocks that rings determines the next event.

Case 1 If the clock that rings is associated to an I individual, the latter is removed. Change her status from I to R and the type of her emanating half-edges accordingly: $I-S$ half-edges become $R-S$ half-edges for example.

Case 2 If the clock that rings is associated with a half $I-S$-edge (with unaffected susceptible alter), an infection occurs.

Step 1 Match randomly the $I-S$-half-edge whose clock has rung to a half-edge of a susceptible: this determines the susceptible becoming infected.

Step 2 Let k be the degree of the newly infected individual. Choose uniformly $k-1$ half edges among the open half-edges of the cluster of I and R individuals ($I-S$ or $R-S$ edges of this cluster, with susceptible alter still unaffected) and among the half edges of susceptible individuals. Let j, ℓ and m be the respective number of $I-S$, $R-S$ and $S-S$ edges chosen among the $k-1$ picks.

Step 3 The chosen half-edges of type $I-S$ and $R-S$ determine the infectious or removed neighbours of the newly infected individual who become the new (infectious) alter of these edges. The remaining m edges of type $S-S$ remain open in the sense that the susceptible neighbour is not fixed.
Change the status of the newly infected from S to I. Change the status of the m (resp. j, ℓ) $S-S$-type (resp. $I-S$-type, $R-S$-type) edges considered to $I-S$-type (resp. $I-I$-type, $R-I$-type). □

We then wait for another clock to ring and repeat the procedure.

From the dynamics described above, we can read that the global force of infection at time t is

$$\lambda N^{\mathrm{IS}}_{t_-}.$$

When an infection occurs, a half-edge of a susceptible individual is chosen and determines who is the contaminated person. Therefore, a given susceptible of degree k has a probability $k/N^{\mathrm{S}}_{t_-}$ to be the next infected individual. So that the rate of infection of a given susceptible of degree k at time t is:

$$\Lambda_{t_-}(k) = \lambda k \frac{N^{\mathrm{IS}}_{t_-}}{N^{\mathrm{S}}_{t_-}} = \lambda k p_I(t_-), \tag{3.3.2}$$

where $p_I(t)$ is defined by

$$p_I(t) = \frac{N^{\mathrm{IS}}_t}{N^{\mathrm{S}}_t},$$

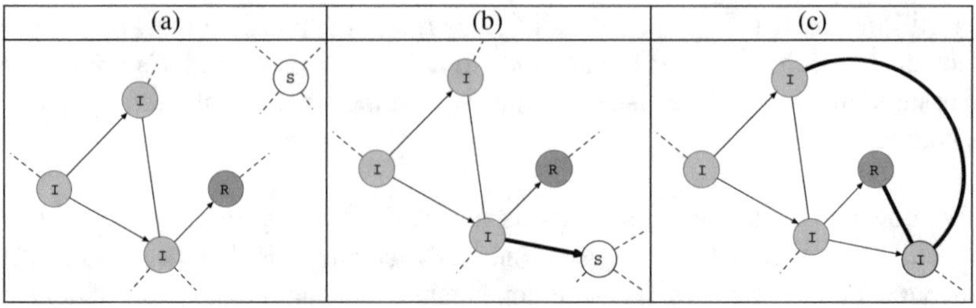

Fig. 3.3.1 *Infection process. Arrows provide the infection tree. Susceptible, infectious and removed individuals are colored in white, grey and dark grey respectively. (a) The degree of each individual is known, and for each infectious (resp. removed) individual, we know his/her number of edges of type* IS *(resp.* RS*). (b) A contaminating half edge is chosen and a susceptible of degree k is infected at time t with the rate $\Lambda_t(k)$ defined in (3.3.13). The contaminating edge is drawn in bold line. The number N^{IS}_{t-} of edges from* I *to* S *momentarily becomes $N^{\mathrm{IS}}_{t-}-1+(k-1)$. (c) Once the susceptible individual has been infected, we determine how many of its remaining arrows are linked to the classes* I *and* R*. If we denote by j and ℓ these numbers, then $N^{\mathrm{IS}}_t = N^{\mathrm{IS}}_{t-}-1+(k-1)-j-\ell$ and $N^{\mathrm{RS}}_t = N^{\mathrm{RS}}_{t-}-\ell$.*

is the proportion of edges linked to susceptible individuals that can transmit the disease. It is the discrete stochastic quantity that we expect will converge to (3.2.5).

Starting from t, and because of the properties of exponential distributions, the next event will take place after an exponentially distributed time with parameter $\lambda N^{\mathrm{IS}}_t + \gamma I_t$. Let T denote the time of this event after t.

Case 1 The next event corresponds to a removal, i.e., a node goes from status I to status R. Choose uniformly $u \in I_{T-}$ (with probability $1/I_{T-}$, then update the measures $\mu^{\mathrm{IS}}_{T_-}$ and $\mu^{\mathrm{RS}}_{T_-}$:

$$\mu^{\mathrm{IS}}_T = \mu^{\mathrm{IS}}_{T-} - \delta_{D_u(\mathrm{S}_{T_-})} \text{ and } \mu^{\mathrm{RS}}_T = \mu^{\mathrm{RS}}_{T-} + \delta_{D_u(\mathrm{S}_{T_-})}.$$

Case 2 The next event corresponds to a new infection. We choose uniformly a half-edge with susceptible alter, and this alter becomes infectious. The new infective has degree k with probability $k\mu^{\mathrm{S}}_{T_-}(k)/N^{\mathrm{S}}_{T_-}$. When the new individual is 'discovered' by the disease, she/he reveals her/his links with other infectious or removed individuals. The probability, given that the degree of the individual is k and that j (resp. ℓ) out of her $k-1$ other half-edges (all but the contaminating IS edge) are chosen to be of type II (resp. IR), according to Step 2', is given by the following multivariate hypergeometric distribution:

$$p_{T_-}(j,\ell\,|\,k-1) = \frac{\binom{N^{\mathrm{IS}}_{T_-}-1}{j}\binom{N^{\mathrm{RS}}_{T_-}}{\ell}\binom{N^{\mathrm{S}}_{T_-}-N^{\mathrm{IS}}_{T_-}-N^{\mathrm{RS}}_{T_-}}{k-1-j-\ell}}{\binom{N^{\mathrm{S}}_{T_-}-1}{k-1}}. \tag{3.3.3}$$

Finally, to update the values of μ^{IS}_T and μ^{RS}_T given k, j and ℓ, we have to choose the infectious and removed individuals to which the newly infectious is linked: some of their edges, which were IS or RS, now become II or RI. We draw two sequences of integers $\underline{n} = (n_1, \dots, n_{I_{T\_}})$ and $\underline{m} = (m_1, \dots, m_{R_{T\_}})$ that will indicate how many links each infectious or removed individual has to the newly contaminated individual. There exist constraints on these sequences: the number of edges recorded for each individual by the vectors $\underline{n}$ and $\underline{m}$ can not exceed the number of existing edges. Let us define the set

$$\mathscr{L} = \bigcup_{m=1}^{+\infty} \mathbb{Z}_+^m, \tag{3.3.4}$$

and for all finite integer-valued measure μ on $\mathbb{Z}_+$, corresponding to a degree distribution as in Section 3.3.1, and whose atoms are labelled say, according to Definition (3.3.2) and for all integer $\ell \in \mathbb{Z}_+$, we define the subset

$$\mathscr{L}(\ell,\mu) = \Big\{ \underline{n} = (n_1, \dots, n_{\langle \mu, \mathbf{1} \rangle}) \in \mathbb{Z}_+^{\langle \mu, \mathbf{1} \rangle} \quad \text{such that} \\ \forall u \in \{1, \dots, \langle \mu, \mathbf{1} \rangle\}, n_u \leq D_u(\mu) \text{ and } \sum_{u=1}^{\langle \mu, \mathbf{1} \rangle} n_u = \ell \Big\}, \tag{3.3.5}$$

where $D_u(\mu)$ stands for the degree of the vertex u, read from the measure μ (see Example 3.3.3). Each sequence $\underline{n} \in \mathscr{L}(\ell,\mu)$ provides a possible configuration of how the ℓ connections of a given individual can be shared between neighbours whose degrees are summed up by μ. The component n_u, for $1 \leq u \leq \langle \mu, 1 \rangle$, provides the number of edges that this individual shares with the individual u. This number is necessarily smaller than the degree $D_u(\mu)$ of individual u. Moreover, the components of the vector $\underline{n}$ sum to ℓ. The probabilities of the draws of $\underline{n}$ and $\underline{m}$ that provide respectively the number of edges $\text{I}-\text{S}$ which become $\text{I}-\text{I}$ per infectious individual and the number of edges $\text{R}-\text{S}$ which become $\text{R}-\text{I}$ per removed individual are given by:

$$\rho(\underline{n} | j+1, \mu_{T\_}^{\text{IS}}) = \frac{\prod_{u \in \text{I}_{T\_}} \binom{D_u(\text{S}_{T\_})}{n_u}}{\binom{N_{T\_}^{\text{IS}}}{j+1}} \mathbf{1}_{\underline{n} \in \mathscr{L}(j+1, \mu_{T\_}^{\text{IS}})}$$

$$\rho(\underline{m} | \ell, \mu_{T\_}^{\text{RS}}) = \frac{\prod_{v \in \text{R}_{T\_}} \binom{D_v(\text{S}_{T\_})}{m_v}}{\binom{N_{T\_}^{\text{RS}}}{\ell}} \mathbf{1}_{\underline{m} \in \mathscr{L}(\ell, \mu_{T\_}^{\text{RS}})}. \tag{3.3.6}$$

Note that $I_{T\_} = \langle \mu_{T\_}^{\text{IS}}, 1 \rangle$ is the total mass of the measure $\mu_{T\_}^{\text{IS}}$ and that $D_u(\text{S}_{T\_})$ corresponds to the degree of the individual u encoded by $\mu_{T\_}^{\text{IS}}$ with the labelling of Definition 3.3.2, i.e. to the number of edges from u to S before time T.

Then, we update the measures as follows:

$$\mu_T^{\text{S}} = \mu_{T-}^{\text{S}} - \delta_k$$
$$\mu_T^{\text{IS}} = \mu_{T-}^{\text{IS}} + \delta_{k-1-j-\ell} + \sum_{u \in \text{I}_{T\_}} \left(\delta_{D_u(\text{S}_{T\_}) - n_u} - \delta_{D_u(\text{S}_{T\_})} \right)$$

$$\mu_T^{\text{RS}} = \mu_{T-}^{\text{RS}} + \sum_{v \in \text{R}_{T-}} \left(\delta_{D_v(\text{S}_{T-}) - m_v} - \delta_{D_v(\text{S}_{T-})} \right). \tag{3.3.7}$$

Here, we propose stochastic differential equations (SDEs) driven by Poisson point measures (PPMs) to describe the evolution of the degree distributions (3.3.1) as in [44].

We consider two Poisson point measures Q^1 and Q^2 on $E_1 := \mathbb{Z}_+ \times \mathbb{R}_+ \times \mathbb{Z}_+ \times \mathbb{Z}_+ \times \mathbb{R}_+ \times \mathscr{L} \times \mathbb{R}_+ \times \mathscr{L} \times \mathbb{R}_+$ and $\mathbb{R}_+ \times \mathbb{Z}_+$ with intensity measures the product of Lebesgue measures on $\mathbb{R}_+$ and the of counting measures on each discrete set. The atoms of the point measure Q^1 are of the form $(s,k,\theta_1,j,\ell,\theta_2,\underline{n},\theta_3,\underline{m},\theta_4)$. They provide possible times s at which an infection may occur, and gives an integer k corresponding to the degree of the susceptible being possibly infected, the numbers $j+1$ and ℓ of edges that this individual has to the sets $\text{I}_{s\_}$ and $\text{R}_{s\_}$. The marks $\underline{n}$ and $\underline{m} \in \mathscr{L}$ are as in the previous section. The marks θ_1, θ_2 and θ_3 are auxiliary variables used for the construction (see (3.3.9)–(3.3.10)) below.
The atoms of the point measure Q^2 are of the form (s,u) and give possible removal times s associated with the label u of the individual that may be removed.

The following SDEs describe the evolution of the epidemic: for all $t \geq 0$,

$$\mu_t^{\text{S}} = \mu_0^{\text{S}} - \int_0^t \int_{E_1} \delta_k \mathbf{1}_{\theta_1 \leq \Lambda_{s\_}(k)\mu_{s\_}^{\text{S}}(k)} \tag{3.3.8}$$
$$\mathbf{1}_{\theta_2 \leq p_{s\_}(j,\ell|k-1)} \mathbf{1}_{\theta_3 \leq \rho(\underline{n}|j+1,\mu_{s\_}^{\text{IS}})} \mathbf{1}_{\theta_4 \leq \rho(\underline{m}|\ell,\mu_{s\_}^{\text{RS}})} \, \mathrm{d}Q^1$$

$$\mu_t^{\text{IS}} = \mu_0^{\text{IS}} + \int_0^t \int_{E_1} \Big(\delta_{k-(j+1+\ell)} + \sum_{u \in \text{I}_{s\_}} \big(\delta_{D_u(\mu_{s\_}^{\text{IS}}) - n_u} - \delta_{D_u(\mu_{s\_}^{\text{IS}})} \big) \Big) \tag{3.3.9}$$
$$\times \mathbf{1}_{\theta_1 \leq \Lambda_{s\_}(k)\mu_{s\_}^{\text{S}}(k)} \mathbf{1}_{\theta_2 \leq p_{s\_}(j,\ell|k-1)} \mathbf{1}_{\theta_3 \leq \rho(\underline{n}|j+1,\mu_{s\_}^{\text{IS}})} \mathbf{1}_{\theta_4 \leq \rho(\underline{m}|\ell,\mu_{s\_}^{\text{RS}})} \, \mathrm{d}Q^1$$
$$- \int_0^t \int_{\mathbb{Z}_+} \delta_{D_u(\mu_{s\_}^{\text{IS}})} \mathbf{1}_{u \in \text{I}_{s\_}} \, \mathrm{d}Q^2$$

$$\mu_t^{\text{RS}} = \mu_0^{\text{RS}} + \int_0^t \int_{E_1} \Big(\sum_{v \in \text{R}_{s\_}} \big(\delta_{D_v(\mu_{s\_}^{\text{RS}}) - m_v} - \delta_{D_v(\mu_{s\_}^{\text{RS}})} \big) \Big) \tag{3.3.10}$$
$$\times \mathbf{1}_{\theta_1 \leq \Lambda_{s\_}(k)\mu_{s\_}^{\text{S}}(k)} \mathbf{1}_{\theta_2 \leq p_{s\_}(j,\ell|k-1)} \mathbf{1}_{\theta_3 \leq \rho(\underline{n}|j+1,\mu_{s\_}^{\text{IS}})} \mathbf{1}_{\theta_4 \leq \rho(\underline{m}|\ell,\mu_{s\_}^{\text{RS}})} \, \mathrm{d}Q^1$$
$$+ \int_0^t \int_{\mathbb{Z}_+} \delta_{D_u(\mu_{s\_}^{\text{IS}})} \mathbf{1}_{u \in \text{I}_{s\_}} \, \mathrm{d}Q^2,$$

where we write $\mathrm{d}Q^1$ and $\mathrm{d}Q^2$ instead of $\mathrm{d}Q^1(s,k,\theta_1,j,\ell,\theta_2,\underline{n},\theta_3,\underline{m},\theta_4)$ and $\mathrm{d}Q^2(s,u)$ to simplify the notation.

Proposition 3.3.4. *For any given initial conditions μ_0^{S}, μ_0^{SI} and μ_0^{RS} that are integer-valued measures on $\mathbb{Z}_+$ and for PPMs Q^1 and Q^2, there exists a unique strong solution to the SDEs (3.3.8)–(3.3.10) in the space $\mathbb{D}(\mathbb{R}_+, (\mathscr{M}_F(\mathbb{Z}_+))^3)$, the Skorokhod space of càdlàg functions with values in $(\mathscr{M}_F(\mathbb{Z}_+))^3$.*

Proof. For the proof, we notice that for every $t \in \mathbb{R}_+$, the measure μ_t^{S} is dominated by μ_0^{S} and the measures μ_t^{IS} and μ_t^{RS} have a mass bounded by $\langle \mu_0^{\text{S}} + \mu_0^{\text{IS}} + \mu_0^{\text{RS}}, 1 \rangle$ and a support included in $[\![0,\max\{\max(\mathrm{supp}(\mu_0^{\mathrm{S}})),\max(\mathrm{supp}(\mu_0^{\mathrm{IS}})),\max(\mathrm{supp}(\mu_0^{\mathrm{RS}}))\}]\!]$. The result then follows the steps of [55] and [105] (Proposition 2.2.6) where a pathwise construction of the solution on the positive real line is given using the Poisson point processes Q^1 and Q^2. □

The course of the epidemic can be deduced from (3.3.8), (3.3.9) and (3.3.10). For the sizes $(S_t,I_t,R_t)_{t\in\mathbb{R}_+}$ of the different classes, for instance, we have with the choice of $f\equiv 1$ that for all $t\geq 0$, $S_t=\langle\mu_t^{\mathrm{S}},\mathbf{1}\rangle$, $I_t=\langle\mu_t^{\mathrm{IS}},\mathbf{1}\rangle$ and $R_t=\langle\mu_t^{\mathrm{RS}},\mathbf{1}\rangle$ (see Notation 0.0.1). Writing the semi-martingale decomposition that results from standard stochastic calculus for jump processes and SDE driven by PPMs (e.g. [55, 62, 63]), we obtain for example:

$$I_t=\langle\mu_t^{\mathrm{IS}},\mathbf{1}\rangle=I_0+\int_0^t\Big(\sum_{k\in\mathbb{Z}_+}\mu_s^{\mathrm{S}}(k)\Lambda_s(k)-\gamma I_s\Big)\,\mathrm{d}s+M_t^{\mathrm{I}},\tag{3.3.11}$$

where M^{I} is a square-integrable martingale that can be written explicitly as a stochastic integral with respect to the compensated PPMs of Q^1 and Q^2, and with predictable quadratic variation given for all $t\geq 0$ by

$$\langle M^{\mathrm{I}}\rangle_t=\int_0^t\sum_{k\in\mathbb{Z}_+}\Big(\mu_s^{\mathrm{S}}(k)\Lambda_s(k)+\gamma I_s\Big)\,\mathrm{d}s.$$

Other quantities of interest are the numbers of edges of the different types NS_t, N_t^{IS}, N_t^{RS}. The latter appear as the first moments of the measures μ_t^{S}, μ_t^{IS} and μ_t^{RS}:

$$NS_t=\langle\mu_t^{\mathrm{S}},\chi\rangle,\quad N_t^{\mathrm{IS}}=\langle\mu_t^{\mathrm{IS}},\chi\rangle\quad\text{and}\quad N_t^{\mathrm{RS}}=\langle\mu_t^{\mathrm{RS}},\chi\rangle.$$

3.3.3 Rescaling

We consider a sequence of larger and larger graphs $(\mathscr{G}_N)_{N\geq 1}$ with $N\to+\infty$. The degree distribution $\mathbf{p}$ underlying these CM graphs remains unchanged with N.
The sequences of measures $(\mu^{\mathrm{N,S}})_{N\in\mathbb{N}}$, $(\mu^{\mathrm{N,IS}})_{N\in\mathbb{N}}$ and $(\mu^{\mathrm{N,RS}})_{n\in\mathbb{N}}$ are defined as

$$\mu_t^{\mathrm{N,S}}=\frac{1}{N}\mu_t^{\mathrm{S}},\qquad\mu_t^{\mathrm{N,IS}}=\frac{1}{N}\mu_t^{\mathrm{IS}},\qquad\mu_t^{\mathrm{N,RS}}=\frac{1}{N}\mu_t^{\mathrm{RS}}\tag{3.3.12}$$

where the measures non-rescaled μ^{S}, μ^{IS} and μ^{RS} are defined as in (3.3.1) and implicitly depend on N:

$$\langle\mu_t^{\mathrm{N,S}},1\rangle+\langle\mu^{\mathrm{N,IS}},1\rangle+\langle\mu^{\mathrm{N,RS}},1\rangle=\frac{N}{N}=1.$$

The proportions S_t^{N}, I_t^{N} and R_t^{N} defined in (3.1.1) can then be rewritten as $S_t^{\mathrm{N}}=\langle\mu^{\mathrm{N,S}},1\rangle$, $I_t^{\mathrm{N}}=\langle\mu^{\mathrm{N,IS}},1\rangle$ and $R_t^{\mathrm{N}}=\langle\mu^{\mathrm{N,RS}},1\rangle$. Also, we have $N_t^{\mathrm{N,S}}=\langle\mu^{\mathrm{N,S}},\chi\rangle$, $N_t^{\mathrm{N,IS}}=\langle\mu^{\mathrm{N,IS}},\chi\rangle$ and $N_t^{\mathrm{N,RS}}=\langle\mu^{\mathrm{N,RS}},\chi\rangle$, the numbers, renormalized by N, of edges with susceptible ego, infectious ego and susceptible alter, removed ego and susceptible alter.

We assume that the initial conditions satisfy:

Assumption 3.3.5. The sequences $(\mu_0^{\text{N,S}})_{n\in\mathbb{N}}$, $(\mu_0^{\text{N,IS}})_{n\in\mathbb{N}}$ and $(\mu_0^{\text{N,RS}})_{n\in\mathbb{N}}$ converge to measures $\bar{\mu}_0^{\text{S}}$, $\bar{\mu}_0^{\text{IS}}$ and $\bar{\mu}_0^{\text{RS}}$ in $\mathscr{M}_F(\mathbb{Z}_+)$ equipped with the topology of weak convergence.

Remark 3.3.6. 1. Assumption 3.3.5 entails that the initial (susceptible and infectious) population size is of order N if $\bar{\mu}_0^{\text{S}}$ and $\bar{\mu}_0^{\text{IS}}$ are nontrivial.
2. If the distributions underlying the measures $\mu_0^{\text{N,S}}$, $\mu_0^{\text{N,IS}}$ and $\mu_0^{\text{N,RS}}$ do not depend on the total number of vertices (e.g. Poisson, power-laws or geometric distributions), Assumption 3.3.5 can be viewed as a law of large numbers. When the distributions depend on the total number of vertices N (as in Erdös-Renyi graphs), there may be scalings under which Assumption 3.3.5 holds. For Erdös-Renyi graphs for instance, if the probability p_N of connecting two vertices satisfies $\lim_{N\to+\infty} Np_N = \lambda$, then we obtain in the limit a Poisson distribution with parameter λ.
3. Notice the appearance in Equation (3.3.2) of the size biased degree distribution. The latter reflects the fact that, in the CM, individuals having large degrees have higher probability to connect than individuals having small degrees. Thus, there is no reason why the degree distributions of the susceptible individuals $\bar{\mu}_0^{\text{S}}/\bar{S}_0$ and the distribution $\sum_{k\in\mathbb{Z}_+} p_k\delta_k$ underlying the CM should coincide. This is developed in Section 3.3.6. □

It is possible to write rescaled SDEs which are the same as the SDEs (3.3.8)–(3.3.10) parameterized by N (see [44] for details). Several semi-martingale decompositions will be useful in the sequel. We focus on $\mu^{\text{N,IS}}$ but similar decompositions hold for $\mu^{\text{N,S}}$ and $\mu^{\text{N,RS}}$, which we do not detail since they can be deduced by direct adaptation of the computation which follows.

Proposition 3.3.7. *Define:*

$$\Lambda_s^N(k) = \lambda k \frac{N_s^{\text{N,IS}}}{N_s^{\text{N,S}}}, \text{ and } p_s^N(j,\ell \mid k-1) = \frac{\binom{N_s^{\text{N,IS}}-1}{j}\binom{N_s^{\text{N,RS}}}{\ell}\binom{N_s^{\text{N,S}}-N_s^{\text{N,IS}}-N_s^{\text{N,RS}}}{k-1-j-\ell}}{\binom{N_s^{\text{N,S}}-1}{k-1}}. \tag{3.3.13}$$

For all $f \in \mathscr{B}_b(\mathbb{Z}_+)$, for all $t \geq 0$,

$$\langle \mu_t^{\text{N,IS}}, f\rangle = \sum_{k\in\mathbb{Z}_+} f(k)\mu_0^{\text{N,IS}}(k) + A_t^{\text{N,IS},f} + M_t^{\text{N,IS},f}, \tag{3.3.14}$$

where the finite variation part $A_t^{\text{N,IS},f}$ of $\langle \mu_t^{\text{N,IS}}, f\rangle$ reads

$$\begin{aligned} A_t^{\text{N,IS},f} = &\int_0^t \sum_{k\in\mathbb{Z}_+} \Lambda_s^N(k)\mu_s^{\text{N,S}}(k) \sum_{j+\ell+1\leq k} p_s^N(j,\ell|k-1) \sum_{\underline{n}\in\mathscr{L}} \rho(\underline{n}|j+1,\mu_s^{\text{N,IS}}) \\ &\times \Big(f(k-(j+1+\ell)) + \sum_{u\in I_s^{\text{N}}} \big(f(D_u(\text{S}_s)-n_u) - f(D_u(\text{S}_s))\big)\Big)\, ds \\ &- \int_0^t \gamma\langle \mu_s^{\text{N,IS}}, f\rangle\, ds, \end{aligned} \tag{3.3.15}$$

and where the martingale part $M_t^{\mathrm{N,IS},f}$ of $\langle \mu_t^{\mathrm{N,IS}}, f\rangle$ is a square integrable martingale starting from 0 with quadratic variation

$$\begin{aligned}\langle M^{N,\mathrm{IS},f}\rangle_t =& \frac{1}{N}\int_0^t \gamma\langle \mu_s^{\mathrm{N,IS}}, f^2\rangle\, ds\\ &+\frac{1}{N}\int_0^t \sum_{k\in\mathbb{Z}_+} \Lambda_s^N(k)\mu_s^{\mathrm{N,S}}(k) \sum_{j+\ell+1\leq k} p_s^N(j,\ell|k-1)\sum_{\underline{n}\in\mathscr{L}} \rho(\underline{n}|j+1,\mu_s^{\mathrm{N,IS}})\\ &\times\Big(f(k-(j+1+\ell)) + \sum_{u\in I_s^{\mathrm{N}}} \big(f\big(D_u(\mu_s^{\mathrm{N,IS}})-n_u\big) - f\big(D_u(\mu_s^{\mathrm{N,IS}})\big)\big)\Big)^2\, ds.\end{aligned}$$

Proof. The proof proceeds from standard stochastic calculus for jump processes, using the SDEs driven by Poisson point processes (see the appendices of Part I of this volume or [44, 62]). □

3.3.4 Large Graph Limit

We prove that the rescaled degree distributions mentioned above can then be approximated for large N, by the solution $(\bar{\mu}_t^{\mathrm{S}}, \bar{\mu}_t^{\mathrm{IS}}, \bar{\mu}_t^{\mathrm{RS}})_{t\geq 0}$ of a system of deterministic measure-valued equations, with initial conditions $\bar{\mu}_0^{\mathrm{S}}$, $\bar{\mu}_0^{\mathrm{IS}}$ and $\bar{\mu}_0^{\mathrm{RS}}$.

We denote by $\bar{S}_t$ (resp. $\bar{I}_t$ and $\bar{R}_t$) the mass of the measure $\bar{\mu}_t^{\mathrm{S}}$ (resp. $\bar{\mu}_t^{\mathrm{IS}}$ and $\bar{\mu}_t^{\mathrm{RS}}$). As for the finite graph, $\bar{\mu}_t^{\mathrm{S}}/\bar{S}_t$ (resp. $\bar{\mu}_t^{\mathrm{IS}}/\bar{I}_t$ and $\bar{\mu}_t^{\mathrm{RS}}/\bar{R}_t$) is the probability degree distribution of the susceptible individuals (resp. the probability distribution of the degrees of the infectious and removed individuals towards the susceptible ones). For all $t\geq 0$, we denote by $\bar{N}_t^{\mathrm{S}} = \langle \bar{\mu}_t^{\mathrm{S}}, \chi\rangle$ (resp. $\bar{N}_t^{\mathrm{IS}} = \langle \bar{\mu}_t^{\mathrm{IS}}, \chi\rangle$ and $\bar{N}_t^{\mathrm{RS}} = \langle \bar{\mu}_t^{\mathrm{RS}}, \chi\rangle$) the continuous number of edges with ego in S (resp. I − S edges, R − S edges). Following Volz [110], pertinent quantities are the proportions $\bar{p}_t^{\mathrm{I}} = \bar{N}_t^{\mathrm{IS}}/\bar{N}_t^{\mathrm{S}}$ (resp. $\bar{p}_t^{\mathrm{R}} = \bar{N}_t^{\mathrm{RS}}/\bar{N}_t^{\mathrm{S}}$ and $\bar{p}_t^{\mathrm{S}} = (\bar{N}_t^{\mathrm{S}} - \bar{N}_t^{\mathrm{IS}} - \bar{N}_t^{\mathrm{RS}})/\bar{N}_t^{\mathrm{S}}$) of edges with infectious (respectively removed, susceptible) alter among those having susceptible ego. We also introduce

$$\theta_t = \exp\Big(-\lambda\int_0^t \bar{p}_s^{\mathrm{I}}\, \mathrm{d}s\Big) \tag{3.3.16}$$

the probability that a degree one node remains susceptible until time t. The limiting measure-valued equation expresses for any bounded real function f on $\mathbb{Z}_+$ as:

$$\langle \bar{\mu}_t^{\mathrm{S}}, f\rangle = \sum_{k\in\mathbb{Z}_+} \bar{\mu}_0^{\mathrm{S}}(k)\,\theta_t^k f(k), \tag{3.3.17}$$

$$\begin{aligned}\langle \bar{\mu}_t^{\mathrm{IS}}, f\rangle =& \langle \bar{\mu}_0^{\mathrm{IS}}, f\rangle - \int_0^t \gamma\langle \bar{\mu}_s^{\mathrm{IS}}, f\rangle\, \mathrm{d}s\\ &+\int_0^t \sum_{k\in\mathbb{Z}_+} \lambda k \bar{p}_s^{\mathrm{I}} \sum_{\substack{j,\ell,m\in\mathbb{Z}_+\\ j+\ell+m=k-1}} \binom{k-1}{j,\ell,m} (\bar{p}_s^{\mathrm{I}})^j (\bar{p}_s^{\mathrm{R}})^\ell (\bar{p}_s^{\mathrm{S}})^m f(m)\bar{\mu}_s^{\mathrm{S}}(k)\, \mathrm{d}s\end{aligned} \tag{3.3.18}$$

$$+\int_0^t \sum_{k\in\mathbb{Z}_+} \lambda k \bar{p}_s^{\mathrm{I}}(1+(k-1)\bar{p}_s^{\mathrm{I}}) \sum_{k'\in\mathbb{N}} \big(f(k'-1)-f(k')\big)\frac{k'\bar{\mu}_s^{\mathrm{IS}}(k')}{\bar{N}_s^{\mathrm{IS}}}\bar{\mu}_s^{\mathrm{S}}(k)\,\mathrm{d}s,$$

$$\langle \bar{\mu}_t^{\mathrm{RS}}, f\rangle = \langle \bar{\mu}_0^{\mathrm{RS}}, f\rangle + \int_0^t \gamma\langle \bar{\mu}_s^{\mathrm{IS}}, f\rangle\,\mathrm{d}s \tag{3.3.19}$$

$$+\int_0^t \sum_{k\in\mathbb{Z}_+} \lambda k \bar{p}_s^{\mathrm{I}}(k-1)\bar{p}_s^{\mathrm{R}} \sum_{k'\in\mathbb{N}} \big(f(k'-1)-f(k')\big)\frac{k'\bar{\mu}_s^{\mathrm{RS}}(k')}{\bar{N}_s^{\mathrm{RS}}}\bar{\mu}_s^{\mathrm{S}}(k)\,\mathrm{d}s.$$

Let us give a heuristic explanation of Equations (3.3.17)–(3.3.19). Notice that the limiting graph is infinite. The probability that an individual of degree k has been infected by none of her k edges is θ_t^k and Equation (3.3.17) follows. In Equation (3.3.18), the first integral corresponds to infectious individuals being removed. In the second integral, $\lambda k \bar{p}_s^{\mathrm{I}}$ is the rate of infection of a given susceptible individual of degree k. Once she gets infected, the multinomial term determines the number of edges connected to susceptible, infectious and removed neighbours. Multi-edges are not encountered in the limiting graph. Each infectious neighbour has a degree chosen according to the size-biased distribution $k'\bar{\mu}^{\mathrm{IS}}(k')/\bar{N}^{\mathrm{IS}}$ and the number of edges to S is reduced by 1. This explains the third integral. Similar arguments explain Equation (3.3.19).

Before stating the theorem, let us introduce the following state space. For any $\varepsilon \geq 0$ and $A > 0$, we define the following closed set of $\mathcal{M}_F(\mathbb{Z}_+)$ as

$$\mathcal{M}_{\varepsilon,A} = \{\nu \in \mathcal{M}_F(\mathbb{Z}_+)\ ;\ \langle \nu, \mathbf{1}+\chi^5\rangle \leq A \text{ and } \langle \nu, \chi\rangle \geq \varepsilon\} \tag{3.3.20}$$

and $\mathcal{M}_{0+,A} = \cup_{\varepsilon>0}\mathcal{M}_{\varepsilon,A}$.

Theorem 3.3.8. *Suppose that Assumption 3.3.5 holds and that there exists an $A > 0$ such that*

$$\big(\mu_0^{N,\mathrm{S}}, \mu_0^{N,\mathrm{IS}}, \mu_0^{N,\mathrm{RS}}\big) \text{ in } (\mathcal{M}_{0,A})^3 \text{ for any } N, \text{ with } \langle \bar{\mu}_0^{\mathrm{IS}}, \chi\rangle > 0. \tag{3.3.21}$$

Then, as N converges to infinity, the sequence $(\mu^{N,\mathrm{S}}, \mu^{N,\mathrm{IS}}, \mu^{N,\mathrm{RS}})_{N\in\mathbb{N}}$ converges in distribution in $\mathbb{D}(\mathbb{R}_+, \mathcal{M}_{0,A}^3)$ to $(\bar{\mu}^{\mathrm{S}}, \bar{\mu}^{\mathrm{IS}}, \bar{\mu}^{\mathrm{RS}})$ which is the unique solution of the deterministic system equations (3.3.17)–(3.3.19) in $\mathscr{C}(\mathbb{R}_+, \mathcal{M}_{0,A} \times \mathcal{M}_{0+,A} \times \mathcal{M}_{0,A})$.

The proof is detailed in Section 3.3.7 and follows standard arguments. First, tightness of the process is proved using the Roelly and Aldous–Rebolledo criteria [99, 66]. Then, the convergence of the generators is studied, which allows us to identify the limit, provided the number of edges S − I remains of order at least εN. For proving uniqueness of the limiting value, we show using Gronwall's lemma that any two solutions of the limiting equation have the same mass and the same moments of order 1 and 2. This allows us to show the uniqueness of the generating function of $\bar{\mu}^{\mathrm{IS}}$ which solves a transport equation.

The assumption of moments of order 5 are needed for the convergence of the generators and discussed in Section 3.3.6.

3.3.5 Ball–Neal and Volz' Equations

Choosing $f(k) = \mathbf{1}_i(k)$, we obtain the following countable system of ordinary differential equations (ODEs).

$$\begin{aligned}
\bar{\mu}_t^{\mathrm{S}}(i) =& \bar{\mu}_0^{\mathrm{S}}(i)\theta_t^i,\\
\bar{\mu}_t^{\mathrm{IS}}(i) =& \bar{\mu}_0^{\mathrm{IS}}(i) - \int_0^t \gamma \bar{\mu}_s^{\mathrm{IS}}(i)\,\mathrm{d}s\\
&+ \int_0^t \lambda \bar{p}_s^{\mathrm{I}} \sum_{j,\ell\geq 0} (i+j+\ell+1)\bar{\mu}_s^{\mathrm{S}}(i+j+\ell+1)\binom{i+j+\ell}{i,j,\ell}(\bar{p}_s^{\mathrm{S}})^i(\bar{p}_s^{\mathrm{I}})^j(\bar{p}_s^{\mathrm{R}})^\ell\,\mathrm{d}s\\
&+ \int_0^t \Big(\lambda(\bar{p}_s^{\mathrm{I}})^2\langle\bar{\mu}_s^{\mathrm{S}},\chi^2-\chi\rangle + \lambda\bar{p}_s^{\mathrm{I}}\langle\bar{\mu}_s^{\mathrm{S}},\chi\rangle\Big)\frac{(i+1)\bar{\mu}_s^{\mathrm{IS}}(i+1) - i\bar{\mu}_s^{\mathrm{IS}}(i)}{\langle\bar{\mu}_s^{\mathrm{IS}},\chi\rangle}\,\mathrm{d}s,\\
\bar{\mu}_t^{\mathrm{RS}}(i) =& \bar{\mu}_0^{\mathrm{RS}}(i)\\
&+ \int_0^t \left\{\beta\bar{\mu}_s^{\mathrm{IS}}(i) + \lambda\bar{p}_s^{\mathrm{I}}\langle\bar{\mu}_s^{\mathrm{S}},\chi^2-\chi\rangle\bar{p}_s^{\mathrm{R}}\frac{(i+1)\bar{\mu}_s^{\mathrm{RS}}(i+1) - i\bar{\mu}_s^{\mathrm{RS}}(i)}{\langle\bar{\mu}_s^{\mathrm{RS}},\chi\rangle}\right\}\mathrm{d}s,
\end{aligned} \tag{3.3.22}$$

It is noteworthy to say that this system corresponds to that in Ball and Neal [13].

The system (3.3.17)–(3.3.19) allows us to recover the equations proposed by Volz [110, Table 3, p. 297] (see also Proposition 3.2.3). The latter are obtained directly from (3.3.17)–(3.3.19) and the definitions of $\bar{S}_t$, $\bar{I}_t$, $\bar{p}_t^{\mathrm{I}}$ and $\bar{p}_t^{\mathrm{S}}$ which relate these quantities to the measures $\bar{\mu}_t^{\mathrm{S}}$ and $\bar{\mu}_t^{\mathrm{IS}}$. Let

$$h(z) = \sum_{k\in\mathbb{Z}_+} \bar{\mu}_0^{\mathrm{S}}(k)z^k \tag{3.3.23}$$

be the generating function for the initial degree distribution of the susceptible individuals $\bar{\mu}_0^{\mathrm{S}}$. This generating function is *a priori* different from the generating function of the degree distribution of the total CM graph: $g(z) = \sum_{k\in\mathbb{Z}_+} p_k z^k$. Let also $\theta_t = \exp(-\lambda\int_0^t \bar{p}_s^{\mathrm{I}}\,\mathrm{d}s)$. Then:

$$\bar{S}_t = \langle\bar{\mu}_t^{\mathrm{S}},\mathbf{1}\rangle = h(\theta_t), \tag{3.3.24}$$

$$\bar{I}_t = \langle\bar{\mu}_t^{\mathrm{IS}},\mathbf{1}\rangle = \bar{I}_0 + \int_0^t \Big(\lambda\bar{p}_s^{\mathrm{I}}\theta_s h'(\theta_s) - \gamma\bar{I}_s\Big)\,\mathrm{d}s, \tag{3.3.25}$$

$$\bar{p}_t^{\mathrm{I}} = \bar{p}_0^{\mathrm{I}} + \int_0^t \Big(\lambda\,\bar{p}_s^{\mathrm{I}}\bar{p}_s^{\mathrm{S}}\theta_s\frac{h''(\theta_s)}{h'(\theta_s)} - \lambda\,\bar{p}_s^{\mathrm{I}}(1-\bar{p}_s^{\mathrm{I}}) - \gamma\bar{p}_s^{\mathrm{I}}\Big)\,\mathrm{d}s, \tag{3.3.26}$$

$$\bar{p}_t^{\mathrm{S}} = \bar{p}_0^{\mathrm{S}} + \int_0^t \lambda\bar{p}_s^{\mathrm{I}}\bar{p}_s^{\mathrm{S}}\Big(1-\theta_s\frac{h''(\theta_s)}{h'(\theta_s)}\Big)\,\mathrm{d}s. \tag{3.3.27}$$

Here, the graph structure appears through the generating function g. In (3.3.25), we see that the classical contamination terms $\lambda\bar{S}_t\bar{I}_t$ (mass action) or $\lambda\bar{S}_t\bar{I}_t/(\bar{S}_t+\bar{I}_t)$ (frequency dependence) of mixing SIR models (e.g. Part I of this volume or [5, 37]) are replaced by $\lambda\bar{p}_t^{\mathrm{I}}\theta_t h'(\theta_t) = \lambda\bar{N}_t^{\mathrm{IS}}$. The fact that new infectious individuals are chosen in the size-biased distribution is hidden in the term $h''(\theta_t)/h'(\theta_t)$.

Proposition 3.3.9. *The system* (3.3.17)–(3.3.19) *implies Volz' equations* (3.3.24)–(3.3.27).

Before proving Proposition 3.3.9, we begin with a corollary of Theorem 3.3.8.

Corollary 3.3.10. *For all* $t \in \mathbb{R}_+$

$$\begin{aligned}
\bar{N}^{\mathrm{S}}_t =&\theta_t h'(\theta_t)\\
\bar{N}^{\mathrm{IS}}_t =&\bar{N}^{\mathrm{IS}}_0 + \int_0^t \lambda \bar{p}^{\mathrm{I}}_s \theta_s h'(\theta_s)\Big((\bar{p}^{\mathrm{S}}_s - \bar{p}^{\mathrm{I}}_s)\theta_s \frac{h''(\theta_s)}{h'(\theta_s)} - 1\Big) - \gamma \bar{N}^{\mathrm{IS}}_s \, ds\\
\bar{N}^{\mathrm{RS}}_t =& \int_0^t \Big(\gamma \bar{N}^{\mathrm{IS}}_s - \lambda \bar{p}^{\mathrm{R}}_s \bar{p}^{\mathrm{I}}_s \theta_s^2 h''(\theta_s)\Big) \, ds.
\end{aligned} \tag{3.3.28}$$

Proof. In the proof of Proposition 3.3.12, we will show below that when $N \to +\infty$, $(N^{N,\mathrm{IS}}_t)_{N\in\mathbb{N}}$ converges uniformly, as $N \to +\infty$ and on compact intervals $[0,T]$, and in probability to the deterministic and continuous solution $\bar{N}^{\mathrm{IS}}$ such that for all t, $\bar{N}^{\mathrm{IS}}_t = \langle \bar{\mu}^{\mathrm{IS}}_t, \chi \rangle$. (3.3.17) with $f = \chi$ reads

$$\bar{N}^{\mathrm{S}}_t = \sum_{k\in\mathbb{Z}_+} \bar{\mu}^{\mathrm{S}}_0(k) k \theta_t^k = \theta_t \sum_{k=1}^{+\infty} \bar{\mu}^{\mathrm{S}}_0(k) k \theta_t^{k-1} = \theta_t h'(\theta_t), \tag{3.3.29}$$

i.e. the first assertion of (3.3.28).

Choosing $f = \chi$ in (3.3.18), we obtain

$$\begin{aligned}
\bar{N}^{\mathrm{IS}}_t = \bar{N}^{\mathrm{IS}}_0 - \int_0^t \gamma \bar{N}^{\mathrm{IS}}_s \, \mathrm{d}s + \int_0^t \sum_{k\in\mathbb{Z}_+} \Lambda_s(k) \sum_{j+\ell\leq k-1} (k-2j-2-\ell)\\
\times \Big[\frac{(k-1)!}{j!(k-1-j-\ell)!\ell!} (\bar{p}^{\mathrm{I}}_s)^j (\bar{p}^{\mathrm{R}}_s)^\ell (\bar{p}^{\mathrm{S}}_s)^{k-1-j-\ell}\Big] \bar{\mu}^{\mathrm{S}}_s(k) \, \mathrm{d}s.
\end{aligned}$$

Notice that the term in the square brackets is the probability of obtaining $(j,\ell,k-1-j-\ell)$ from a draw in the multinomial distribution of parameters $(k-1,(\bar{p}^{\mathrm{I}}_s, \bar{p}^{\mathrm{R}}_s, \bar{p}^{\mathrm{S}}_s))$. Hence,

$$\sum_{j+\ell\leq k-1} j \times \Big(\frac{(k-1)!}{j!(k-1-j-\ell)!\ell!} (\bar{p}^{\mathrm{I}}_s)^j (\bar{p}^{\mathrm{R}}_s)^\ell (\bar{p}^{\mathrm{S}}_s)^{k-1-j-\ell}\Big) = (k-1)\bar{p}^{\mathrm{I}}_s$$

as we recognize the mean number of edges to I_s of an individual of degree k. Other terms are treated similarly. Hence, with the definition of $\Lambda_s(k)$, (3.3.2),

$$\begin{aligned}
\bar{N}^{\mathrm{IS}}_t = \bar{N}^{\mathrm{IS}}_0 + \int_0^t \lambda \, \bar{p}^{\mathrm{I}}_s \Big(\langle \bar{\mu}^{\mathrm{S}}_s, \chi^2 - 2\chi \rangle - (2\bar{p}^{\mathrm{I}}_s + \bar{p}^{\mathrm{R}}_s)\langle \bar{\mu}^{\mathrm{S}}_s, \chi(\chi-1)\rangle\Big) \, \mathrm{d}s\\
- \int_0^t \gamma \bar{N}^{\mathrm{IS}}_s \, \mathrm{d}s.
\end{aligned}$$

But since

$$\langle \bar{\mu}_t^{\mathrm{S}}, \chi(\chi-1)\rangle = \sum_{k\in\mathbb{Z}_+} \bar{\mu}_0^{\mathrm{S}}(k)k(k-1)\theta_t^k = \theta_t^2 h''(\theta_t)$$

$$\langle \bar{\mu}_t^{\mathrm{S}}, \chi^2-2\chi\rangle = \langle \bar{\mu}_t^{\mathrm{S}}, \chi(\chi-1)\rangle - \langle \bar{\mu}_t^{\mathrm{S}}, \chi\rangle = \theta_t^2 h''(\theta_t) - \theta_t h'(\theta_t),$$

we obtain by noticing that $1-2\bar{p}_s^{\mathrm{I}} - \bar{p}_s^{\mathrm{R}} = \bar{p}_s^{\mathrm{S}} - \bar{p}_s^{\mathrm{I}}$,

$$\bar{N}_t^{\mathrm{IS}} = \bar{N}_0^{\mathrm{IS}} + \int_0^t \lambda\, \bar{p}_s^{\mathrm{I}}\Big((\bar{p}_s^{\mathrm{S}} - \bar{p}_s^{\mathrm{I}})\theta_s^2 h''(\theta_s) - \theta_s h'(\theta_s)\Big)\,\mathrm{d}s - \int_0^t \gamma \bar{N}_s^{\mathrm{IS}}\,\mathrm{d}s, \quad (3.3.30)$$

which is the second assertion of (3.3.28). The third equation is obtained similarly. □

We are now ready to prove Volz' equations:

Proof of Proposition 3.3.9. We begin with the proof of (3.3.24) and (3.3.25). Fix again $t \geq 0$. For the size of the susceptible population, taking $f = \mathbf{1}$ in (3.3.17) gives (3.3.24). For the size of the infective population, setting $f = \mathbf{1}$ in (3.3.18) entails

$$\begin{aligned}
\bar{I}_t =& \bar{I}_0 + \int_0^t \Big(\sum_{k\in\mathbb{Z}_+} \lambda k \bar{p}_s^{\mathrm{I}} \bar{\mu}_s^{\mathrm{S}}(k) - \gamma \bar{I}_s\Big)\,\mathrm{d}s \\
=& \bar{I}_0 + \int_0^t \Big(\lambda \bar{p}_s^{\mathrm{I}} \sum_{k\in\mathbb{Z}_+} \bar{\mu}_0^{\mathrm{S}}(k) k \theta_s^k - \gamma \bar{I}_s\Big)\,\mathrm{d}s \\
=& \bar{I}_0 + \int_0^t \Big(\lambda \bar{p}_s^{\mathrm{I}} \theta_s h'(\theta_s) - \gamma \bar{I}_s\Big)\,\mathrm{d}s
\end{aligned}$$

by using (3.3.17) with $f = \chi$ for the second equality.

Let us now consider the probability that an edge with a susceptible ego has an infectious alter. Both equations (3.3.24) and (3.3.25) depend on $\bar{p}_t^{\mathrm{I}} = \bar{N}_t^{\mathrm{IS}}/\bar{N}_t^{\mathrm{S}}$. It is thus important to obtain an equation for this quantity. In Volz [110], this equation also leads to introduce the quantity $\bar{p}_t^{\mathrm{S}}$.
From Corollary 3.3.10, we see that $\bar{N}^{\mathrm{S}}$ and $\bar{N}^{\mathrm{IS}}$ are differentiable and:

$$\begin{aligned}
\frac{\mathrm{d}\bar{p}_t^{\mathrm{I}}}{\mathrm{d}t} =& \frac{\mathrm{d}}{\mathrm{d}t}\Big(\frac{\bar{N}_t^{\mathrm{IS}}}{\bar{N}_t^{\mathrm{S}}}\Big) = \frac{1}{\bar{N}_t^{\mathrm{S}}}\frac{\mathrm{d}}{\mathrm{d}t}(\bar{N}_t^{\mathrm{IS}}) - \frac{\bar{N}_t^{\mathrm{IS}}}{(\bar{N}_t^{\mathrm{S}})^2}\frac{\mathrm{d}}{\mathrm{d}t}(\bar{N}_t^{\mathrm{S}}) \\
=& \Big(\lambda \bar{p}_t^{\mathrm{I}}(\bar{p}_t^{\mathrm{S}} - \bar{p}_t^{\mathrm{I}})\theta_t \frac{h''(\theta_t)}{h'(\theta_t)} - \lambda \bar{p}_t^{\mathrm{I}} - \gamma \bar{p}_t^{\mathrm{I}}\Big) \\
&- \Big(\frac{\bar{p}_t^{\mathrm{I}}}{\theta_t h'(\theta_t)}\big(-\lambda \bar{p}_t^{\mathrm{I}}\theta_t h'(\theta_t) + \theta_t h''(\theta_t)(-\lambda \bar{p}_t^{\mathrm{I}}\theta_t)\big)\Big) \\
=& \lambda \bar{p}_t^{\mathrm{I}} \bar{p}_t^{\mathrm{S}} \theta_t \frac{h''(\theta_t)}{h'(\theta_t)} - \lambda \bar{p}_t^{\mathrm{I}}(1 - \bar{p}_t^{\mathrm{I}}) - \gamma \bar{p}_t^{\mathrm{I}},
\end{aligned}$$

by using (3.3.28) for the derivatives of $\bar{N}^{\mathrm{S}}$ and $\bar{N}^{\mathrm{IS}}$ in the second line. This achieves the proof of (3.3.26).

For (3.3.27), we notice that $\bar{p}_t^{\mathrm{S}} = 1 - \bar{p}_t^{\mathrm{I}} - \bar{p}_t^{\mathrm{R}}$ and achieve the proof by showing that

$$\bar{p}_t^{\mathrm{R}} = \int_0^t \left(\gamma \bar{p}_s^{\mathrm{I}} - \lambda \bar{p}_s^{\mathrm{I}} \bar{p}_s^{\mathrm{R}}\right) \mathrm{d}s \tag{3.3.31}$$

by using arguments similar as for $\bar{p}_t^{\mathrm{I}}$. □

3.3.6 Degree Distribution of the "Initial Condition"

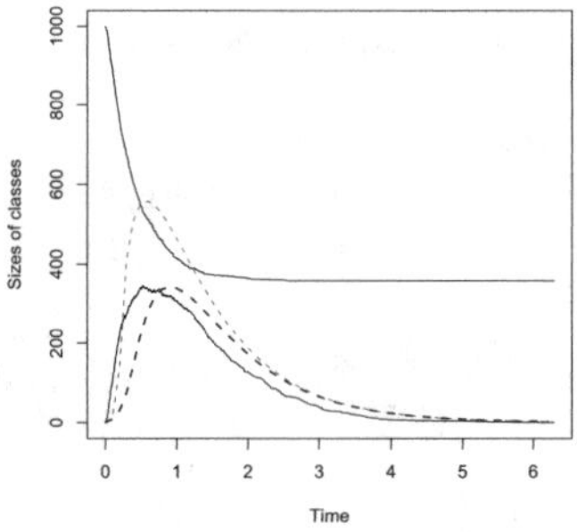

The assumption of moments of order 5 in the Theorem 3.3.8 may seem restrictive. Janson et al. [65] showed that this assumption was not necessary if Volz' equations are established by considering the process $(S_t^{\mathrm{N}}, I_t^{\mathrm{N}}, R_t^{\mathrm{N}}, N_t^{\mathrm{N,S}}, N_t^{\mathrm{N,I}}, N_t^{\mathrm{N,R}})_{t\in\mathbb{R}_+}$ where $N_t^{\mathrm{N,S}} = \langle \mu_t^{\mathrm{N,S}}, k\rangle$, $N_t^{\mathrm{N,I}}$ and $N_t^{\mathrm{N,R}}$ are respectively the numbers of half-edges of the susceptible, infectious and removed individuals that are not attached to the cluster. This process contains less information than the process $(\mu_t^{\mathrm{N,S}}, \mu_t^{\mathrm{N,IS}}, \mu_t^{\mathrm{N,RS}})_{t\in\mathbb{R}_+}$, and an assumption on the existence of moments of order 2 uniformly bounded in N is sufficient. Janson and coauthors emphasize that if we allow the CM graph to have self-loops and multiple edges, then only the uniform integrability of the degree distribution of an individual chosen at random is needed, which seems to be the minimal assumption...

However, when considering the beginning of the epidemics, it appears that the assumption corresponding to Equation (3.3.21) is not so restrictive. Indeed, we emphasize that it should be distinguished between the degree distribution of the graph $\mathbf{p}$, associated with the generating function g, and the degree distribution of the S individuals when the proportion of infectious individuals has reached a non-negligible value, and which we associate with the generating function h. If we consider the degree distribution of the susceptible individuals, we see that the individuals with highest degrees will be infected first, since individuals are chosen in the size-biased distribution (1.2.1) when pairing the half-edges at random. After the $[\varepsilon N]$ first infections, with $\varepsilon > 0$, when the Theorem 3.3.8 starts to apply, all the susceptible individuals of highest degree have disappeared from $\mu^{\mathrm{N,S}}$. Then, $\mu^{\mathrm{N,S}}$ will even admit exponential moments.

For a population of size N, whose individuals have degrees $D_1,\dots D_N$, let us define, for all $k\in\mathbb{Z}_+$, the number of vertices with degree k among them by

$$N_k^{\mathrm{N}} = \mathrm{Card}\{u\in\{1,\dots,N\},\ D_u=k\}.$$

To each of the D_u half-edges of individual u, we associate an independent uniform random variable on $[0,1]$. The vertex u is infected before the vertex v if the minimal value Z_u of the random variables attached to its half-edges is smaller than the minimal value Z_v of the random variables attached to the half-edges of v. This construction has been used by Riordan [97] and is related to size-biased orderings.

Proposition 3.3.11. *(i) The degree distribution $(\widehat{p}_k^{\varepsilon,\mathrm{N}})_{k\geq 1}$ of the remaining susceptible individuals after the $[\varepsilon N]$ first infections is:*

$$\widehat{p}_k^{\varepsilon,\mathrm{N}} = \frac{1}{N-[\varepsilon N]}\sum_{u=1}^{N}\mathbf{1}_{D_u=k}\mathbf{1}_{Z_u>Z_{([\varepsilon N])}} \tag{3.3.32}$$

where $(Z_{(1)},\dots,Z_{(N)})$ are the order statistics of $(Z_1,\dots,Z_N)$, and where

$$\mathbb{P}(Z_u\leq z\,|\,D_u) = 1-(1-z)^{D_u}.$$

(ii) For $z\in(0,1)$, let $M(z)$ be the survival function of the distribution of the Z_i and let $M_N(z)$ be the empirical survival function of $(Z_1,\dots,Z_N)$:

$$M_N(z) = \frac{1}{N}\sum_{u=1}^{N}\mathbf{1}_{Z_u>z}, \quad \textit{and} \quad M(z)=\sum_{k\geq 0}p_k(1-z)^k = g(1-z),$$

where $g(z)=\sum_{k\geq 0}p_k z^k$ is the generating function of the degree distribution $\mathbf{p}$ of the CM graph. Let ε defined by $z^\varepsilon = \inf\{z\in(0,1),\ M(z)\geq\varepsilon\}$ be the quantile of order ε of the Z_u. Then, provided M is continuous and strictly increasing at z^ε,

$$\lim_{N\to+\infty} Z_{[\varepsilon N]} = z^\varepsilon \qquad \textit{almost surely.}$$

(iii) For such an ε, the degree distribution of the remaining susceptible individuals after the $[\varepsilon N]$ first infections converges weakly to:

$$\lim_{N\to+\infty}\sum_{k\geq 0}\widehat{p}_k^{\varepsilon,\mathrm{N}}\delta_k = \frac{1}{1-\varepsilon}\sum_{k\geq 0}p_k(1-z^\varepsilon)^k\,\delta_k, \tag{3.3.33}$$

where z^ε is solution of $1-\varepsilon = g(1-z^\varepsilon)$. Moreover, we have convergence of the moments of order 5:

$$\lim_{N\to+\infty}\sum_{k\geq 0}k^5\widehat{p}_k^{\varepsilon,\mathrm{N}} = \frac{1}{1-\varepsilon}\sum_{k\geq 0}k^5 p_k(1-z^\varepsilon)^k < +\infty. \tag{3.3.34}$$

In particular, the limiting distribution (3.3.33) admits moments of all orders.

Proof. Let us prove (ii). Let $z \in [0,1]$. The proportion of vertices of degree k whose minimal value of the Z_u is smaller than z is $M_k^N(z) = \frac{1}{N}\sum_{u=1}^N \mathbf{1}_{D_u=k}\mathbf{1}_{Z_u>z}$. By the law of large numbers, $\lim_{N\to+\infty} M_k^N(z) = p_k(1-z)^k$ a.s., which implies that

$$\lim_{N\to+\infty} \frac{1}{N}\sum_{u=1}^N \mathbf{1}_{Z_u>z}\delta_{D_u} = \sum_{k\geq 0} p_k(1-z)^k\delta_k$$

for the weak convergence.

Assume that $\varepsilon > 0$ is such that M is continuous and strictly increasing at z^ε. Then, $M(z^\varepsilon) = \varepsilon$. Let $\delta > 0$ and

$$\eta = \min(|M(z^\varepsilon - \delta) - M(z^\varepsilon)|, |M(z^\varepsilon + \delta) - M(z^\varepsilon)|).$$

By the Kolmogorov–Smirnov theorem: $\lim_{N\to+\infty} \|M_N - M\|_\infty = 0$. Then, there exists $\mathbb{P}(d\omega)$-a.s. an integer $N_0(\omega)$ sufficiently large such that for all $N \geq N_0$, $\|M_N - M\|_\infty < \eta/2$. Since M is non-decreasing and since $Z_{[\varepsilon N]}$ is such that $M_N(Z_{[\varepsilon N]}) = \frac{[\varepsilon N]}{N}$, then,

$$\begin{aligned}\big|M(Z_{([\varepsilon N])}) - \varepsilon\big| \leq & \big|M(Z_{([\varepsilon N])}) - M_N(Z_{([\varepsilon N])})\big| + \big|M_N(Z_{([\varepsilon N])}) - \varepsilon\big| \\ \leq & \frac{\eta}{2} + \Big|\frac{[\varepsilon N]}{N} - \varepsilon\Big|.\end{aligned}$$

Thus, for $N \geq \max(N_0, 2/\eta)$, $|M(Z_{[\varepsilon N]}) - \varepsilon| < \eta$ and hence $Z_{[\varepsilon N]} \in (z^\varepsilon - \delta, z^\varepsilon + \delta)$ a.s. This implies that $(Z_{[\varepsilon N]})_{N\geq 1}$ converges a.s. to z^ε.

If $(\widehat{p}_k^{\varepsilon,N})_{k\in\mathbb{Z}_+}$ is the degree distribution after the $[\varepsilon N]$ first infections, then

$$\lim_{N\to+\infty} \sum_{k\geq 0} \widehat{p}_k^{\varepsilon,N}\delta_k = \frac{1}{1-\varepsilon}\sum_{k\geq 0} p_k(1-z^\varepsilon)^k\delta_k. \tag{3.3.35}$$

The convergence, for every $k \in \mathbb{Z}_+$, of $\widehat{p}_k^{\varepsilon,N}$ to $p_k(1-z^\varepsilon)^k/(1-\varepsilon)$ implies the convergence of (3.3.35) for the vague topology. Because (3.3.35) deals with probability measures, the criterion of [76, Proposition 2] implies that the convergence also holds for the weak topology.

Since

$$\begin{aligned}&\lim_{N\to+\infty} \mathbb{E}\Big(\frac{1}{N}\sum_{i=1}^N \big|\mathbf{1}_{Z_i>Z_{[\varepsilon N]}} - \mathbf{1}_{Z_i>z^\varepsilon}\big|\mathbf{1}_{d_i=k}\Big) \\ &\qquad = \lim_{N\to+\infty} \mathbb{P}\Big(Z_1 \in [Z_{[\varepsilon N]} \wedge z^\varepsilon, Z_{[\varepsilon N]} \vee z^\varepsilon],\ d_1 = k\Big) = 0, \end{aligned}\tag{3.3.36}$$

and since $N/(N - [\varepsilon N])$ converges to $1/(1-\varepsilon)$, we obtain (3.3.33).

For the convergence of the moments of order 5, we notice that for large $K \in \mathbb{N}$,

$$\begin{aligned}&\mathbb{E}\Big(\Big|\sum_{k\geq 0} k^5 M_k^N(Z_{[\varepsilon N]}) - \sum_{k\geq 0} k^5 p_k(1-z^\varepsilon)^k\Big|\Big)\\ \leq&\mathbb{E}\Big(\Big|\sum_{k\leq K} k^5\big(M_k^N(Z_{[\varepsilon N]}) - p_k(1-z^\varepsilon)^k\big)\Big|\Big) + \mathbb{E}\Big(\sum_{k>K} k^5 M_k^N(Z_{[\varepsilon N]})\Big) + \sum_{k>K} k^5 p_k(1-z^\varepsilon)^k.\end{aligned}$$

The first term converges to 0 with the preceding arguments. The third term is controlled for K sufficiently large. For the second term, we use that for all $z \in (0,1)$,

$$\mathbb{E}\big(\sum_{k>K} k^5 M_k^N(z)\big) = \sum_{k>K} k^5 p_k(1-z)^k$$

and that $Z_{[\varepsilon N]}$ converges a.s. to z^ε. □

3.3.7 Proof of the Limit Theorem

We now prove Theorem 3.3.8.

In the proof, we will see that the epidemic remains large and described by a deterministic equation provided the number of edges from I to S remains of the order of N. Let us thus define, for all $\varepsilon > 0$, $\varepsilon' > 0$ and $n \in \mathbb{N}$,

$$t_{\varepsilon'} := \inf\{t \geq 0, \langle \bar{\mu}_t^{\text{IS}}, \chi\rangle < \varepsilon'\} \tag{3.3.37}$$

and:

$$\tau_\varepsilon^N = \inf\{t \geq 0,\, \langle \mu_t^{\text{N,IS}}, \chi\rangle < \varepsilon\}. \tag{3.3.38}$$

In the sequel, we choose $0 < \varepsilon < \varepsilon' < \langle \bar{\mu}_0^{\text{IS}}, \chi\rangle$.

Step 1 Let us prove that $(\mu^{\text{N,S}}, \mu^{\text{N,IS}}, \mu^{\text{N,RS}})_{N\in\mathbb{N}}$ is tight. Let $t \in \mathbb{R}_+$ and $N \in \mathbb{N}$. By hypothesis, we have that

$$\begin{aligned}&\langle \mu_t^{\text{N,S}}, \mathbf{1}+\chi^5\rangle + \langle \mu_t^{\text{N,IS}}, \mathbf{1}+\chi^5\rangle + \langle \mu_t^{\text{N,RS}}, \mathbf{1}+\chi^5\rangle\\ &\qquad\leq \langle \mu_0^{\text{N,S}}, \mathbf{1}+\chi^5\rangle + \langle \mu_0^{\text{N,IS}}, \mathbf{1}+\chi^5\rangle \leq 2A.\end{aligned} \tag{3.3.39}$$

Thus the sequences of marginals $(\mu_t^{\text{N,S}})_{N\in\mathbb{N}}$, $(\mu_t^{\text{N,IS}})_{N\in\mathbb{N}}$ and $(\mu_t^{\text{N,RS}})_{N\in\mathbb{N}}$ are tight for each $t \in \mathbb{R}_+$. Now by the criterion of Roelly [99], it remains to prove that for each bounded function f on $\mathbb{Z}_+$, the sequence $((\langle \mu_\cdot^{\text{N,S}}, f\rangle, \langle \mu_\cdot^{\text{N,IS}}, f\rangle, \langle \mu_\cdot^{\text{N,RS}}, f\rangle)_{N\in\mathbb{N}}$ is tight in $\mathbb{D}(\mathbb{R}_+, \mathbb{R}^3)$. Since we have the semi-martingale decompositions of these processes, it is sufficient, by using the Rebolledo criterion, to prove that the finite variation part and the bracket of the martingale satisfy the Aldous criterion (see e.g. [66]). We only prove that $\langle \mu_\cdot^{\text{N,IS}}, f\rangle$ is tight. The computations are similar for the other components.

The Rebolledo–Aldous criterion is satisfied if for all $\alpha > 0$ and $\eta > 0$ there exists $N_0 \in \mathbb{Z}_+$ and $\delta > 0$ such that for all $N > N_0$ and for all stopping times S_N and T_N such that $S_N < T_N < S_N + \delta$,

$$\mathbb{P}\big(|A_{T_N}^{\text{N,IS},f} - A_{S_N}^{\text{N,IS},f}| > \eta\big) \leq \alpha, \quad \text{and} \tag{3.3.40}$$

$$\mathbb{P}\big(|\langle M^{\mathrm{N,IS},f}\rangle_{T_N} - \langle M^{\mathrm{N,IS},f}\rangle_{S_N}| > \eta\big) \leq \alpha.$$

For the finite variation part,

$$\mathbb{E}\Big[|A^{\mathrm{N,IS},f}_{T_N} - A^{\mathrm{N,IS},f}_{S_N}|\Big] \leq \mathbb{E}\left[\int_{S_N}^{T_N} \gamma\|f\|_\infty \langle \mu^{\mathrm{N,IS}}_s, 1\rangle \,\mathrm{d}s\right]$$
$$+\mathbb{E}\left[\int_{S_N}^{T_N} \sum_{k\in\mathbb{Z}_+} \Lambda^N_s(k)\mu^{\mathrm{N,S}}_s(k) \sum_{j+\ell\leq k-1} p^N_s(j,\ell|k-1)(2j+3)\|f\|_\infty \,\mathrm{d}s\right].$$

The term $\sum_{j+\ell\leq k-1} jp^N_s(j,\ell|k-1)$ is the mean number of links to $\mathrm{I}^N_{s\_}$ that the newly infected individual has, given that this individual is of degree k. It is bounded by k. Then, with (3.3.13),

$$\mathbb{E}\Big[|A^{\mathrm{N,IS},f}_{T_N} - A^{\mathrm{N,IS},f}_{S_N}|\Big] \leq \delta\mathbb{E}\Big[\beta\|f\|_\infty(S^{\mathrm{N}}_0 + I^{\mathrm{N}}_0) + \lambda\|f\|_\infty\langle \mu^{\mathrm{N,S}}_0, 2\chi^2+3\chi\rangle\Big],$$

by using that the number of infectives is bounded by the size of the population and that $\mu^{\mathrm{N,S}}_s(k) \leq \mu^{\mathrm{N,S}}_0(k)$ for all k and $s\geq 0$. From (3.3.21), the r.h.s. is finite. Using Markov's inequality,

$$\mathbb{P}\big(|A^{\mathrm{N,IS},f}_{T_N} - A^{\mathrm{N,IS},f}_{S_N}| > \eta\big) \leq \frac{(5\lambda+2\gamma)A\delta\|f\|_\infty}{\eta},$$

which is smaller than α for δ small enough.

We use the same arguments for the bracket of the martingale:

$$\begin{aligned}\mathbb{E}\big[|\langle M^{\mathrm{N,IS},f}\rangle_{T_N} - \langle M^{\mathrm{N,IS},f}\rangle_{S_N}|\big]&\\ \leq \mathbb{E}\Big[\frac{\delta\gamma\|f\|^2_\infty(S^{\mathrm{N}}_0+I^{\mathrm{N}}_0)}{N} &+ \frac{\delta\lambda\|f\|^2_\infty\langle\mu^{\mathrm{N,S}}_0, \chi(2\chi+3)^2\rangle}{N}\Big]\\ \leq \frac{(25\lambda+2\gamma)A\delta\|f\|^2_\infty}{N}&,\end{aligned} \tag{3.3.41}$$

using Assumption 3.3.5 and (3.3.21). The r.h.s. can be made smaller than $\eta\alpha$ for a small enough δ, so the second inequality of (3.3.40) follows again from Markov's inequality. By [99], this provides the tightness in $\mathbb{D}(\mathbb{R}_+, \mathscr{M}^3_{0,A})$, with $\mathscr{M}_{0,A}$ defined in (3.3.20).

By Prohorov's theorem (e.g. [52], p. 104) and Step 1, we obtain that the distributions of $(\mu^{\mathrm{N,S}}, \mu^{\mathrm{N,IS}}, \mu^{\mathrm{N,RS}})$, for $N\in\mathbb{N}$, form a relatively compact family of bounded measures on $\mathbb{D}(\mathbb{R}_+, \mathscr{M}^3_{0,A})$, and so do the laws of the stopped processes $(\mu^{\mathrm{N,S}}_{.\wedge\tau^N_\varepsilon}, \mu^{\mathrm{N,IS}}_{.\wedge\tau^N_\varepsilon}, \mu^{\mathrm{N,RS}}_{.\wedge\tau^N_\varepsilon})_{N\in\mathbb{N}}$ (recall (3.3.38)). Because of the moment assumptions for the degree distributions, the limiting process is continuous. Let $\bar{\mu} := (\bar{\mu}^{\mathrm{S}}, \bar{\mu}^{\mathrm{IS}}, \bar{\mu}^{\mathrm{RS}})$ be a limiting point in $\mathscr{C}(\mathbb{R}_+, \mathscr{M}^3_{0,A})$ of the sequence of stopped processes and let us consider a subsequence again denoted by $\mu^N := (\mu^{\mathrm{N,S}}, \mu^{\mathrm{N,IS}}, \mu^{\mathrm{N,RS}})_{N\in\mathbb{N}}$, with an abuse of notation, and that converges to $\bar{\mu}$. Because the limiting values are continuous, the convergence of $(\mu^N)_{N\in\mathbb{N}}$ to $\bar{\mu}$ holds for the uniform convergence on every compact subset of $\mathbb{R}_+$ (e.g. [24] p. 112).

Now, let us define for all $t \in \mathbb{R}_+$ and for all bounded functions f on $\mathbb{Z}_+$, the mappings $\Psi_t^{\mathrm{S},f}$, $\Psi_t^{\mathrm{IS},f}$ and $\Psi_t^{\mathrm{RS},f}$ from $\mathbb{D}(\mathbb{R}_+,\mathcal{M}_{0,A}^3)$ into $\mathbb{D}(\mathbb{R}_+,\mathbb{R})$ such that (3.3.17)–(3.3.19) read

$$\begin{aligned}&(\langle\bar{\mu}_t^{\mathrm{S}},f\rangle,\langle\bar{\mu}_t^{\mathrm{IS}},f\rangle,\langle\bar{\mu}_t^{\mathrm{RS}},f\rangle)\\&=\left(\Psi_t^{\mathrm{S},f}\left(\bar{\mu}^{\mathrm{S}},\bar{\mu}^{\mathrm{IS}},\bar{\mu}^{\mathrm{RS}}\right),\Psi_t^{\mathrm{IS},f}\left(\bar{\mu}^{\mathrm{S}},\bar{\mu}^{\mathrm{IS}},\bar{\mu}^{\mathrm{RS}}\right),\Psi_t^{\mathrm{RS},f}\left(\bar{\mu}^{\mathrm{S}},\bar{\mu}^{\mathrm{IS}},\bar{\mu}^{\mathrm{RS}}\right)\right).\end{aligned}\quad(3.3.42)$$

Our purpose is to prove that the limiting values are the unique solution of (3.3.17)–(3.3.19).
Before proceeding to the proof, a remark is in order. A natural way of reasoning would be to prove that $\Psi^{\mathrm{S},f}$, $\Psi^{\mathrm{IS},f}$ and $\Psi^{\mathrm{RS},f}$ are Lipschitz continuous in some spaces of measures. To avoid doing so by considering the set of measures with moments of any order, which is a set too small for applications, we circumvent this difficulty by first proving that the mass and the first two moments of any solutions of the system are the same. Then, we prove that the generating functions of these measures satisfy a partial differential equation known to have a unique solution.

Step 2 We now prove that the differential system (3.3.17)–(3.3.19) has at most one solution in $\mathscr{C}(\mathbb{R}_+,\mathcal{M}_{0,A}\times\mathcal{M}_{0+,A}\times\mathcal{M}_{0,A})$. Let $T>0$. Let $\bar{\mu}^i=(\bar{\mu}^{\mathrm{S},i},\bar{\mu}^{\mathrm{IS},i},\bar{\mu}^{\mathrm{RS},i})$, $i\in\{1,2\}$ be two solutions of (3.3.17)–(3.3.19), started with the same initial conditions in $\mathcal{M}_{0,A}\times\mathcal{M}_{\varepsilon,A}\times\mathcal{M}_{0,A}$ for some small $\varepsilon>0$. Set

$$\begin{aligned}\Upsilon_t=&\sum_{j=0}^{3}|\langle\bar{\mu}_t^{\mathrm{S},1},\chi^j\rangle-\langle\bar{\mu}_t^{\mathrm{S},2},\chi^j\rangle|\\&+\sum_{j=0}^{2}\left(|\langle\bar{\mu}_t^{\mathrm{IS},1},\chi^j\rangle-\langle\bar{\mu}_t^{\mathrm{IS},2},\chi^j\rangle|+|\langle\bar{\mu}_t^{\mathrm{RS},1},\chi^j\rangle-\langle\bar{\mu}_t^{\mathrm{RS},2},\chi^j\rangle|\right).\end{aligned}$$

Let us first remark that for all $0\le t<T$, $\bar{N}_t^{\mathrm{S}}\ge\bar{N}_t^{\mathrm{IS}}>\varepsilon$ and then

$$\begin{aligned}|\bar{p}_t^{\mathrm{I},1}-\bar{p}_t^{\mathrm{I},2}|=&\left|\frac{\bar{N}_t^{\mathrm{IS},1}}{\bar{N}_t^{\mathrm{S},1}}-\frac{\bar{N}_t^{\mathrm{IS},2}}{\bar{N}_t^{\mathrm{S},2}}\right|\le\frac{A}{\varepsilon^2}\left|\bar{N}_t^{\mathrm{S},1}-\bar{N}_t^{\mathrm{S},2}\right|+\frac{1}{\varepsilon}\left|\bar{N}_t^{\mathrm{IS},1}-\bar{N}_t^{\mathrm{IS},2}\right|\\=&\frac{A}{\varepsilon^2}\left|\langle\bar{\mu}_t^{\mathrm{S},1},\chi\rangle-\langle\bar{\mu}_t^{\mathrm{S},2},\chi\rangle\right|+\frac{1}{\varepsilon}\left|\langle\bar{\mu}_t^{\mathrm{IS},1},\chi\rangle-\langle\bar{\mu}_t^{\mathrm{IS},2},\chi\rangle\right|\le\frac{A}{\varepsilon^2}\Upsilon_t.\end{aligned}\quad(3.3.43)$$

The same computations show a similar result for $|\bar{p}_t^{\mathrm{S},1}-\bar{p}_t^{\mathrm{S},2}|$.

Using that $\bar{\mu}^i$ are solutions to (3.3.17)–(3.3.18) let us show that Υ satisfies a Gronwall inequality which implies that it is equal to 0 for all $t\le T$. For the degree distributions of the susceptible individuals, we have for $p\in\{0,1,2,3\}$ and $f=\chi^p$ in (3.3.17):

$$\begin{aligned}|\langle\bar{\mu}_t^{S,1},\chi^p\rangle-\langle\bar{\mu}_t^{S,2},\chi^p\rangle|=&\Big|\sum_{k\in\mathbb{Z}_+}\bar{\mu}_0^S(k)k^p\big(e^{-\lambda\int_0^t\bar{p}_s^{I,1}ds}-e^{-\lambda\int_0^t\bar{p}_s^{I,2}ds}\big)\Big|\\ \le&\lambda\sum_{k\in\mathbb{Z}_+}k^p\bar{\mu}_0^S(k)\int_0^t|\bar{p}_s^{I,1}-\bar{p}_s^{I,2}|ds\le\lambda\frac{A^2}{\varepsilon^2}\int_0^t\Upsilon_s ds,\end{aligned}$$

by using (3.3.43) and the fact that $\bar{\mu}_0^S\in\mathscr{M}_{0,A}$.
For $\bar{\mu}^{IS}$ and $\bar{\mu}^{RS}$, we use (3.3.18) and (3.3.19) with the functions $f=\chi^0=\mathbf{1}$, $f=\chi$ and $f=\chi^2$. We proceed here with only one of the computations, others can be done similarly. From (3.3.18):

$$\begin{aligned}&\langle\bar{\mu}_t^{IS,1},\mathbf{1}\rangle-\langle\bar{\mu}_t^{IS,2},\mathbf{1}\rangle=\\ &\qquad\gamma\int_0^t\langle\bar{\mu}_s^{IS,1}-\bar{\mu}_s^{IS,2},\mathbf{1}\rangle\,\mathrm{d}s+\lambda\int_0^t\big(\bar{p}_s^{I,1}\langle\bar{\mu}_s^{S,1},\chi\rangle-\bar{p}_s^{I,2}\langle\bar{\mu}_s^{S,2},\chi\rangle\big)\,\mathrm{d}s.\end{aligned}$$

Hence, with (3.3.43),

$$\Big|\langle\bar{\mu}_t^{IS,1}-\bar{\mu}_t^{IS,2},\mathbf{1}\rangle\Big|\le C(\lambda,\gamma,A,\varepsilon)\int_0^t\Upsilon_s\,\mathrm{d}s.$$

By analogous computations for the other quantities, we show that

$$\Upsilon_t\le C'(\lambda,\gamma,A,\varepsilon)\int_0^t\Upsilon_s\,\mathrm{d}s,$$

hence $\Upsilon\equiv 0$. It follows that for all $t<T$, and for all $j\in\{0,1,2\}$,

$$\langle\bar{\mu}_t^{S,1},\chi^j\rangle=\langle\bar{\mu}_t^{S,2},\chi^j\rangle\quad\text{and}\quad\langle\bar{\mu}_t^{IS,1},\chi^j\rangle=\langle\bar{\mu}_t^{IS,2},\chi^j\rangle,\tag{3.3.44}$$

and in particular, $\bar{N}_t^{S,1}=\bar{N}_t^{S,2}$ and $\bar{N}_t^{IS,1}=\bar{N}_t^{IS,2}$. This implies that $\bar{p}_t^{S,1}=\bar{p}_t^{S,2}$, $\bar{p}_t^{I,1}=\bar{p}_t^{I,2}$ and $\bar{p}_t^{R,1}=\bar{p}_t^{R,2}$. From (3.3.17), we have that $\bar{\mu}^{S,1}=\bar{\mu}^{S,2}$.

Our purpose is now to prove that $\bar{\mu}^{IS,1}=\bar{\mu}^{IS,2}$. Let us introduce the following generating functions: for any $t\in\mathbb{R}_+$, $i\in\{1,2\}$ and $\eta\in[0,1)$,

$$\mathscr{G}_t^i(\eta)=\sum_{k\ge 0}\eta^k\bar{\mu}_t^{IS,i}(k).$$

Since we already know that these measures have the same total mass, it remains to prove that $\mathscr{G}^1\equiv\mathscr{G}^2$. Let us define

$$\begin{aligned}H(t,\eta)=&\int_0^t\sum_{k\in\mathbb{Z}_+}\lambda k\bar{p}_s^I\sum_{\substack{j,\ell,m\in\mathbb{Z}_+\\ j+\ell+m=k-1}}\binom{k-1}{j,\ell,m}(\bar{p}_s^I)^j(\bar{p}_s^R)^\ell(\bar{p}_s^S)^m\eta^m\bar{\mu}_s^S(k)\,ds,\\ K_t=&\sum_{k\in\mathbb{Z}_+}\lambda k\bar{p}_t^I(k-1)\bar{p}_t^R\frac{\bar{\mu}_t^S(k)}{\bar{N}_t^{IS}}.\end{aligned}\tag{3.3.45}$$

The latter quantities are respectively of class $\mathscr{C}^1$ and $\mathscr{C}^0$ with respect to time t and are well-defined and bounded on $[0,T]$. Moreover, H and K do not depend on the chosen solution because of (3.3.44). Applying (3.3.18) to $f(k)=\eta^k$ yields

$$\begin{aligned}\mathscr{G}_t^i(\eta) =&\mathscr{G}_0^i(\eta)+H(t,\eta)+\int_0^t \Big(K_s\sum_{k'\in\mathbb{N}}(\eta^{k'-1}-\eta^{k'})k'\bar{\mu}_s^{\mathrm{IS},i}(k')-\gamma\mathscr{G}_s^i(\eta)\Big)ds\\ =&\mathscr{G}_0^i(\eta)+H(t,\eta)+\int_0^t \Big(K_s(1-\eta)\partial_\eta\mathscr{G}_s^i(\eta)-\gamma\mathscr{G}_s^i(\eta)\Big)ds.\end{aligned}$$

Then, the functions $t\mapsto\widetilde{\mathscr{G}_t^i}(\eta)$ defined by $\widetilde{\mathscr{G}_t^i}(\eta)=e^{\beta t}\mathscr{G}_t^i(\eta)$, $i\in\{1,2\}$, are solutions of the following transport equation (of unknown function g):

$$\partial_t g(t,\eta)-(1-\eta)K_t\,\partial_\eta g(t,\eta)=\partial_t H(t,\eta)e^{\beta t}. \tag{3.3.46}$$

In view of the regularity of H and K, it is known that this equation admits a unique solution (see e.g. [53]). Hence $\mathscr{G}_t^1(\eta)=\mathscr{G}_t^2(\eta)$ for all $t\in\mathbb{R}_+$ and $\eta\in[0,1)$. The same method applies to $\bar{\mu}^{\mathrm{RS}}$. Thus there is at most one solution to the differential system (3.3.17)–(3.3.19).

Step 3 We now show that μ^N nearly satisfies (3.3.17)–(3.3.19) as N gets large. Recall (3.3.14) for a bounded function f on $\mathbb{Z}_+$. To identify the limiting values, we establish that for all $N\in\mathbb{N}$ and all $t\geq 0$,

$$\langle\mu^{\mathrm{N,IS}}_{t\wedge\tau_\varepsilon^N},f\rangle=\Psi^{\mathrm{IS},f}_{t\wedge\tau_\varepsilon^N}(\mu^N)+\Delta^{\mathrm{N},f}_{t\wedge\tau_\varepsilon^N}+M^{\mathrm{N,IS},f}_{t\wedge\tau_\varepsilon^N}, \tag{3.3.47}$$

where $M^{N,\mathrm{IS},f}$ is defined in (3.3.14) and where $\Delta^{N,f}_{.\wedge\tau_\varepsilon^N}$ converges to 0 when $N\to+\infty$, in probability and uniformly in t on compact time intervals.

Let us fix $t\in\mathbb{R}_+$. Computation similar to (3.3.41) give:

$$\mathbb{E}\big((M_t^{\mathrm{N,IS},f})^2\big)=\mathbb{E}\big(\langle M^{\mathrm{N,IS},f}\rangle_t\big)\leq\frac{(25\lambda+2\gamma)At\|f\|_\infty^2}{N}. \tag{3.3.48}$$

Hence the sequence $(M_t^{\mathrm{N,IS},f})_{N\in\mathbb{Z}_+}$ converges in L^2 and in probability to zero.

We now consider the finite variation part of (3.3.14), given in (3.3.15). The sum in (3.3.15) corresponds to the links to I that the new infected individual has. We separate this sum into cases where the new infected individual only has simple edges to other individuals of I, and cases where multiple edges exist. The latter term is expected to vanish for large populations.

$$A_t^{\mathrm{N,IS},f}=B_t^{\mathrm{N,IS},f}+C_t^{\mathrm{N,IS},f}, \tag{3.3.49}$$

where

$$B_t^{\mathrm{N,IS},f} = -\int_0^t \gamma\langle \mu_s^{\mathrm{N,IS}}, f\rangle \,\mathrm{d}s$$
$$+\int_0^t \sum_{k\in\mathbb{Z}_+} \Lambda_s^N(k)\mu_s^{\mathrm{N,S}}(k) \sum_{j+\ell+1\leq k} p_s^N(j,\ell|k-1)\Bigg\{ f(k-(j+1+\ell))$$
$$+ \sum_{\substack{u\in\mathscr{L}(j+1,\mu_s^{\mathrm{N,IS}});\\ \forall u\leq I_{s_-}^{\mathrm{N}},\, n_u\leq 1}} \rho(\underline{n}|j+1,\mu_s^{\mathrm{N,IS}}) \sum_{u\in I_{s_-}^{\mathrm{N}}} \left(f\left(D_u(\mu_{s_-}^{\mathrm{N,IS}})-n_u\right) - f\left(D_u(\mu_{s_-}^{\mathrm{N,IS}})\right)\right) \Bigg\}\,\mathrm{d}s \tag{3.3.50}$$

and

$$C_t^{\mathrm{N,IS},f} = \int_0^t \sum_{k\in\mathbb{Z}_+} \Lambda_s^N(k)\mu_s^{\mathrm{N,S}}(k) \sum_{j+\ell+1\leq k} p_s^N(j,\ell|k-1)$$
$$\times \sum_{\substack{\underline{n}\in\mathscr{L}(j+1,\mu_s^{\mathrm{N,IS}});\\ \exists u\leq I_{s_-}^{\mathrm{N}},\, n_u>1}} \rho(\underline{n}|j+1,\mu_s^{\mathrm{N,IS}}) \sum_{u\in I_{s_-}^{\mathrm{N}}} \left(f\left(D_u(\mu_{s_-}^{\mathrm{N,IS}})-n_u\right) - f\left(D_u(\mu_{s_-}^{\mathrm{N,IS}})\right)\right)\,\mathrm{d}s. \tag{3.3.51}$$

We first show that $C_t^{\mathrm{N,SI},f}$ is a negligible term. Let $q_{j,\ell,s}^N$ denote the probability that the newly infected individual at time s has a double (or of higher order) edge to some alter in $I_{s_-}^{\mathrm{N}}$, given j and ℓ. The probability to have a multiple edge to a given infectious i is less than the number of pairs of edges linking the newly infected to i, times the probability that these two particular edges linking i to a susceptible alter at time s_- actually lead to the newly infected. Hence,

$$\begin{aligned} q_{j,\ell,s}^N &= \sum_{\substack{\underline{n}\in\mathscr{L}(j+1,\mu_s^{\mathrm{N,IS}});\\ \exists u\in I_{s_-}^{\mathrm{N}},\, n_u>1}} \rho(\underline{n}|j+1,\mu_s^{\mathrm{N,IS}}) \\ &\leq \binom{j}{2} \sum_{u\in I_{s_-}^{\mathrm{N}}} \frac{D_u(\mathrm{S}_{s_-}^{\mathrm{N}})(D_u(\mathrm{S}_{s_-}^{\mathrm{N}})-1)}{N_{s_-}^{\mathrm{N,IS}}(N_{s_-}^{\mathrm{N,IS}}-1)} = \binom{j}{2}\frac{1}{N}\frac{\langle \mu_{s_-}^{\mathrm{N,IS}},\chi(\chi-1)\rangle}{\frac{N_{s_-}^{\mathrm{N,IS}}}{N}\left(\frac{N_{s_-}^{\mathrm{N,IS}}}{N}-\frac{1}{N}\right)} \\ &\leq \binom{j}{2}\frac{1}{N}\frac{A}{\varepsilon(\varepsilon-1/N)} \qquad \text{if } s<\tau_\varepsilon^N \text{ and } N>1/\varepsilon. \end{aligned} \tag{3.3.52}$$

Then, since for all $u\in\mathscr{L}(j+1,\mu_s^{\mathrm{N,IS}})$,

$$\left|\sum_{u\in I_{s_-}^{\mathrm{N}}} \left(f\left(D_u(\mu_{s_-}^{\mathrm{N,IS}})-n_u\right) - f\left(D_u(\mu_{s_-}^{\mathrm{N,IS}})\right)\right)\right| \leq 2(j+1)\|f\|_\infty, \tag{3.3.53}$$

we have by (3.3.52) and (3.3.53), for $N>1/\varepsilon$,

$$
\begin{aligned}
&|C^{\mathrm{N,IS},f}_{t\wedge\tau^N_\varepsilon}| &(3.3.54)\\
&\leq \int_0^{t\wedge\tau^N_\varepsilon} \sum_{k\in\mathbb{Z}_+} \lambda k \mu^{\mathrm{N,S}}_s(k) \sum_{j+\ell+1\leq k} p^N_s(j,\ell|k-1)2(j+1)\|f\|_\infty \frac{j(j-1)A}{2N\varepsilon(\varepsilon-1/N)}\,\mathrm{d}s\\
&\leq \frac{A\lambda t\|f\|_\infty}{N\varepsilon(\varepsilon-1/N)}\langle \mu^{\mathrm{N,S}}_0,\chi^4\rangle,
\end{aligned}
$$

which tends to zero in view of (3.3.21) and thanks to the fact that $\mu^{\mathrm{N,S}}_s$ is dominated by $\mu^{\mathrm{N,S}}_0$ for all $s\geq 0$ and $N\in\mathbb{N}$.

We now aim at proving that $B^{\mathrm{N,IS},f}_{.\wedge\tau^N_\varepsilon}$ is close to $\Psi^{\mathrm{IS},f}_{.\wedge\tau^N_\varepsilon}(\mu^N)$. First, notice that

$$
\begin{aligned}
&\sum_{\substack{\underline{n}\in\mathscr{L}(j+1,\mu^{\mathrm{N,IS}}_s);\\ \forall u\in I^{\mathrm{N}}_{s_-},\, n_u\leq 1}} \rho(u|j+1,\mu^{\mathrm{N,IS}}_s) \sum_{i\in I^{\mathrm{N}}_{s_-}} \left(f\left(D_u(\mu^{\mathrm{N,IS}}_{s_-})-n_u\right)-f\left(D_u(\mu^{\mathrm{N,IS}}_{s_-})\right)\right)\\
&= \sum_{u_0\neq\cdots\neq u_j\in I^{\mathrm{N}}_{s_-}} \left(\frac{\prod_{k=0}^j D_{u_k}(\mathrm{S}^{\mathrm{N}}_s)}{N^{\mathrm{N,IS}}_{s_-}\ldots(N^{\mathrm{N,IS}}_{s_-}-(j+1))}\right)\\
&\qquad\times\sum_{m=0}^{j}\left(f\left(D_{u_m}(\mathrm{S}^{\mathrm{N}}_{s_-})-1\right)-f\left(D_{u_m}(\mathrm{S}^{\mathrm{N}}_{s_-})\right)\right)\\
&= \sum_{m=0}^{j}\sum_{u_0\neq\cdots\neq u_j\in I^{\mathrm{N}}_{s_-}} \left(\frac{\prod_{k=0}^j D_{u_k}(\mathrm{S}^{\mathrm{N}}_s)}{N^{\mathrm{N,IS}}_{s_-}\ldots(N^{\mathrm{N,IS}}_{s_-}-(j+1))}\right)\\
&\qquad\times\left(f\left(D_{u_m}(\mathrm{S}^{\mathrm{N}}_{s_-})-1\right)-f\left(D_{u_m}(\mathrm{S}^{\mathrm{N}}_{s_-})\right)\right) &(3.3.55)\\
&= \sum_{m=0}^{j}\left(\sum_{x\in I^{\mathrm{N}}_{s_-}}\frac{D_x(\mathrm{S}^{\mathrm{N}}_{s_-})}{N^{\mathrm{N,IS}}_{s_-}}\left(f\left(D_x(\mathrm{S}^{\mathrm{N}}_{s_-})-1\right)-f\left(D_x(\mathrm{S}^{\mathrm{N}}_{s_-})\right)\right)\right)\\
&\qquad\times\left(\sum_{u_0\neq\cdots\neq u_{j-1}\in I^{\mathrm{N}}_{s_-}\setminus\{x\}}\frac{\prod_{k=0}^{j-1} D_{u_k}(\mathrm{S}^{\mathrm{N}}_s)}{(N^{\mathrm{N,IS}}_{s_-}-1)\ldots(N^{\mathrm{N,IS}}_{s_-}-(j+1))}\right)\\
&= (j+1)\frac{\langle\mu^{\mathrm{N,IS}}_{s_-},\chi(\tau_1 f-f)\rangle}{N^{\mathrm{N,IS}}_{s_-}}\left(1-q^N_{j-1,\ell,s}\right),
\end{aligned}
$$

where we recall (see Notation 0.0.1) that $\tau_1 f(k)=f(k-1)$ for every function f on $\mathbb{Z}_+$ and $k\in\mathbb{Z}_+$. In the third equality, we split the term u_m from the other terms $(u_{m'})_{m'\neq m}$. The last sum in the r.h.s. of this equality is the probability of drawing j different infectious individuals that are not u_m and that are all different, hence $1-q^N_{j-1,\ell,s}$.

Define for $t>0$ and $N\in\mathbb{Z}_+$,

$$
p^{\mathrm{N,I}}_t=\frac{\langle\mu^{\mathrm{N,IS}}_t,\chi\rangle-1}{\langle\mu^{\mathrm{N,S}}_t,\chi\rangle-1},
$$

$$p_t^{N,R} = \frac{\langle \mu_t^{N,RS}, \chi \rangle}{\langle \mu_t^{N,S}, \chi \rangle - 1},$$
$$p_t^{N,S} = \frac{\langle \mu_t^{N,S}, \chi \rangle - \langle \mu_t^{N,IS}, \chi \rangle - \langle \mu_t^{N,RS}, \chi \rangle}{\langle \mu_t^{N,S}, \chi \rangle - 1},$$

the proportion of edges with infectious (resp. removed and susceptible) alters and susceptible egos among all the edges with susceptible egos but the contaminating edge. For all integers j and ℓ such that $j+\ell \le k-1$ and $N \in \mathbb{N}$, denote by

$$\tilde{p}_t^N(j,\ell \mid k-1) = \frac{(k-1)!}{j!(k-1-j-\ell)!\ell!}(p_t^{N,I})^j (p_t^{N,R})^\ell (p_t^{N,S})^{k-1-j-\ell},$$

the probability that the multinomial variable counting the number of edges with infectious, removed and susceptible alters, among $k-1$ given edges, equals $(j,\ell,k-1-j-\ell)$. We have that

$$|\Psi^{IS,f}_{t\wedge\tau_\varepsilon^N}(\mu^N) - B^{N,IS,f}_{t\wedge\tau_\varepsilon^N}| \le |D^{N,IS,f}_{t\wedge\tau_\varepsilon^N}| + |E^{N,IS,f}_{t\wedge\tau_\varepsilon^N}|, \tag{3.3.56}$$

where

$$D_t^{N,IS,f} = \int_0^t \sum_{k\in\mathbb{Z}_+} \Lambda_s^N(k)\mu_s^{N,S}(k) \sum_{j+\ell+1\le k} \left(p_s^N(j,\ell|k-1) - \tilde{p}_s^N(j,\ell|k-1)\right)$$
$$\times \left(f(k-(j+\ell+1)) + (j+1)\frac{\langle \mu_{s_-}^{N,IS}, \chi(\tau_1 f - f)\rangle}{N_{s_-}^{N,IS}} \right) ds,$$
$$E_t^{N,IS,f} = \int_0^t \sum_{k\in\mathbb{Z}_+} \Lambda_s^N(k)\mu_s^{N,S}(k)$$
$$\times \sum_{j+\ell+1\le k} p_s^N(j,\ell|k-1)(j+1)\frac{\langle \mu_{s_-}^{N,IS}, \chi(\tau_1 f - f)\rangle}{N_{s_-}^{N,IS}} q^N_{j-1,\ell,s}\, ds.$$

First,

$$|D^{N,IS,f}_{t\wedge\tau_\varepsilon^N}| \le \int_0^{t\wedge\tau_\varepsilon^N} \sum_{k\in\mathbb{Z}_+} \lambda k \alpha_s^N(k) \|f\|_\infty \left(1+\frac{2kA}{\varepsilon}\right) \mu_s^{N,S}(k)\, ds, \tag{3.3.57}$$

where for all $k \in \mathbb{Z}_+$

$$\alpha_t^N(k) = \sum_{j+\ell+1\le k} \left| p_t^N(j,\ell|k-1) - \tilde{p}_t^N(j,\ell|k-1) \right|.$$

The multinomial probability $\tilde{p}_s^N(j,\ell|k-1)$ approximates the hypergeometric one, $p_s^N(j,\ell|k-1,s)$, as N increases to infinity, in view of the fact that the total population size, $\langle \mu_0^{N,S}, \mathbf{1}\rangle + \langle \mu_0^{N,IS}, \mathbf{1}\rangle$, is of order n. Hence, the r.h.s. of (3.3.57) vanishes by dominated convergence.

On the other hand, using (3.3.52),

$$|E^{N,\mathrm{IS},f}_{t\wedge\tau^N_\varepsilon}| \leq \int_0^{t\wedge\tau^N_\varepsilon} \sum_{k\in\mathbb{Z}_+} \lambda k^2 \mu^{N,\mathrm{S}}_s(k) \frac{2\|f\|_\infty A}{\varepsilon} \frac{k^2 A}{2N\varepsilon(\varepsilon-1/N)}\,\mathrm{d}s$$
$$\leq \frac{A^3\,\lambda t\|f\|_\infty}{N\varepsilon^2(\varepsilon-1/N)}, \tag{3.3.58}$$

in view of (3.3.21). Gathering (3.3.48), (3.3.49), (3.3.54), (3.3.56), (3.3.57) and (3.3.58) concludes the proof that the rest of (3.3.47) vanishes in probability uniformly over compact intervals.

As a consequence, the sequence $(\Psi^{\mathrm{IS},f}_{.\wedge\tau^N_\varepsilon}(\mu^N))_{N\in\mathbb{N}}$ is also tight in $\mathbb{D}(\mathbb{R}_+,\mathscr{M}_{0,A}\times\mathscr{M}_{\varepsilon,A}\times\mathscr{M}_{0,A})$.

Step 4 Recall that in this proof, $\bar{\mu}=(\bar{\mu}^{\mathrm{S}},\bar{\mu}^{\mathrm{IS}},\bar{\mu}^{\mathrm{RS}})$ is the limit of the sequence $(\mu^N_{.\wedge\tau^N_\varepsilon})_{N\in\mathbb{N}}=(\mu^{N,\mathrm{S}}_{.\wedge\tau^N_\varepsilon},\mu^{N,\mathrm{IS}}_{.\wedge\tau^N_\varepsilon},\mu^{N,\mathrm{RS}}_{.\wedge\tau^N_\varepsilon})_{N\in\mathbb{N}}$, and recall that these processes take values in the closed set $\mathscr{M}^3_{0,A}$. Our purpose is now to prove that $\bar{\mu}$ satisfies (3.3.17)–(3.3.19). Using Skorokhod's representation theorem, there exists, on the same probability space as $\bar{\mu}$, a sequence, again denoted by $(\mu^N_{.\wedge\tau^N_\varepsilon})_{N\in\mathbb{N}}$ with an abuse of notation, with the same marginal distributions as the original sequence, and that converges a.s. to $\bar{\mu}$.

The maps $\nu_. := (\nu^1_.,\nu^2_.,\nu^3_.)\mapsto\langle\nu^1_.,\mathbf{1}\rangle/(\langle\nu^1_0,\mathbf{1}\rangle+\langle\nu^2_0,\mathbf{1}\rangle+\langle\nu^3_0,\mathbf{1}\rangle)$ (respectively $\langle\nu^2_.,\mathbf{1}\rangle/(\langle\nu^1_0,\mathbf{1}\rangle+\langle\nu^2_0,\mathbf{1}\rangle+\langle\nu^3_0,\mathbf{1}\rangle)$ and $\langle\nu^3_.,\mathbf{1}\rangle/(\langle\nu^1_0,\mathbf{1}\rangle+\langle\nu^2_0,\mathbf{1}\rangle+\langle\nu^3_0,\mathbf{1}\rangle)$) are continuous from $\mathscr{C}(\mathbb{R}_+,\mathscr{M}_{0,A}\times\mathscr{M}_{\varepsilon,A}\times\mathscr{M}_{0,A})$ into $\mathscr{C}(\mathbb{R}_+,\mathbb{R})$.
Using the moment assumption (3.3.21), the following mappings are also continuous for the same spaces: $\langle\nu^1_.,\chi\rangle/\langle\nu^2_.,\chi\rangle$, $\nu_.\mapsto\mathbf{1}_{\langle\nu^1_.,\chi\rangle>\varepsilon}/\langle\nu^2_.,\chi\rangle$ and $\nu_.\mapsto\langle\nu^2_.,\chi(\tau_1 f-f)\rangle$, for bounded function f on $\mathbb{Z}_+$ and where we recall that $\tau_1 f(k)=f(k-1)$ for every $k\in\mathbb{Z}_+$ (see Notation 0.0.1). Thus, using the continuity of the mapping $y\in\mathbb{D}([0,t],\mathbb{R})\mapsto\int_0^t y_s\,\mathrm{d}s$, we obtain the continuity of the mapping Ψ^f_t defined in (3.3.42) on $\mathbb{D}(\mathbb{R}_+,\mathscr{M}_{0,A}\times\mathscr{M}_{\varepsilon,A}\times\mathscr{M}_{0,A})$.

By (3.3.21), the process $(N^{N,\mathrm{IS}}_{.\wedge\tau^N_\varepsilon})_{N\in\mathbb{N}}$ converges in distribution to $\bar{N}^{\mathrm{IS}}_.=\langle\bar{\mu}^{\mathrm{IS}}_.,\chi\rangle$. Since the latter process is continuous, the convergence holds in $(\mathbb{D}([0,T],\mathbb{R}_+),\|\cdot\|_\infty)$ for any $T>0$ (see [24, p. 112]). As $y\in\mathbb{D}(\mathbb{R}_+,\mathbb{R})\mapsto\inf_{t\in[0,T]}y(t)\in\mathbb{R}$ is continuous, we have a.s. that:

$$\inf_{t\in[0,T]}\bar{N}^{\mathrm{IS}}_t=\lim_{N\to+\infty}\inf_{t\in[0,T]}N^{N,\mathrm{IS}}_{t\wedge\tau^N_\varepsilon}\quad(\geq\varepsilon).$$

Analogously to (3.3.37), we consider $\bar{t}_{\varepsilon'}=\inf\{t\in\mathbb{R}_+,\bar{N}^{\mathrm{IS}}_t\leq\varepsilon'\}$ for $\varepsilon'>\varepsilon>0$. A difficulty lies in the fact that we do not know yet whether this time is deterministic. We have a.s.:

$$\varepsilon'\leq\inf_{t\in[0,T]}\bar{N}^{\mathrm{IS}}_{t\wedge\bar{t}_{\varepsilon'}}=\lim_{N\to+\infty}\inf_{t\in[0,T]}N^{N,\mathrm{IS}}_{t\wedge\tau^N_\varepsilon\wedge\bar{t}_{\varepsilon'}}. \tag{3.3.59}$$

Hence, using Fatou's lemma:

$$\begin{aligned}1 =&\mathbb{P}\Big(\inf_{t\in[0,\bar{t}_{\varepsilon'}]}\bar{N}_t^{\mathrm{IS}}>\varepsilon\Big)\\ \leq& \lim_{N\to+\infty}\mathbb{P}\Big(\inf_{t\in[0,T\wedge\bar{t}_{\varepsilon'}]}N^{\mathrm{N,IS}}_{t\wedge\tau^N_\varepsilon}>\varepsilon\Big)=\lim_{N\to+\infty}\mathbb{P}\Big(\tau^N_\varepsilon>T\wedge\bar{t}_{\varepsilon'}\Big).\end{aligned}\tag{3.3.60}$$

We have hence

$$\Psi^{\mathrm{IS},f}_{.\wedge\tau^N_\varepsilon\wedge\bar{t}_{\varepsilon'}\wedge T}(\mu^N)=\Psi^{\mathrm{IS},f}_{.\wedge\tau^N_\varepsilon\wedge T}(\mu^N)\mathbf{1}_{\tau^N_\varepsilon\leq\bar{t}_{\varepsilon'}\wedge T}+\Psi^{\mathrm{IS},f}_{.\wedge\bar{t}_{\varepsilon'}\wedge T}(\mu^N_{.\wedge\tau^N_\varepsilon})\mathbf{1}_{\tau^N_\varepsilon>\bar{t}_{\varepsilon'}\wedge T}.\tag{3.3.61}$$

From the estimates of the different terms in (3.3.47), $\Psi^{\mathrm{IS},f}_{.\wedge\tau^N_\varepsilon\wedge T}(\mu^N)$ is upper bounded by a moment of μ^N of order 4. In view of (3.3.21) and (3.3.60), the first term in the r.h.s. of (3.3.61) converges in L^1 and hence in probability to zero. Using the continuity of $\Psi^{\mathrm{IS},f}$ on $\mathbb{D}(\mathbb{R}_+,\mathscr{M}_{0,A}\times\mathscr{M}_{\varepsilon,A}\times\mathscr{M}_{0,A})$, $\Psi^{\mathrm{IS},f}(\mu^N_{.\wedge\tau^N_\varepsilon})$ converges to $\Psi^{\mathrm{IS},f}(\bar{\mu})$ and therefore, $\Psi^{\mathrm{IS},f}_{.\wedge\bar{t}_{\varepsilon'}\wedge T}(\mu^N_{.\wedge\tau^N_\varepsilon})$ converges to $\Psi^{\mathrm{IS},f}_{.\wedge\bar{t}_{\varepsilon'}\wedge T}(\bar{\mu})$. Thanks to this and (3.3.60), the second term in the r.h.s. of (3.3.61) converges to $\Psi^{\mathrm{IS},f}_{.\wedge\bar{t}_{\varepsilon'}\wedge T}(\bar{\mu})$ in $\mathbb{D}(\mathbb{R}_+,\mathbb{R})$. Then, the sequence $\big(\langle\mu^{\mathrm{N,IS}}_{.\wedge\tau^N_\varepsilon\wedge\bar{t}_{\varepsilon'}\wedge T},f\rangle-\Psi^{\mathrm{IS},f}_{.\wedge\tau^N_\varepsilon\wedge\bar{t}_{\varepsilon'}\wedge T}(\mu^N)\big)_{N\in\mathbb{N}}$ converges in probability to $\langle\bar{\mu}^{\mathrm{IS}}_{.\wedge\bar{t}_{\varepsilon'}\wedge T},f\rangle-\Psi^{\mathrm{IS},f}_{.\wedge\bar{t}_{\varepsilon'}\wedge T}(\bar{\mu})$. From (3.3.47), this sequence also converges in probability to zero.

By identification of these limits, $\bar{\mu}^{\mathrm{IS}}$ solves (3.3.18) on $[0,\bar{t}_{\varepsilon'}\wedge T]$. If $\langle\bar{\mu}_0^{\mathrm{RS}},\chi\rangle>0$ then similar techniques can be used. Else, the result is obvious since for all $t\in[0,t_{\varepsilon'}\wedge T]$, $\langle\mu_t^{\mathrm{N,IS}},\chi\rangle>\varepsilon$ and the term $p_t^N(j,\ell|k-1)$ is negligible when $\ell>0$. Thus $\bar{\mu}$ coincides a.s. with the only continuous deterministic solution of (3.3.17)–(3.3.19) on $[0,\bar{t}_{\varepsilon'}\wedge T]$. This implies that $\bar{t}_{\varepsilon'}\wedge T=t_{\varepsilon'}\wedge T$ and yields the convergence in probability of $(\mu^N_{.\wedge\tau^N_\varepsilon})_{N\in\mathbb{N}}$ to $\bar{\mu}$, uniformly on $[0,t_{\varepsilon'}\wedge T]$ since $\bar{\mu}$ is continuous.

We finally prove that the non-localized sequence $(\mu^N)_{N\in\mathbb{N}}$ also converges uniformly and in probability to $\bar{\mu}$ in $\mathbb{D}([0,t_{\varepsilon'}],\mathscr{M}_{0,A}\times\mathscr{M}_{\varepsilon,A}\times\mathscr{M}_{0,A})$. For a small positive η,

$$\begin{aligned}\mathbb{P}\Big(\sup_{t\in[0,t_{\varepsilon'}]}\Big|\langle\mu_t^{\mathrm{N,IS}},f\rangle-\Psi_t^{\mathrm{IS},f}(\bar{\mu})\Big|>\eta\Big)&\\ \leq\mathbb{P}\Big(\sup_{t\in[0,t_{\varepsilon'}]}\Big|\Psi^{\mathrm{IS},f}_{t\wedge\tau^N_\varepsilon}(\mu^N)-\Psi_t^{\mathrm{IS},f}(\bar{\mu})\Big|>\frac{\eta}{2}\,;\,\tau^n_\varepsilon\geq t_{\varepsilon'}\Big)&\\ +\mathbb{P}\Big(\sup_{t\in[0,t_{\varepsilon'}]}\Big|\Delta^{\mathrm{N},f}_{t\wedge\tau^N_\varepsilon}+M^{\mathrm{N,IS},f}_{t\wedge\tau^N_\varepsilon}\Big|>\frac{\eta}{2}\Big)+\mathbb{P}\Big(\tau^N_\varepsilon<t_{\varepsilon'}\Big).&\end{aligned}\tag{3.3.62}$$

Using the continuity of Ψ^f and the uniform convergence in probability proved above, the first term in the r.h.s. of (3.3.62) converges to zero. We can show that the second term converges to zero by using Doob's inequality together with the estimates of the bracket of $M^{\mathrm{N,IS},f}$ (similar to (3.3.41)) and of $\Delta^{\mathrm{N},f}$ (Step 2). Finally, the third term vanishes in view of (3.3.60).

The convergence of the original sequence $(\mu^N)_{N\in\mathbb{N}}$ is then implied by the uniqueness of the solution to (3.3.17)–(3.3.19) proved in Step 2.

Step 5 When $N \to +\infty$, by taking the limit in (3.3.12), $(\mu^{\mathrm{N,S}})_{N\in\mathbb{N}}$ converges in $\mathbb{D}(\mathbb{R}_+, \mathscr{M}_{0,A})$ to the solution of the following transport equation: for every bounded function $f : (k,t) \mapsto f_t(k) \in \mathscr{C}_b^{0,1}(\mathbb{Z}_+ \times \mathbb{R}_+, \mathbb{R})$ of class $\mathscr{C}^1$ with bounded derivative with respect to t,

$$\langle \bar{\mu}_t^{\mathrm{S}}, f_t\rangle = \langle \bar{\mu}_0^{\mathrm{S}}, f_0\rangle - \int_0^t \langle \bar{\mu}_s^{\mathrm{S}}, \lambda\chi\bar{p}_s^{\mathrm{I}} f_s - \partial_s f_s\rangle \, \mathrm{d}s. \tag{3.3.63}$$

Choosing $f(k,s) = \varphi(k)\exp\big(-\lambda k \int_0^{t-s} \bar{p}^{\mathrm{I}}(u)du\big)$, we obtain that

$$\langle \bar{\mu}_t^{\mathrm{S}}, \varphi\rangle = \sum_{k\in\mathbb{Z}_+} \varphi(k)\theta_t^k \bar{\mu}_0^{\mathrm{S}}(k). \tag{3.3.64}$$

where $\theta_t = \exp\big(-\lambda \int_0^t \bar{p}^{\mathrm{I}}(u)du\big)$ is the probability that a given degree 1 node remains susceptible at time t. This is the announced Equation (3.3.17).

The proof of Theorem 3.3.8 is now completed. □

Recall that the time $t_{\varepsilon'}$ has been defined in (3.3.37). We end this section with a lower bound of the time $t_{\varepsilon'}$ until which we proved that the convergence to Volz' equations holds.

Proposition 3.3.12. *Under the assumptions of Theorem 3.3.8,*

$$t_{\varepsilon'} > \bar{\tau}_{\varepsilon'} := \frac{\log\big(\langle \bar{\mu}_0^{\mathrm{S}}, \chi^2\rangle + \bar{N}_0^{\mathrm{IS}}\big) - \log\big(\langle \bar{\mu}_0^{\mathrm{S}}, \chi^2\rangle + \varepsilon'\big)}{\max(\gamma,\lambda)}. \tag{3.3.65}$$

Proof. Because of the moment Assumption 3.3.5 and (3.3.21), we can prove that (3.3.47) also holds for $f = \chi$. This is obtained by replacing in (3.3.48), (3.3.54), (3.3.57) and (3.3.58) $\|f\|_\infty$ by k and using the Assumption of boundedness of the moments of order 5 in (3.3.54) and (3.3.58). This shows that $(N^{\mathrm{N,IS}})_{N\in\mathbb{N}}$ converges, uniformly on $[0, t_{\varepsilon'}]$ and in probability, to the deterministic and continuous solution $\bar{N}^{\mathrm{IS}} = \langle \bar{\mu}^{\mathrm{IS}}, \chi\rangle$. We introduce the event $\mathscr{A}_\xi^N = \{|\, N_0^{\mathrm{N,IS}} - N\bar{N}_0^{\mathrm{IS}} \,| \leq \xi\}$ where their differences are bounded by $\xi > 0$. Recall the definition (3.3.38) and let us introduce the number of edges Z_t^N that were IS at time 0 and that have been removed before t. For $t \geq \tau_{\varepsilon'}^N$, we have necessarily that $Z_t^N \geq N_0^{\mathrm{N,IS}} - N\varepsilon'$. Thus,

$$\begin{aligned}\mathbb{P}\big(\{\tau_{\varepsilon'}^N \leq t\} \cap \mathscr{A}_\xi^N\big) \leq& \mathbb{P}\big(\{Z_t^N > N_0^{\mathrm{N,IS}} - N\varepsilon'\} \cap \mathscr{A}_\xi^N\big)\\ \leq& \mathbb{P}\Big(\big\{Z_t^N > N(\bar{N}_0^{\mathrm{IS}} - \varepsilon') - \xi\big\} \cap \mathscr{A}_\xi^N\Big).\end{aligned} \tag{3.3.66}$$

When susceptible (resp. infectious) individuals of degree k are contaminated (resp. removed), at most k I − S-edges are lost. Let $X_t^{N,k}$ be the number of edges that, at time 0, are I − S with susceptible alter of degree k, and that have transmitted the disease before time t. Let $Y_t^{N,k}$ be the number of initially infectious individuals x with $d_x(\mathrm{S}_0) = k$ and who have been removed before time t. $X_t^{N,k}$ and $Y_t^{N,k}$ are bounded by $k\mu_0^{N,S}(k)$ and $\mu_0^{N,IS}(k)$. Thus:

$$Z_t^N \leq \sum_{k\in\mathbb{Z}_+} k\big(X_t^{N,k}+Y_t^{N,k}\big). \tag{3.3.67}$$

Let us stochastically bound Z_t^N from above. Since each I – S-edge transmits the disease independently at rate λ, $X_t^{N,k}$ is stochastically dominated by a binomial r.v. of parameters $k\mu_0^{N,S}(k)$ and $1-e^{-\lambda t}$. We proceed similarly for $Y_t^{N,k}$. Conditional on the initial condition, $X_t^{N,k}+Y_t^{N,k}$ is thus stochastically dominated by a binomial r.v. $\tilde{Z}_t^{N,k}$ of parameters $(k\mu_0^{N,S}(k)+\mu_0^{N,IS}(k))$ and $1-e^{-\max(\lambda,\gamma)t}$. Then (3.3.66) and (3.3.67) give:

$$\mathbb{P}\big(\{\tau_{\varepsilon'}^N \leq t\}\cap\mathscr{A}_\xi^N\big) \leq \mathbb{P}\Big(\sum_{k\in\mathbb{Z}_+}\frac{k\tilde{Z}_t^{N,k}}{N} > \bar{N}_0^{IS}-\varepsilon'-\frac{\xi}{N}\Big). \tag{3.3.68}$$

Thanks to Assumption 3.3.5 and (3.3.21), the series $\sum_{k\in\mathbb{Z}_+} k\tilde{Z}_t^{N,k}/N$ converges in L^1 and hence in probability to $(\langle\bar{\mu}_0^S,\chi^2\rangle+\bar{N}_0^{IS})(1-e^{-\max(\lambda,\gamma)t})$ when $N\to+\infty$. Thus, for sufficiently large N,

$$\mathbb{P}\big(\{\tau_{\varepsilon'}^N \leq t\}\cap\mathscr{A}_\xi^N\big) = 1 \text{ if } t>\bar{\tau}_{\varepsilon'} \text{ and } 0 \text{ if } t<\bar{\tau}_{\varepsilon'}.$$

For all $t<\bar{\tau}_{\varepsilon'}$, it follows from Assumption 3.3.5, (3.3.21) and Lemma A.0.4 that:

$$\lim_{N\to+\infty}\mathbb{P}\Big(\tau_{\varepsilon'}^N \leq t \leq \lim_{N\to+\infty}\mathbb{P}\big(\{\tau_{\varepsilon'}^N \leq t\}\cap\mathscr{A}_\xi^N\big)\Big)+\mathbb{P}\big((\mathscr{A}_\xi^N)^c\big)=0,$$

so that by Theorem 3.3.8

$$1=\lim_{N\to+\infty}\mathbb{P}(\tau_{\varepsilon'}^N \geq \bar{\tau}_{\varepsilon'}) = \lim_{n\to+\infty}\mathbb{P}\Big(\inf_{t\leq\bar{\tau}_{\varepsilon'}} N_t^{N,IS} \geq \varepsilon'\Big) = \mathbb{P}\Big(\inf_{t\leq\bar{\tau}_{\varepsilon'}} \bar{N}_t^{IS} \geq \varepsilon'\Big).$$

This shows that $t_{\varepsilon'} \geq \bar{\tau}_{\varepsilon'}$ a.s., which concludes the proof. □

Chapter 4

Statistical Description of Epidemics Spreading on Networks: The Case of Cuban HIV

In this section, we turn our attention to epidemics spreading on networks. Probability models have been described in Section 1.4. We now deal with the statistical treatment of data obtained from diseases propagating on networks. The statistical methods described here are illustrated on the sexual network obtained from the Cuban HIV contact-tracing system that we now describe. For a complete description of the Cuban network, we refer to [35]. The Cuban graph is available as supplementary material of this book.

Since 1986, a contact-tracing detection system has been set up in Cuba in order to bring the spread of the HIV epidemic under control. It has also enabled the gathering of a considerable amount of detailed epidemiological data at the individual level. In the resulting database, any individual tested as HIV positive is indexed and anonymized for confidentiality reasons. Information related to uninfected individuals is not recorded in the data, and of course infected individuals not diagnosed yet are also absent. The network only consists of detected HIV+ individuals. However, note that the network is age-structured and data related to the infectious population of the first six years of the epidemic seems to show (e.g. [37]) that this population has been discovered by now.
Individuals in the database are described through several attribute variables: gender and sexual orientation, way of detection, age at detection, date of detection, area of residence, etc. In the sequel, we will mainly focus on the gender/sexual orientation, for which three modalities are identified: 'woman', 'heterosexual man', 'MSM' (Men who have Sex with Men; men who reported at least one sexual contact with another man in the two years preceding HIV detection). Because Female-to-female transmission is neglected, no sexual orientation is distinguished for women (e.g. [30]). It is worth recalling that in Cuba HIV spreads essentially through sexual transmission. Infection by blood transfusion or related to drug use are neglected. We refer to [8] for a preliminary overview of the HIV/AIDS epidemics in Cuba, as well as a description and the context of the construction of the database used in the present study and the context in which it was constructed.

T. Britton, E. Pardoux (eds.), *Stochastic Epidemic Models with Inference*, Lecture Notes in Mathematics 2255, https://doi.org/10.1007/978-3-030-30900-8_11

Importantly, for each HIV+ individual that is detected, the list of indices corresponding to the sexual partners appearing in the database she/he possibly named for contact-tracing is also available. In [33, 34, 35] the graph of sexual partners that have been diagnosed HIV positive on the Cuban data repository is reconstructed and an exploratory statistical analysis of the resulting sexual contact network is carried. The network is composed of 5,389 vertices, or nodes, that correspond to the individuals diagnosed as HIV positive between 1986 and 2006 in Cuba, i.e. 1,109 women (20.58%) and 4,280 men (79.42%); 566 (10.50%) of which are heterosexual and 3,714 (68.92%) are MSMs. Individuals declared as sexual contacts but who are not HIV positive are not listed in the database: the only observed vertices correspond to individuals who have been detected as HIV positive or AIDS. The vertices that depict the fact that two individuals have been sexual partners during the two years that preceded the detection of either one are linked by 4,073 edges. Only edges between observed HIV cases are hence observed, but the degree (total number of sexual partners) is known. Also, some information is documented on who infects whom, giving access to a partial infection tree. Our data exhibit a "giant component", counting 2,386 nodes. The second largest component has only 17 vertices and there are about 2000 isolated individuals or couples. It is remarkable that in the existing literature on sexually transmitted diseases graph networks are generally smaller and/or do not exhibit such a large connected component and/or contain a very small number of infected persons (e.g. [102, 116]).

In Section 4.2, using graph-mining techniques, the connectivity/communication properties of the sexual contact network are described to understand the impact of heterogeneity (with respect to the attributes observed) in the graph structure. Particular attention is paid to the graphical representation of the data, as conventional methods cannot be used with databases of the size of the one used in this study. A clustering of the population is performed so as to represent structural information in an interpretable way. Beyond global graph visualization, the task of partitioning the network into groups, with dense internal links and low external connectivity, is known as clustering. In contrast to standard multivariate analysis, in which the network structure of the data is ignored, our method has shed light on how different mechanisms (e.g. social behaviour, detection system) have affected the epidemics of HIV in the past, and provide a way of predicting the future evolution of this disease. This study paves the way for building more realistic network models in the field of mathematical modelling of infectious diseases.

4.1 Modularity and Assortative Mixing

Assortative mixing coefficients can be computed to highlight the possible existence of selective linking in the network structure. Various measures have been proposed in the literature for quantifying the tendency for individuals to have connections with other individuals that are similar in regards to certain attributes, depending on the nature of the latter (quantitative vs. qualitative). For a partition of J classes, $\mathscr{P} =$

$C_1, \ldots, C_J$, one may calculate the proportion $m_{i,j}$ of edges in the graph connecting a node lying in group i to another one in group j, $1 \le i \le j \le J$ and build the $J \times J$ mixing matrix $\mathscr{M} = (m_{i,j})$ (notice it is symmetric since edges are not directed here). We can then define the modularity coefficient $Q_{\mathscr{P}}$ (e.g. [84]) by:

$$Q_{\mathscr{P}} = \mathrm{Tr}(\mathscr{M}) - ||\mathscr{M}^2|| = \sum_i \left\{ m_{i,i} - \left(\sum_{j=1}^{N} m_{i,j} \right)^2 \right\}, \qquad (4.1.1)$$

where $||A|| = \sum_i \sum_j a_{i,j}$ denotes the sum of all the entries of a matrix $A = (a_{i,j})$ and $\mathrm{Tr}(A)$ its trace when the latter is square.

We can define the assortative coefficient as

$$r = Q_{\mathscr{P}} / (1 - ||\mathscr{M}^2||).$$

As pointed out in [87], large values of r indicate "selective linking": values around 0 correspond to randomly mixed network, whereas values close to 1 are associated with perfectly assortative network. The assortative coefficient can also be negative.

Ego is a	Alter is a woman	Alter is a heterosexual man	Alter is an MSM	Total
Woman	77 (*1.9%*)	157 (*3.9%*)	408 (*10.0%*)	642 (*15.8%*)
HT man	282 (*6.9%*)	4 (*0.1%*)	20 (*0.5%*)	306 (*7.5%*)
MSM	800 (*19.6%*)	25 (*0.6%*)	2300 (*56.5%*)	3125 (*76.7%*)
Total	1159 (*28.5%*)	186 (*4.6%*)	2728 (*67.0%*)	

Table 4.1.1 *Sexual orientation of egos and alters for the edges in the whole graph. The figures presented here account for the direction of the edges: egos are detected first and alters are the partners they refer to during the contact-tracing interviews. Frequencies are given together with row and column proportions between brackets. The diagonal of the contingency table represents 58,46% of the whole edges. The assortative mixing coefficient is* $r = 0.0512$. *The independence between the sexual orientation of egos and alters is rejected by a* χ^2*-test with a p-value smaller than* $2.2\,10^{-16}$. *In theory, there should be no sexual contact between two heterosexual men or between a heterosexual man and an MSM. The semantic of the database also exclude sexual contact between women. However, those events actually occur in the dataset.*

A first class of partitions are constituted by nodes taking the same modalities of qualitative variables: area of residence, sexual orientation, age, detection mode... Let us comment on the partition defined by the gender/sexual orientation variable (see Table 4.1.1). As edges correspond to sexual contacts in the present graph, the gender/sexual orientation of adjacent vertices cannot be arbitrary of course. More than a half of the edges (56.47%) link two MSM. Links between MSM and women make 1,208 edges (29.66%) and there are 439 edges (10.78%) between women and heterosexual men. Looking at the infection tree provided similar proportions: 1,202 edges (52.56%), 667 edges (29.16%) and 375 edges (16.40%) respectively. Figures reveal an asymmetry in HIV infection: among (oriented) infection edges involving women, the latter are more often alters than egos (66.13% of the edges shared with heterosexual men and 74.21% of the edges shared with MSM). The declarative degree shows a smaller mean degree for heterosexual men and comparable degree distributions between women and MSM. MSM are expected to contribute most to the connectivity of the graph, especially bisexual men who act as contact points between women and MSM who declare only contacts with men.

Of course, a natural question is to see whether we can define other partitions that are more closely related to the modularity defined in (4.1.1). This is the topic of the next section, which is related with visual-mining and modularity clustering.

4.2 Visual-mining

Graph visualization techniques are used routinely to gain insights about medium size graph structures, but their practical relevance is questionable when the number of vertices and the density of the graph are high both for computational issues (as many graph drawing algorithms have high complexities) and for readability issues [22, 59]. We illustrate the clustering and visualization on the Cuba HIV data where the situation is borderline as the giant component of the graph contains 2,386 vertices and 3,168 edges (respectively 44.28% and 77.78% of the global quantities). As the graph is of medium size from a computational point of view and has a low density, it is a reasonable candidate for state-of-the-art global and detailed visualization techniques. We use the optimised force directed placement algorithm proposed in [108]. It recasts the classical force directed paradigm [56] into a nonlinear optimization problem in which the following energy is minimised over the vertex positions in the euclidean plane, $(z_1,\dots,z_n)$,

$$\mathscr{E}(z_1,\dots,z_n) = \sum_{1\leq i\neq j\leq n} \left(a_{i,j}\frac{1}{3\delta}\|z_i - z_j\|^3 - \delta^2 \ln \|z_i - z_j\| \right),$$

where, δ is a free parameter that is roughly proportional to the expected average distance between vertices in the plane at the end of the optimization process, $a_{i,j}$ are the terms of the adjacency matrix of the network and $\|\cdot\|$ denotes the Euclidean distance in the plane.

However, the structure of the graph under study, in particular its uneven density, has adverse effects on the readability of its global representation. We rely therefore on the classical simplification approach [59] that consists in building a clustering of the vertices of the graph and in representing the simpler graph of the clusters. More precisely, the general idea is to define a partition composed of groups with dense internal links but low inter-group connectivity. Each group can then be considered as a vertex of a new graph: two such vertices are connected if there is at least one pair of original vertices in each group that are connected in the original graph.

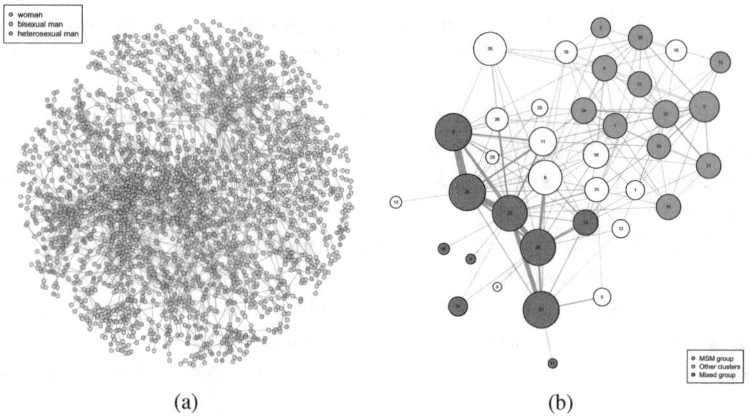

Fig. 4.2.1 *(a): Raw view of the giant component for the Cuban HIV epidemics. (b) Modularity clustering of the giant component in 37 classes.*

Following [34, 33, 101], we compute a maximal modularity clustering [84] as the obtained clusters are well adapted to subsequent visual representation, as shown in [89]. Maximizing $Q_{\mathscr{P}}$ over all the partitions $\mathscr{P}$ provides an optimal J classes partition. This is an NP-Hard and can only be solved via some heuristics. As in [101], we use a modified version of the multi-level greedy merging approach proposed in [90]: our modification guarantees that the final clusters are connected. The optimization process is carried out on the partitions for a given number of clusters J but also over the number of clusters J itself which is then automatically selected. This makes the method essentially parameter free.

It should be noted however that one can find partitions with a rather high modularity even in completely random graphs (configuration model graphs where vertices have different degrees but are paired independently) where no modular structure actually exists (see [95] for an estimation of the expected value of this spurious modularity in the limit of large and dense graphs). To check that the modular structure found in a network cannot be explained by this phenomenon, we use the simulation approach proposed in [35, 101]. Using a Markov Chain Monte Carlo (MCMC) approach inspired by [98], we generate configuration model graphs with exactly the same size and degree distribution as the epidemics graph. Using the above algorithm, we compute a maximal modularity clustering on each of those graphs. The modularities of the clustering provide an estimate of the distribution of the maximal modularity in random graphs with our degree distribution. If a partition of this graph exhibits a higher modularity, we conclude that it must be the result of some actual modular structure rather than a random outcome.

The maximal modularity clustering is visualised using the force directed placement algorithm described above. In addition to giving a general idea of the global structure of the graph, the obtained visual representation can be used to display distributions of covariates at the cluster level. Homogeneity tests are performed in order to assess possible significant differences between these statistical subpopulations.

However, as demonstrated in [54], finding the maximal modularity clustering can lead to ignoring small modular structures that fall below the resolution limit of the modularity measure. It is then recommended in [54] to recursively apply maximal modularity clustering to the original clusters in order to investigate potential smaller scale modules. We follow this strategy coupled with the MCMC approach described above: each cluster is tested for substructure by applying the maximal modularity clustering technique from [101] and by assessing the actual significance of a potential sub-structure via comparison with similar random graphs.

To sum up, we recall the procedure that we recommend for clustering a large network:

- maximization of the modularity (4.1.1) (see [84]).
  - this favours dense clusters and produces interesting partitions for visualization (Fortunato 2010)
  - the optimisation is an NP-hard problem but high quality sub-optimal solutions can be obtained by annealing (Rossi Villa-Vialaneix 2010) or other methods (Noak Rotta, 2009)
- Clustering significance:
  - compute the modularity of the partition that is obtained,
  - test the significance of the obtained partition by simulating configuration models with same degree distribution and compute modularity.
- **Hierarchical clustering:** if the first clustering is relevant, and if the classes have large sizes, we can refine the partition.
  - Reiterate the clustering for each element of the partition, without taking inter-cluster connections.
  - Test the significance of the cluster's partition
  - Test the significance of the global clustering of the graph.
- **Coarsening:** merge clusters that induce the least reduction in modularity as long as we remain above the original graph.
- **Visualization:** use the Fruchterman–Reingold algorithm to display the network of clusters

4.3 Analysis of the "Giant Component"

The network density is globally low and very heterogeneous. But although the connectivity of the network seems fragile at first glance, density may be locally very high. The harmonic average of the geodesic path lengths equals 10.24 and 12.2 for the directed graph (taking into account the information of who mentions whom). Most of the graph connectivity is concentrated in the largest component (3,168

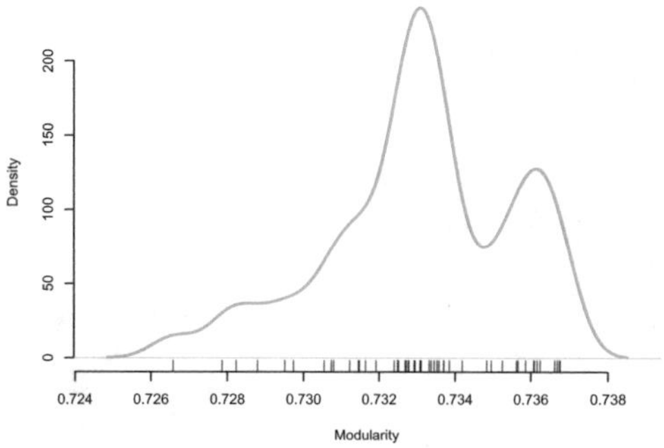

Fig. 4.2.2 *In Figure 4.2.1, a modularity clustering is performed on the Cuban HIV data. The modularity of the partition obtained is* $\simeq 0.85$. *To test the significancy of this partition, 100 configuration model graphs with same size and same degree distribution as the observed one are simulated. The empirical distribution of the random modularity obtained by these simulations is depicted with small black bars on the abscissa axis and has a support bounded by* 0.74. *This shows that the partition obtained by maximizing the modularity is significant (at level 95% for instance).*

edges out of 4,073). The largest component has a diameter of 26 (36 when taking into account the direction of the infections) and the harmonic average of the geodesic path lengths are the same inside the largest component. These values are slightly higher than those of other real networks mentioned in [88] but remain well below the number of vertices and compatible with the logarithmic scaling related to the so-termed small world effect.

Figure 4.2.1 (b) seems quite clear, with what appears to be two parts in the graph: the lower part of the graph (on the figure) seems to be dominated by MSM while the upper part gathers almost all persons from the giant component that have only heterosexual contacts. However, the upper part is quite difficult to read as it seems denser than the lower part. The layout shows what might be interpreted as cycles and also a lot of small trees connected to denser parts. The actual connection patterns between the upper part and the lower part are also very unclear. Because of these crowding effects, structural properties of the network from Figure 4.2.1 appears quite difficult and probably misleading. We rely therefore on the simplification technique outlined in Section 4.2 leveraging a clustering of the giant component to get an insight into its general organization.

A graphical representation of the partition obtained by the method from [101] is displayed in Figure 4.3.1 (a). The clustering thus produced exhibits a modularity of 0.8522 and is made up of 37 clusters. This modularity is very high compared to the random level and strongly supports the hypothesis of a specific ("non-random") underlying community structure. For comparison purpose, the average maximal modularity attained by random graphs built from a configuration model with the same size and degree distribution as those of the giant component observed over a collection of 100 simulated replications (using the same partitioning method) is of the order 0.74, with a maximum of 0.7435.

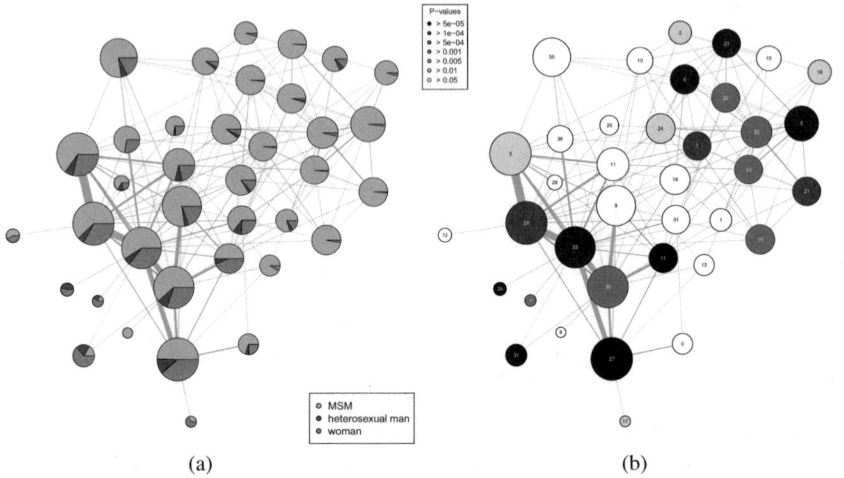

Fig. 4.3.1 *The giant component divided into 37 clusters. (a) Each disk of representation corresponds to one cluster and has an area proportional to the number of persons (original vertices) gathered in the associated cluster. The pie chart of the disk displays the percentage of MSM (green), of heterosexual men (blue) and of women (red) in the cluster. Links between clusters summarise the connectivity pattern between members of the clusters. The thinnest edge width corresponds to only one connection between a member of one cluster and another person in the connected cluster (the corresponding edges are drawn using dâshed segments). Thicker edges have a width proportional to the number of connected persons. (b) Disk areas and edges thicknesses are chosen as in (a). The grey level of a disk encode the p-value of a* χ^2 *test of homogeneity in which the distribution of the sexual orientations in the associated cluster is compared to the distribution in the giant component.*

Considering that the modules are meaningful, the visual representation provided by Figure 4.3.1 (a) is more faithful to the underlying graphical structure than the finer displays of Figure 4.2.1 (b). That said, the two graphs tend to agree as the pie charts of Figure 4.3.1 clearly show two parts in the network: the lower left part seems to gather most of the women and heterosexual men (as the upper part of Figure 4.2.1 (b)), while the upper right part contains clusters made almost entirely of MSM, as the lower part of Figure 4.2.1 (b). While the display of Figure 4.3.1 (a) might seem cluttered, it is in fact very readable if one considers that only 328 edges of the giant component connect persons from different clusters while 2,840 connections happen inside clusters. Then most of the edges on Figure 4.3.1 (a) could be disregarded as they corresponds to only one pair of connected persons (this is the case of 94 of such edges out of 142 and the former are represented as dashed segments). Taken this aspect into account, it appears that the MSM part of the giant component (upper right part) is made of loosely connected clusters while the bulk of the connectivity between clusters is gathered in the mixed part of the component, in which most women and heterosexual men are gathered. The fact that the mixed part is more dense was already visible in Figure 4.2.1 (b), but Figure 4.3.1 (a) provides a much stronger demonstration.

The pie chart based visualization of Figure 4.3.1 (a) shows the sexual orientation distribution in the clusters and hence sheds light on its relationship with the graphical structure. In Figure 4.3.1 (b), a visual representation of the corresponding p-values is given. The darker the node, the more statistically significant the difference between the cluster distribution of sexual orientation and the distribution of the giant component.

Combining Figures 4.3.1 (a) and (b) is very useful: Figure (b) highlights atypical clusters while Figure (a) identifies why they are atypical. It appears that among the 37 clusters, 22 exhibit a χ^2 p-value below 5%. They will be abusively referred to as "atypical clusters" in the following. The set of those clusters can be split into two subsets, depending on the percentage of MSM in the cluster: above or below the global value of 76% (the percentage in the giant component), as illustrated by Figure 4.3.1 (b). Almost two thirds (67%) of the individuals of the largest connected component lie in the atypical clusters. Among the latter, 774 individuals belong to the 12 clusters which display a large domination of MSM (denoted the MSM group of clusters in the sequel) and 825 to the 10 clusters that contain an unexpectedly large number of heterosexual persons (denoted the mixed group of clusters in the sequel).

According to Figure 4.3.1, the two subsets of atypical clusters seem to be almost disconnected. This is confirmed by a detailed connectivity analysis. There are indeed 864 internal connections in the MSM group, 1,276 in the heterosexual group, and only 10 links between pairs of individuals belonging to the two different groups. This asymmetry was expected, given the quality of the clustering with only 328 inter-cluster connections. Nevertheless, the number of connections between the two groups of clusters is also small compared to connections between the clusters of the groups: 129 connections between persons of distinct clusters in the group of mixed clusters and 55 in the group of MSM clusters. Finally, there are 83 connections from persons in the group of mixed clusters to persons in non-atypical clusters, and 36 connections from persons in the group of MSM clusters to persons in non-atypical clusters. Mean geodesic distances inside the MSM group are larger than in the mixed group (respectively 9.95 and 7.28, computed without orientation). To conclude, the two groups are weakly connected to the outside, with a small number of direct connections, and rather internally more connected than expected.

4.4 Descriptive Statistics for Epidemics on Networks

We now review some basic descriptive statistics for networks. Exhaustive statistical exploration of networks has been described by Newman [88] for example.

4.4.1 Estimating Degree Distributions

For the Cuban HIV data, we want to calculate for instance the degree distribution $(p_k : k \in \mathbb{N})$ using the number of declared sexual partners in the two years preceding detection, where p_k is the proportion of vertices having declared k sexual partners.

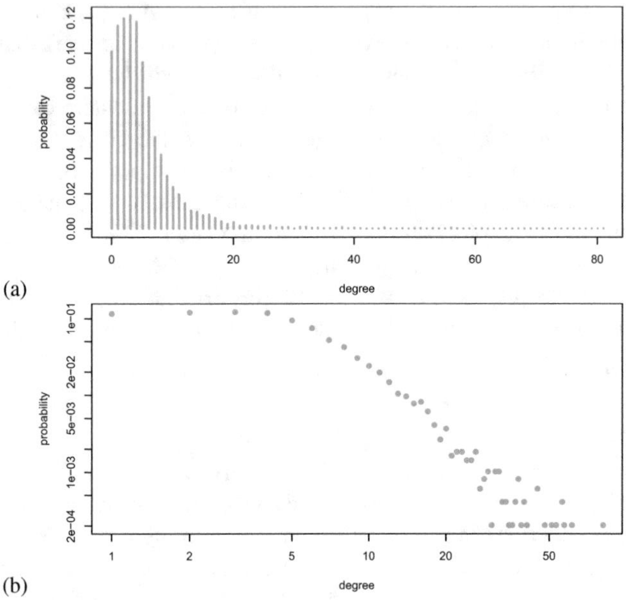

Fig. 4.4.1 *(a) Distribution of the declared number of sexual partners for the HIV+ individuals detected and present in the Cuban database. (b) Preceding degree distribution plotted in a log-log scale: the graph exhibits a power-law behaviour.*

The degree distributions of most real-world networks, referred to as scale-free networks, often exhibit a power-law behaviour in their right tails (see [49]), i.e.

$$p_k \sim k^{-\alpha}, \text{ as } k \text{ becomes large,}$$

for some exponent $\alpha > 1$ (notice that $\sum_{k=1}^{\infty} 1/k^{\alpha} < \infty$ in this case). Roughly speaking, this describes the situations where the majority of vertices have few connections, but a small fraction of the vertices are highly connected (e.g. Chapter 4 in [83] for further details). We propose to fit a power-law exponent and consider two methods for this purpose, see also [32]. First, we minimize, over $\alpha > 1$, the following measure of dissimilarity between the observed degree distribution and the power-law distribution with exponent α based on degree values larger than k_0

$$\mathcal{K}_{k_0}(p,\alpha) = \sum_{k \geq k_0} \frac{p_k}{c_{p,k_0}} \log\left(\frac{C_\alpha \cdot p_k}{c_{p,k_0} \cdot k^{-\alpha}}\right), \tag{4.4.1}$$

where log denotes the natural logarithm, $c_{p,k_0} = \sum_{k \geq k_0} p_k$ and $C_\alpha = \sum_{k \geq k_0} 1/k^\alpha$. Notice that, when k_0 is larger than the maximum observed degree distribution $k_{\max}$, we have $\mathcal{K}_{k_0}(p, \alpha) = 0$ no matter the exponent α. Also, the computation of (4.4.1) involves summing a finite number of terms only, since the empirical frequency p_k is equal to zero for any degree k sufficiently large. The criterion $\mathcal{K}_{k_0}(p, \alpha)$ is known as the Kullback–Leibler divergence between the empirical and theoretical conditional distributions given that the degree is larger than k_0. Incidentally, we point out that other dissimilarity measures could be considered for the purpose of fitting a power-law, such as the χ^2-distance for instance. For a fixed threshold $k_0 \geq 1$, it is natural to select the value of the power-law exponent that provides the best fit, that is:

$$\widehat{\alpha}_{k_0} = \arg\min_{\alpha > 1} \mathcal{K}_{k_0}(p, \alpha).$$

Choosing k_0 precisely being a challenging question to statisticians. Following in the footsteps of the heuristic selection procedures proposed in the context of heavy-tailed continuous distributions (see Chapter 4 in [96]), when possible, we suggest to choose $\widehat{\alpha}_{k_0}$ with k_0 in a region where the graph $\{(k, \widehat{\alpha}_k) : k = 1, \ldots, k_{\max}\}$ is becoming horizontal, or at least shows an inflexion point. For completeness, we also compute the Hill estimator:

$$\widetilde{\alpha}_m = \left(\frac{1}{m} \sum_{j=1}^{m} \frac{k_{(j)}}{k_{(m)}} \right)^{-1},$$

where n is the number of vertices of the graph under study, $1 \leq m \leq n$ and $k_{(1)} = k_{\max}, k_{(2)}, \ldots, k_{(m)}$ denote the m largest observed degrees sorted in decreasing order of their magnitude. The tuning parameter m is selected graphically, by plotting the graph $\{(m, \widetilde{\alpha}_m) : m = 1, \ldots, n\}$. In the case when the degrees of the vertices of the graph are independent, as for the configuration model [85], this statistic can be viewed as a conditional maximum likelihood estimator and arguments based on asymptotic theory supports its pertinence in this situation, see [60].

Let us consider the declared degree distribution in the Cuban database (see Fig. 4.4.1). Among the 5,389 individuals appearing in the database, 483 declared no sexual partners during this period. Degree distributions for the whole population exhibit a clear power-law behaviour. Power laws are fitted to the declared degree distributions, for the whole population and for the strata defined by the variable gender/sexual orientation respectively. Both methods present similar results. The resulting estimates (see Table 4.4.1) reveal the thickness of the upper tails: the smaller the tail exponent α, the heavier the distribution tail. Women correspond to the heaviest tail, followed by MSM and heterosexual men. However, an ANOVA reveals no statistically significant impact of the covariates gender/sexual orientation. All the same, using the observed degree distribution, we obtain $(k_0, \alpha) = (3, 2.99)$ which is very close to the result when using the number of neighbours having been detected positive.

All the tail exponent estimates are below the critical value of $\alpha_c = 3.4788$, below which a giant component exists in scale-free networks generated by means of the configuration model, and above the value 2, below which the whole graph reduces to the giant component with probability one (see [79, 88]).

	$\widehat{k}_0$	$\widehat{\alpha}_{k_0}$	Mean	Std dev.	Min	Max
Whole population	7	3.06	6.17	5.54	1	82
Women	6	2.71	5.88	5.03	1	39
Heterosexual men	7	3.36	4.98	4.11	1	30
MSM	7	3.02	6.43	5.84	1	82

Table 4.4.1 Degree distribution for the Cuban HIV+ network, for the whole population and by sexual orientation.

For completeness, we can also compare with the Hill estimator (4.4.1) to the estimator (4.4.1) in each case, obtained by plotting the curves $(m, \widetilde{\alpha}_m)$ in Fig. 4.4.2: reassuringly, we found that both estimation methods yield similar results.

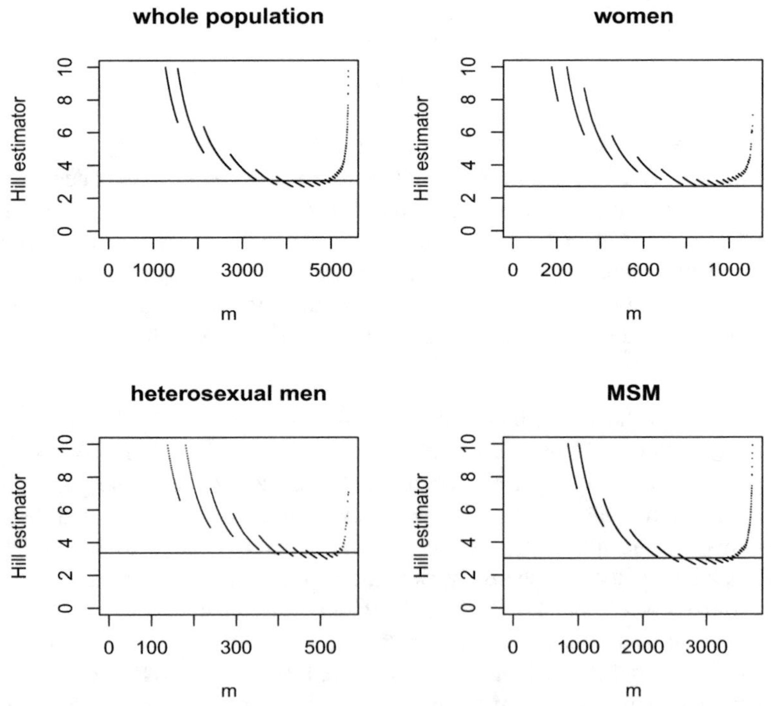

Fig. 4.4.2 *Graph of* $(m, \widetilde{\alpha}_m)$ *for* $m \in \{1, \ldots, n\}$*. This graph allows us to choose the Hill estimator. The horizontal line* $y = \widehat{\alpha}_{k_0}$ *permits to visualize the estimator* $\widehat{\alpha}_{k_0}$ *and compare it with the Hill estimator.*

4.4.2 Joint Degree Distribution of Sexual Partners

The independence assumption between the degrees of adjacent vertices does not hold here, see Fig. 4.4.3, in contrast to what is assumed for the vast majority of graph-based SIR models of epidemic disease, e.g. [49, 88]. Indeed, the linear correlation coefficient between the degree distributions of alters and egos is equal to 0.68. Testing the significance of this coefficient, that describes the correlation of these degree distributions, allows us to test the independence of the latter. Independence between the degree distributions of alters and egos is rejected by a χ^2-test with a p-value of $6.85\,10^{-6}$. In particular, highly connected vertices tend to be connected to vertices with a high number of connections too. From the perspective of mathematical modeling, this suggests to consider graph models with a dependence structure between the degrees of adjacent nodes, in opposition to most percolation processes on (configuration model) networks used to describe the spread of epidemics [79, 13, 110, 44, 58]. However, it is worth noticing that, if we restrict our analysis to some specific, more homogeneous, subgroups, the independence assumption may be grounded in evidence. So if assumptions such that the network is generated by a configuration model do not hold globally, they may be valid for smaller clusters, which is another motivation for clustering.

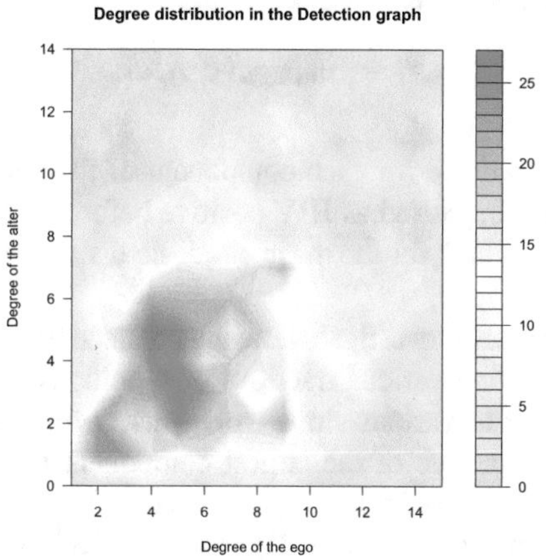

Fig. 4.4.3 *Joint degree distribution of the number of contacts for connected vertices.*

4.4.3 Computation of Geodesic Distances and Other Connectivity Properties

There is a large literature on describing the social networks on which epidemics might propagate (see Newman [88] for a more exhaustive list of descriptive statistics, and [35, 36] for an application to the Cuban HIV epidemics). Here, we mention some of them, related to community and connexity. All results presented here are obtained with the R-package `igraph` [42].

A set of connected vertices with the corresponding edges, constitutes a component of the graph. The collection of components forms a partition of the graph. We identify the components of the network and compute their respective sizes. When the size of the largest component is much larger than the size of the second largest component, see section IV A in [88] and the references therein, one then refers to the notion of giant component.

A geodesic path between two connected vertices x and y is a path with shortest length that connects them, its length $d(x,y)$ being the geodesic distance between x and y. One also defines the mean geodesic distance:

$$\mathscr{L} = \frac{1}{n(n+1)} \sum_{(x,y)\in\mathscr{V}^2} d(x,y),$$

where $\mathscr{V}$ denotes the set of all vertices of the connected graph and n its size. For non-connected graphs, one usually computes a harmonic average. Mean geodesic distances measure "how far" two randomly chosen vertices are, given the network structure. When $\mathscr{L}$ is much smaller than n, one says that a "small-world effect" is observed. In this regard, the diameter of a connected graph, that is to say the length of the longest geodesic path, is also a quantity of major interest:

$$\delta = \max_{(x,y)\in\mathscr{V}^2} d(x,y).$$

Computations have been made for each component of the network of sexual contacts among individuals diagnosed as HIV positive before 2006 in Cuba, using the dedicated "burning algorithm" for the mean geodesic distances, see [4].

Along these lines, we also investigate how the connectivity properties of the network evolve when removing various fractions of specific strata of the population: we studied the resilience to various strata (robustness of certain statistics such as mean geodesic distance or size of the largest component to deletion of points in these strata), the clustering coefficients (defined as the number of triangles over the number of connected triples of vertices) and the articulation points (points that disconnect the component they belong to into two components when removed; see Section 6 of [36]). Indicators show an apparent weak resilience: 1,157 articulation points (out of 2,386 nodes), only 187 cliques (among them 177 triangles) and low assortative mixing coefficients. Global statistics thus indicate a low density of the graph (many articulation points, resilient structure, low clustering coefficients), the clustering emphasised the important heterogeneity in the network, with some dense regions that are internally more connected than average and with few links to the outside. We found subgroups with atypical covariate distributions, each reflecting a different stage of the evolution of the epidemic. Clustering the graph also allows us to unfold the complex structure of the Cuban HIV contact-tracing network. As a byproduct, the clustering indicates sub-structures that may be considered as random graphs resulting from configuration models, bridging the gap between the modelling papers whose assumptions on network structures do not often match reality.

Appendix: Finite Measures on $\mathbb{Z}_+$

First, some notation is needed in order to clarify the way the atoms of a given element of $\mathcal{M}_F(\mathbb{Z}_+)$ are ranked. For all $\mu \in \mathcal{M}_F(\mathbb{Z}_+)$, let F_μ be its cumulative distribution function and F_μ^{-1} be its right inverse defined as

$$\forall x \in \mathbb{R}_+, F_\mu^{-1}(x) = \inf\{i \in \mathbb{Z}_+, F_\mu(i) \geq x\}. \tag{A.0.2}$$

Let $\mu = \sum_{n\in\mathbb{Z}_+} a_n\delta_n$ be an integer-valued measure of $\mathcal{M}_F(\mathbb{Z}_+)$, i.e. such that the a_n's are themselves integers. Then, for each atom $n \in \mathbb{Z}_+$ of μ such that $a_n > 0$, we duplicate the atom n with multiplicity a_n, and we rank the atoms of μ by increasing values, sorting arbitrarily the atoms having the same value. Then, we denote for any $i \leq \langle \mu, \mathbf{1}\rangle$,

$$\gamma_i(\mu) = F_\mu^{-1}(i), \tag{A.0.3}$$

the level of the ith atom of the measure, when ranked as described above. We refer to Example 3.3.3 for a simple illustration.

We now make precise a few topological properties of spaces of measures and measure-valued processes. For $T > 0$ and a Polish space (E, d_E), we denote by $\mathbb{D}([0,T],E)$ the Skorokhod space of càdlàg (right-continuous and left-limited) functions from $[0,T]$ into E (e.g. [24, 66]) equipped with the Skorokhod topology induced by the metric

$$d_T(f,g) := \inf_{\alpha\in\Delta([0,T])} \left\{ \sup_{\substack{(s,t)\in[0,T]^2,\\ s\neq t}} \left|\log \frac{\alpha(s)-\alpha(t)}{s-t}\right| + \sup_{t\leq T} d_E\left(f(t), g(\alpha(t))\right) \right\}, \tag{A.0.4}$$

where the infimum is taken over the set $\Delta([0,T])$ of continuous increasing functions $\alpha : [0,T] \to [0,T]$ such that $\alpha(0) = 0$ and $\alpha(T) = T$.

Limit theorems are heavily dependent on the topologies considered. We introduce here several technical lemmas on the space of measures related to these questions. For any fixed $0 \leq \varepsilon < A$, recall the definition of $\mathcal{M}_{\varepsilon,A}$ in (3.3.20). Note that for any $\nu \in \mathcal{M}_{\varepsilon,A}$, and $i \in \{0,\dots,5\}$, $\langle \nu, \chi^i \rangle \le A$ since the support of ν is included in $\mathbb{Z}_+$.

Lemma A.0.1. *Let $\mathfrak{I}$ be an arbitrary set and consider a family $(\nu_\tau, \tau \in \mathfrak{I})$ of elements of $\mathcal{M}_{\varepsilon,A}$. Then, for any real-valued function f on $\mathbb{Z}_+$ such that $f(k) = o(k^5)$, we have that*

$$\lim_{K\to\infty} \sup_{\tau\in\mathfrak{I}} |\langle \nu_\tau, f\mathbf{1}_{[K,\infty)}\rangle| = 0.$$

Proof. By Markov inequality, for any $\tau \in \mathfrak{I}$, for any K, we have

$$\sum_{k\ge K} |f(k)|\nu_\tau(k) \le A \sup_{k\ge K} \frac{|f(k)|}{k^5},$$

hence

$$\lim_{K\to\infty} \sup_{\tau\in\mathfrak{I}} |\langle \nu_\tau, f\rangle| \le A \limsup_{k\to\infty} \frac{|f(k)|}{k^5} = 0.$$

The proof is thus complete. □

Lemma A.0.2. *For any $A > 0$, the set $\mathcal{M}_{\varepsilon,A}$ is a closed subset of $\mathcal{M}_F(\mathbb{Z}_+)$ embedded with the topology of weak convergence.*

Proof. Let $(\mu_n)_{n\in\mathbb{N}}$ be a sequence of $\mathcal{M}_{\varepsilon,A}$ converging to $\mu \in \mathcal{M}_F(\mathbb{Z}_+)$ for the weak topology, Fatou's lemma for sequences of measures implies

$$\langle \mu, \chi^5 \rangle \le \liminf_{n\to\infty} \langle \mu_n, \chi^5 \rangle.$$

Since $\langle \mu_n, \mathbf{1} \rangle$ tends to $\langle \mu, \mathbf{1} \rangle$, we have that $\langle \mu, \mathbf{1} + \chi^5 \rangle \le A$.

Furthermore, by uniform integrability (Lemma A.0.1), it is also clear that

$$\varepsilon \le \lim_{n\to\infty} \langle \mu_n, \chi \rangle = \langle \mu, \chi \rangle,$$

which shows that $\mu \in \mathcal{M}_{\varepsilon,A}$. □

Lemma A.0.3. *The traces on $\mathcal{M}_{\varepsilon,A}$ of the total variation topology and of the weak topology coincide.*

Proof. It is well known that the total variation topology is coarser than the weak topology. In the reverse direction, assume that $(\mu_n)_{n\in\mathbb{N}}$ is a sequence of weakly converging measures all belonging to $\mathcal{M}_{\varepsilon,A}$. Since,

$$d_{TV}(\mu_n, \mu) \le \sum_{k\in\mathbb{Z}_+} |\mu_n(k) - \mu(k)|.$$

according to Lemma A.0.1, it is then easily deduced that the right-hand side converges to 0 as n goes to infinity. □

Lemma A.0.4. *If the sequence $(\mu_n)_{n\in\mathbb{N}}$ of $\mathcal{M}_{\varepsilon,A}^{\mathbb{N}}$ converges weakly to the measure $\mu \in \mathcal{M}_{\varepsilon,A}$, then $(\langle \mu_n, f \rangle)_{n\in\mathbb{N}}$ converges to $\langle \mu, f \rangle$ for all function f such that $f(k) = o(k^5)$ for all large k.*

Proof. The triangle inequality implies that:

$$|\langle \mu_n, f\rangle - \langle \mu, f\rangle| \le |\langle \mu_n, f\mathbf{1}_{[0,K]}\rangle - \langle \mu, f\mathbf{1}_{[0,K]}\rangle| \\ + |\langle \mu, f\mathbf{1}_{(K,+\infty)}\rangle| + |\langle \mu_n, f\mathbf{1}_{(K,+\infty)}\rangle|.$$

We then conclude by uniform integrability and weak convergence. □

Recall that $\mathscr{M}_{\varepsilon,A}$ can be equipped with the total variation distance topology, hence the topology on $\mathbb{D}([0,T], \mathscr{M}_{\varepsilon,A})$ is induced by the distance

$$\rho_T(\mu_., \nu_.) = \inf_{\alpha \in \Delta([0,T])} \left(\sup_{\substack{(s,t)\in[0,T]^2,\\ s\neq t}} \left| \log \frac{\alpha(s) - \alpha(t)}{s-t} \right| + \sup_{t\le T} d_{TV}(\mu_t, \nu_{\alpha(t)}) \right).$$

References for Part III

1. E. Abbe. Community detection and stochastic block models: recent development. *Journal of Machine Learning Research*, 18:1–86, 2018.
2. L. Addario-Berry, N. Broutin and C. Goldschmidt, Critical random graphs: limiting constructions and distributional properties, *Electronic Journal of Probability*, 15(25):741–775, 2010.
3. L. Addario-Berry, N. Broutin and C. Goldschmidt, The continuum limit of critical random graphs, *Probability Theory and Related Fields*, 152(3-4):367–406, 2012.
4. R. Ahuja, T. Magnanti and J. Orlin, *Network flows: theory, algorithms and applications*, Prentice Hall, New Jersey, 1993.
5. H. Anderson and T. Britton, *Stochastic Epidemic models and Their Statiatical Analysis*, volume 151 of *Lecture Notes in Statistics*, Springer, New York, 2000.
6. H. Andersson, Limit theorems for a random graph epidemic model, *Annals of Applied Probability*, 8(4):1331–1349, 1998.
7. H. Andersson, Epidemic models and social networks, *Mathematical Scientist*, 24(2):128–147, 1999.
8. H. De Arazoza, J. Joanes, R. Lounes, C. Legeai, S. Clémencon, J. Perez and B. Auvert, The HIV/AIDS epidemic in Cuba: description and tentative explanation of its low prevalence, *BMC Infectious Disease*, 7:130, 2007.
9. F. Ball, T. Britton and D. Sirl, A network with tunable clustering, degree correlation and degree distribution, and an epidemic thereon, *Journal of Mathematical Biology*, 66(4-5):979–1019, 2013.
10. F. Ball and D. Clancy, The final size and severity of a generalised stochastic multitype epidemic model, *Advances in Applied Probability*, 25(4):721–736, 1993.
11. F. Ball and P. Donnelly, Strong approximations for epidemic models, *Stochastic Processes and their Applications*, 55(1):1–21, 1995.
12. F. Ball, D. Mollison and G. Scalia-Tomba, Epidemics with two levels of mixing, *The Annals of Applied Probability*, 7:46–89, 1997.
13. F. Ball and P. Neal, Network epidemic models with two levels of mixing, *Mathematical Biosciences*, 212:69–87, 2008.
14. F. Ball, L. Pellis and P. Trapman, Reproduction numbers for epidemic models with households and other social structures. I. Definition and calculation of R_0, *Mathematical Biosciences*, 235(1):85–97, 2012.
15. F. Ball, L. Pellis and P. Trapman, Reproduction numbers for epidemic models with households and other social structures II: Comparisons and implications for vaccination, *Mathematical Biosciences*, 274:108–139, 2016.
16. F. Ball, D. Sirl and P. Trapman, Epidemics on random intersection graphs, *Annals of Applied Probability*, 24(3):1081–1128, 2014.
17. F. Ball, L. Pellis and P. Trapman, Reproduction numbers for epidemic models with households and other social structures II: comparisons and implications for vaccination, to appear in Math. Biosci.; arXiv preprint arXiv:1410.4469, 2016.

18. S. Bansal, B.T. Grenfell and L.A. Meyers, When individual behaviour matters: homogeneous and network models in epidemiology, *Journal of the Royal Society Interface*, 4(16):879–891, 08 2007.
19. A.D. Barbour and G. Reinert, Approximating the epidemic curve, *Electronic Journal of Probability*, 18(54):2557, 2013.
20. M. Barthélemy, A. Barrat, R. Pastor-Satorras and A. Vespignani, Dynamical patterns of epidemic outbreaks in complex heterogeneous networks, *Journal of Theoretical Biology*, 235:275–288, 2005.
21. M.S. Bartlett, *Stochastic Population Models in Ecology and Epidemiology*, London, methuen edition, 1960.
22. G. Di Battista, P. Eades, R. Tamassia and I.G. Tollis, *Graph Drawing: Algorithms for the Visualization of Graphs*, Prentice Hall, 1999.
23. N.G. Becker and K. Dietz, The effect of household distribution on transmission and control of highly infectious diseases, *Math. Biosci.*, 127(2):207–219, 1995.
24. P. Billingsley, *Convergence of Probability Measures*, John Wiley & Sons, New York, 1968.
25. B. Bollobás, *Random graphs*, Cambridge University Press, 2 edition, 2001.
26. C. Borgs, J. Chayes, L. Lovász, V. Sós and K. Vesztergombi, Limits of randomly grown graph sequences, *European Journal of Combinatorics*, 32(7):985–999, 2011.
27. T. Britton, M. Deijfen, A.N. Lagerås and M. Lindholm, Epidemics on random graphs with tunable clustering, *Journal of Applied Probability*, 45:743–756, 2008.
28. T. Britton, S. Janson, and A. Martin-Löf, Graphs with specified degree distributions, simple epidemics, and local vaccination strategies, *Adv. Appl. Probab.*, 39(4):922–948, 2007.
29. N. Champagnat, S. Méléard and V.C. Tran, Stochastic analysis of emergence of evolutionary cyclic behavior in population dynamics with transfer, arXiv:1901.02385, 2019.
30. S.K. Chan, L.R. Thornton, K.J. Chronister, J. Meyer, M. Wolverton, C.K. Johnson, R.R. Arafat, P. Joyce, W.M. Switzer, W. Heneine, A. Shankar, T. Granade, S. Michele Owen, P. Sprinkle and V. Sullivan, Likely Female-to-Female sexual transmission of HIV-Texas, *Morbidity and Mortality Weekly Report*, 63(10):209–212, 2014, Centers for Disease Control and Prevention.
31. S. Chatterjee, *Large Deviations for Random Graphs*, volume 2197 of *Lecture Notes in Mathematics, Ecole d'Eté de Probabilités de Saint-Flour XLV - 2015*, Springer, Cham, 1 edition, 2017.
32. A. Clauset, C. Shalizi and M. Newman, Power-law distributions in empirical data, *SIAM Review*, 51:661–703, 2009.
33. S. Clémencon, H. De Arazoza, F. Rossi and V.C. Tran, Hierarchical clustering for graph vizualization, In *Proceedings of XVIIIth European Symposium on Artificial Neural Networks (ESANN 2011)*, pages 227–232, Bruges, Belgium, April 2011, `http://hal.archives-ouvertes.fr/hal-00603639/fr/`.
34. S. Clémencon, H. De Arazoza, F. Rossi and V.C. Tran, Visual mining of epidemic networks, In *Proceedings of the International Work conference of Artificial Neural Networks (IWANN)*, volume 6692 of *Lecture Notes in Computer Sciences*, pages 276–283. Springer, June 2011.
35. S. Clémencon, H. De Arazoza, F. Rossi and V.C. Tran, A statistical network analysis of the hiv/aids epidemics in cuba, *Social Network Analysis and Mining*, 5:Art.58, 2015.
36. S. Clémencon, H. De Arazoza, F. Rossi and V.C. Tran, Supplementary materias for "a statistical network analysis of the HIV/AIDS epidemics in Cuba", *Social Network Analysis and Mining*, 5, 2015. Supplementary materials.
37. S. Clémencon, V.C. Tran and H. De Arazoza, A stochastic SIR model with contact-tracing: large population limits and statistical inference, *Journal of Biological Dynamics*, 2(4):391–414, 2008.
38. A. Cori, A.J. Valleron, F. Carrat, G. Scalia-Tomba, G. Thomas and P.Y. Boëlle, Estimating influenza latency and infectious period durations using viral excretion data, *Epidemics*, 4(3):132–138, 2012.
39. E. Coupechoux and M. Lelarge, How clustering affects epidemics in random networks, *Advances in Applied Probability*, 46:985–1008, 2014.
40. E. Coupechoux and M. Lelarge, Contagions in random networks with overlapping communities, *Advances in Applied Probability*, 47(4):973–988, 2015.

41. A. Cousien, V.C. Tran, S. Deuffic-Burban, M. Jauffret-Roustide, G. Mabileau, J.S. Dhersin and Y. Yazdanpanah, Effectiveness and cost-effectiveness of interventions targeting harm reduction and chronic hepatitis c cascade of care in people who inject drugs: the case of France, *Journal of Viral Hepatitis*, 25(10):1197–1207, 2018.
42. G. Csardi and T. Nepusz, The igraph software package for complex network research, *Inter-Journal*, Complex Systems:1695, 2006.
43. L. Danon, A.P. Ford, T. House, C.P. Jewell, M.J. Keeling, G.O. Roberts, J.V. Ross and M.C. Vernon, Networks and the epidemiology of infectious disease, In *Interdisciplinary Perspectives on Infectious Diseases*, volume 2011, pages 1–28, 2011.
44. L. Decreusefond, J.-S. Dhersin, P. Moyal and V.C. Tran, Large graph limit for a sir process in random network with heterogeneous connectivity, *Annals of Applied Probability*, 22(2):541–575, 2012.
45. Demographic, Nigeria, Health survey (NDHS), *Problems in accessing health care. NDHS/National Population Commission*, page 140, 2003.
46. O. Diekmann, M. Gyllenberg, J.A.J. Metz and H.R. Thieme, On the formulation and analysis of general deterministic structured population models. I. Linear theory, *Journal of Mathematical Biology*, 36(4):349–388, 1998.
47. O. Diekmann, H. Heesterbeek and T. Britton, *Mathematical Tools for Understanding Infectious Disease Dynamics*, Princeton Series in Theoretical and Computational Biology. Princeton University Press, New Jersey, 2012.
48. O. Diekmann, M. Gyllenberg, J.A.J. Metz and H.R. Thieme, On the formulation and analysis of general deterministic structured population models. I. Linear theory, *J. Math. Biol.*, 36(4):349–388, 1998.
49. R. Durrett, *Random graph dynamics*, Cambridge University Press, New York, 2007.
50. K.T.D. Eames and M.J. Keeling, Modelling dynamic and network heterogeneities in the spread of sexually transmitted diseases, *Proceedings of the National Academy of Sciences of the United States of America*, 99(20):13330–13335, 2002.
51. J. Enright and R.R. Kao, Epidemics on dynamic networks, *Epidemics*, 24:88–97, 2018.
52. S.N. Ethier and T.G. Kurtz, *Markov Processus, Characterization and Convergence*. John Wiley & Sons, New York, 1986.
53. L.C. Evans, *Partial Differential Equations*, volume 19 of *Graduate Studies in Mathematics*, American Mathematical Society, 1998.
54. S. Fortunato and M. Barthélemy, Resolution limit in community detection, *Proceedings of the National Academy of Sciences*, 104(1):36–41, 2007.
55. N. Fournier and S. Méléard, A microscopic probabilistic description of a locally regulated population and macroscopic approximations, *Ann. Appl. Probab.*, 14(4):1880–1919, 2004.
56. T. Fruchterman and B. Reingold, Graph drawing by force-directed placement, *Software-Practice and Experience*, 21:1129–1164, 1991.
57. E. Goldstein, K. Paur, C. Fraser, E. Kenah, J. Wallinga and M. Lipsitch, Reproductive numbers, epidemic spread and control in a community of households, *Mathematical Biosciences*, 221(1):11–25, 2009.
58. M. Graham and T. House, Dynamics of stochastic epidemics on heterogeneous networks, *Journal of Mathematical Biology*, 68(7):1583–1605, 2014.
59. I. Herman, G. Melancon and M. Scott Marshall, Graph visualization and navigation in information visualisation, *IEEE Transactions on Visualization and Computer Graphics*, 6(1):24–43, 2000.
60. B. Hill, A simple general approach to inference about the tail of a distribution, *Annals of Statistics*, 3(5):1163–1174, 01 1975.
61. T. House, Modelling epidemics on networks, *Contemporary Physics*, 53(3):213–225, 2012.
62. N. Ikeda and S. Watanabe, *Stochastic Differential Equations and Diffusion Processes*, volume 24, North-Holland Publishing Company, 1989, Second Edition.
63. J. Jacod and A.N. Shiryaev, *Limit Theorems for Stochastic Processes*, Springer-Verlag, Berlin, 1987.
64. P. Jagers, *Branching Processes with Biological Applications*, Wiley Series in Probability and Mathematical Statistics, Wiley-Interscience, London-New York-Sydney, 1975.
65. S. Janson, M. Luczak and P. Windridge, Law of large numbers for the SIR epidemic on a random graph with given degrees, *Annals of Applied Probability*, 2014, accepted.

66. A. Joffe and M. Métivier, Weak convergence of sequences of semimartingales with applications to multitype branching processes, *Advances in Applied Probability*, 18:20–65, 1986.
67. W.O. Kermack and A.G. McKendrick, A contribution to the mathematical theory of epidemics, *Proc. Roy. Soc. Lond. A*, 115:700–721, 1927.
68. I.Z. Kiss, L. Berthouze, J.C. Miller and P.L. Simon, Mapping out emerging network structures in dynamic network models coupled with epidemics, In *Temporal Network Epidemiology*, Theoretical Biology, pages 267–289. Springer, 2017.
69. I.Z. Kiss, D.M. Green and R.R. Kao, Infectious disease control using contact tracing in random and scale-free networks, *J. R. Soc. Interface*, 3(6):55–62, 2013.
70. I.Z. Kiss, J.C. Miller and P. Simon, *Mathematics of Epidemics on Networks*, volume 46 of *Interdisciplinary Applied Mathematics*, Springer, 1 edition, 2017.
71. A. Kleczkowski and B.T. Grenfell, Mean-field-type equations for spread of epidemics: The small world model, *Physica A*, 274:355–360, 1999.
72. M. Kretzschmar and M. Morris, Measures of concurrency in networks and the spread of infectious disease, *Math. Biosci.*, 133:165–195, 1996.
73. L. Lovàsz and B. Szegedy, Limits of dense graph sequences, *Journal of Combinatorial Theory, Series B*, 96:933–957, 2006.
74. T.L. Mah and J.D. Shelton, Concurrency revisited: increasing and compelling epidemiological evidence, *Journal of the International AIDS Society*, 14(33), 2011.
75. R.M. May and A.L. Lloyd, Infection dynamics on scale-free networks, *Phys. Rev. E*, 64:066112, 2001.
76. S. Méléard and S. Roelly, Sur les convergences étroite ou vague de processus à valeurs mesures, *CRAS de l'Acad. des Sci. Paris*, t. 317, Série I, 785–788, 1993.
77. S. Méléard and V.C. Tran, Trait substitution sequence process and canonical equation for age-structured populations, *Journal of Mathematical Biology*, 58(6):881–921, 2009.
78. J.C. Miller, A note on a paper by Erik Volz: SIR dynamics in random networks, *Journal of Mathematical Biology*, 62(3):349–358, 2011, `http://arxiv.org/abs/0909.4485`.
79. M. Molloy and B. Reed, A critical point for random graphs with a given degree sequence, *Random structures and algorithms*, 6:161–180, 1995.
80. M. Molloy and B. Reed, The size of the giant component of a random graph with a given degree sequence, *Combinatorics probability and computing*, 7(3):295–305, 1998.
81. C. Moore and M.E.J. Newman, Epidemics and percolation in small-world networks, *Phys. Rev. E*, 61:5678–5682, 2000.
82. M. Morris and M. Kretzschmar, Concurrent partnerships and transmission dynamics in networks, *Social Networks*, 17:299–318, 1995.
83. M. Newman, A. Barabási and D. Watts, *The structure and dynamics of networks*, Princeton University Press, 2006.
84. M. Newman and M. Girvan, Finding and evaluating community structure in network., *Physical Review E*, 69:026113, 2004.
85. M. Newman, S. Strogatz and D. Watts, Random graphs with arbitrary degree distributions and their applications, *Physical Review E*, 64(2):026118, 2001.
86. M.E.J. Newman, The spread of epidemic disease on networks, *Physical Reviews E*, 66, 2002.
87. M.E.J. Newman, Mixing patterns in networks, *Phys. Rev. E*, 67:026126, 2003.
88. M.E.J. Newman, The structure and function of complex networks, *SIAM Review*, 45:167–256, 2003.
89. A. Noack, Modularity clustering is force-directed layout, *Physical Review E*, 79:026102, 2009.
90. A. Noack and R. Rotta, Multi-level algorithms for modularity clustering, In *SEA '09: Proceedings of the 8th International Symposium on Experimental Algorithms*, pages 257–268,Springer-Verlag, Berlin, Heidelberg, 2009.
91. R. Pastor-Satorras and A. Vespignani, Epidemics and immunization in scale-free networks, In *Handbook of Graphs and Networks: From the Genome to the Internet*, pages 113–132, Berlin, 2002. Wiley-VCH.
92. L. Pellis, T. House and M.J. Keeling, Exact and approximate moment closures for non-Markovian network epidemics, *Journal of Theoretical Biology*, 382:160–177, 2015.
93. L. Pellis, S.E.F. Spencer and T. House, Real-time growth rate for general stochastic sir epidemics on unclustered networks, *Mathematical biosciences*, 265:65–81, 2015.

94. L. Pellis, N.M. Ferguson and C. Fraser, Epidemic growth rate and household reproduction number in communities of households, schools and workplaces, *J. Math. Biol.*, 63(4):691–734, 2011.
95. J. Reichardt and S. Bornholdt, Partitioning and modularity of graphs with arbitrary degree distribution, *Physical Review E*, 76(1):015102, 2007.
96. S. Resnick, *Heavy-tail phenomena*, Springer, 2007.
97. O. Riordan, The phase transition in the configuration model, *Combinatorics, Probability and Computing*, 21(1-2):265–299, 2012.
98. J.M. Roberts Jr., Simple methods for simulating sociomatrices with given marginal totals, *Social Networks*, 22(3):273–283, 2000.
99. S. Roelly, A criterion of convergence of measure-valued processes: Application to measure branching processes, *Stochastics*, 17:43–65, 1986.
100. D.A. Rolls, P. Wang, R. Jenkinson, P.E. Pattison, G.L. Robins, R. Sacks-Davis, G. Daraganova, M. Hellard and E. McBryde, Modelling a disease-relevant contact network of people who inject drugs, *Social Networks*, 35(4):699–710, 2013.
101. F. Rossi and N. Villa-Vialaneix, Représentation d'un grand réseau à partir d'une classification hiérarchique de ses sommets, *Journal de la Société Francaise de Statistique*, 152(3):34–65, 2011.
102. R.B. Rothenberg, D.E. Woodhouse, J.J. Potterat, S.Q. Muth, W.W. Darrow and A.S. Klovdahl, Social networks in disease transmission: The Colorado Springs study, In R.H. Needle, S.L. Coyle, S.G. Genser and R.T. Trotter II, editors, *Social networks, drug abuse and HIV transmission*, volume 151 of *Research Monographs*, pages 3–18. National Instit, 1995.
103. B.V. Schmid and M. Kretzschmar, Determinants of sexual network structure and their impact on cumulative network measures, *PLoS Computational Biology*, 8(4):e1002470, 2012.
104. Statistics Sweden, *Statistical Yearbook of Sweden 2014*, Statistics Sweden, 2014.
105. V.C. Tran, *Modèles particulaires stochastiques pour des problèmes d'évolution adaptative et pour l'approximation de solutions statistiques*, Phd thesis, Université Paris X - Nanterre, 12 2006, `http://tel.archives-ouvertes.fr/tel-00125100`.
106. V.C. Tran, *Une ballade en forêts aléatoires. Théorèmes limites pour des populations structurées et leurs généalogies, étude probabiliste et statistique de modèles SIR en épidémiologie, contributions à la géométrie aléatoire*, Habilitation à diriger des recherches, Université de Lille 1, 11 2014, `http://tel.archives-ouvertes.fr/tel-01087229`.
107. P. Trapman, F. Ball, J.-S. Dhersin, V.C. Tran, J. Wallinga and T. Britton. Inferring r0 in emerging epidemics-the effect of common population structure is small, *Journal of the Royal Society Interface*, 13:20160288, 2016.
108. D. Tunkelang, *A Numerical Optimization Approach to General Graph Drawing*. PhD thesis, School of Computer Science, Carnegie Mellon University, 01 1999.
109. R. Van der Hofstad, *Random Graphs and Complex Networks*, volume 1 of *Cambridge Series in Statistical and Probabilistic Mathematics*, Cambridge University Press, Cambridge, 2017.
110. E. Volz, SIR dynamics in random networks with heterogeneous connectivity, *Mathematical Biology*, 56:293–310, 2008.
111. E. Volz and L. Ancel Meyers, Susceptible-infected-recovered epidemics in dynamic contact networks, *Proceeding of the Royal Society B*, 274:2925–2933, 2007.
112. J. Wallinga and M. Lipsitch, How generation intervals shape the relationship between growth rates and reproductive numbers, *Proceedings of the Royal Society B: Biological Sciences*, 274(1609):599–604, 2007.
113. J. Wallinga, P. Teunis and M. Kretzschmar, Using data on social contacts to estimate age-specific transmission parameters for respiratory-spread infectious agents, *Am. J. Epidemiol.*, 164(10):936–944, 2006.
114. W. Whitt, Blocking when service is required from several facilities simultaneously, *AT&T Tech. J.*, 64:1807–1856, 1985.
115. WHO Ebola Response Team, Ebola virus disease in West Africa – the first 9 months of the epidemic and forward projections, *N Engl J Med*, 371:1481–1495, 2014.
116. J.L. Wylie and A. Jolly, Patterns of Chlamydia and Gonorrhea infection in sexual networks in Manitoba, Canada, *Sexually transmitted diseases*, 28(1):14–24, January 2001.

Part IV
Statistical Inference for Epidemic Processes in a Homogeneous Community

Catherine Larédo (with Viet Chi Tran in Chapter 4)

Catherine Larédo, INRA
e-mail: catherine.laredo@inra.fr

Introduction

Mathematical modeling of epidemic spread and estimation of key parameters from data provided much insight in the understanding of public health problems related to infectious diseases. These models are naturally parametric models, where the present parameters rule the evolution of the epidemics under study.

Multidimensional continuous-time Markov jump processes $(\mathscr{Z}(t))$ on $\mathbb{Z}^p$ form a usual set-up for modeling epidemics on the basis of compartmental approaches as for instance the SIR-like (Susceptible-Infectious-Removed) epidemics (see Part I of these notes and also [2], [35], [83]). However, when facing incomplete epidemic data, inference based on $(\mathscr{Z}(t))$ is not easy to be achieved.

There are different situations where missing data are present. One situation concerns Hidden Markov Models, which are in most cases Markov processes observed with noise. It corresponds for epidemics to the fact that the exact status of all the individuals within a population are not observed, or that detecting the status has some noise (see [22] for instance). Another situation comes from the fact that observations are performed at discrete times. They can also be aggregated (e.g. number of infected per day). A third case, for multidimensional processes, is that some coordinates cannot be observed in practice. While the statistical inference has a longstanding theory for complete data, this is no longer true for many cases that occur in practice. Many methods have been proposed to fill this gap starting from the Expectation-Maximization algorithm ([34], [90]) up to various Bayesian methods ([25], [106]), Monte Carlo methods ([51], [104]), based on particle filtering ([41], [42]), Approximate Bayesian Computation methods ([9], [15], [114], [120]), maximum iterating filtering ([70]), Sequential Monte Carlo or Particle MCMC ([3], [37]), see also the R package POMP ([89]). Nevertheless, these methods do not completely circumvent the issues related to incomplete data. Indeed, as summarized in [19], there are some limitations in practice due to the size of missing data and to the various tuning parameters to be adjusted.

The aim of this part is to provide some tools to estimate the parameters ruling the epidemic dynamics on the basis of available data. We begin with a chapter about inferential methodology for stochastic processes which is not specific to applications to epidemics but is the backbone of the various inference methods detailed in the next chapters of this part.

The methods used to build estimators are linked with the precise nature of the observations, each kind of observations generating a different statistical problem. We detail these facts in the first chapter. We have intentionally omitted in this chapter the additional problem of noisy observations, which often occurs in practice. This is another layer which comes on top. It entails Hidden Markov Models and State space Models (see [22] or [124]) and also the R-package Pomp ([89]).

Chapter 2 is devoted to the statistical inference for Markov chains. Indeed, discrete time Markov chains models are interesting here because many questions that arise for more complex epidemic models can be illustrated in this set-up.

We had rather focus here on parametric inference since epidemic models always include in their dynamics parameters that need to be estimated in order to derive predictions. At the early stage of an outbreak, a good approximation for the epidemic dynamics is to consider that the population of Susceptible is infinite and that Infected individuals evolve according to a branching process (see Part I, Section 1.2 of these notes). We also present in this chapter some classical statistical results in this domain.

As detailed in Part I, Chapter 1, epidemics in a close population of size N are naturally modeled by pure jump processes $(\mathscr{Z}^N(t))$. However, inference for such models requires that all the jumps (i.e. times of infection and recovery for the *SIR* model) are observed. Since these data are rarely available in practice, statistical methods often rely on data augmentation, which allows us to complete the data and add in the analysis all the missing jumps. For moderate to large populations, the complexity increases rapidly, becoming the source of additional problems. Various approaches were developed during the last years to deal with partially observed epidemics. Data augmentation and likelihood-free methods such as the Approximate Bayesian Computation (ABC) opened some of the most promising pathways for improvement (see e.g. [18], [101]). Nevertheless, these methods do not completely circumvent the issues related to incomplete data. As stated also in [19], [27], there are some limitations in practice, due to the size of missing data and to the various tuning parameters to be adjusted (see also [2], [105]).

In this context, it appears that diffusion processes satisfactorily approximating epidemic dynamics can be profitably used for inference of model parameters for epidemic data, due to their analytical power (see e.g. [45], [109]). More precisely, when normalized by N, $(Z^N(t) = N^{-1}\mathscr{Z}^N(t))$ satisfies an ODE as the population size N goes to infinity and moreover, in the first part of these notes, it is proved that the Wasserstein L_1-distance between $(Z^N(t))$ and a multidimensional diffusion process with diffusion coefficient proportional to $1/\sqrt{N}$ is of order $o(N^{-1/2})$ on a finite interval $[0,T]$ (see Part I, Sections 2.3 and 2.4). Hence, in the case of a major outbreak in a large community, epidemic dynamics can be described using multidimensional diffusion processes $(X^N(t))_{t\geq 0}$ with a small diffusion coefficient proportional to $1/\sqrt{N}$. We detail in Chapter 3 the parametric inference for epidemic dynamics described using multidimensional diffusion processes $(X^N(t))_{t\geq 0}$ with a small diffusion coefficient proportional to $1/\sqrt{N}$ based on discrete observations. Since epidemics are usually observed over limited time periods, we consider the parametric inference based on observations of the epidemic dynamics on a fixed interval $[0,T]$.

The last chapter is devoted to the inference for the continuous time *SIR* model. We present several algorithms which address the problem of incomplete data in this set-up: Expectation-Maximization algorithm, Monte Carlo methods and Approximate Bayesian Computation methods. Finally, all the classical statistical results required for this part are detailed in the Appendix.

Chapter 1
Observations and Asymptotic Frameworks

Multidimensional continuous-time Markov jump processes $(\mathscr{Z}(t))$ on $\mathbb{Z}^p$ form a usual set-up for modeling epidemics on the basis of compartmental approaches as for instance the *SIR*-like (Susceptible-Infectious-Removed) epidemics (see Part I of these notes and also [2], [35], [83]). However, when facing incomplete epidemic data, inference based on $(\mathscr{Z}(t))$ is not easy to be achieved.

Assume that a stochastic process $(\mathscr{Z}(t), t \in [0, T])$ models the epidemic dynamics with parameters associated with this process (transition kernels depending on a parameter θ for Markov chains, drift and diffusion coefficients for a diffusion process, infinitesimal generator for a Markov pure jump process). The observed process corresponds to the value θ_0 of this parameter. This value θ_0 is called the true (unknown) parameter value. Our concern here is the estimation of θ_0 from the observations that are available and the study of their properties. The methods used to build estimators are linked with the precise nature of the observations, each kind of observations generating a different statistical problem. We detail these facts in the next sections. We have intentionally omitted in this chapter the additional problem of noisy observations, which often occurs in practice. This is another layer which comes on top. It entails Hidden Markov Models and State space Models (see [22] or [124]) and also the R-package Pomp ([89]).

1.1 Various Kinds of Observations and Asymptotic Frameworks

As developed in Part I of these notes, the epidemic dynamics is modeled by a stochastic process $(\mathscr{Z}(t))$ defined on $[0, T]$ with values in $\mathbb{R}^p$, which describes at each time t the number of individuals in each of the p health states (e.g. $p = 3$ for the *SIR* model). Inference for epidemic models is complicated by the fact that collected observations usually do not contain all the information on the whole path of $(\mathscr{Z}(t), 0 \leq t \leq T)$. Moreover, the inference method relies on an asymptotic framework which allows us to control the properties of estimators. We detail here in a general set-up these facts, which are not specific to the inference for epidemic dy-

© Springer Nature Switzerland AG 2019
T. Britton, E. Pardoux (eds.), *Stochastic Epidemic Models with Inference*,
Lecture Notes in Mathematics 2255, https://doi.org/10.1007/978-3-030-30900-8_12

namics, but rely on general properties of inference for stochastic processes, this knowledge being useful for applications to epidemics.

1.1.1 Observations

Historically, continuous observation of $(\mathscr{X}(t), 0 \le t \le T)$ was systematically assumed in the literature concerning the statistics of continuous time stochastic processes (see [68], [96], [97]). It is justified by the property that theoretical results can be obtained. However, many various cases can occur in practice. Among them, including the complete case, the more frequent are
Case (a). Continuous observation of $(\mathscr{X}(t))$ on $[0,T]$.
Case (b). Discrete observations: $(\mathscr{X}(t_1), \dots, \mathscr{X}(t_n))$ with $0 \le t_1 < t_2 < \dots < t_n \le T$.
Case (c). Aggregated observations $(J_0, \dots, J_{n-1})$ with $J_i = \int_{t_i}^{t_{i+1}} \mathscr{X}(s)ds$.
Case (d). Model with latent variables: Some coordinates of $(\mathscr{X}(t), t \in [0,T])$ are unobserved.

Case (a) corresponds to complete data. For the *SIR* epidemics, it means that the times of infection and recovery are observed for each individual in the population. Case (b) corresponds to the fact that observations are made at successive known times (one observation per day or per week during the epidemic outburst (see [12], [26], [18], [27]). Case (c) occurs in epidemics when the available observations are the number of Infected individuals and Removed per week for instance. Case (d) deals with the fact that, in routinely collected observations of epidemic models, one or several model variables are unobserved (or latent) (see e.g. [22], [41] for general references and [18], [19], [70], [71], [106], [120] for applications to epidemics).

1.1.2 Various Asymptotic Frameworks

Taking into account an asymptotic framework is necessary to study and compare the properties of different estimators. It is also a preliminary step for the study of non-asymptotic properties. While for i.i.d. observations, the natural asymptotic framework is that the number n of observations goes to infinity, for stochastic processes various approaches are used according to the model properties or to the available observations. Two different situations need to be considered according to the time interval of observation $[0,T]$, where T either goes to infinity or is fixed.

1.1.2.1 Increasing Time of Observation $[0,T]$ with $T \to \infty$

If $(\mathscr{X}(t))$ on $[0,T]$ is continuously observed, a general theory is available for ergodic processes and for stationary mixing processes. Inference can also be performed for some special models but does no longer rely on a general theory. This occurs for supercritical branching processes and for the explosive $AR(1)$ process.

Let us consider the case of discrete observations of a continuous time process with regular sampling Δ. The observations are: $(\mathscr{X}(t_1), \mathscr{X}(t_2), \ldots, \mathscr{X}(t_n))$ with $t_i = i\Delta$ and $T = n\Delta$.
Two distinct cases arise from the study of parametric inference for diffusion processes
(1) The sampling interval Δ is fixed ($T = n\Delta$ and $n \to \infty$).
(2) The sampling interval $\Delta = \Delta_n \to 0$ with $T = n\Delta_n \to \infty$ as $n \to \infty$.
Since the likelihood is not explicit and difficult to compute, it raises many theoretical problems. References for the inference in these cases are Kessler [85], [86] followed by many others [87].

In practice, when a sampling interval Δ is present in the data collecting, it might be important to take it explicitly into account. Deciding whether Δ is small or not depends more on the time scale than on its precise value. However this parameter Δ explicitly enters in the estimators, and some estimators with apparently good properties for Δ fixed might explode for small Δ. It corresponds in theory to different rates of convergence for the various coordinates of the unknown parameter θ as $n \to \infty$. This typically occurs for discrete observations of a diffusion process (see Section 1.2).

1.1.2.2 Fixed Observation Time $[0, T]$

Several asymptotic frameworks are used.

(1) *Discrete observations on [0,T] with* $T = n\Delta_n$ *fixed*
The sampling interval $\Delta_n \to 0$ while the number of observations n tends to infinity. For diffusion processes, only parameters in the diffusion coefficient can be estimated (see [48], [73]).

(2) *Observation of k i.i.d. sample paths of* $(\mathscr{X}^i(t), 0 \le t \le T)$, $i = 1, \ldots k$ *with* $k \to \infty$.
Observations of $(\mathscr{X}^i(t))$ can be continuous or discrete.This framework is relevant for panel data which describe for instance the dynamics of several epidemics in different locations. It allows us to include covariates or additional random effects in the model. The assumption is that the number of paths k goes to infinity (see e.g [59]).

(3) *Presence of a "Small parameter"* $\varepsilon > 0 : (\mathscr{X}^\varepsilon(t), 0 \le t \le T)$, *and* $\varepsilon \to 0$.
Inference is studied in the set-up of a family of stochastic models $(\mathscr{X}^\varepsilon(t), 0 \le t \le T)$ depending on a parameter $\varepsilon > 0$. Such a family of processes naturally appears in the theory of "Small perturbations of dynamical systems", where $(X^\varepsilon(t))$ denotes a diffusion process with small diffusion coefficient $\varepsilon\sigma(\cdot)$ (see e.g. [44]). The presence of a small parameter occurs in the study of epidemics in large closed populations of size N, when they are density dependent. The small parameter ε is associated to the population size N by the relation $\varepsilon = 1/\sqrt{N}$ leading to the family of processes

$\mathscr{Z}^{\varepsilon}(t) = \varepsilon^2 \mathscr{Z}(t)$ (normalization by the population size of the process). From a probability perspective, we refer to Part I, Sections 2.3 and 2.4 (see also [39, Chapter 8]). For statistical purposes, we investigate in Chapter 3 of this part the asymptotic framework "$\varepsilon \to 0$" and, for discrete observations, the cases where the sampling interval Δ can be fixed or $\Delta = \Delta_n \to 0$.

(4) *Asymptotics on the initial population number.*
It consists in assuming that one coordinate of $(\mathscr{Z}(t))$ at time 0 satisfies that $\mathscr{Z}^i(0) = M \to \infty$. The parametric inference for the continuous time *SIR* model is performed in this framework (see the results recalled in Section 4.2 or [2]). This is also used for subcritical branching processes where the initial number of ancestors goes to ∞ (see e.g.[59]).

1.1.3 Various Estimation Methods

As pointed out in the introduction of this part, we are mainly concerned by the problem of parametric inference. There exist several estimation methods.

Maximum Likelihood Estimation
This entails that one can compute the likelihood of the observation. For a continuously observed process, this is generally possible, but for a discrete time observation of a continuous-time process or for other kinds of incomplete observations, it is often intractable. This opens the whole domain of stochastic algorithms which aim at completing the data in order to estimate parameters with Maximum Likelihood methods. In particular, the well-known Expectation-Maximisation algorithm ([34]) and other related algorithms (see e.g. [3], [90], [106]) are based on the likelihood. For regular statistical models, Maximum Likelihood Estimators (MLE) are consistent and efficient (best theoretical variance).

Minimum Contrast Estimation or Estimating Functions
When it is difficult to use the accurate (exact) likelihood, pseudo-likelihoods (contrast functions; approximate likelihoods,..), or pseudo -score functions (approximations of the score function, estimating functions) are often used. When they are well designed, these methods lead to consistent estimators converging at the right rate. They might loose the efficiency property of MLE in regular statistical models (see e.g. [123] for the general theory and [31], [67] for stochastic processes).

Empirical and non-parametric Methods
This comprises all the methods that rely on limit theorems (such as the ergodic theorem) associated with various functionals of the observations. Among these methods, we can refer to Moments methods and Generalized Moment Methods (see e.g. [123] for the general theory and [64] for discrete observation of continuous-time Markov processes).

Algorithmic Methods
Many methods have been developed to perform estimation for incomplete data. It is difficult to be exhaustive. Let us quote [3], [37] for Particle Markov Monte Carlo methods; [10], [15], [17], [114], [120] for Approximate Bayesian Computation; [25], [101] for Bayesian MCMC; [70], [89] for iterated filtering and the R-package POMP. In the last chapter of this part, MCMC and ABC methods are detailed for the *SIR* model.

1.2 An Example Illustrating the Inference in these Various Situations

Let us investigate here the consequences of these various situations for the statistical inference on a simple stochastic model for describing a population dynamics: the AR(1) model which is a simple model for describing dynamics in discrete time, its continuous time description corresponding to the Ornstein–Uhlenbeck diffusion process. Besides studying a simplified population model, the main interest of this example lies in the property that computations are explicit for the various inference approaches listed in the previous section.

1.2.1 A Simple Model for Population Dynamics: AR(1)

The AR(1) model is a classical model for describing population dynamics in discrete time. On $(\Omega, \mathscr{F}, \mathbb{P})$ a probability space, let (ε_i) be a sequence of i.i.d. random variables on $\mathbb{R}$ with distribution $\mathscr{N}(0,1)$. Consider the autoregressive process on $\mathbb{R}$ defined, for $i \geq 0$,

$$X_{i+1} = aX_i + \gamma\varepsilon_{i+1}, \quad X_0 = x_0. \tag{1.2.1}$$

In order to compare this model with its continuous time version, the Ornstein–Uhlenbeck diffusion process, we assume that $a > 0$ and that x_0 is deterministic and known. The observations are $(X_i, i = 1, \ldots, n)$ and the unknown parameters $(a, \gamma) \in (0, +\infty)^2$. The distribution $\mathbb{P}^n_{a,\gamma}$ of the n-tuple $(X_1, \ldots, X_n)$ is easy to compute, since the random variables $(X_i - aX_{i-1}, i = 1, \ldots, n)$ are independent and identically distributed $\mathscr{N}(0, \gamma^2)$. If λ_n denotes the Lebesgue measure on $\mathbb{R}^n$, then

$$\frac{d\mathbb{P}^n_{a,\gamma}}{d\lambda_n}(x_i, i = 1, \ldots, n) = \frac{1}{(\gamma\sqrt{2\pi})^n} \exp\Big(-\frac{1}{2\gamma^2}\sum_{i=1}^n (x_i - ax_{i-1})^2\Big).$$

Hence, the loglikelihood function is

$$\log L_n(a, \gamma) = \ell_n(a, \gamma) = -\frac{n}{2}\log(2\pi) - \frac{n}{2}\log\gamma^2 - \frac{1}{2\gamma^2}\sum_{i=1}^n (X_i - aX_{i-1})^2. \tag{1.2.2}$$

The maximum likelihood estimators are

$$\hat{a}_n = \frac{\sum_{i=1}^n X_{i-1}X_i}{\sum_{i=1}^n X_{i-1}^2}; \quad \hat{\gamma}_n^2 = \frac{1}{n}\sum_{i=1}^n (X_i - \hat{a}_n X_{i-1})^2. \tag{1.2.3}$$

The properties of $(\hat{a}_n, \hat{\gamma}_n^2)$ can be studied as $n \to \infty$: $(\hat{a}_n, \hat{\gamma}_n^2)$ is strongly consistent:

$$(\hat{a}_n, \hat{\gamma}_n^2) \to (a, \gamma^2) \text{ a. s. under } \mathbb{P}_{a,\gamma} \text{ as } n \to \infty.$$

The rates of convergence differ according to the probabilistic properties of (X_i).
(1) If $0 < a < 1$, (X_i) is a Harris recurrent Markov chain with stationary distribution $\mu_{a,\gamma}(dx) = \mathcal{N}(0, \frac{\gamma^2}{1-a^2})$. The estimators $\hat{a}_n, \hat{\gamma}_n^2$ are asymptotically independent and satisfy

$$\begin{pmatrix} \sqrt{n}(\hat{a}_n - a) \\ \sqrt{n}(\hat{\gamma}_n^2 - \gamma^2) \end{pmatrix} \to \mathcal{N}_2\left(0, \begin{pmatrix} 1-a^2 & 0 \\ 0 & 2\gamma^4 \end{pmatrix}\right). \tag{1.2.4}$$

(2) If $a = 1$, (X_i) is a null recurrent random walk and $n(\hat{a}_n - 1)$ converges to a non-Gaussian distribution, while $\hat{\gamma}_n^2$ has the properties of Case (1).
(3) If $a > 1$ and $x_0 = 0$, (X_i) is explosive. One can prove that $a^n(\hat{a}_n - a)$ converges to a random variable $Y = \eta Z$, where η, Z are two independent random variables, $Z \sim \mathcal{N}(0,1)$ and η is an explicit positive random variable. The estimator $\hat{\gamma}_n^2$ keeps the properties of Case (1).

1.2.2 Ornstein–Uhlenbeck Diffusion Process with Increasing Observation Time

This section is based on Chapter 1 of [47] where all the statistical inference is detailed. It is presented here as a starting point for problems that arise when dealing with epidemic data. In order to investigate the various situations detailed in Section 1.1, let us now consider the continuous time version of the $AR(1)$ population model, the Ornstein–Uhlenbeck diffusion process defined by the stochastic differential equation

$$d\xi_t = \theta \xi_t dt + \sigma dW_t; \; \xi_0 = x_0. \tag{1.2.5}$$

where $(W_t, t \geq 0)$ denotes a standard Brownian motion on $(\Omega, \mathcal{F}, P)$, and x_0 is either deterministic or is a random variable independent of (W_t). Then, $(\xi_t, t \geq 0)$ is a diffusion process on $\mathbb{R}$ with continuous sample paths. This equation can be solved, setting $Y_t = e^{-\theta t}\xi_t$, so that

$$\xi_t = x_0 e^{\theta t} + e^{\theta t}\int_0^t e^{-\theta s} dW_s. \tag{1.2.6}$$

Let us first consider the case where (ξ_t) is observed with regular sampling intervals Δ. The observations $(\xi_{t_i}; i = 1, \ldots, n)$ with $t_i = i\Delta$ satisfy

$$\xi_{t_{i+1}} = e^{\theta\Delta}\xi_{t_i} + \sigma e^{\theta(i+1)\Delta}\int_{i\Delta}^{(i+1)\Delta} e^{-\theta s} dW_s. \tag{1.2.7}$$

Hence, $(\xi_{t_{i+1}} - e^{\theta\Delta}\xi_{t_i})$ is independent of $\mathscr{F}_{t_i}$, where $\mathscr{F}_t = \sigma(\xi_0, W_s, s \le t)$ and the sequence $(\xi_{t_i}, i \ge 0)$ is the autoregressive model $AR(1)$ defined in (1.2.1) setting

$$X_i = \xi_{t_i}, \quad a = e^{\theta\Delta}, \quad \gamma^2 = \frac{\sigma^2}{2\theta}(e^{2\theta\Delta} - 1), \tag{1.2.8}$$

since the random variables $((\sigma e^{\theta(i+1)\Delta} \int_{i\Delta}^{(i+1)\Delta} e^{-\theta s} dW_s), 1 \le i \le n)$ are independent Gaussian $\mathscr{N}(0, \gamma^2)$.

Cases (1), (2), (3) of the $AR(1)$ are respectively $\{\theta < 0\}$, $\{\theta = 0\}$ and $\{\theta > 0\}$.

Case (a) Continuous observation on $[0,T]$.

Let us first start with the parametric inference associated with the complete observation of (ξ_t) on $[0,T]$. The space of observations is $(C_T, \mathscr{C}_T)$, the space of continuous functions from $[0,T]$ into $\mathbb{R}$ and $\mathscr{C}_T$ is the Borel σ-algebra. associated with the topology of uniform convergence on $[0,T]$. Let $\mathbb{P}_{\theta,\sigma^2}$ denote the probability distribution on $(C_T, \mathscr{C}_T)$ of the observation $(\xi_t, 0 \le t \le T)$ satisfying (1.2.5) . It is well known that if $\sigma^2 \neq \tau^2$, the distributions $\mathbb{P}_{\theta,\sigma^2}$ and $\mathbb{P}_{\theta,\tau^2}$ are singular on $(C_T, \mathscr{C}_T)$ (see e.g. [96]). Indeed, the quadratic variations of (ξ_t) satisfy, as $\Delta_n = t_i - t_{i-1} \to 0$,

$$\sum_{i=1}^{n} (\xi_{t_i} - \xi_{t_{i-1}})^2 \to \sigma^2 T \text{ in } \mathbb{P}_{\theta,\sigma^2}\text{-probability}.$$

Therefore, the set $A = \{\omega, \sum_{i=1}^{n} (\xi_{t_i} - \xi_{t_{i-1}})^2 \to \sigma^2 T\}$ satisfies $\mathbb{P}_{\theta,\sigma^2}(A) = 1$ and $\mathbb{P}_{\theta,\tau^2}(A) = 0$ for $\tau^2 \neq .\sigma^2$.
A statistical consequence is that the diffusion coefficient is identified when (ξ_t) is continuously observed.

We assume that σ is fixed and known and omit it in this section. Let $\mathbb{P}_{0,\sigma^2} = \mathbb{P}_0$ the distribution associated with $\theta = 0$ (i.e $d\xi_t = \sigma dW_t$). The Girsanov formula gives an expression of the likelihood function on $[0,T]$,

$$L_T(\theta) = \frac{d\mathbb{P}_\theta}{d\mathbb{P}_0}(\xi_t, 0 \le t \le T) = \exp\left(\frac{\theta}{\sigma^2}\int_0^T \xi_t \, d\xi_t - \frac{\theta^2}{2\sigma^2}\int_0^T \xi_t^2 dt\right). \tag{1.2.9}$$

Substituting (ξ_t) by its expression in (1.2.5), the MLE is

$$\hat{\theta}_T = \frac{\int_0^T \xi_t d\xi_t}{\int_0^T \xi_t^2 dt} = \theta + \sigma \frac{\int_0^T \xi_t dW_t}{\int_0^T \xi_t^2 dt}. \tag{1.2.10}$$

The estimator $\hat{\theta}_T$ defined in (1.2.10) reads as

$$\hat{\theta}_T = \theta + \frac{M_T}{\langle M \rangle_T} \text{ with } M_t = \frac{1}{\sigma}\int_0^t \xi_s dW_s. \tag{1.2.11}$$

where (M_t) is a $(\mathscr{F}_t)$-martingale in L^2 with angle bracket $\langle M \rangle_t$ (i.e. the process such that $(M_t^2 - \langle M \rangle_t)$ is a martingale). Noting that $\langle M \rangle_T \to \infty$ as $T \to \infty$, the law of large

numbers yields that $\frac{M_T}{\langle M\rangle_T} \to 0$. Hence the MLE defined by (1.2.10) is consistent.
As for the $AR(1)$- model, the rate of convergence of $\hat{\theta}_T$ to θ depends on the properties of (M_t). Three different cases can be listed as $T \to \infty$:
(1) $\{\theta < 0\}$: (ξ_t) is a positive recurrent process with stationary distribution $\mathscr{N}(0, \frac{\sigma^2}{2|\theta|})$ and $\sqrt{T}(\hat{\theta}_T - \theta) \to_{\mathscr{L}} \mathscr{N}(0, 2|\theta|)$.
(2) $\{\theta = 0\}$: (ξ_t) is a null recurrent diffusion; $T\hat{\theta}_T$ converges to a fixed distribution.
(3) $\{\theta > 0\}$: (ξ_t) is a transient diffusion; $e^{\theta T}(\hat{\theta}_T - \theta)$ converges in distribution to $Y = \eta\, Z$, where η, Z are two independent random variables, $Z \sim \mathscr{N}(0,1)$ and η is an explicit a positive random variable.

Case (b)-1 Discrete observations with sampling interval Δ fixed.
Let $t_i = i\Delta, T = n\Delta$ and assume that the number of observations $n \to \infty$.
Using (1.2.8), $(X_i = \xi_{t_i})$ is an AR(1) with $a = e^{\theta\Delta}$,$\gamma^2 = \sigma^2 v(\theta)$ with $v(\theta) = \frac{1}{2\theta}(e^{2\theta\Delta} - 1)$.

Let $\phi_\Delta : (0, +\infty)^2 \to \mathbb{R} \times (0, +\infty)$

$$\phi_\Delta \; : m = \begin{pmatrix} a \\ \gamma^2 \end{pmatrix} \to \begin{pmatrix} \theta = \frac{\log a}{\Delta} \\ \sigma^2 = \frac{a^2-1}{2\log a}\Delta\gamma^2 \end{pmatrix}.$$

This is a C^1-diffeomorphism and the MLE for θ and σ^2 can be deduced from $(\hat{a}_n, \hat{\gamma}_n^2)$ obtained in Section 1.2.1. This yields

$$\hat{\theta}_n = \frac{1}{\Delta}\log\left(\frac{\sum_{i=1}^n X_{i-1}X_i}{\sum_{i=1}^n X_{i-1}^2}\right); \quad \hat{\sigma}_n^2 = \frac{1}{n}\sum_{i=1}^n (X_i - \exp(\hat{\theta}_n\Delta)\, X_{i-1})^2.$$

These two estimators inherit the asymptotic properties of the maximum likelihood estimators $(\hat{a}_n, \hat{\gamma}_n^2)$ obtained in Subsection 1.2.1, their asymptotic variance is obtained using Theorem A.1.1 stated in the Appendix, Section A.1.2 (see also [123], Theorem 3.1). Therefore, $(\hat{\theta}_n, \hat{\sigma}_n^2)$ is consistent and, using that $a_n(\hat{m}_n - m)$ converges to a random variable Y yields

$$a_n \begin{pmatrix} \hat{\theta}_n - \theta \\ \hat{\sigma}_n^2 - \sigma^2 \end{pmatrix} \to_{\mathscr{L}} \nabla_x \phi_\Delta(m) Y, \tag{1.2.12}$$

where a_n is respectively for Cases (1), (2), (3) the matrix

$$\begin{pmatrix} \sqrt{n} & 0 \\ 0 & \sqrt{n} \end{pmatrix}, \quad \begin{pmatrix} n & 0 \\ 0 & \sqrt{n} \end{pmatrix}, \quad \begin{pmatrix} e^{n\Delta\theta} & 0 \\ 0 & \sqrt{n} \end{pmatrix}.$$

In particular, for Case (1) where $Y \sim \mathscr{N}_2(0, \Sigma)$, the limit distribution $\mathscr{N}_2(0, \nabla_x\phi_\Delta(m)\Sigma(\nabla_x\phi(m))^*)$ where Σ is the matrix obtained in (1.2.4).

Looking precisely at the theoretical asymptotic variance of $\hat{\theta}_n$ obtained in (1.2.12), we can observe that, for small Δ, this variance is $\frac{2|\theta|}{\Delta}$ and therefore explodes. It corresponds to the property that $\sqrt{n}$ is not the right rate of convergence of θ for small Δ.

Case (b)-2 Discrete observations with sampling interval $\Delta = \Delta_n \to 0$

We just detail Case (1), which corresponds to the ergodic Ornstein–Uhlenbeck process, first studied in [85]. Under the condition $n\Delta_n^2 \to 0$, the estimators $\hat{\theta}_n, \hat{\sigma}_n^2$ are consistent and converge at different rates under $\mathbb{P}_\theta$,

$$\begin{pmatrix} \sqrt{n\Delta_n}(\hat{\theta}_n - \theta) \\ \sqrt{n}(\hat{\sigma}_n^2 - \sigma^2) \end{pmatrix} \overset{\mathscr{L}}{\to} \mathscr{N}_2\left(0, \begin{pmatrix} 2|\theta| & 0 \\ 0 & 2\sigma^4 \end{pmatrix}\right). \tag{1.2.13}$$

Case (c)-1 Aggregated observations on intervals $[i\Delta, (i+1)\Delta]$ with Δ fixed.

Assume now that the available observations are aggregated data on successive intervals, (J_i) with

$$J_i = \int_{t_i}^{t_{i+1}} \xi_s \, ds. \tag{1.2.14}$$

The inference problem has first been studied by [55], [54] for an ergodic stationary diffusion process. It entails that $\theta < 0$ and that X_0 is random, independent of $(W_t, t \geq 0)$, distributed according to the stationary distribution of (ξ_t), $\mathscr{N}(0, \frac{\sigma^2}{2|\theta|})$.

The process $(J_i)_{i \geq 0}$ is a non-Markovian strictly stationary centered Gaussian process. Using (1.2.6) and (1.2.14), J_i and J_{i+1} are linked by the relation

$$J_{i+1} - e^{\theta\Delta} J_i = \frac{\sigma}{\theta} \int_{i\Delta}^{(i+1)\Delta} (e^{\theta\Delta} - e^{\theta((i+1)\Delta - s)}) dW_s \tag{1.2.15}$$
$$+ \frac{\sigma}{\theta} \int_{(i+1)\Delta}^{(i+2)\Delta} (e^{\theta((i+2)\Delta - s)} - 1) dW_s.$$

Hence, for all $i \geq 1$, $(J_{i+1} - e^{\theta\Delta} J_i)$ is independent of $(J_0, \ldots, J_{i-1})$ and (J_i) possesses the structure of an ARMA(1,1) process, for which the statistical inference is derived with other tools. Indeed,

$$\mathrm{Var}(J_i) = \sigma^2 r_0(\theta) \;;\; \mathrm{Cov}(J_i, J_j) = \sigma^2 r_{i-j}(\theta) \quad \text{with}$$
$$r_0(\theta) = \frac{1}{\theta^2}\left(\Delta + \frac{1 - e^{\theta\Delta}}{\theta}\right) \;;\; r_k(\theta) = -\frac{1}{2\theta^3} e^{-\theta\Delta}(e^{\theta\Delta} - 1)^2 \, e^{\theta\Delta|k|} \text{ if } k \neq 0.$$

Its spectral density has also an explicit expression, $f_{\theta,\sigma^2}(\lambda) = \sigma^2 f_\theta(\lambda)$.

The likelihood function is known theoretically but its exact expression is intractable. Instead of the exact likelihood, a well-known method to derive estimators is to use the Whittle contrast $U_n(\theta, \sigma^2)$ which provides efficient estimators. It is based on the periodogram: if j denotes now the complex number $j^2 = -1$,

$$U_n(\theta, \sigma^2) = \frac{1}{2\pi} \int_{-\pi}^{\pi} \left(\log f_{\theta,\sigma^2}(\lambda) + \frac{I_n(\lambda)}{f_{\theta,\sigma^2}(\lambda)}\right) d\lambda, \text{ with } I_n(\lambda) = \frac{1}{n} |\sum_{k=0}^{n-1} J_k e^{-jk\lambda}|^2.$$

The estimators are then defined as any solution of $U_n(\tilde{\theta}_n, \tilde{\sigma}_n^2) = \inf_{\theta,\sigma^2} U_n(\theta, \sigma^2)$. This yields consistent and asymptotically Gaussian estimators at rate $\sqrt{n}$.

Case (c)-2 Aggregated observations on intervals $[i\Delta,(i+1)\Delta]$ with $\Delta = \Delta_n \to 0$.
Let us now consider the case of $\Delta = \Delta_n \to 0, T = n\Delta_n \to \infty$ as $n \to \infty$. Let $J_{i,n} = \int_{i\Delta_n}^{(i+1)\Delta_n} \xi_s ds$. Assume that $\theta < 0$. The diffusion is positive recurrent with stationary measure $\mu_{\theta,\sigma^2}(dx) \sim \mathcal{N}(0, \frac{\sigma^2}{2|\theta|})$. The following two convergences hold in probability (see [55]).

$$\frac{1}{n}\sum_{i=0}^{n-1}(\Delta_n^{-1}J_{i+1,n} - \Delta_n^{-1}J_{i,n})^2 \to \frac{2}{3}\sigma^2, \text{ while}$$

$$\frac{1}{n}\sum_{i=0}^{n-1}(\xi_{(i+1)\Delta_n} - \xi_{i\Delta_n})^2 \to \sigma^2.$$

Hence, for small Δ_n, the heuristics $\frac{1}{\Delta_n}J_{i,n} \sim \xi_{i\Delta_n}$ is too rough and does not yield good statistical results. The two processes corresponding to these two kinds of observations are structurally distinct: $(\xi_{i\Delta_n})$ is an AR(1) process while $(\frac{1}{\Delta_n}J_{i,n})$ is ARMA(1,1). Ignoring this can lead to biased estimators.

1.2.3 Ornstein–Uhlenbeck Diffusion with Fixed Observation Time

Case (a) Continuous observation on $[0,T]$
As in Section 1.2.2 Case **(a)**, the parameter σ^2 is identified from the continuous observation of (ξ_t). Therefore we assume that σ^2 is known. The expression for the likelihood (1.2.9) holds. We get that, without additional assumptions, as for instance the presence of a small parameter ε, the MLE given in (1.2.10) $\hat{\theta}_T$ has a fixed distribution. On a fixed time interval, parameters in the drift term of a diffusion cannot be consistently estimated.

Case (b)-1 Discrete observations with fixed sampling Δ
The number of observations n is fixed. Without additional assumptions, neither θ nor σ^2 can be consistently estimated.

Case (b)-2 Discrete observations with sampling $\Delta_n \to 0$
Let $\Delta = \Delta_n = T/n \to 0$ as $n \to \infty$. Equation (1.2.7) holds and (1.2.2) is the likelihood. The maximum likelihood estimator $\hat{\theta}_n$ satisfies

$$\hat{\theta}_n = \frac{1}{\Delta_n}\log\left(1 + \Delta_n \frac{\sum_{i=1}^n \xi_{t_{i-1}}(\xi_{t_i} - \xi_{t_{i-1}})}{\Delta_n \sum_{i=1}^n \xi_{t_{i-1}}^2}\right). \tag{1.2.16}$$

Since $t_i = i\frac{T}{n}$, using the property of stochastic integrals and the Lebesgue integral yields that, under $\mathbb{P}_\theta$,

$$\sum_{i=1}^n \xi_{t_{i-1}}(\xi_{t_i} - \xi_{t_{i-1}}) \to \int_0^T \xi_s d\xi_s \text{ in probability;} \quad \sum_{i=1}^n \Delta_n\, \xi_{t_{i-1}}^2 \to \int_0^T \xi_s^2 ds \text{ a.s.}$$

Therefore, as $n \to \infty$, $\hat{\theta}_n$ converges to the random variable $\theta_T = \frac{\int_0^T \xi_s d\xi_s}{\int_0^T \xi_s^2 ds}$. Hence $\hat{\theta}_n$ is not consistent. Note that θ_T is precisely the MLE for θ obtained for continuous observation, which possesses good properties only if $T \to \infty$.
The story is different for the estimation of σ^2. The normalized quadratic variations of (ξ_t) is a consistent estimator of σ^2 and $\sum(\xi_{t_i} - \xi_{t_{i-1}})^2 \to \sigma^2 T$ in probability. Moreover,

$$\tilde{\sigma}^2 = \frac{1}{T}\sum_{i=1}^{n}(\xi_{t_i} - \xi_{t_{i-1}})^2 \text{ satisfies that } \sqrt{n}(\tilde{\sigma}^2 - \sigma^2) \to \mathcal{N}(0, 2\sigma^4). \tag{1.2.17}$$

Note that this result holds whatever the value of θ.

Case (c)-1 Aggregated observations on intervals $[i\Delta, (i+1)\Delta]$ with Δ fixed
As in Case (b)-1, θ and σ^2 cannot be consistently estimated.

Case (c)-2 Aggregated observations on intervals $[i\Delta, (i+1)\Delta]$ with $\Delta = \Delta_n \to 0$
This has been studied in [55]. Then, as $\Delta_n \to 0$, in probability,

$$\sum_{i=0}^{n-1}(\Delta_n^{-1} J_{i+1,n} - \Delta_n^{-1} J_{i,n})^2 \to \frac{2}{3}\sigma^2 T \quad \text{while} \quad \sum_{i=0}^{n-1}(\xi_{(i+1)\Delta_n} - \xi_{i\Delta_n})^2 \to \sigma^2 T.$$

Here again, the heuristics $\frac{1}{\Delta_n} J_{i,n} \sim \xi_{i\Delta_n}$ is too rough and does not yield good statistical results.

1.2.4 Ornstein–Uhlenbeck Diffusion with Small Diffusion Coefficient

This asymptotic framework is "$\varepsilon \to 0$". It naturally occurs for diffusion approximations of epidemic processes. The equation under study is now

$$d\xi_t = \theta \xi_t dt + \varepsilon \sigma dW_t \;\; \xi_0 = x_0. \tag{1.2.18}$$

We detail the results for fixed observation time $[0, T]$.

Case (a) Continuous observation on $[0, T]$
As before, we assume that σ^2 is known and omit it. Let $\mathbb{P}_\theta^\varepsilon$ the distribution on $(C_T, \mathcal{C}_T)$ of (ξ_t) satisfying (1.2.18). The likelihood is now

$$L_{T,\varepsilon}(\theta) = \frac{d\mathbb{P}_\theta^\varepsilon}{dP_0^\varepsilon}(\xi_s, 0 \le s \le T) = \exp\Big(\frac{\theta}{\varepsilon^2\sigma^2}\int_0^T \xi_s \, d\xi_s - \frac{\theta^2}{2\varepsilon^2\sigma^2}\int_0^T \xi_s^2 ds\Big). \tag{1.2.19}$$

$$\hat{\theta}_{T,\varepsilon} = \theta + \varepsilon\sigma \frac{\int_0^T \xi_t dW_t}{\int_0^T \xi_t^2 dt}. \tag{1.2.20}$$

Therefore $\hat{\theta}_{T,\varepsilon} \to \theta$ in probability under P_θ^ε as $\varepsilon \to 0$. Moreover, using results of [91]),

$$\varepsilon^{-1}(\hat{\theta}_{T,\varepsilon} - \theta) \to_{\mathscr{L}} \mathscr{N}(0, \tau^2), \quad \text{with } \tau^2 = \frac{2\theta\sigma^2}{x_0^2(e^{2\theta T} - 1)}.$$

Case (b)-1 Discrete observations with fixed sampling interval Δ
If Δ is fixed, only θ can be consistently estimated (see [60]). This is detailed in Chapter 3, Section 3.5. Setting $a = e^{\theta\Delta}$, and $X_i = \xi_{i\Delta}$, then, using (1.2.1),

$$X_i = aX_{i-1} + \varepsilon\gamma\eta_i, \quad \text{where} \quad \gamma^2 = \frac{e^{2\theta\Delta} - 1}{2\theta}\sigma^2,$$

and (η_i) i.i.d. $\mathscr{N}(0,1)$ random variables. Using (1.2.2) and (1.2.3) yields

$$\hat{a}_{\varepsilon,\Delta} = a + \varepsilon\gamma \frac{\sum_{i=1}^n X_{i-1}\eta_i}{\sum_{i=1}^n X_{i-1}^2}.$$

Therefore, as $\varepsilon \to 0$, $\hat{a}_{\varepsilon,\Delta}$ is consistent and

$$\varepsilon^{-1}(\hat{a}_{\varepsilon,\Delta} - a) \to \mathscr{N}(0, V_\Delta), \quad \text{with } V_\Delta = \gamma^2 \frac{e^{2\theta\Delta} - 1}{x_0^2(e^{2\theta T} - 1)} = \sigma^2 \frac{(e^{2\theta\Delta} - 1)^2}{2x_0^2\theta(e^{2\theta T} - 1)}.$$

Note that for small Δ, $V_\Delta \sim \frac{\Delta}{x_0^2(e^{2\theta T} - 1)}\sigma^2$.

Case (b)-2 Discrete observations with sampling $\Delta = \Delta_n \to 0$
This was first studied in [56], [118] and is detailed in Chapter 3. Let $T = n\Delta_n$ (the number of observations $n \to \infty$ as $\Delta_n \to 0$). Both θ and σ can be estimated from discrete observations. One can prove that they converge at different rates: under $\mathbb{P}_\theta$ as $\varepsilon \to 0, n \to \infty$,

$$\begin{pmatrix} \varepsilon^{-1}(\hat{\theta}_{\varepsilon,n} - \theta \\ \sqrt{n}(\hat{\sigma}_n^2 - \sigma^2 \end{pmatrix} \to \mathscr{N}_2\left(0, \begin{pmatrix} \frac{2\theta\sigma^2}{x_0^2(e^{2\theta T} - 1)} & 0 \\ 0 & 2\sigma^4 \end{pmatrix}\right). \tag{1.2.21}$$

1.2.5 Conclusions

This detailed example based on the Ornstein–Uhlenbeck diffusion studied under various asymptotic frameworks and various kinds of observations shows that, before estimating parameters ruling the process under study, one has to carefully consider how the available observations are obtained from the process and to study their properties. Some approximations are relevant and keep good statistical properties, while other ones lead to estimators which are not even consistent.

Chapter 2
Inference for Markov Chain Epidemic Models

In order to present an overview of the statistical problems, we first detail the statistical inference for Markov chains. Indeed, discrete time Markov chains models are interesting here because many questions that can arise for more complex models can be illustrated in this set-up. Moreover, continuous-time stochastic models are often observed in practice at discrete times, which might sum up to a Markov chain model. Therefore, this point of view allows us to illustrate some classical statistical methods for stochastic models used in epidemics. We have rather focus here on parametric inference since epidemic models always include in their dynamics parameters that need to be estimated in order to derive predictions. A recap on parametric inference for Markov chains is given in the Appendix, Section A.2.1, together with some notations and basic definitions. We apply in this chapter these results on some classical stochastic models used in epidemics (see Part I, Chapter 1 and also [2], [35]).

2.1 Markov Chains with Countable State Space

Markov chain models occur when assuming that a latent period of fixed length follows the receipt of infection by any susceptible. According to the epidemic model, the state space of the Markov chain can be finite if the epidemics takes place in a fixed finite population, countable (birth and death processes, branching processes, open Markov Models detailed in Part I, Chapter 4 of these notes), or continuous (see e.g. the simple AR(1) dynamic model).

Let us first consider a Markov chain (X_n) with finite state space $E = \{0, \ldots, N\}$ and transition matrix $(Q(i,j), i,j \in E)$. Assume that $X_0 = x_0$ is deterministic and known. Our aim is to estimate the transition matrix Q, which corresponds to $q = N(N+1)$ parameters since, for all $i \in E$, $\sum_{j=0}^{N} Q(i,j) = 1$.
Following the definitions recalled in Section A.2 in the Appendix, denote by $\mathbb{P}_Q$ the distribution on $(E^{\mathbb{N}}, \mathscr{E}^{\mathbb{N}})$ of (X_n) and $\mathscr{F}_n = \sigma(X_0, \ldots, X_n)$. Let $\mu_n = \otimes_{k=1}^{n} \nu_k$ with $\nu_k(\cdot)$ the measure on E such that $\nu_k(i) = 1$ for $i \in E$.

T. Britton, E. Pardoux (eds.), *Stochastic Epidemic Models with Inference*,
Lecture Notes in Mathematics 2255, https://doi.org/10.1007/978-3-030-30900-8_13

For A a subset of E, let $\delta_A(\cdot)$ denote the Dirac function: $\delta_A(x) = 1$ if $x \in A$, $\delta_A(x) = 0$ if $x \notin A$. Define

$$N_n^{ij} = \sum_{k=1}^{n} \delta_{\{i,j\}}(X_{k-1}, X_k); \quad N_n^{i\cdot} = \sum_{k=1}^{n} \delta_{\{i\}}(X_{k-1}). \tag{2.1.1}$$

Using (2.1.1), the likelihood and the loglikelihood read as

$$L_n(Q) = \frac{d\mathbb{P}_Q}{d\mu_n}(X_k, k=1,\ldots,n) = \prod_{k=1}^{n} Q(X_{k-1}, X_k) = \prod_{i,j \in E} Q(i,j)^{N_{ij}^n}, \tag{2.1.2}$$

$$\ell_n(Q) = \sum_{i,j \in E} N_n^{ij} \log Q(i,j). \tag{2.1.3}$$

The computation of the Maximum Likelihood Estimator, $(\hat{Q}_n(i,j,), i,j \in E)$, corresponds to the maximization of $\ell_n(Q)$ under the $(N+1)$ constraints $\{\sum_{j=0}^{N} Q(i,j) - 1 = 0\}$. This yields that

$$\hat{Q}_n(i,j) = \frac{N_n^{ij}}{N_n^{i\cdot}}. \tag{2.1.4}$$

Since the random variables $(N_n^{ij}, i \neq j)$ are equal to the number of transitions from i to j up to time n and $N_n^{i\cdot}$ is the time spent in state i up to time n, the estimators $\hat{Q}_n(i,j)$ are equal to the empirical estimates of the transitions.

To study the properties of the MLE, we assume

(H1) The Markov chain (X_n) with transition matrix Q is positive recurrent aperiodic on E.

Denote by $\lambda_Q(\cdot)$ the stationary distribution of (X_n). Then, the following holds.

Proposition 2.1.1. *Under (H1), the MLE $(\hat{Q}_n(i,j), i,j \in E)$ is strongly consistent and, under $\mathbb{P}_Q$,*

$$\sqrt{n}\left(\hat{Q}_n(i,j) - Q(i,j)\right)_{0 \le i \le N, 0 \le j \le N-1} \to_{\mathscr{L}} \mathscr{N}_q(0, \Sigma) \text{ with } q = N(N+1),$$

$$\Sigma_{ij,ij} = \frac{Q(i,j)(1-Q(i,j))}{\lambda_Q(i)}; \quad \Sigma_{ij,ij'} = -\frac{Q(i,j)Q(i,j')}{\lambda_Q(i)}; \quad \Sigma_{ij,i'j'} = 0 \text{ if } i' \neq i.$$

Proof. Under (H1), successive applications of the ergodic theorem yield that, almost surely under $\mathbb{P}_Q$,
$\frac{1}{n}N_n^{ij} \to \lambda_Q(i)Q(i,j)$, $\frac{1}{n}N_n^{i\cdot} \to \lambda_Q(i)$ so that $\hat{Q}_n(i,j) \to Q(i,j)$.
Let us study $(\hat{Q}_n(i,j) - Q(i,j))$. For $0 \le i \le N, 0 \le j \le N-1$, define

$$Y_k^{ij} = \left(\delta_{\{j\}}(X_k) - Q(i,j)\right)\delta_{\{i\}}(X_{k-1}), \quad M_n^{ij} = \sum_{k=1}^{n} Y_k^{ij}. \tag{2.1.5}$$

Then

$$\hat{Q}_n(i,j) - Q(i,j) = \frac{N_n^{ij} - Q(i,j)N_n^{i.}}{N_n^{i.}} = \frac{M_n^{ij}}{N_n^{i.}} = \frac{\sum_{k=1}^n Y_k^{ij}}{N_n^{i.}}. \tag{2.1.6}$$

Clearly, $E_Q(Y_k^{ij}|\mathscr{F}_{k-1}) = 0$ and (M_n^{ij}) is a centered $\mathscr{F}_n$-martingale with values in $\mathbb{R}^q$. Its angle bracket is the random matrix $\langle M \rangle_n$ with indices $(ij),(i'j')$

$$\langle M \rangle_n^{ij,i'j'} = \sum_{k=1}^n E_Q(Y_k^{ij} Y_i^{i'j'}|\mathscr{F}_{k-1}).$$

Straightforward computations yield that

$$E_Q(Y_k^{ij} Y_k^{ij}|\mathscr{F}_{k-1})) = Q(i,j)(1-Q(i,j))\delta_{\{i\}}(X_{k-1}),$$
$$E_Q(Y_k^{ij} Y_k^{ij'}|\mathscr{F}_{k-1})) = -Q(i,j)Q(i,j')\delta_{\{i\}}(X_{k-1}) \text{ if } j' \neq j \text{ and}$$
$$E_Q(Y_k^{ij} Y_i^{i'j'}|\mathscr{F}_{k-1}) = 0 \text{ if } i' \neq i.$$

Define the q-dimensional matrix J_Q by

$$J_Q(ij,ij) = Q(i,j)(1-Q(i,j))\lambda_Q(i),$$
$$J_Q(ij,ij') = -Q(i,j)Q(i,j')\lambda_Q(i) \text{ for } j' \neq j \text{ and}$$
$$J_Q(ij,i'j') = 0 \text{ if } i' \neq i.$$

Then, the ergodic theorem yields that $\frac{1}{n}\langle M \rangle_n^{ij,i'j'} \to J_Q(ij,i'j')$ a.s. under $\mathbb{P}_Q$. Applying the Central Limit Theorem for multidimensional martingales (see Appendix, Section A.4.2) yields that, under $\mathbb{P}_Q$, $\frac{1}{\sqrt{n}} M_n \to \mathscr{N}(0,J_Q)$ in distribution. Finally, using that $\frac{1}{n} N_n^{i.} \to \lambda_Q(i)$ a.s., an application of Slutsky's lemma to (2.1.6) achieves the proof of Proposition 2.1.1. □

2.1.1 Greenwood Model

This is a basic model which was introduced by Greenwood [58] to study measles epidemics in United Kingdom. It is an *SIR* epidemic in a finite population of size N. The latent period is fixed and equal 1 with infectiousness confined to a single time point. At the moment of infectiousness of any given infective, the chance of contact with any specified susceptible, sufficient or adequate to transmit the infection is $p = 1 - q$. Infected individuals are removed from the infection chain. At time 0, assume that the number of Susceptible S_0 and Infected I_0 verify $S_0 + I_0 = N$.
Denote by S_n, I_n the number of Susceptible and Infected at time n. Then, for all $n \geq 0$,

$$S_n = I_{n+1} + S_{n+1}, \tag{2.1.7}$$

and, at each generation the actual number of new cases has a Binomial distribution depending on the parameter p. In the Greenwood model, the chance of a susceptible of being infected depends only on the presence of some infectives and not on their actual number. Hence, if $I_n = 0$, the epidemic terminates immediately since there is no further infectives. If $I_n \geq 1$, the conditional distribution of I_{n+1} given the past $\mathscr{F}_n = \sigma((S_i, I_i), i = 0, \ldots n)$ is

$$\mathscr{L}(I_{n+1}|\mathscr{F}_n) = \text{Bin}(S_n, p) \quad \text{and } S_{n+1} = S_n - I_{n+1}.$$

The process keeps going on up to the time where there is no longer Infected in the population. Noting that $\mathscr{F}_n = \sigma(S_i, i = 0, \ldots n)$, (S_n) is a Markov chain on $\{0, \ldots, S_0\}$ with transition matrix

$$Q_p(i,j) = \binom{i}{i-j} p^{i-j}(1-p)^j \text{ if } 0 \leq j \leq i \leq S_0; \quad Q_p(i,j) = 0 \text{ otherwise.} \tag{2.1.8}$$

Parametric inference

Assume that the successive numbers of Susceptible $(s_0, s_1, \ldots, s_n)$ have been observed up to time n. In this model, (S_n) decreases with n, and extinction occurs after a geometric number of generations. Therefore, the inference framework is to assume that S_0 (hence N) $\to \infty$.

Let $\mathbb{P}_p$ the probability associated to the Markov chain with transition Q_p and initial condition s_0. The likelihood associated with parameter p and observations $(s_1, \ldots, s_n)$ is, if $s_0 \geq s_1 \cdots \geq s_n$,

$$L_n(p; s_1, \ldots, s_n) = \prod_{k=1}^{n} \mathbb{P}_p(S_k = s_k | S_{k-1} = s_{k-1}) = C(s_0, \ldots, s_n) p^{s_0 - s_n} (1-p)^{\sum_{k=1}^{n} s_n}. \tag{2.1.9}$$

All the quantities independent of p have been gathered in the term $C(s_0, , \ldots, s_n)$. They depend on the model and the observations, and therefore have no influence on the estimation of p. Elementary computations yield that the value of p that maximizes the likelihood is

$$\hat{p}_n = \frac{s_0 - s_n}{\sum_{k=0}^{n-1} s_k} = \frac{1}{\text{“mean time to infection”}}.$$

Another approach for estimating parameters of a stochastic process is the Conditional Least Squares (CLS) method. This is the analog of the traditional Least Squares method for i.i.d. observations. It is especially relevant when computing the likelihood is intractable. Noting that $\mathbb{E}_p(S_k|\mathscr{F}_{k-1}) = (1-p)S_{k-1}$, it reads as

$$U_n(p, S_1, \ldots, S_n) = \sum_{k=1}^{n} (S_k - \mathbb{E}_p(S_k|\mathscr{F}_{k-1}))^2 = \sum_{k=1}^{n} (S_k - (1-p)S_{k-1}))^2. \tag{2.1.10}$$

The associated Conditional Least Squares estimator is

$$\tilde{p}_n = 1 - \frac{\sum_{k=1}^{n} s_{k-1} s_k}{\sum_{k=1}^{n} s_{k-1}^2}. \tag{2.1.11}$$

A concern in statistics is to answer the question: how does such an estimator (or other ones) behave according to the asymptotic framework (here $S_0 \to \infty$). Is one of these two estimators better?

2.1.2 Reed–Frost Model

It is also a chain Binomial *SIR* model relevant to model the evolution of an ordinary influenza in a small group of individuals. The latent period is long with respect to a short infectious period and new infections occur at successive generations separated by latent periods. It is assumed that latent periods are equal to 1, contacts between Susceptibles and Infected are independent, and that the probability of contact between a Susceptible and an Infected is $p = 1 - q$. Therefore the probability of a Susceptible escaping infection given I Infected is q^I, and if $\mathscr{F}_n = \sigma((S_0, I_0), \ldots, (S_n, I_n))$,

$$\mathscr{L}(I_{n+1}|\mathscr{F}_n) = \text{Bin}(S_n, p_n) \text{ with } p_n = 1 - q^{I_n} \quad \text{and } S_{n+1} = S_n - I_{n+1}.$$

Then (S_n, I_n) is a Markov chain on $\mathbb{N}^2$ with probability transitions,

$$\begin{aligned} Q_q((s_n, i_n), (s_{n+1}, i_{n+1})) &= \binom{s_n}{s_{n+1}} (q^{i_n})^{s_{n+1}} (1 - q^{i_n})^{i_{n+1}} \text{ if } s_{n+1} + i_{n+1} = s_n, \\ &= 0 \text{ otherwise.} \end{aligned}$$

Parametric inference

Assume that the successive numbers of Susceptible and Infected have been observed up to time n and consider the estimation of $q = 1 - p$. Denote $\mathbb{P}_q$ the probability associated with the Markov chain with transition Q_q and initial condition (s_0, i_0). Then, if $s_{k+1} + i_{k+1} = s_k$ for $k = 0, \ldots, n-1$,

$$L_n(q; (s_1, i_1 \ldots, (s_n, i_n)) = \prod_{k=0}^{n-1} \binom{s_k}{s_{k+1}} (q^{i_k})^{s_{k+1}} (1 - q^{i_k})^{i_{k+1}}. \tag{2.1.12}$$

Therefore, $\log L_n(q) = C((s_k, i_k)) + \sum_{k=0}^{n-1} (s_{k+1} i_k \log q + i_{k+1} \log(1 - q^{i_k}))$. Differentiating with respect to q yields

$$\frac{d \log L_n}{dq} = \frac{1}{q} \sum_{k=0}^{n-1} \frac{i_k}{1 - q^{i_k}} (s_{k+1} - s_k q^{i_k}).$$

The maximum likelihood estimator $\hat{q}_n$ of q is a solution of the equation

$$\sum_{k=0}^{n-1} \frac{i_k}{1 - q^{i_k}} (s_{k+1} - s_k q^{i_k}) = 0.$$

Its properties can be studied as the number of observations increases (implying that the initial population grows to infinity).

Here a problem which occurs in practice already appears in this simple model, the case of "Partially Observed Markov Processes": it corresponds to the fact that both coordinates (S_n, I_n) are not observed, but only the successive numbers of Infected individuals $(I_k, k = 0, \ldots, n-1)$ are available. In the special case of Hidden Markov Models (see the Appendix, Section A.1.2 for the definition of H.M.M.), the theory for inference is now well known ([22], [124]), while there is no general theory for partially observed Markov processes. Many methods and algorithms have been proposed to deal with it in practice (see e.g. [37], [42], [70]). For applications specific to epidemics, many authors have addressed this problem (see e.g. [25], [29], [66], [70], together with the development of packages (see R package POMP [88])

2.1.3 Birth and Death Chain with Re-emerging

We consider now the example of an epidemic model with re-emerging in a large infinite population. It can be described by a birth and death chain on $\mathbb{N}$ with reflection at 0. This models for instance farm animals epidemics when infection can also be produced by the environment. Let p, q denote the birth rate and death rates with $\{0 < p, q < 1, p+q < 1\}$. We assume that $I_0 = i_0 \geq 1$ and that (I_n), the number of infected at time n, evolves as follows:

- if $k \geq 1$, then $\mathbb{P}(I_{n+1} = k+1 | I_n = k) = p$, $\mathbb{P}(I_{n+1} = k-1 | I_n = k) = q$, $\mathbb{P}(I_{n+1} = k | I_n = k) = 1 - p - q$;
- if $k = 0$, then $\mathbb{P}(I_{n+1} = 1 | I_n = 0) = p$, $\mathbb{P}(I_{n+1} = 0 | I_n = 0) = 1 - p$ (re-emerging probability).

The Markov chain (I_n) is irreducible aperiodic on $\mathbb{N}$ and, if $p < q$, (I_n) is positive recurrent with stationary distribution

$$\lambda_{(p,q)}(i) = \left(1 - \frac{p}{q}\right)\left(\frac{p}{q}\right)^i.$$

<u>Parametric inference</u>

Let $\Theta = \{(p,q), 0 < p < q < 1 \text{ with } p+q < 1\}$ and let θ_0 be the true parameter value. Assume that $I_0 = i_0 > 0$ is non-random and fixed and consider the estimation of $\theta = (p,q) \in \Theta$ based on the observation of the successive numbers of Infected up to time n.

Let $(Q_\theta(i,j), i, j \in \mathbb{N})$ denote the transition kernel (I_n):

- if $i \neq 0$, then $Q_\theta(i,j) = p\delta_{\{i+1\}}(j) + q\delta_{\{i-1\}}(j) + (1-p-q)\delta_{\{i\}}(j)$,
- if $i = 0$, then $Q_\theta(0,j) = p\delta_1(j) + (1-p)\delta_0(j)$.

Noting that for $j \neq \{i-1, i, i+1\}$, $N_n^{ij} = 0$, the loglikelihood $\ell_n(\theta)$ satisfies

$$\ell_n(\theta) = \sum_{i,j \in N} N_n^{ij} \log Q_\theta(i,j)$$
$$= B_n \log p + D_n \log q + R_n \log(1-p-q) + N_n^{0,0} \log(1-p), \text{ with}$$

$$B_n = \sum_{i \geq 0} N_n^{i,i+1},\ D_n = \sum_{i \geq 1} N_n^{i,i-1},\ R_n = \sum_{i \geq 1} N_n^{i,i}. \tag{2.1.13}$$

Since the Markov chain (I_n, I_{n+1}) is positive recurrent on $\mathbb{N}^2$ with stationary measure $\lambda_\theta(i) Q_\theta(i,j)$, we can study directly the limit behaviour of $\ell_n(\theta)$. Applying the ergodic theorem to (I_n, I_{n+1}) yields that, almost surely under $\mathbb{P}_{\theta_0}$,

$$\frac{1}{n} N_n^{i,i+1} \to p_0 \lambda_{\theta_0}(i) \text{ for } i \geq 1,$$
$$\frac{1}{n} N_n^{i,i-1} \to q_0 \lambda_{\theta_0}(i),$$
$$\frac{1}{n} N_n^{i,i} \to r_0 \lambda_{\theta_0}(i),$$
$$\frac{1}{n} N_n^{0,0} \to (1 - \frac{p_0}{q_0})(1-p_0).$$

Therefore, using (2.1.13),

$$\frac{1}{n} B_n \to p_0,$$
$$\frac{1}{n} D_n \to q_0 \times \frac{p_0}{q_0} = p_0,$$
$$\frac{1}{n} R_n \to \frac{r_0 p_0}{q_0},$$
$$\frac{1}{n} N_n^{0,0} \to (1 - \frac{p_0}{q_0})(1-p_0).$$

Joining these results, under P_{θ_0}, as $n \to \infty$,

$$\frac{1}{n} \ell_n(\theta) \to p_0 \log p + p_0 \log q + \frac{r_0 p_0}{q_0} \log r + (1 - \frac{p_0}{q_0})(1-p_0) \log(1-p) := J(\theta_0, \theta).$$

We can check directly that $\theta \to J(\theta_0, \theta)$ possesses a unique global maximum at θ_0. The associated maximum likelihood estimator $\hat{\theta}_n$ is

$$\hat{p}_n = \frac{1}{n} B_n; \quad \hat{q}_n = \frac{B_n}{D_n + R_n}(1 - \frac{1}{n} B_n). \tag{2.1.14}$$

Successive applications of the ergodic theorem yield that $(\hat{p}_n, \hat{q}_n)$ converges $\mathbb{P}_{\theta_0}$ a.s. to (p_0, q_0).

To study the limit distribution of $(\hat{p}_n, \hat{q}_n)$, we use the results of Section A.2.1.1 in the Appendix. Let $Q = (Q(i,j))$ denote the (unnormalized) transition kernel on $\mathbb{N} \times \mathbb{N}$:

$$Q(i,i+1) = 1 = Q(i,i) \text{ for } i \in \mathbb{N} \text{ and}$$
$$Q(i,i-1) = 1 \text{ for } i \geq 1.$$

According to (A.2.1), the family $(Q_\theta, \theta \in \Theta)$ is dominated by Q with associated function $f_\theta(i,j)$:

$$\begin{aligned} f_\theta(i,i+1) &= p \text{ for } i \geq 0, \\ f_\theta(i,i-1) &= q \text{ for } i \geq 1, \\ f_\theta(i,i) &= 1-p-q, \\ f_\theta(0,0) &= 1-p. \end{aligned}$$

Except the compactness assumption of Θ (only required for the consistency of the MLE), the Markov chain satisfies Assumptions (H1)–(H8) of Section A.2.1.1, Therefore, under $\mathbb{P}_{\theta_0}$,

$$\sqrt{n}\begin{pmatrix} \hat{p}_n - p_0 \\ \hat{q}_n - q_0 \end{pmatrix} \to_{\mathscr{L}} \mathscr{N}(0, I^{-1}(\theta_0)),$$

with, using Definition (A.2.5),

$$I(\theta_0) = \sum_{i \geq 0} \lambda_{\theta_0}(i) \sum_{j \geq 0} \frac{\nabla_\theta f_{\theta_0}(i,j) \nabla_\theta^* f_{\theta_0}(i,j)}{f_{\theta_0}(i,j)^2} Q_{\theta_0}(i,j).$$

Hence $I(\theta_0)$ can be explicitly computed: for $\theta = (p,q)$, we get

$$I(p,q) = \begin{pmatrix} \frac{r+p^2}{p(1-p)r} & \frac{p}{qr} \\ \frac{p}{qr} & \frac{p(1-p)}{rq^2} \end{pmatrix} \Rightarrow I^{-1}(p,q) = \begin{pmatrix} p(1-p) & -pq \\ -pq & \frac{q^2(p^2+r)}{p(1-p)} \end{pmatrix}. \tag{2.1.15}$$

2.1.4 Modeling an Infection Chain in an Intensive Care Unit

This example is taken from Chapter 4 of [35]. It aims at describing nosocomial infections (i.e. infections acquired in a hospital). The incidence of these infections is highest in an Intensive Care Unit, which is characterized by a small number of beds (about 10 beds at most) and rapid turnover of patients by way of admission and discharge. There are two routes for infection (colonization) for a patient.

- The endogenous route (α mechanism): bacteria are already present in a newly admitted patient but at low undetectable levels and resistant bacteria develop because of antibiotic treatments during the stay. Let $e^{-\alpha} = (1-a)$ the probability per individual per time unit of getting infected by this route.
- The exogenous route (β transmission): it models the probability of infection of a Susceptible by an Infected in the ICU per time unit, $e^{-\beta} = (1-b)$.

To describe the composition of the ICU in terms of Infected and Susceptible individuals on long time intervals, a Markov chain model can be used as follows.

Each patient has probability d of being discharged by unit of time. Discharge and admission take place every day at noon; new admitted individuals are susceptible. Observations are obtained from a bookkeeping scheme that concerns the state of the ICU immediately after discharge (12h05).

Consider the simplest example, an ICU with two beds. It corresponds to three possible states: State 0 (both patients are Susceptible), State 1 (one Susceptible, one Infected) and 2 (both are Infected). Denote by X_n the composition of the ICU at time n. Let us compute according to $\theta = (a,b,d)$ the transition matrix Q_θ of (X_n). Introduce $\bar{X}_{n+1}$ the state of the ICU just before discharge (at 11h55) on the next day. If $X_n = 0$, $\mathbb{P}(\bar{X}_{n+1} = 0) = a^2$, $\mathbb{P}(\bar{X}_{n+1} = 1) = 2a(1-a)$ and $\mathbb{P}(\bar{X}_{n+1} = 2) = (1-a)^2$. If $X_n = 1$, $\mathbb{P}(\bar{X}_{n+1} = 1) = ab$, and $\mathbb{P}(\bar{X}_{n+1} = 2) = (1-ab)$. Finally, if $X_n = 2$, $\mathbb{P}(\bar{X}_{n+1} = 2) = 1$. This yields that, after discharge (12h05), $X_{n+1} = 0,1,2$ with respective probabilities,

$$Q_\theta = \begin{pmatrix} (a+(1-a)d)^2 & 2(1-a)(1-d)(a+(1-a)d) & (1-a)^2(1-d)^2 \\ abd+(1-ab)d^2 & 2(1-ab)d(1-d)+ab(1-d) & (1-ab)(1-d)^2 \\ d^2 & 2d(1-d) & (1-d)^2 \end{pmatrix}.$$

Let $\Theta = (0,1)^3$. Assume that the states (X_i) of the ICU after discharge have been observed up to time n. The maximum likelihood estimator of θ reads, using (2.1.1),

$$\begin{aligned} \ell_n(\theta) &= \sum_{k=1}^{n} \log Q_\theta(X_{k-1},X_k) = \sum_{i,j\in\{0,1,2\}} N_n^{ij} \log Q_\theta(i,j), \\ \hat{\theta}_n &= \operatorname{argsup}_{\theta\in\Theta} \ell_n(\theta). \end{aligned}$$

Since (X_n) is a positive recurrent Markov chain on $\{0,1,2\}$, we can apply the results stated in the Appendix, Section A.2. The MLE $\hat{\theta}_n$ is consistent and converges at rate $\sqrt{n}$ to a Gaussian law $\mathcal{N}_3(0, I^{-1}(\theta))$, where $I(\theta)$ is the Fisher information matrix defined in (A.2.5).

Assume now that there is no systematic control of the exact status of the patients after discharge, but that each patient is tested with probability p. Then, the observations are no longer (X_n), but (Y_n), with conditional transition matrix $(T_p(i,j) = P(Y_n = j | X_n = i), 0 \le i,j \le 2)$,

$$T_p = \begin{pmatrix} (1-p)^2 & 2p(1-p) & p^2 \\ p(1-p) & p^2+(1-p)^2 & p(1-p) \\ p^2 & 2p(1-p) & (1-p)^2 \end{pmatrix}.$$

If only (Y_n) is observed, we have to deal with a Hidden Markov Model (X_n, Y_n) as defined in the Appendix, Section A.1.2. The estimation of θ or (θ, p) has to take into account this additional noise to be efficient (see e.g [22]).

2.2 Two Extensions to Continuous State and Continuous Time Markov Chain Models

2.2.1 A Simple Model for Population Dynamics

The $AR(1)$ model is a classical model of population dynamics with continuous state space and allows us to illustrate explicitly various inference questions. Consider the autoregressive process on $\mathbb{R}$s introduced in Section 1.2.1 defined by

$$X_0 = x_0; \qquad \text{and for } i \geq 1, X_i = aX_{i-1} + \gamma \varepsilon_i,$$

where (ε_i) is a sequence of i.i.d. random variables on $\mathbb{R}$ with distribution $f_\theta(x)dx$, independent of X_0.
This is a Markov chain on $(\mathbb{R}, \mathscr{B}(\mathbb{R}))$ with transition kernel $Q_{\theta,a}(x,dy) = f_\theta(y-ax)dy$. If X_0 is known, choosing as dominating kernel the Lebesgue measure on $\mathbb{R}$, the likelihood reads as

$$L_n(a,\theta) = \prod_{i=1}^{n} f_\theta(X_i - aX_{i-1}).$$

The Gaussian $AR(1)$ corresponds to $\varepsilon_i \sim \mathscr{N}(0,\gamma^2)$:

$$\begin{aligned} Q_{a,\gamma^2}(x,dy) &= \frac{1}{\gamma\sqrt{2\pi}} \exp -(\frac{1}{2\gamma^2}(y-ax)^2)dy, \text{ and} \\ L_n(a,\gamma^2) &= \prod_{i=1}^{n} \frac{1}{\gamma\sqrt{2\pi}} \exp(-\frac{1}{2\gamma^2}(X_i - aX_{i-1})^2), \\ \ell_n(a,\gamma^2) &= -(n/2)\log\gamma^2 - 1/(2\gamma^2)\sum_{i=1}^{n}(X_i - aX_{i-1})^2. \end{aligned}$$

The properties of the MLE have been presented in Chapter 1.

2.2.2 Continuous Time Markov Epidemic Model

We just recall here results for the SIR Markov jump process (see Section 4.2). Assume that the jump process $(\mathscr{Z}^N(t))$ is continuously observed on $[0,T]$. Its dynamics is described by the two parameters (λ,γ). The Maximum Likelihood Estimator $(\hat{\lambda},\hat{\gamma})$ is explicit (see [2] or Section 4.2). Indeed, let (T_i) denote the successive jump times and set $J_i = 0$ if we have an infection and $J_i = 1$ if we have a recovery. Let $K_N(T) = \sum_{i\geq 0} 1_{T_i \leq T}$. Then

$$\hat{\lambda}_N = \frac{1}{N}\frac{\sum_{i=1}^{K_N(T)}(1-J_i)}{\int_0^T S^N(t)I^N(t)dt} = \frac{1}{N}\frac{\#\text{ Infections}}{\int_0^T S^N(t)I^N(t)dt},$$

$$\hat{\gamma}_N = \frac{1}{N} \frac{\sum_{i=1}^{K_N(T)} J_i}{\int_0^T I^N(t)dt} = \frac{\#\,\text{Recoveries}}{\text{“Mean infectious period”}}.$$

As the population size N goes to infinity, $(\hat{\lambda}_N, \hat{\gamma}_N)$ is consistent and

$$\sqrt{N}\begin{pmatrix} \hat{\lambda}_N - \lambda \\ \hat{\gamma}_N - \gamma \end{pmatrix} \to \mathcal{N}_2\left(0, I^{-1}(\lambda,\gamma)\right), \text{ where } I(\lambda,\gamma) = \begin{pmatrix} \frac{\int_0^T s(t)i(t)dt}{\lambda} & 0 \\ 0 & \frac{\int_0^T i(t)dt}{\gamma} \end{pmatrix},$$

and $(s(t), i(t))$ is the solution of the ODE associated with the limit behaviour of the normalized process $(\mathcal{Z}^N(t)/N)$: $\frac{ds}{dt} = -\lambda s(t)i(t)$; $\frac{di}{dt} = \lambda s(t)i(t) - \gamma i(t)$.

The matrix $I(\lambda,\gamma)$ is the Fisher information matrix of this statistical model.

2.3 Inference for Branching Processes

At the early stage of an outbreak, a good approximation for the epidemic dynamics is to consider that the population of Susceptible is infinite and that Infected individuals evolve according to a branching process (see Section 1.2 of Part I). We present here some classical statistical results in this domain. This Markov chain model is an example of non-ergodic processes which leads to different statistical results.

2.3.1 Notations and Preliminary Results

Some basic facts on discrete time branching processes (or Bienaymé–Galton–Watson processes) are given in Part I, Section A.1 of these notes (see also the classical monographs on branching processes [6] or [78]). We complete these facts with some properties useful for the inference.

Consider an ancestor $Z_0 = 1$ has ξ_0 children according to an offspring law G defined by

$$\mathbb{P}(\xi_0 = k) = p_k, \; k \geq 0 \text{ and } \sum_{k\geq 0} p_k = 1.$$

Let $m = \mathbb{E}(\xi_0)$ and $g(s) = \mathbb{E}(s^{\xi_0})$. The i-th of those children has $\xi_{1,i}$ children, where the random variables $\{\xi_{k,i}, k \geq 0, i \geq 1\}$ are i.i.d. with distribution G. Let Z_n denote the number of individuals in generation n. Then,

$$Z_{n+1} = \sum_{i=1}^{Z_n} \xi_{n,i}. \tag{2.3.1}$$

Denote by $E = \{\exists\, n,\; Z_n = 0\}$ the set of extinction.
If $m \leq 1$ and if $p_1 \neq 1$, the process Z_n has a probability $q = 1$ of extinction.

If $m > 1$, the process is supercritical and has a probability of extinction $q < 1$, which is the smallest solution of the equation $g(s) = s$ on $[0,1]$. The set E^c is equal to $\{\omega, Z_n(\omega) \to \infty\}$.

This extinction probability is an important parameter for the early stages of an epidemic. It corresponds to the probability of a minor outbreak.
We complete the results given in Part I, Section A.1. Let $\mathscr{F}_n = \sigma(Z_0, \dots, Z_n)$ and define $W_n = m^{-n} Z_n$. Then (W_n) is a $\mathscr{F}_n$-martingale.

Theorem 2.3.1. *Assume that $m > 1$ and that the offspring law G has finite variance σ^2. Then, there is a non-negative random variable W such that*

(i) $W_n \to W$ as $n \to \infty$ a.s. and in L^2.
(ii) $\{W > 0\} = \{Z_n \to \infty\} = E^c$ and $\{W = 0\} = \{\lim_n Z_n = 0\} = E$.
(iii) Moreover, $\mathbb{E}W = 1$, $\mathrm{var}(W) = \frac{\sigma^2}{m(m-1)}$.

Corollary 2.3.2. *If $m > 1$, then, almost surely*

$$\frac{1}{m^n} \sum_{i=1}^{n} Z_i \to \frac{m}{m-1} W; \quad \frac{1}{m^n} \sum_{i=1}^{n} Z_{i-1} \to \frac{1}{m-1} W. \tag{2.3.2}$$

Proof. We write $\sum_{i=1}^n Z_i = \sum_{i=1}^n m^i \frac{Z_i}{m^i}$. Using Theorem 2.3.1, $\frac{Z_n}{m^n} \to W$ a.s. An application of the Toeplitz lemma stated below and some algebra yield the two results.

Lemma 2.3.3. *(Toeplitz Lemma) Let (a_n) a sequence of non-negative real numbers and (x_n) a sequence on $\mathbb{R}$. If $\sum_{i=1}^n a_i \to \infty$ and if $(x_n) \to x \in \mathbb{R}$ as $n \to \infty$, then*

$$\frac{\sum_{i=1}^n a_i x_i}{\sum_i^n a_i} \to x \text{ as } n \to \infty.$$

□

Assume that the offspring distribution $G_\theta(\cdot)$ depends on a parameter θ with finite mean $m(\theta) > 1$ and finite variance $\sigma^2(\theta)$. Denote by $\mathbb{P}_\theta$ the law on $(\mathbb{N}^{\mathbb{N}}, \mathscr{B}(N^{\mathbb{N}}))$ of the branching process (Z_n) with offspring law $G_\theta(\cdot)$. Then $(Z_n, n \geq 0)$ is a Markov chain with state space $\mathbb{N}$, initial condition $Z_0 = 1$ and transition matrix,

$$Q_\theta(i,j) = G_\theta^{\star i}(j), \tag{2.3.3}$$

where $\star$ denotes the convolution product of two functions and $f^{\star i}$ is the i-fold convolution product of $f(\cdot)$. Let μ_i denote the measure $\mu_i(k) = 1$ for all $k \in \mathbb{N}$, $\lambda_n = \otimes_{i=1}^n \mu_i$. Then, the likelihood reads as

$$\frac{d\mathbb{P}_\theta}{d\lambda_n}(Z_0, \dots, Z_n) = L_n(\theta) = \prod_{i=1}^{n} G_\theta^{\star Z_{i-1}}(Z_i); \quad \ell_n(\theta) = \sum_{i=1}^{n} \log(G_\theta^{\star Z_{i-1}}(Z_i)). \tag{2.3.4}$$

Under this expression, studying the likelihood for general offspring laws is intractable. We detail in the next section a framework where it is possible to study this likelihood, and in the next section another method based on Weighted Conditional Least Squares.

2.3.2 *Inference when the Offspring Law Belongs to an Exponential Family*

Among parametric families of distributions, exponential families of distributions, widely used in statistics, provide here a nice framework to study this likelihood. A short recap is given in the Appendix Section A.1.2 (see e.g. the classical monograph [11] for the complete exposition).

Assume that the offspring law is a power series distribution:

$$p(k) = A(\zeta)^{-1}\, a_k\, \zeta^k, \quad \text{with } A(\zeta) = \sum_{k\geq 0} a_k \zeta^k. \tag{2.3.5}$$

Setting $\theta = \log\zeta$, $\Theta = \{\theta \in \mathbb{R},\ A(e^\theta) < \infty\}$, $h : k \to h(k) = a_k$ and $\phi : \theta \to \phi(\theta) = \log A(\log(e^\theta))$, we get that it is a special case of an exponential family of distributions on $\mathbb{N}$ with $T(X) = X$ and

$$p(\theta, k) = h(k) \exp\left(k\theta - \phi(\theta)\right). \tag{2.3.6}$$

The random variable X satisfies that

$$m(\theta) := \mathbb{E}_\theta(X) = \nabla_\theta \phi(\theta); \quad \sigma^2(\theta) := Var_\theta(X) = \nabla^2_\theta \phi(\theta). \tag{2.3.7}$$

Moreover, if $X_1, \ldots, X_n$ are i.i.d. with distribution (2.3.5), then

$$\mathbb{P}(X_1 + \cdots + X_n = k) = H(n,k) \exp(k\theta - n\phi(\theta)) \ \text{ where } H(n,k) = h^{*n}(k). \tag{2.3.8}$$

Therefore for offspring distributions satisfying (2.3.5) or (2.3.6), the transition kernel is

$$Q_\theta(i,k) = H(i,k) \exp(k\theta - i\phi(\theta)).$$

Let us note that several families of classical distributions on $\mathbb{N}$ are included in this set-up:

- Geometric distributions on $\mathbb{N}^*$ with parameter p (i.e. $P(X = k) = p(1-p)^{k-1}$): $\theta = \log(1-p)$; $h(k) = 1$ and $\phi(\theta) = \log \frac{e^\theta}{1-e^\theta}$.
- Binomial distributions ($\mathscr{B}(N,p), p \in (0,1)$) with N fixed: $\theta = \log \frac{p}{1-p}$, $h(k) = \frac{N!}{k!(N-k)!}$ and $\phi(\theta) = N\log(1+e^\theta)$.
- Poisson distributions $\mathscr{P}(\lambda)$: $\theta = \log\lambda$, $h(k) = \frac{1}{k!}$ and $\phi(\theta) = e^\theta$.

- Negative Binomial distributions ($\mathcal{NB}(r,p), p \in (0,1)$) with r fixed (i.e. $P(X=k) = \frac{\Gamma(k+r)}{\Gamma(r)k!} p^r (1-p)^k$:
  $\theta = \log(1-p)$, $h(k) = \frac{(k+r)\dots(r+1)}{k!}$ and $\phi(\theta) = r\log(1-e^\theta)$).

Let us come back to the likelihood (2.3.4). Let $\theta_0 \in \Theta$ be the true value of the parameter. We assume

(A1) The offspring distribution G_θ belongs to an exponential power series family: For all $k \in \mathbb{N}$, $G_\theta(k) = h(k)\exp(k\theta - \phi(\theta))$.
(A2) Θ is a compact subset of $\{\theta, \sum_{k\geq 0} h(k)e^{\theta k} < \infty\}$, $\theta_0 \in \text{Int}(\Theta)$.
(A3) For all $\theta \in \Theta$, $m(\theta) > 1$ and $\sigma^2(\theta)$ finite.
(A4) There exists a $\delta > 0$ such that $E(Y^{2+\delta}) = \mu_{2+\delta} < \infty$ where $Y \sim G_\theta$.

Consider the estimation of θ when the successive generation sizes $(Z_1, \dots Z_n)$ are observed. Under (A1)–(A3), the loglikelihood is, using (2.3.8),

$$\ell_n(\theta) = C(Z_0, \dots, Z_n) + \sum_{i=1}^{n} (\theta Z_i - \phi(\theta) Z_{i-1}), \tag{2.3.9}$$

with $C(Z_0, \dots, Z_n) = \sum_{i=1}^n \log H(Z_{i-1}, Z_i)$. The constant $C(Z_0, \dots., Z_n)$ depends only on the observations and brings no information on θ.

The M.L.E $\hat{\theta}_n$, defined as any solution of $\nabla_\theta \ell_n(\theta) = 0$, satisfies

$$\sum_{i=1}^{n} Z_i - \nabla_\theta \phi(\hat{\theta}_n) \sum_{i=1}^{n} Z_{i-1} = 0.$$

Using that $\nabla_\theta \phi(\theta) = m(\theta)$ (see (2.3.7)), $\hat{\theta}_n$ satisfies

$$m(\hat{\theta}_n) = \frac{\sum_{i=1}^n Z_i}{\sum_{i=1}^n Z_{i-1}}. \tag{2.3.10}$$

By Theorem 2.3.1, $m(\theta_0)^{-n} Z_n$ converges a.s. and in L^2 under $\mathbb{P}_{\theta_0}$ to a random variable W such that $W > 0$ on E^c, the non-extinction set, which satisfies $\mathbb{P}_{\theta_0}(E^c) = 1 - q > 0$ under (A3).

Theorem 2.3.4. *Assume (A1)–(A4).Then, on E^c, $m(\hat{\theta}_n)$ satisfies*

(i) $m(\hat{\theta}_n) \to m(\theta_0)$ *a.s. under* $\mathbb{P}_{\theta_0}$.
(ii) $m(\theta_0)^{n/2}(m(\hat{\theta}_n) - m(\theta_0)) \to_{\mathcal{L}} \sqrt{(m(\theta_0)-1)\sigma^2(\theta_0)}\, \eta^{-1} N$, *where* η, N *are independent r.v.s,* $N \sim \mathcal{N}(0,1)$, *and* η *is the positive variable defined by* $\eta^2 = W$ *on* E^c.

Clearly, $m(\theta)$ is the parameter that is naturally estimated here.

Proof. Let us write

$$m(\hat{\theta}_n) = \frac{\frac{\sum_{i=1}^n Z_i}{m^n}}{\frac{\sum_{i=1}^n Z_{i-1}}{m^n}}.$$

Using Corollary 2.3.2, both terms of the above fraction converge a.s. so that $m(\hat{\theta}_n) \to m(\theta_0)$ a.s.

Let us prove (ii). The score function reads as

$$\nabla_\theta \ell_n(\theta) = \sum_{i=1}^n Z_i - m(\theta) \sum_{i=1}^n Z_{i-1} = \sum_{i=1}^n (Z_i - m(\theta) Z_{i-1}).$$

Under $\mathbb{P}_{\theta_0}$, $\nabla_\theta \ell_n(\theta_0)$ is a centered $\mathscr{F}_n$-martingale (M_n) with increments $X_i = Z_i - m(\theta_0)Z_{i-1}$. Conditionally on $\mathscr{F}_{i-1}$, X_i is the sum of Z_{i-1} independent centered random variables so that

$$\mathbb{E}_{\theta_0}(X_i^2 | \mathscr{F}_{i-1}) = \sigma^2(\theta_0) Z_{i-1}; \quad \langle M \rangle_n = \sigma^2(\theta_0) \sum_{i=1}^n Z_{i-1}.$$

Hence

$$s_n^2(\theta_0) = \mathbb{E}_{\theta_0}(\langle M \rangle_n) = \sigma^2(\theta_0) \sum_{i=1}^n m(\theta_0)^{i-1} = \sigma^2(\theta_0) \frac{m(\theta_0)^n - 1}{m(\theta_0) - 1}.$$

Therefore $s_n^2(\theta_0) \to \infty$ as $n \to \infty$ and

$$\frac{s_n^2(\theta_0)}{m(\theta_0)^n} \to \frac{\sigma^2(\theta_0)}{m(\theta_0) - 1}. \tag{2.3.11}$$

Let us check the conditions of the Central limit theorem for martingales (see A.4.1) recalled in the Appendix Under (A3), (M_n) is a square integrable centered $\mathscr{F}_n$-martingale such that $\mathbb{E}_{\theta_0}(\langle M_n \rangle) = s_n(\theta_0)^2 \to \infty$. Let us check (H2). We have

$$\frac{1}{s_n(\theta_0)^2} \langle M_n \rangle = \frac{m^n(\theta_0)}{s_n^2(\theta_0)} \frac{\sigma^2(\theta_0)}{m^n(\theta_0)} \sum_{i=1}^n Z_{i-1}.$$

Hence according to Corollary 2.3.2 and Theorem 2.3.1, $\frac{1}{s_n(\theta_0)^2} \langle M_n \rangle \to W$ in probability under $\mathbb{P}_{\theta_0}$ with $W > 0$ on E^c and $E_{\theta_0}(W) = 1$. Therefore we can set $W = \eta^2$ and obtain (H2).

It remains to check the asymptotic negligibility Assumption (H1'). We have, for $X_i = Z_i - m(\theta_0)Z_{i-1}$,

$$\mathbb{E}_{\theta_0}(|X_i|^{2+\delta} | \mathscr{F}_{i-1}) = Z_{i-1} \mathbb{E}_{\theta_0}(|Y - m(\theta_0)|^{2+\delta}).$$

Under (A4), using that $\mathbb{E}_{\theta_0}(|Y - m(\theta_0)|^{2+\delta}) \le C(\mu_{2+\delta} + m(\theta_0)^{2+\delta}) < \infty$ yields

$$\frac{1}{s_n^{2+\delta}} \sum_i^n \mathbb{E}_{\theta_0}(|X_i|^{2+\delta} | \mathscr{F}_{i-1}) = (\frac{1}{s_n^\delta}) \mathbb{E}_{\theta_0}(|Y - m(\theta_0)|^{2+\delta}) (\frac{1}{s_n^2} \sum_{i=1}^n Z_{i-1}). \tag{2.3.12}$$

Using Corollary 2.3.2 and (2.3.11) yields that the last term of (2.3.12) is bounded in probability under $\mathbb{P}_{\theta_0}$. Since $\delta > 0$, the first term of (2.3.12) tends to 0, which achieves the proof of (H1').

Therefore, we get that on the non-extinction set , under $\mathbb{P}_{\theta_0}$,

$$\left(\frac{M_n}{s_n}, \frac{\langle M\rangle_n}{s_n^2}\right) \to_{\mathscr{L}} (\eta N, \eta^2), \tag{2.3.13}$$

with η, N independent, $\eta = W^{1/2}$ and $N \sim \mathscr{N}(0,1)$.
To study the limit distribution of $\hat{m}_n$, we write

$$\hat{m}_n - m(\theta_0) = \frac{\sum_{i=1}^n (Z_i - m(\theta_0)Z_{i-1})}{\sum_{i=1}^n Z_{i-1}} = \sigma^2(\theta_0)\frac{M_n}{\langle M_n\rangle}.$$

This yields that

$$m(\theta_0)^{n/2}(\hat{m}_n - m(\theta_0)) = \sigma^2(\theta_0)\frac{m(\theta_0)^{n/2}}{s_n}\frac{\frac{M_n}{s_n}}{\frac{\langle M_n\rangle}{s_n^2}}.$$

Using (2.3.11) and (2.3.13) achieves the proof of (ii). □

Let us stress that here, contrary to the previous models, the Fisher information, $E_\theta\langle M\rangle_n = \sigma^2(\theta)\frac{m(\theta)^n - 1}{m(\theta) - 1}$ converges to infinity at a much faster rate than "usually" for $m(\theta) > 1$. Indeed, the information contained in $(Z_1, \ldots, Z_n)$ is of the same order as the information in the last observation Z_n. In that respect, the model is explosive in terms of growth of information.

Note that this result could be obtained using the MLE Heuristics presented in the Appendix, substituting $\sqrt{n}$ by s_n and using that
$\nabla_\theta^2 \ell_n(\theta) = -\nabla_\theta^2 \phi(\theta)\sum_{i=1}^n Z_{i-1} = -\sigma^2(\theta)\sum_{i=1}^n Z_{i-1} = -\langle M(\theta)\rangle_n$.

Now we have estimated $m(\theta)$ instead of θ. To estimate θ, we just have to consider the application $\theta \to m(\theta)$. Assuming that there exists ϕ differentiable such that $\phi(y) = \theta = m^{-1}(y)$, an application of Theorem A.1.1 yields the result for θ.

2.3.3 Parametric Inference for General Galton–Watson Processes

We assume now that the offspring distribution $G(\cdot)$ has mean m and finite variance σ^2 and consider the Galton–Watson process with initial condition $Z_0 = 1$ and offspring distribution G. We assume

(B1) The offspring law G satisfies $m > 1$ and $\sigma^2 < \infty$.
(B2) The offspring law G has a finite moment of order 4: $E(Y^4) = \mu_4 < \infty$ where $Y \sim G$.

On the basis on the successive population sizes $(Z_1, \ldots, Z_n)$, we are concerned with the estimation of $\theta = (m, \sigma^2)$. Denote by $\mathbb{P}_\theta$ the distribution on $(\mathbb{N}^{\mathbb{N}}, \mathscr{B}(N^{\mathbb{N}}))$ of (Z_n). Under (B1), the branching process is supercritical ($m > 1$) and the non-extinction set E^c has a positive probability. Clearly, studying estimators based on

(2.3.4) is intractable. Therefore, we had rather study estimators based on Conditional Least Square methods. The conditional mean and variance of Z_n with respect to $\mathscr{F}_{n-1}$ write

$$\mathbb{E}_\theta(Z_n|\mathscr{F}_{n-1}) = mZ_{n-1}; \quad Var_\theta(Z_n|\mathscr{F}_{n-1}) = \sigma^2 Z_{n-1}. \tag{2.3.14}$$

On the non-extinction set E^c, let us consider the contrast function (which is a weighted Conditional Least Square method):

$$U_n(\theta) = \sum_{i=1}^{n} \frac{1}{Z_{i-1}} (Z_i - mZ_{i-1})^2. \tag{2.3.15}$$

Note that $U_n(\theta)$ only depends on m and therefore σ^2 cannot be estimated using U_n. Define $\tilde{m}_n$ as a solution of

$$U_n(\tilde{m}_n) = min_{\theta\in\Theta} U_n(\theta).$$

Hence it satisfies $\nabla_\theta U_n(\tilde{m}_n) = 0$, which yields

$$\tilde{m}_n = \frac{\sum_{i=1}^n Z_i}{\sum_{i=1}^n Z_{i-1}}. \tag{2.3.16}$$

The simplest approach for estimating σ^2 is to use the residual variance:

$$\tilde{\sigma}_n^2 = \frac{1}{n} \sum_{i=1}^{n} \frac{1}{Z_{i-1}} (Z_i - \tilde{m}_n Z_{i-1})^2. \tag{2.3.17}$$

Then the following holds.

Theorem 2.3.5. *Assume (B1)–(B2). Then, on the non-extinction set E^c, the estimators $(\tilde{m}_n, \tilde{\sigma}_n^2)$ defined in* (2.3.16)–(2.3.17) *satisfy, as $n \to \infty$, under $\mathbb{P}_\theta$,*

(i) *$\tilde{m}_n \to m$ almost surely.*
(ii) *$m^{n/2}(\tilde{m}_n - m) \to_{\mathscr{L}} \sqrt{(m-1)\sigma^2}\, \eta^{-1} N$, where η, N are independent r.v.s, $N \sim \mathscr{N}(0,1)$, η is the positive variable defined by $\eta^2 = W$.*
(iii) *$\tilde{\sigma}_n^2 \to \sigma^2$ in probability under $\mathbb{P}_\theta$.*
(iv) *$\sqrt{n}(\tilde{\sigma}_n^2 - \sigma^2) \to_{\mathscr{L}} \mathscr{N}(0, 2\sigma^4)$.*

Proof. The study of the asymptotic properties of $\tilde{m}_n$ is similar to the previous section, since $\tilde{m}_n$ has the same expression with respect to the observations that $\hat{m}_n(\theta)$. The proofs of (iii) and (iv) are derived from [59], Chapter 3. Let us prove (iii). We have $\tilde{\sigma}_n^2 - \sigma^2 = \frac{1}{n}(A_n^1 + A_n^2 + A_n^3)$ with

$$A_n^2 = (m - \tilde{m}_n)^2 (\sum_{i=1}^{n} Z_{i-1}),$$

$$A_n^3 = 2(m - \tilde{m}_n) \sum_{i=1}^{n} (Z_i - mZ_{i-1}) \text{ and}$$

$$A_n^1 = \sum_{i=1}^{n} X_i \quad \text{with } X_i = \frac{1}{Z_{i-1}}(Z_i - mZ_{i-1})^2 - \sigma^2. \tag{2.3.18}$$

Let us study the first term A_n^1. It is a centered $\mathscr{F}_n$-martingale under $\mathbb{P}_\theta$. The computation of $\mathbb{E}_\theta(X_i^2|\mathscr{F}_{i-1})$ relies on the property that, for i.i.d. random variables Y_i with $\mathbb{E}(Y_i) = m$, $\mathrm{Var}Y_i = \sigma^2$ and finite fourth moment $\mathbb{E}(Y^4) = \mu_4$, $\bar{Y} = \frac{1}{n}\sum_{i=1}^n Y_i$ satisfies

$$\mathbb{E}(\bar{Y} - m)^4 = \frac{3\sigma^4}{n^2} + \frac{1}{n^3}(\mu_4 - 3\sigma^4).$$

Hence on the non-extinction set E^c,

$$\langle A^1 \rangle_n = \sum_{i=1}^{n}(2\sigma^4 + \frac{1}{Z_{i-1}}(\mu_4 - 3\sigma^4)). \tag{2.3.19}$$

Hence $\mathrm{Var}(A_1^n) \le 2n(\sigma^4 + \mu^4)$. Therefore, applying a strong law of large numbers for martingales ([63], Theorem 2.18) yields $\frac{1}{n}A_n^1 \to 0$ $\mathbb{P}_\theta$-a.s.
The second term is $A_n^2 = \left(m^n(\tilde{m}_n - m)^2\right)\left(\frac{1}{m^n}\sum_{i=1}^n Z_{i-1}\right)$. By (ii) and Corollary 2.3.2, we get that these two terms converge in distribution so that A_n^2 is bounded in probability.
Noting that $M_n = \sum_{i=1}^n (Z_{i-1} - mZ_{i-1})$ is the martingale studied in the previous section yields that $A_n^3 = [m^{n/2}(m - \tilde{m}_n)][\frac{1}{m^{n/2}}M_n]$. By (ii) $[m^{n/2}(m - \tilde{m}_n)]$ converges in distribution. The CLT for (M_n) stated in (2.3.13) yields that $m^{n/2}M_n$ converges in distribution. Hence, A_n^3 is also bounded in probability. Joining these results yields that $\frac{1}{n}(A_n^1 + A_n^2 + A_n^3) \to 0$, which achieves the proof of (iii).

Let us prove (iv). The previous computations yield that $n^{-1/2}A_n^2$ and $n^{-1/2}A_n^3$ both converge to 0. The martingale (A_n^1) is centered square integrable and $s_n^2 = E_\theta \langle M \rangle_n$ satisfies $\frac{1}{n}s_n^2 \to 2\sigma^4$. Condition (H1') is satisfied assuming the existence of a moment of order $4 + \delta$ with $\delta > 0$ for the offspring law G. Therefore, the CLT for martingales (see Theorem A.4.1) yields that $\frac{1}{n}\langle M \rangle_n \to 2\sigma^4$ a.s. Joining these results achieves the proof of (iv). □

With similar arguments, one can prove the asymptotic independence of $(\tilde{m}_n, \tilde{\sigma}_n^2)$.

The extinction probability is an important parameter in many applications. In the early stages of an epidemic, the extinction probability corresponds to the probability of a minor outbreak. However, unless the extinction probability q is a function of m and σ^2 only, it cannot be consistently estimated observing the generation sizes. A parametric setting $(G_\theta, \theta \in \Theta)$ is required for the offspring law. Let $g(\theta, s)$ denote the generating function of G_θ and define

$$\tilde{q}_n = \inf\{s, g(s, \tilde{\theta}_n) = s\}.$$

Then, according to [59], under additional regularity assumptions, $\tilde{q}_n$ is consistent if $\tilde{\theta}_n$ is consistent, and converges at the same rate $m(\theta_0)^{n/2}$ as $\tilde{\theta}_n$.

2.3.4 Examples

Example 1. Let us consider the supercritical branching process with offspring law $\mathscr{P}oi(\lambda)$ with $\lambda > 1$ and initial condition $Z_0 = 1$. Theorem 2.3.4 applies here and yields that, under $\mathbb{P}_{\lambda_0}$, on the non-extinction set E^c,

$$\hat{\lambda}_n = \frac{\sum_{i=1}^n Z_i}{\sum_{i=1}^n Z_{i-1}} \to \lambda_0 \quad \text{a.s.},$$

$$\lambda_0^{n/2}(\hat{\lambda}_n - \lambda_0) \to \sqrt{(\lambda_0 - 1)\lambda_0}\; \eta^{-1} N, \text{ with } \eta, N \text{ independent } N \sim \mathscr{N}(0,1), \eta^2 = W,$$

where $W > 0$ on E^c, $EW = 1, \mathrm{Var}W = \frac{1}{\lambda_0 - 1}$.

Example 2. Consider now the supercritical branching process with offspring law the Geometric distribution G on N^* with parameter p ($G(k) = p(1-p)^{k-1}, k \geq 1$). First, note that $\mathbb{P}_p(E) = 0$ and if $Y \sim G$, $\mathbb{E}(Y) = 1/p$ and $\mathrm{Var}Y = \frac{1-p}{p^2}$. Assume that $0 < p < 1$ and that $Z_0 = 1$. Theorem 2.3.4 yields that, under $\mathbb{P}_{p_0}$,

$$\frac{1}{\hat{p}_n} = \frac{\sum_{i=1}^n Z_i}{\sum_{i=1}^n Z_{i-1}} \to \frac{1}{p_0} \quad \text{a. s.},$$

$$p_0{}^{-n/2}\left(\frac{1}{\hat{p}_n} - \frac{1}{p_0}\right) \to \sqrt{\frac{(1-p_0)^2}{p_0^3}}\; \eta^{-1} N \text{ with } \eta^2 = W, \mathbb{E}(W) = 1, \mathrm{Var}W = 1.$$

To estimate p, an application of Theorem A.1.1 with $\phi(y) = 1/y$ yields that, under $\mathbb{P}_{\theta_0}$,

$$\hat{p}_n = \frac{\sum_{i=1}^n Z_{i-1}}{\sum_{i=1}^n Z_i} \to p_0, \quad p_0^{-n/2}(\hat{p}_n - p_0) \to \sqrt{p_0}(1 - p_0)\; \eta^{-1} W.$$

Example 3. Consider the general fractional linear branching process with offspring law G: $G(0) = a, G(k) = (1-a)p(1-p)^{k-1}, k \geq 1$. Then the mean offspring is $m = \frac{1-a}{p}$ and $\sigma^2 = \frac{(1-a)}{p^2}(1 - p + a)$. Assume that $m > 1$, the extinction set has probability $q = \frac{a}{1-p}$. On E^c, m is estimated at rate $m^{n/2}$ while σ^2 is estimated at rate $\sqrt{n}$. Therefore, $\hat{q}_n$, which depends on $\hat{m}_n$ and $\hat{\sigma}_n^2$, is estimated at rate $\sqrt{n}$.

2.3.5 Variants of Branching Processes

A large class of branching processes are used for modeling Epidemic dynamics. It encompasses subcritical or critical branching processes (a), branching processes with immigration (b), multitype branching processes with immigration, Crump–Mode–Jagers branching process, which are continuous time branching processes which are no longer Markov if the time between successive generations is not exponential (c).

Case (a) can be studied either assuming that the initial population size $\{Z_0 \to \infty\}$ or conditionally on late extinction (leading to quasi-stationary distributions). Cases (b) and (c) can be studied along similar lines than the ones in the previous section. Stating all these results is beyond the scope of these notes. We had rather choose to present accurately the simplest case, which already contains many problems arising in these other models.

Chapter 3
Inference Based on the Diffusion Approximation of Epidemic Models

3.1 Introduction

The contents of this chapter is mainly based on the three papers [60], [61] and [62].

In the first part of these notes, several mathematical models have been proposed to describe Epidemic dynamics in a closed homogeneous community. The properties of the stochastic $SEIR$ model have been studied in the first part of these notes. Several mathematical formalisms were proposed to describe transitions of individuals between states: ODE/PDE ([35]), difference equations and continuous or discrete-time stochastic processes (see Part I of these notes and also [32], [35]), such as point processes, Pure jump processes, renewal processes, branching processes, diffusion processes. When data are available, key parameters can be estimated using these models through likelihood-based or M-estimation methods sometimes coupled to Bayesian methods (see e.g. [35]). However, these data are most often partially observed (e.g. infection and recovery dates are not observed for all individuals during the outbreak, not all the infectious individuals are reported) and also temporally and/or spatially aggregated. In this case, estimation via likelihood-based approaches is rarely straightforward, regardless to the mathematical formalism.

For instance, the natural modeling of epidemics by pure jump processes presents systematically the drawback that inference for such models requires that all the jumps are observed. Since these data are rarely available in practice, statistical methods rely on data augmentation in order to complete the data and add in the analysis all the missing jumps. For moderate to large populations, the complexity increases rapidly, becoming the source of additional problems. Various approaches were developed during the last years to deal with partially observed epidemics. Data augmentation and likelihood-free methods such as the Approximate Bayesian Computation (ABC) opened some of the most promising pathways for improvement (see e.g.[18], [101]). Nevertheless, these methods do not completely circumvent the issues related to incomplete data. As stated also in [27], [19], there are some limitations in practice, due to the size of missing data and to the various tuning parameters to be adjusted (see also [2], [105]). Moreover, identifiability issues are rarely

T. Britton, E. Pardoux (eds.), *Stochastic Epidemic Models with Inference*,
Lecture Notes in Mathematics 2255, https://doi.org/10.1007/978-3-030-30900-8_14

addressed.

In this context, it appears that diffusion processes, satisfactorily approximating epidemic dynamics (see e.g. [45], [109]), can be profitably used for inference of model parameters from epidemiological data. In Part I, Sections 2.2 and 2.3, the Markov jump process $(\mathscr{Z}^N(t))$ in a closed population of size N, when normalized by N, $(Z^N(t) = N^{-1}\mathscr{Z}^N(t))$ satisfies an ODE as the population size N goes to infinity. In Section 2.4, it is proved the Wasserstein L_1-distance between $(Z^N(t))$ and a multidimensional diffusion process with diffusion coefficient proportional to $1/\sqrt{N}$ is of order $o(N^{-1/2})$ on a finite interval $[0,T]$. Hence, epidemic dynamics can be described using multidimensional diffusion processes $(X^N(t))_{t\geq 0}$ with a small diffusion coefficient proportional to $1/\sqrt{N}$. Since epidemics are usually observed over limited time periods, we consider in what follows the parametric inference based on observations of the epidemic dynamics on a fixed interval $[0,T]$. Let us stress that this approach assumes a major outbreak in a large community.

Historically, statistics for diffusions were developed for continuously observed processes which renders possible getting an explicit formulation of the likelihood ([91], [96]). In this context, two asymptotics exist for estimating parameters in the drift coefficient of a diffusion continuously observed on a time interval $[0,T]$: $T \to \infty$ for recurrent diffusions and $\{T$ fixed and the diffusion coefficient tends to $0\}$. As mentioned above, in practice, epidemic data are not continuous, but partial, with various mechanisms underlying the missingness and leading to intractable likelihoods: trajectories can be discretely observed with a sampling interval (low frequency or high frequency observations, i.e. $n \to \infty$); discrete observations can correspond to integrated processes; some coordinates can be unobserved. Since the 1990s, statistical methods associated to the first two types of data have been developed (e.g. [48], [49], [54]), [86]). Recently proposed approaches for multidimensional diffusions are based on the filtering theory ([41], [50]). Concerning diffusions with small diffusion coefficient from discrete observations, it was first studied in [46], [56], [118], and more devoted to epidemic dynamics in [60], [61]. Statistical inference for diffusion processes entails some special features, that we recall for sake of clarity in A.3. It reveals that, in the context of discrete observations, it is important to distinguish parameters in the drift and parameters in the diffusion coefficients because they are not estimated at the same rate. We detail and extend here some recent work ([60], [61], [62]) where we focus on the parametric inference in the drift coefficient $b(\alpha, X^\varepsilon(t))$ and in the diffusion coefficient $\varepsilon\sigma(\beta, X^\varepsilon(t))$ of a multidimensional diffusion model $(X^\varepsilon(t))_{t\geq 0}$ with small diffusion coefficient, when it is observed at discrete times on a fixed time interval in the asymptotics $\varepsilon \to 0$.

Section 3.2 presents the diffusion approximation of the Markov jump process describing the epidemic dynamics starting from its Q- matrix and detail these approximations for several epidemic models studied in Part I of these notes, where another method is used to get these approximations (see Part I, Sections 2.3 and 2.4). We then consider the parametric inference when the epidemic dynamics is observed at discrete times on a finite interval, which corresponds to one outbreak of the epidemics. The inference is studied for small sampling intervals (Section 3.4) and fixed sampling intervals (Section 3.5). On simulated data sets of two epidemic models, the *SIR* and the *SIRS* with seasonal forcing (see [83, Chapter 5]), we study the properties of our estimators based on discrete observations of these two jump Markov processes, and compare our results to the optimal inference for these jump processes, which is obtained when all the jumps (i.e. observations of all the times of infection and recovery within the population) are observed (Section 3.6).

It often occurs that in practice some components of the epidemics are not observed. In the *SIR* epidemics, the successive numbers of Susceptible for instance might be unobserved and the data consist of the successive increments of the number of Infected on each time interval. We study in Section 3.7 the inference when one coordinate of the process is observed at discrete times. We detail the results on two examples, the 2-dimensional Ornstein–Uhlenbeck diffusion process and the diffusion approximation of the *SIR*-model when only the successive numbers of Infected are available (Section 3.7.2.1). Finally, Section 3.7.2.2 is devoted to the estimation based on the real data set on Influenza epidemics, which is described by an *SIRS* epidemic model.

3.2 Diffusion Approximation of Jump Processes Modeling Epidemics

This section starts from the definition of the stochastic epidemic model by a Pure jump Markov process $(\mathscr{Z}^N(t))$ on $\mathbb{Z}^d$ specified by its Q - matrix. We detail how to get the diffusion approximation of $(\mathscr{Z}^N(t))$ from this description, which is another way for getting the diffusion process obtained in Part I, Section 2.4 of these notes. Using limit theorems for stochastic processes, we characterize the limiting Gaussian process. Then, based on the theory of small perturbations of dynamical systems ([44]), we link the normalized process to a diffusion process with small diffusion coefficient. These approximations are then applied to *SIR*, *SEIR*, and *SIRS* models for epidemic dynamics.

3.2.1 Approximation Scheme Starting from the Jump Process Q-matrix

Let $(\mathscr{Z}^N(t))$ a multidimensional Markov jump process with state space $E \subset \mathbb{Z}^p$ which describes the epidemic dynamics in a closed population of size N, the integer "p" corresponding to the number of health states in the infection dynamics model.

This process is described by an initial distribution on E and a collection of non-negative functions $(\beta_j(t,\cdot) : E \to \mathbb{R}^+)$ indexed by $j \in \mathbb{Z}^p$, $j \neq (0,\dots,0)$, that satisfy,

$$\forall i \in E, 0 < \sum_{j \in \mathbb{Z}^p} \beta_j(t,i) = \beta(t,i) < \infty. \qquad (3.2.1)$$

These functions are the transition rates of the process $(\mathscr{Z}^N(t))$ with $Q(t)$-matrix having as elements

$$q_{i,i+j}(t) = \beta_j(t,i) \text{ if } j \neq 0, \text{ and } q_{i,i}(t) = -\beta(t,i) \text{ for } i, i+j \in E. \qquad (3.2.2)$$

Another useful description of $(\mathscr{Z}^N(t))$ is based on the joint distribution of its jump chain and holding times. The process stays in each state $i \in E$ during an exponential time $\mathscr{E}(\beta(t,i))$, and then jumps to the state $i+j$ according to a Markov chain (X_n) with transition probabilities $\mathbb{P}(X_{n+1} = i+j \mid X_n = i) = \beta_j(t,i)/\beta(t,i)$.

We consider the class of density dependent Markov jump processes $(\mathscr{Z}^N(t))$ which possess a limit behaviour when normalized by the population size N. Let us define the two sets

$$E = \{0,\dots,N\}^p \quad E^- = \{-N,\dots,N\}^p. \qquad (3.2.3)$$

The state space of $(\mathscr{Z}^N(t))$ is E and its jumps belong to E^-.
From the original jump process $(\mathscr{Z}^N(t))$ on $E = \{0,\dots,N\}^p$, let

$$Z^N(t) = \frac{\mathscr{Z}^N(t)}{N} \text{ with state space } E_N = \{N^{-1}i, i \in E\}. \qquad (3.2.4)$$

Its jumps are now $y = j/N$ and transition rates from $z \in E_N$ to $z + j/N$ at time t defined using (3.2.2),

$$q^N_{z,z+y}(t) = \beta_{Ny}(t,Nz). \qquad (3.2.5)$$

Denote for $x = (x_1,\dots,x_p) \in \mathbb{R}^d$, $[x] = ([x_1],\dots,[x_p]) \in \mathbb{Z}^p$, where $[x_i]$ is the integer part of x_i.

We assume in the sequel that $(\mathscr{Z}^N(t))$ is density dependent, i.e. there exist a collection of functions $\beta_j : \mathbb{R}^+ \times [0,1]^p \to \mathbb{R}^+$ such that,

(H1) $\forall j$, $\forall z \in [0,1]^p$ $\frac{1}{N}\beta_j(t,[Nz]) \to \beta_j(t,z)$ as $N \to \infty$ locally uniformly in t.
(H2) $\forall j \in E^-$, $\beta_j(t,z) \in C^2(\mathbb{R}^+,[0,1]^p)$.

Then, define the two functions $b^N(t,z)$ and $b(t,z) : \mathbb{R}^+ \times [0,1]^p \to \mathbb{R}^p$ and the two $p \times p$ positive symmetric matrices Σ^N and Σ (with the notation $M^\star$ for the transposition of a matrix or of a column vector j in E),

$$b^N(t,z) = \frac{1}{N}\sum_{j \in E^-}\beta_j(t,[Nz])j; \quad b(t,z) = \sum_{j \in E^-}\beta_j(t,z)j; \qquad (3.2.6)$$

$$\Sigma^N(t,z) = \frac{1}{N}\sum_{j \in E^-}\beta_j(t,[Nz])jj^\star; \quad \Sigma(t,z) = \sum_{j \in E^-}\beta_j(t,z)jj^\star. \qquad (3.2.7)$$

Under (H1) the functions $b(t,z)$ and $\Sigma(t,z)$ are well defined and $b(t,z)$ is Lipschitz under (H2). Therefore, there exists a unique smooth solution $z(t)$ to the ODE

$$\frac{dz}{dt} = b(t,z(t))dt ; \quad z(0) = x. \qquad (3.2.8)$$

Let $\nabla_z b(t,z)$ denote the gradient of $b(t,z)$

$$\nabla_z b(t,z) = \big(\frac{\partial b_i}{\partial z_j}(t,z)\big)_{1\le i,j\le p}\,. \tag{3.2.9}$$

The resolvent matrix $\Phi(t,u)$ associated with (3.2.8) is defined as the solution

$$\frac{d\Phi}{dt}(t,s) = \nabla_z b(t,z(t))\Phi(t,s); \quad \Phi(s,s) = I_p. \tag{3.2.10}$$

Under (H1), (H2) the following holds: if $Z^N(0) \to x$ as $N \to \infty$, then, locally uniformly in t,

$$\forall t \ge 0, \lim_{N\to\infty} \parallel Z^N(t) - z(t) \parallel = 0 \text{ a.s.} \tag{3.2.11}$$

where $z(t)$ is solution of (3.2.8).
Let $(D,\mathscr{D})$ denote the space of "cadlag" functions $\{f : \mathbb{R}^+ \to \mathbb{R}^p\}$ endowed with the Skorokhod topology. Then,

$$\sqrt{N}(Z^N(t) - z(t))_{t\ge 0} \to (G(t))_{t\ge 0} \text{ in distribution in } (D,\mathscr{D}), \tag{3.2.12}$$

where $(G(t))$ is a centered p-dimensional Gaussian process with covariance matrix

$$\mathrm{Cov}(G(t),G(r)) = \int_0^{t\wedge r} \Phi(t,u)\Sigma(u,z(u))\,\Phi^\star(r,u)du. \tag{3.2.13}$$

The proofs of these results are given under a general form in Part I, Sections 2.2 and 2.3 of these notes, and based on this presentation in [60], [61].

Heuristically, there is an approach which yields the diffusion approximation of $(Z^N(t))$; it rests on an expansion of the generator $\mathscr{A}_N$ of $(Z^N(t))$ (3.2.4). For $f \in C^2(\mathbb{R}^+ \times \mathbb{R}^p, \mathbb{R})$, it reads as

$$\mathscr{A}_N f(t,z) = \sum_{j\in E^-} \beta_j(t,Nz)(f(t,z+\frac{j}{N}) - f(t,z)).$$

A Taylor expansion of $\mathscr{A}_N f(t,z)$ yields, using (H1), (H2) and (3.2.6), for $j = (j_1,\ldots,j_p)^* \in E^-$,

$$\begin{aligned}\mathscr{A}_N f(t,z) &= \sum_{j\in E^-} N\beta_j(t,z)(f(t,z+\frac{j}{N}) - f(t,z)) + o(1/N)\\ &= (\nabla_z f(t,z))^\star\, b(t,z) + \frac{1}{2N}\left(\sum_{j\in E^-} \beta_j(t,z) \sum_{k,l=1}^{d} j_k\, j_l\, \nabla^2_{z_k z_l} f(t,z)\right)\\ &\qquad + o(1/N)\\ &= (\nabla_z f(t,z))^\star\, b(t,z) + \frac{1}{2N}\sum_{k,l=1}^{d} \Sigma_{kl}(t,z)\,\nabla^2_{z_k z_l} f(t,z) + o(1/N),\end{aligned}$$

where the last equality is obtained using (3.2.7). The first two terms of the last expression correspond to the generator of a diffusion process on $\mathbb{R}^p$ with drift coefficient $b(t,\cdot)$ and diffusion matrix $\frac{1}{N}\Sigma(t,\cdot)$,

$$dX^N(t) = b(t,X^N(t))dt + \frac{1}{\sqrt{N}}\sigma(t,X^N(t))dB(t)\ ;\ X^N(0) = x, \tag{3.2.14}$$

where $(B(t)_{t\geq 0})$ is a Brownian motion on $\mathbb{R}^p$ defined on a probability space $(\Omega,(\mathscr{F}_t)_{t\geq 0},\mathbb{P})$ independent of $X^N(0)$, and $\sigma(t,\cdot)$ is a square root of $\Sigma(t,\cdot)$: $\sigma(t,z)\,\sigma(t,z)^\star = \Sigma(t,z)$.

These approaches can be connected together a posteriori using the theory of random perturbations of dynamical systems ([7], [44]) and the following theorem.

Theorem 3.2.1. *Setting $\varepsilon = 1/\sqrt{N}$, the paths of $X^N(\cdot)$ satisfy, as $\varepsilon \to 0$,*

$$X^N(t) = X^\varepsilon(t) = z(t) + \varepsilon g(t) + \varepsilon^2 R^\varepsilon(t),\ \textit{with}\ \sup_{t\leq T} \parallel \varepsilon R^\varepsilon(t) \parallel \to 0\ \textit{in probability}, \tag{3.2.15}$$

where $z(t)$ is the solution of (3.2.8)*, $B(t)$ is a p-dimensional Brownian motion and $(g(t))$ is the process satisfying the SDE*

$$dg(t) = \nabla_z b(t,z(t))g(t)dt + \sigma(t,z(t))dB(t),\ \ g(0) = 0.$$

This stochastic differential equation can be solved explicitly and we get, using (3.2.10), that

$$g(t) = \int_0^t \Phi(t,s)\sigma(s,z(s))dB(s). \tag{3.2.16}$$

Hence, $(g(t))$ is a centered Gaussian process having the same covariance matrix (3.2.13) as the process $(G(t))$ defined in (3.2.12). Therefore, for $\varepsilon = 1/\sqrt{N}$, $\sqrt{N}(Z_t^N - z(t))_{t\geq 0}$ and $\varepsilon^{-1}(Z^\varepsilon(t) - z(t))_{t\geq 0}$ converge to a Gaussian process having the same distribution.

It is moreover proved in Part I, Section 2.4 of these notes, that the Wasserstein L^1 distance between $(Z^N(t))$ and $(X^N(t))$ converges to 0.

3.2.2 Diffusion Approximation of Some Epidemic Models

3.2.2.1 The Diffusion Approximation Applied to the SIR Epidemic Model

We apply first the generic method leading successively to $b(\cdot)$, $\Sigma(\cdot)$ and (X^N) described in 3.2.1 to the *SIR* model introduced iin Part I, Chapter 1 of these notes through the 2-dimensional continuous-time Markov jump process $\mathscr{Z}^N(t) = (S(t),I(t))$ to build the associated *SIR* diffusion process. Along to its initial state $\mathscr{Z}^N(0) = (S(0),I(0))$, the Markov jump process is characterized by two transitions, $(S,I) \xrightarrow{\frac{\lambda}{N}SI} (S-1,I+1)$ and $(S,I) \xrightarrow{\gamma I} (S,I-1)$. Parameters λ and $\gamma = 1/d$ represent the transmission rate and the recovery rate (or the inverse of the mean infection duration d), respectively. The rate $\lambda SI/N$ translates two main assumptions: the population mix homogeneously (same λ for each pair between one S and one I) and the transmission is proportional to the fraction of infectious individuals in the population, I/N (frequency-dependent formulation of the transmission term).

The diffusion approximation of the process$(\mathscr{Z}^N(t))$ describing the epidemic dynamics can be summarized by three steps. The original *SIR* jump process in a closed population has state space $\{0,\dots,N\}^2$, the jumps j are $(-1,1)$ and $(0,-1)$ with transition rates,

$$q_{(S,I),(S-1,I+1)} = \lambda S\,\frac{I}{N} = \beta_{(-1,1)}(S,I); \quad q_{(S,I),(S,I-1)} = \gamma I = \beta_{(0,-1)}(S,I).$$

Normalizing $(\mathscr{Z}^N(t))$ by the population size N, we obtain, setting $z=(s,i)\in[0,1]^2$, as $N\to\infty$,

$$\frac{1}{N}\beta_{(-1,1)}([Nz]) \to \beta_{(-1,1)}(s,i) = \lambda si; \quad \frac{1}{N}\beta_{(0,-1)}([Nz]) \to \beta_{(0,-1)}(s,i) = \gamma i.$$

These two limiting functions clearly satisfy (H1)–(H2). Finally, the two functions given in (3.2.6), (3.2.7) are well defined and now depend on (λ,γ).
Set $\theta=(\lambda,\gamma)$ and denote by $b(\theta,z)$ and $\Sigma(\theta,z)$ the associated functions. We get

$$b(\theta,(s,i)) = \begin{pmatrix} -\lambda si \\ \lambda si-\gamma i \end{pmatrix}; \quad \Sigma(\theta,(s,i)) = \begin{pmatrix} \lambda si & -\lambda si \\ -\lambda si & \lambda si+\gamma i \end{pmatrix}. \tag{3.2.17}$$

Assume that $\mathscr{Z}^N(0)$ satisfies $(N^{-1}S(0),N^{-1}I(0)) \to x=(s_0,i_0)$ with $s_0>0$, $i_0>0$, $s_0+i_0\le 1$ as $N\to\infty$. Then the associated ODE is, using (3.2.8),

$$\frac{ds}{dt} = -\lambda si\,; \quad \frac{di}{dt} = \lambda si-\gamma i\,; \quad (s(0),i(0)) = (s_0,i_0). \tag{3.2.18}$$

The diffusion approximation of the *SIR* epidemics obtained in (3.2.14) is the solution of the SDE

$$\begin{aligned} dS^N(t) &= -\lambda S^N(t)I^N(t)dt + \frac{1}{\sqrt{N}}\sqrt{\lambda S^N(t)I^N(t)}\,dB_1(t), \quad S^N(0)=s_0, \\ dI^N(t) &= (\lambda S^N(t)I^N(t)-\gamma I^N(t))dt - \frac{1}{\sqrt{N}}\left(\sqrt{\lambda S^N(t)I^N(t)}\,dB_1(t) - \sqrt{\gamma I^N(t)}\,dB_2(t)\right), \\ &\quad I^N(0)=i_0, \end{aligned}$$

where $(B(t))$ is standard two-dimensional Brownian motion and $\sigma(\theta,z)$ corresponds to the Choleski decomposition of $\Sigma(\theta,z)=\sigma(\theta,z)\sigma^\star(\theta,z)$,

$$\sigma(\theta,(s,i)) = \begin{pmatrix} \sqrt{\lambda si} & 0 \\ -\sqrt{\lambda si} & \sqrt{\gamma i} \end{pmatrix}.$$

In order to visualize the influence of the population size N on the sample paths of the normalized jump process $Z_N(t)=\mathscr{Z}^N(t)/N$, several trajectories have been simulated using an *SIR* model with parameters $(\lambda, \gamma) = (0.5, 1/3)$, so that $R_0 = \lambda/\gamma = 1.5$. Results are displayed in Figure 3.2.1. We observe that, as the population size increases, the stochasticity of sample paths decreases. However, it still keeps a non-negligible stochasticity for a large population size ($N = 10000$). Since the peak of $I^N(t)$ is quite small (about 0.08 here), this can be explained by a moderate size of the ratio "signal over noise" even for large N (here of order $0.08/0.01$).

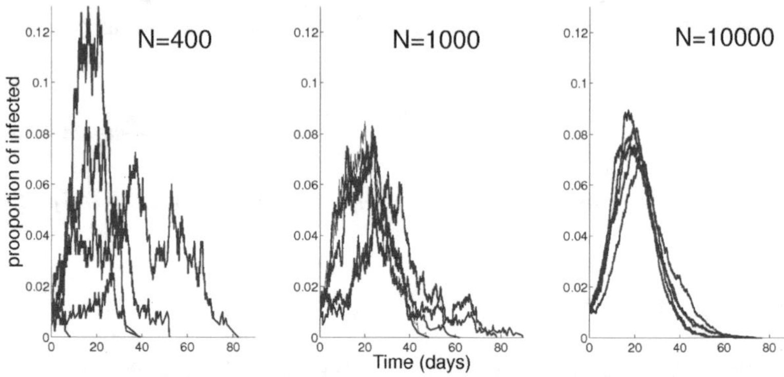

Fig. 3.2.1 Five simulated trajectories of the proportion of infectious individuals over time using the *SIR* Markov jump process for $(s_0, i_0) = (0.99, 0.01)$ $(\lambda, \gamma) = (0.5, 1/3)$ and for each $N = \{400, 1000, 10000\}$ (from left to right).

3.2.2.2 The Diffusion Approximation Applied to the *SIRS* Epidemic Model with Seasonal Forcing

Another important class of epidemics models is the *SIRS* model, which allows possible reinsertion of removed individuals into S class. The additional transition reads as $(S,I) \overset{\delta(N-S-I)}{\longrightarrow} (S+1,I)$, where δ is the average rate of immunity waning. To mimic recurrent epidemics, additional mechanisms need to be considered. Indeed, to avoid that successive epidemics cycles die out, one way is to introduce an external immigration flow. Hence, one possible model to describe recurrent epidemics is the *SIRS* model with seasonal transmission (at rate $\lambda(t)$), external immigration flow in the I class (at rate η) and, when the time-scale of study is large, demography (with birth and death rates equal to μ for a stable population of size N). Seasonality in transmission is captured using a time non-homogeneous transmission rate, expressed under a periodic form

$$\lambda(t) := \lambda_0(1 + \lambda_1 \sin(2\pi t/T_{per})) \tag{3.2.19}$$

where λ_0 is the baseline transition rate, λ_1 the intensity of the seasonal effect on transmission and T_{per} is introduced to model an annual or t seasonal trend (see [83], Chapter 5). Typically for modeling Influenza epidemics, we fixed it at $T = 365$.

Assuming again a constant population size, we obtain a new two-dimensional system with four transitions for the corresponding Markov jump process:

$$(S,I) \overset{\frac{\lambda(t)}{N}S(I+N\eta)}{\longrightarrow} (S-1,I+1)\ ; \quad (S,I) \overset{\mu S}{\longrightarrow} (S-1,I);$$
$$(S,I) \overset{(\gamma+\mu)I}{\longrightarrow} (S,I-1)\ ; \quad (S,I) \overset{\mu N+\delta(N-S-I)}{\longrightarrow} (S+1,I).$$

Figure 3.2.2 illustrates the dynamics of the *SIRS* model (in ODE formalism) which is forced using sinusoidal terms. In particular, given the parameter values we have chosen, we can notice two distinct regimes: one with annual cycles (top graph) and the other with biennial dynamics (middle graph). The qualitative changes in model dynamics are explored by modifying a control parameter or *bifurcation parameter* (here λ_1) and constructing a *bifurcation diagram.*

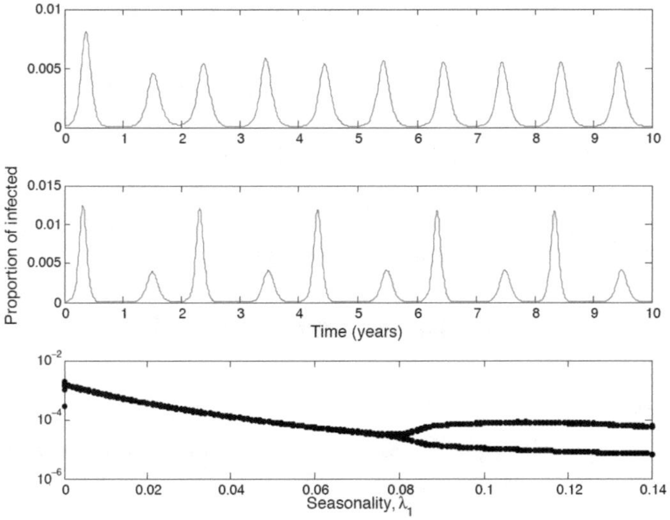

Fig. 3.2.2 Proportion of infected individuals, $I(t)$, over time (top and middle panels) simulated using the ODE variant of the *SIRS* model with $N = 10^7$, $T_{per} = 365$, $\mu = 1/(50\times T_{per})$, $\eta = 10^{-6}$, $(s_0,i_0) = (0.7,10^{-4})$ and $(\lambda_0,\gamma,\delta) = (0.5,1/3,1/(2\times 365))$. The top panel corresponds to $\lambda_1 = 0.05$, the middle panel to $\lambda_1 = 0.1$. The bottom panel represents the bifurcation diagram with respect to λ_1.

The diffusion approximation is built following the same generic scheme of Section 3.2.1 as for the *SIR* model in Section 3.2.2.1. The four jumps j corresponding to functions β_j are $j^* = (-1,1);(-1,0);(0,-1);(1,0)$ leading to

$$\beta_{(-1,1)}(t,S,I) = \frac{\lambda(t)}{N}S(I+N\eta), \quad \beta_{(0,-1)}(t,S,I) = (\gamma+\mu)S,$$
$$\beta(0,-1)(t,S,I) = (\gamma+\mu)S, \quad \beta_{(1,0)}(t,S,I) = \mu N+\delta(N-S-I)S.$$

The jump process is time-dependent and so we have to check (H1b)–(H2). Straightforward computations yield that they are satisfied since, for $(s,i) \in [0,1]^2$,

$$\beta_{(-1,1)}(t,(s,i)) = \lambda(t)s(i+\eta); \quad \beta_{(-1,0)}(t,(s,i)) = \mu s;$$
$$\beta_{(0,-1)}(t,(s,i)) = (\gamma+\mu)i; \qquad \beta_{(1,0)}(t,(s,i)) = \mu + \delta(1-s-i).$$

Finally, setting $\theta = (\lambda_0, \lambda_1, \gamma, \delta, \eta, \mu)$, the associated drift function $b(\theta,t,(s,i))$ and diffusion matrix $\Sigma(\theta,t,(s,i))$ are

$$b(\theta,t,(s,i)) = \begin{pmatrix} -\lambda(t)s(i+\eta) + \delta(1-s-i) + \mu(1-s) \\ \lambda(t)s(i+\eta) - (\gamma+\mu)i \end{pmatrix}, \tag{3.2.20}$$

$$\Sigma(\theta,t,(s,i)) = \begin{pmatrix} \lambda(t)s(i+\eta) + \delta(1-s-i) + \mu(1+s) & -\lambda(t)s(i+\eta) \\ -\lambda(t)s(i+\eta) & \lambda(t)s(i+\eta) + (\gamma+\mu)i \end{pmatrix}. \tag{3.2.21}$$

Therefore, the associated ODE is, using (3.2.20),

$$\frac{ds}{dt} = -\lambda(t)s(i+\eta) + \delta(1-s-i) + \mu(1-s), \quad s(0) = s_0;$$
$$\frac{di}{dt} = \lambda(t)s(i+\eta) - (\gamma+\mu)i, \quad i(0) = i_0.$$

Choosing $\sigma(\theta,t,(s,i))$ such that $\sigma(\theta,t,(s,i))\sigma(\theta,t,(s,i))^\star = \Sigma(\theta,t,(s,i))$, we obtain that the approximating diffusion $X_N(t)$ satisfies

$$dX^N(t) = b(\theta,t,(S_N,I_N))dt + \frac{1}{\sqrt{N}}\sigma(\theta,t(S^N,I^N)); \; X^N(0) = x. \tag{3.2.22}$$

3.2.2.3 A Minimal Model for Ebola Transmission with Temporal Transition Rate

According to [20], a basic model for Ebola dynamics consists in a *SEIR* model with temporal transmission rate. In a rough approximation, assuming homogeneous mixing in a size N community yields, setting $\mathscr{X}^N(t) = (S,E,I)$,

$$(S,E,I) \overset{\lambda(t)\frac{SI}{N}}{\longrightarrow} (S-1,E+1,I);$$
$$(S,E,I) \overset{\nu E}{\longrightarrow} (S,E-1,I+1);$$
$$(S,E,I) \overset{\gamma I}{\longrightarrow} (S,E,I-1).$$

The diffusion approximation has drift and diffusion matrix given by, for $z = (s,e,i)$,

$$b(\theta,t,z) = \begin{pmatrix} -\lambda(t)si \\ \lambda(t)si - \nu e \\ \nu e - \gamma i \end{pmatrix}; \quad \Sigma(\theta,t,z) = \begin{pmatrix} \lambda(t)si & -\lambda(t)si & 0 \\ -\lambda(t)si & \lambda(t)si + \nu e & -\nu e \\ 0 & -\nu e & \nu e + \gamma i \end{pmatrix}.$$

Two questions concerning the inference arise in this model: the non-parametric estimation of $\lambda(\cdot)$ and the presence of random effects since the dynamics are observed in different locations.

3.2.2.4 Two Variants of the *SEIRS* Model with Demography

In Part I, Chapter 2 of these notes, an example of *SEIRS* model with demography is proposed (see Example 2.2.2). Removed individuals loose their immunity at rate δ; there is an influx of susceptible at rate μN and individuals, whichever type, die at rate μ. Hence, 9 jumps are present in this model, for (s,e,i,r), which yields for $Z=(S,E,I)$,

$$(S,E,I) \xrightarrow{\lambda \frac{SI}{N}} (S-1,E+1,I), \quad (S,E,I) \xrightarrow{\nu E} (S,E-1,I+1),$$

$$(S,E,I) \xrightarrow{\mu N+\delta(N-S-E-I)} (S+1,E,I), \quad (S,E,I) \xrightarrow{\mu I+\gamma I} (S,E,I-1).$$

$$(S,E,I) \xrightarrow{\mu S} (S-1,E,I), \quad (S,E,I) \xrightarrow{\mu E} (S,E-1,I), \quad (S,E,I) \xrightarrow{\mu(N-S-E-I)} (S,E,I).$$

This yields, setting $z=(s,e,i)$ and $\theta=(\lambda,\nu,\gamma,\delta,\mu)$

$$b(\theta,z) = \begin{pmatrix} -\lambda si+\mu(1-s)+\delta(1-s-i-e) \\ \lambda si-(\mu+\nu)e \\ \nu e-(\gamma+\nu)i \end{pmatrix};$$

$$\Sigma(\theta,z) = \begin{pmatrix} \lambda si+\mu(1+s)+\delta(1-s-i-e) & -\lambda si & 0 \\ -\lambda si & \lambda si+(\mu+\nu)e & -\nu e \\ 0 & -\nu e & \nu e+(\gamma+\nu)i \end{pmatrix}.$$

3.3 Inference for Discrete Observations of Diffusions on [0,T]

Our concern here is parametric inference for these models. Statistical inference for discretely observed diffusion processes present some specific properties (see Section A.3 in the Appendix) that lead us to consider distinct parameters in the drift coefficient (here α) and in the diffusion coefficient (β). The state space of the diffusion is $\mathbb{R}^p$, and the parameter set Θ is a subset of $\mathbb{R}^a \times \mathbb{R}^b$, with $\alpha \in \mathbb{R}^a, \beta \in \mathbb{R}^b$. For instance, the *SIR* diffusion approximation corresponds to $p=2$ and $\alpha=\beta=(\lambda,\gamma)$.

In order to deal with general epidemics, we consider time-dependent diffusion processes on $\mathbb{R}^p$ with small diffusion coefficient $\varepsilon = 1/\sqrt{N}$ satisfying the stochastic differential equation (SDE):

$$dX(t) = b(\alpha,t,X(t))dt + \varepsilon\sigma(\beta,t,X(t))\,dB(t)\,; \quad X(0)=x, \tag{3.3.1}$$

where $(B(t)_{t\geq 0})$ is a p-dimensional Brownian motion defined on a probability space $(\Omega,(\mathscr{F}_t)_{t\geq 0},\mathbb{P})$, $b(\alpha,t,\cdot):\mathbb{R}^p \to \mathbb{R}^p$ and $\sigma(\beta,t,\cdot):\mathbb{R}^p \to \mathbb{R}^p \times \mathbb{R}^p$ and x is non-random fixed.

Since epidemic dynamics are usually observed at discrete times, our aim is to study the estimation of $\theta = (\alpha, \beta)$ based on the observations

$$(X(t_k), k = 1\ldots n) \text{ with } t_k = k\Delta;\ T = n\Delta \quad \text{(sampling interval } \Delta). \tag{3.3.2}$$

For observations on a fixed time interval, $[0,T]$, there are distinct asymptotic results according to Δ.

(1) High frequency sampling $\Delta = \Delta_n \to 0$: The number of observations $n = T/\Delta_n$ goes to ∞ while $T = n\Delta_n$ is fixed. There is a double asymptotic framework: $\varepsilon \to 0$ and $\Delta \to 0$ (or $n = T/\Delta \to \infty$) simultaneously. Let us stress that we shall use both notations for this second asymptotics $n \to \infty$ or $\Delta \to 0$. Although it might be confusing, it is sometimes better to state results according to the number of observations and sometimes according to the sampling interval Δ.

(2) Low frequency sampling Δ is fixed: It leads to a finite number of observations $n = T/\Delta$. Results are obtained in the asymptotic framework $\varepsilon \to 0$.

At first glance, the low frequency sampling seems a priori a suitable framework for epidemic data. However, both high and low frequency observations could be appropriate in practice because the choice of the statistical framework depends more on the relative magnitudes between T, Δ and the population size N $(= \varepsilon^{-2})$ than on their accurate values.

From a statistical point of view, the sequence $(X(t_k))$ is a time-dependent Markov chain and therefore the likelihood depends on its transition probabilities. However, the link between the parameters present in the SDE and the transition probabilities of $(X(t_k))$ is generally not explicit, which leads to intractable likelihoods. This is a well known problem for discrete observations of diffusion processes. Alternative approaches based on M-estimators or contrast functions (see e.g. [123] for independent random variables, [87] for stochastic processes) have to be investigated (see also the recap presented in Section A.3 in the Appendix of this part).

After the statement of some preliminary results, we present successively the statistical inference for high frequency sampling, where the asymptotics is $\varepsilon = 1/\sqrt{N} \to 0$, $\Delta_n = T/n \to 0$ (Section 3.4), and for the low frequency sampling, $\varepsilon = 1/\sqrt{N} \to 0$, Δ fixed (Section 3.5).

3.3.1 Assumptions, Notations and First Results

Let θ_0 be the true value of the parameter and Θ the parameter set. Denote by $\mathscr{M}_p(\mathbb{R})$ the set of $p \times p$ matrices. We first assume that $b(\alpha,t,z)$ and $\sigma(\beta,t,z)$ are measurable in (t,z), Lipschitz continuous with respect to the second variable and satisfy a linear growth condition: for all $t \geq 0, z, z' \in \mathbb{R}^p$, there exists a global constant K such that

(S1): $\forall\theta \in \Theta$, $\| b(\alpha,t,z) - b(\alpha,t,z') \| + \| \sigma(\beta,t,z) - \sigma(\beta,t,z') \| \leq K \| z - z' \|$.

(S2): $\forall(\alpha,\beta)\in\Theta, \| b(\alpha;t,z) \|^2 + \| \sigma(\beta;t,z) \|^2 \leq K(1+ \| z \|^2)$.
(S3): $\forall(\beta,t,z)$, $\Sigma(\beta;t,z) = \sigma(\beta;t,z)\sigma^\star(\beta;t,z)$ is non-singular.

Assumptions (S1)–(S3) are classical assumptions that ensure that, for all θ, (3.3.1) admits a unique strong solution (see e.g. [82, Chapter 5.2.B]).

Another set of assumptions is required for the inference:

(S4): $\Theta = K_a \times K_b$ is a compact set of $\mathbb{R}^{a+b}$, $\theta_0 \in \text{Int}(\Theta)$.
(S5): For all $t \geq 0$, $b(\alpha;t,z) \in C^3(K_a \times \mathbb{R}^+ \times \mathbb{R}^p, \mathbb{R}^p)$ and $\sigma(\beta;t,z) \in C^2(K_b \times \mathbb{R}^+ \times \mathcal{M}_p(\mathbb{R}))$.
(S6): $\alpha \neq \alpha' \Rightarrow b(t;\alpha,z(\alpha,t)) \not\equiv b(t;\alpha',z(\alpha',t))$.
(S7): $\beta \neq \beta' \Rightarrow \Sigma(t;\beta,z(\alpha_0,t)) \not\equiv \Sigma(t;\beta',z(\alpha_0,t))$.

Assumptions **(S4)–(S5)** are classical for the inference for diffusion processes. Usually, it is sufficient in **(S5)** to deal with C^2 functions. The additional differentiability condition comes from regularity conditions required on $\alpha \to \Phi(\alpha,t,s)$. Indeed, **(S5)** on $b(\alpha,t,z)$ ensures that the function $\Phi(\alpha,t,t_0)$ belongs to $C^2(K_a \times [0,T]^2, \mathcal{M}_p)$. Assumption **(S6)** is the usual identifiability assumption for a diffusion continuously observed on $[0,T]$ and **(S7)** is an identifiability assumption for parameters in the diffusion coefficient.

Since $(X(t))$ is a diffusion process on $(\Omega, (\mathscr{F}_t)_{t\geq 0}, \mathbb{P})$, the space of observations is $(C_T = C([0,T],\mathbb{R}^p), \mathscr{C}_T)$ where $\mathscr{C}_T$ is the Borel σ-algebra on $C([0,T],\mathbb{R}^p)$. Let $\mathbb{P}_\theta = \mathbb{P}_{\alpha,\beta}$ the probability distribution on $(C_T, \mathscr{C}_T)$ of $(X(t)), 0 \leq t \leq T)$ satisfying (3.3.1). Let $\mathscr{G}_k^n$ denote the σ-algebra $\sigma(X(s), s \leq \frac{kT}{n})$.

For $g(\theta,t,z) : \Theta \times [0,T] \times \mathbb{R}^p \to \mathbb{R}^p$, $\nabla_z g(\cdot)$ is the $\mathcal{M}_p$ matrix

$$\nabla_z g(\cdot) = (\frac{\partial g_i}{\partial z_j}(\theta,t,z))_{1\leq i,j\leq p} \quad \text{and} \quad \nabla_\theta g(\cdot) = (\frac{\partial g_i}{\partial \theta_j}(\theta,t,z)) \tag{3.3.3}$$

If $z = z(\theta,t)$, then

$$\nabla_\theta\left(g(\theta,t,z(\theta,t))\right) = \nabla_\theta g(\cdot) + \nabla_z g(\cdot)\nabla_\theta z(\cdot). \tag{3.3.4}$$

Quantities are indexed by θ (resp. α or β) when they depend on both α,β (resp.α or β). Introducing the dependence with respect to t,θ in (3.2.8), (3.2.10), (3.2.16) yields,

$$\begin{array}{l} \frac{\partial z}{\partial t}(\alpha,t) = b(\alpha,t,z(\alpha,t)); \quad z(\alpha,0) = x_0, \\ g(\alpha,\beta,t) = \int_0^t \Phi(\alpha,t,u)\sigma(\beta,u,z(\alpha,u))dB(u), \quad \text{with } \Phi(\alpha,\cdot) \text{ such that} \\ \frac{\partial \Phi}{\partial t}(\alpha,t,u) = \nabla_z b(\alpha,t,z(\alpha,t))\Phi(\alpha,t,u)\ ,\ \Phi(\alpha,u,u) = I_p. \end{array} \tag{3.3.5}$$

The expansion (3.2.15) holds for time-dependent diffusion processes.

Proposition 3.3.1. *Assume (S1)–(S5). Then, under* $\mathbb{P}_\theta$, $(X(t), 0 \le t \le T)$ *satisfies that, uniformly with respect to* θ,

$$\begin{array}{c} X(t) = z(\alpha,t) + \varepsilon g(\theta,t) + \varepsilon^2 R^\varepsilon(\theta,t), \quad \textit{with} \\ \lim_{\varepsilon\to 0, r\to\infty} \mathbb{P}_\theta(\sup_{t\le T} \parallel R^\varepsilon(\theta,t) \parallel > r) = 0 \\ \sup_{t\le T} \parallel R^\varepsilon(\theta,t) \parallel \ \textit{has uniformly bounded moments.} \end{array} \tag{3.3.6}$$

Proposition 3.3.2. *Under (S1)–(S5), the process* $(g(\theta,t))$ *satisfies using (3.3.5)*

$$\forall s < t, \quad g(\theta,t) = \Phi(\alpha,t,s)g(\theta,s) + \int_s^t \Phi(\alpha,t,u)\sigma(\beta,u,z(\alpha,u))dB(u),$$

where the two terms of the r.h.s. above are independent random variables.

Proposition 3.3.3. *Assume (S1)–(S2). If moreover* $b(\alpha,\cdot)$ *and* $\sigma(\beta,\cdot)$ *have uniformly bounded derivatives, there exist constants only depending on* T *and* θ *such that*

(i) $\forall t \in [0,T]$, $\mathbb{E}_\theta(\|R^\varepsilon(\theta,t)\|^2 < C_1$,
(ii) $\forall t \in [0,T]$, *as* $h \to 0$, $\mathbb{E}_\theta(\|R^\varepsilon(\theta,t+h) - R^\varepsilon(\theta,t)\|^2) < C_2 h$.

We refer to [7], [44], and [56] for the proofs of these propositions for θ fixed. Assumption (S4) allows us to extend these results to $\theta \in \Theta$.

3.3.2 Preliminary Results

Let us define using (3.3.5) the random variables,

$$B_k(\alpha,X) = X(t_k) - z(\alpha,t_k) - \Phi(\alpha,t_k,t_{k-1})\left[X(t_{k-1}) - z(\alpha,t_{k-1})\right]. \tag{3.3.7}$$

Then the following holds.

Lemma 3.3.4. *Assume (S1)–(S4). Then, under* $\mathbb{P}_\theta$, *as* $\varepsilon \to 0$,

$$B_k(\alpha,X) = \varepsilon\sqrt{\Delta}\, T_k(\theta) + \varepsilon^2 D_k^\varepsilon(\theta,\Delta) \quad \textit{with} \ \sup_k \mathbb{E}_\theta ||D_k^\varepsilon(\theta,\Delta)||^2 \le C\Delta, \ \textit{and}$$

$$T_k(\theta) = \frac{1}{\sqrt{\Delta}} \int_{t_{k-1}}^{t_k} \Phi(\alpha,t_k,u)\sigma(\beta,u,z(\alpha,u))dB(u),$$

where C *a constant independent of* $\theta, \varepsilon, \Delta$.

Therefore, the random variables $T_k(\theta)$ are p-dimensional $\mathcal{G}_k^n$-measurable independent Gaussian random variables with covariance matrix

$$S_k(\alpha,\beta) = S_k(\theta) = \frac{1}{\Delta}\int_{t_{k-1}}^{t_k} \Phi(\alpha,t_k,s)\Sigma(\beta,s,z(\alpha,s))\Phi^\star(\alpha,t_k,s)ds. \tag{3.3.8}$$

Proof. Using Propositions 3.3.1 and 3.3.2 yields that

$$\begin{aligned}D_k^\varepsilon(\theta,\Delta) &= R^\varepsilon(\theta,t_k) - \Phi(\alpha,t_k,t_{k-1})R^\varepsilon(\theta,t_{k-1})\\ &= R^\varepsilon(\theta,t_k) - R^\varepsilon(\theta,t_{k-1}) - (\Phi(\alpha,t_k,t_{k-1}) - I_p)R^\varepsilon(\theta,t_{k-1})\\ &= R^\varepsilon(\theta,t_k) - R^\varepsilon(\theta,t_{k-1}) - \Delta\nabla_z b(\alpha,t_{k-1},z(\alpha,t_{k-1}))R^\varepsilon(\theta,t_{k-1})\\ &\quad +\Delta^2 O_P(1).\end{aligned}$$

An application of Proposition 3.3.3 together with (S4) yields the result. □

Define the two random matrices

$$\Sigma_k(\beta) = \Sigma(\beta,t_k,X(t_k)), \quad \sigma_k(\beta) = \sigma(\beta,t_k,X(t_k)). \tag{3.3.9}$$

Then, for small Δ, we have using (3.3.9)

Lemma 3.3.5. *Assume (S1)–(S5). Then, under $\mathbb{P}_\theta$, as $\varepsilon,\Delta \to 0$,*

$$||S_k(\theta) - \Sigma_{k-1}(\beta)|| \le K\varepsilon \sup_{\theta,t\le T} ||g(\theta,t)|| + \Delta \sup_{\theta,z} ||\nabla_z \Sigma(\beta,s,z)|| \le \varepsilon C_1 O_P(1) + C_2\Delta.$$

The proof is straightforward using (S1), (S5) and Proposition (3.3.6).

Let us now state some preliminary results on the random variables $B_k(\alpha,X)$ defined in (3.3.7) useful for the inference.

Under $\mathbb{P}_{\theta_0}$, Proposition 3.3.1 yields that $B_k(\alpha,X)$ converges to $B_k(\alpha,z(\alpha_0,\cdot))$ and that $B_k(\alpha_0,X)$ converges to $B_k(\alpha_0,z(\alpha_0,\cdot)) = 0$ a.s. Let us define on $[0,T]$

$$\Gamma(\alpha_0,\alpha,t) = b(\alpha_0,t,z(\alpha_0,t)) - b(\alpha,t,z(\alpha,t)) - \nabla_z b(\alpha,t,z(\alpha,t))(z(\alpha_0,t) - z(\alpha,t)). \tag{3.3.10}$$

The sequence $B_k(\alpha,z(\alpha_0,\cdot))$ satisfies:

Lemma 3.3.6. *Assume (S1), (S2), (S4). Then, as $\Delta \to 0$, there exists a constant C such that*

$$\frac{1}{\Delta} B_k(\alpha,z(\alpha_0,\cdot)) = \Gamma(\alpha_0,\alpha,t_{k-1}) + \Delta\,\|\alpha - \alpha_0\|\, r_k(\alpha_0,\alpha)$$

with $\sup_{k,\alpha\in K_a} \|r_k(\alpha_0,\alpha)\| \le C$.

Proof. Using (3.3.7), (3.3.10) and that $\Phi(\alpha,t_k,t_{k-1}) = I_p + \Delta\nabla_z b(\alpha,t_{k-1},z(\alpha,t_{k-1})) + \Delta^2 O(1)$, yields

$$\begin{aligned}B_k(\alpha,z(\alpha_0,\cdot)) &= \int_{t_{k-1}}^{t_k} (b(\alpha_0,s,z(\alpha_0,s)) - b(\alpha,s,z(\alpha,s)))ds\\ &\qquad + (I_p - \Phi(\alpha,t_k,t_{k-1}))\,(z(\alpha_0,t_{k-1}) - z(\alpha,t_{k-1}))\\ &= \Delta\Gamma(\alpha_0,\alpha,t_{k-1}) + \Delta^2\,\|\alpha - \alpha_0\|\, r_k(\alpha_0,\alpha).\end{aligned}$$

Assumptions (S1), (S2) and (S4) ensure that the remainder term has order Δ^2 uniformly in k,α. □

Consider now the random variables $B_k(\alpha,X)$

Lemma 3.3.7. *Assume (S1)–(S5). Then, under $\mathbb{P}_{\theta_0}$, as $\varepsilon,\Delta \to 0$, the following holds for all $k \leq n$,*

$$\frac{1}{\Delta}(B_k(\alpha,X)-B_k(\alpha_0,X)) = \frac{1}{\Delta}B_k(\alpha,z(\alpha_0,\cdot))+\varepsilon||\alpha-\alpha_0||\eta_k(\alpha_0,\alpha,\varepsilon,\Delta)$$
$$= \Gamma(\alpha_0,\alpha,t_{k-1})+||\alpha-\alpha_0||(\Delta O(1)+\varepsilon O_P(1)),$$

where $\eta_k=\eta_k(\alpha_0,\alpha,\varepsilon,\Delta)$ is $\mathscr{G}^n_{k-1}$-measurable and uniformly bounded in probability .

Proof. Using (3.3.6) and (3.3.7), we get that

$$B_k(\alpha,X)-B_k(\alpha_0,X) =$$
$$B_k(\alpha,z(\alpha_0,\cdot))+\varepsilon(\Phi(\alpha_0,t_k,t_{k_1})-\Phi(\alpha,t_k,t_{k_1}))(g(\theta_0,t_{k-1})+\varepsilon R^{\varepsilon}(\theta_0,t_{k-1})).$$

By (S1)–(S5),

$$\left\|\Phi(\alpha_0,t_k,t_{k_1})-\Phi(\alpha,t_k,t_{k_1})\right\|$$
$$\leq 2\Delta\left\|\nabla_z b(\alpha_0,,t_{k-1},z(\alpha_0,t_{k-1}))-\nabla_z b(\alpha,,t_{k-1},z(\alpha,t_{k-1}))\right\|.$$

Now, this term is bounded by $K\Delta||\alpha-\alpha_0||$ since $(t,\alpha)\to\nabla_z b(\alpha,z(\alpha,t))$ is uniformly continuous on $[0,T]\times K_a$. Using now Proposition 3.3.1 yields that $(g(\theta_0,t_{k-1})+\varepsilon R^{\varepsilon}(\theta_0,t_{k-1}))$ is bounded in $\mathbb{P}_{\theta_0}$-probability and $\mathscr{G}^n_{k-1}$-measurable. □

The next lemma concerns the properties of $B_k(\alpha_0,X)$.

Lemma 3.3.8. *Assume (S1)–(S5). Then, using (3.3.9), as $\varepsilon,\Delta\to 0$, under $\mathbb{P}_{\theta_0}$,*

- **(i)** $B_k(\alpha_0,X)=\varepsilon\sigma_{k-1}(\beta_0)(B(t_k)-B(t_{k-1}))+E_k(\theta_0,\varepsilon,\Delta)$, *where* $E_k=E_k(\theta_0,\varepsilon,\Delta)$ *satisfies that, for* $m\geq 2$, $\mathbb{E}_{\theta_0}(||E_k||^m|\mathscr{G}^n_{k-1})\leq C\varepsilon^m\Delta^m$.
- **(ii)** *If (V_k) is a sequence of $\mathscr{G}^n_{k-1}$-measurable random variables in $\mathbb{R}^p$ uniformly bounded in probability, then $\sum_{k=1}^{n} V_k^* B_k(\alpha_0,X)\to 0$ in probability.*

Proof. Let us first prove (i) and study the term E_k. We have $E_k=E_k^1+E_k^2$ with

$$E_k^1 = \int_{t_{k-1}}^{t_k}(b(\alpha_0,t,X(t))-b(\alpha_0,t,z(\alpha_0,t)))\,dt$$
$$+(I_p-\Phi(\alpha_0,t_k,t_{k-1}))(X(t_{k-1})-z(\alpha_0,t_{k-1})) \text{ and}$$
$$E_k^2 = \varepsilon\int_{t_{k-1}}^{t_k}(\sigma(\beta_0,s,X(s))-\sigma(\beta_0,s,X(t_{k-1})))\,dB(s).$$

Set in (3.3.6), $R_1^{\varepsilon}(\theta,t)=g(\theta,t)+\varepsilon R^{\varepsilon}(\theta,t)$. Using that $(t,x)\to b(\alpha,t,x)$ is uniformly Lipschitz, we obtain,

$$\begin{aligned}\left\|E_k^1\right\| \leq & \Delta C \sup_{t\in[t_{k-1};t_k]} \|X(t)-z(\alpha_0,t)\| \\ & + \Delta\varepsilon \left\|\left(\int_0^1 \nabla_z b(\alpha_0,z(\alpha_0,t)))\Phi(\alpha_0,t,t_{k-1})dt\right)R_1^\varepsilon(\theta_0,t_{k-1})\right\| \\ \leq & C'\varepsilon\Delta \sup_{t\in[t_{k-1};t_k]} \|R_1^\varepsilon(\theta_0,t)\|\end{aligned}$$

The proof for E_k^2 follows the sketch given in [56, Lemma 1]. We first prove this result based on the stronger condition Σ and b bounded. Then, similarly to [56, Proposition 1], this assumption can be relaxed. We use sequentially the Burkhölder–Davis–Gundy (see e.g. [82]) and Jensen inequalities to obtain

$$\begin{aligned}& \mathbb{E}_{\theta_0}(\left\|E_k^2\right\|^m |\mathcal{G}_{k-1}^n) \\ & \leq C\varepsilon^m \mathbb{E}_{\theta_0}\left(\left(\int_{t_{k-1}}^{t_k} \|\sigma(\beta_0,s,X(s))-\sigma(\beta_0,t_{k-1},X(t_{k-1})\|^2 ds\right)^{m/2} |\mathcal{G}_{k-1}^n\right) \quad (3.3.11)\end{aligned}$$

$$\leq C\varepsilon^m \Delta^{m/2-1}\int_{t_{k-1}}^{t_k} \mathbb{E}_{\theta_0}\left(\|\sigma(\beta_0,s,X(s))-\sigma(\beta_0,t_{k-1},X(t_{k-1}))\|^m |\mathcal{G}_{k-1}^n\right) |ds. \quad (3.3.12)$$

Then, using that $(t,x) \to \sigma(\beta,t,x)$ is Lipschitz, we obtain:

$$\begin{aligned}& \mathbb{E}_{\theta_0}^\varepsilon(\left\|E_k^2\right\|^m |\mathcal{G}_{k-1}^n) \leq C'\varepsilon^m \Delta^{m/2-1}\int_{t_{k-1}}^{t_k} \mathbb{E}_{\theta_0}^\varepsilon(\|X(s)-X(t_{k-1})\|^m)ds \\ & \leq C'\varepsilon^m \Delta^{m/2-1}\int_{t_{k-1}}^{t_k} \mathbb{E}_{\theta_0}^\varepsilon\left[\left\|\int_{t_{k-1}}^s (b(\alpha_0,u,X(u))du + \varepsilon\sigma(\beta_0,u,X(u))dB(u))\right\|\right]^m ds.\end{aligned}$$

Since b is bounded on $\mathcal{U}$, $\left\|\int_{t_{k-1}}^s b(\alpha_0,u,X(u))du\right\| \leq K|s-t_{k-1}|$ and Itô's isometry yields

$$\begin{aligned}\mathbb{E}_{\theta_0}\left(\left\|\int_{t_{k-1}}^s \sigma(\beta_0,u,X(u))dB(u)\right\|^m\right) & \leq \mathbb{E}_{\theta_0}\left(\left\|\int_{t_{k-1}}^s \Sigma(\beta_0,u,X(u))du\right\|\right)^{m/2} \\ & \leq K|s-t_{k-1}|^{m/2}.\end{aligned}$$

Thus, $\mathbb{E}_{\theta_0}(\left\|E_k^2(\theta_0)\right\|^m |\mathcal{G}_{k-1}^n) \leq C''\varepsilon^m \Delta^{m/2-1}\int_{t_{k-1}}^{t_k} |s-t_{k-1}|^{m/2}ds \leq C'''\varepsilon^m\Delta^m$.

The proof of (ii) relies on the Lemma A.4.3 for triangular arrays stated in Section A.4. Set $\zeta_k^n = V_k^* B_k(\alpha_0,X)$. Using (i), we have

$$\mathbb{E}_{\theta_0}(\zeta_k^n|\mathcal{G}_{k-1}^n) = V_k^*\mathbb{E}_{\theta_0}^\varepsilon(E_k(\theta_0,\varepsilon,\Delta)|\mathcal{G}_{k-1}^n)$$

with $\mathbb{E}_{\theta_0}^\varepsilon(\|E_k(\theta_0,\varepsilon,\Delta)\| |\mathcal{G}_{k-1}^n) \leq C\varepsilon\Delta$.
Since $\sup_{k\leq n}\|V_k\|$ is bounded in probability, $\sum_{k=1}^n \mathbb{E}_{\theta_0}(\zeta_k^n|\mathcal{G}_{k-1}^n) \leq C\varepsilon T \to 0$.
Therefore condition (i) of Lemma A.4.3 is satisfied with $U=0$.
Now, $\mathbb{E}_{\theta_0}[(\zeta_k^n)^2|\mathcal{G}_{k-1}^n)] = V_k^*\mathbb{E}_{\theta_0}(B_k(\alpha_0,X)B_k^*(\alpha_0,X)|\mathcal{G}_{k-1}^n)V_k$.

Using (i) of Lemma 3.3.8 yields that

$$\begin{aligned}\mathbb{E}_{\theta_0}(B_k(\alpha_0,X)B_k^*(\alpha_0,X)|\mathcal{G}_{k-1}^n) &= \varepsilon^2\Delta\Sigma_{k-1}(\beta_0)+\mathbb{E}_{\theta_0}(E_kE_k^*|\mathcal{G}_{k-1}^n)\\ &\leq K_1\varepsilon^2\Delta+C_2\varepsilon^2\Delta^2.\end{aligned}$$

Hence, $\sum_{k=1}^n \mathbb{E}_{\theta_0}((\zeta_k^n)^2|\mathcal{G}_{k-1}^n)\to 0$. Therefore, applying Lemma A.4.3 achieves the proof. □

A last lemma concerns the terms $(\nabla_{\alpha_i}B_k)$ for $i=1,\dots,a$.

Lemma 3.3.9. *Assume (S1)–(S6). Then, under* $\mathbb{P}_{\theta_0}$, *for all* $i,j\leq a$, *for all* $\alpha\in K_a$, *as* $\varepsilon,\Delta\to 0$,

(i) $\frac{1}{\Delta}\nabla_{\alpha_i}B_k(\alpha,X)=-\nabla_{\alpha_i}b(\alpha,t_{k-1},z(\alpha,t_{k-1}))+M_k^i(\alpha)[(z(\alpha_0,t_{k-1})-z(\alpha,t_{k-1}))+\varepsilon Z_{k-1}^{\varepsilon}(\theta_0)]+\Delta O_P(1)$, *where* $M_k^i(\alpha)$ *are uniformly bounded matrices and* $Z_{k-1}^{\varepsilon}(\theta_0)$ *are* $\mathcal{G}_{k-1}^n$*-measurable r.v.s uniformly bounded in probability.*

(ii) For all $k\leq n$, $\frac{1}{\Delta}\left\|\nabla^2_{\alpha_i,\alpha_j}B_k(\alpha,X)\right\|$ *is bounded uniformly in probability.*

Proof. We have, using (3.3.6) and (3.3.7),

$$\begin{aligned}B_k(\alpha,X)=&(X(t_k)-X(t_{k-1}))-(z(\alpha,t_k)-z(\alpha,t_{k-1}))\\ &+(I_p-\Phi(\alpha,t_k,t_{k-1}))(X(t_{k-1})-z(\alpha,t_{k-1})).\end{aligned}$$

Therefore,

$$\nabla_{\alpha_i}B_k(\alpha,X)=E_{k,i}+\varepsilon\Delta M_k^i(\alpha)Z_{k-1}(\theta_0)$$

with $M_k^i(\alpha)=-\frac{1}{\Delta}\nabla_{\alpha_i}\Phi(\alpha,t_k,t_{k-1})$, $Z_{k-1}(\theta_0)=g(\theta_0,t_{k-1})+\varepsilon R^{\varepsilon}(\theta_0,t_{k-1})$ and

$$\begin{aligned}E_{k,i}=&-\nabla_{\alpha_i}(z(\alpha,t_k)-z(\alpha,t_{k-1}))+(\Phi(\alpha,t_k,t_{k-1})-I_p)\nabla_{\alpha_i}z(\alpha,t_{k-1})\\ &-\nabla_{\alpha_i}\Phi(\alpha,t_k,t_{k-1})(z(\alpha_0,t_{k-1})-z(\alpha,t_{k-1})).\end{aligned}$$

Proposition 3.3.1 yields the result for $Z_k(\theta_0)$.

Now, $\Phi(\alpha,t_k,t_{k-1})=\exp\{\int_{t_{k-1}}^{t_k}\nabla_z b(\alpha,s,z(\alpha,s))ds\}$ so that

$$M_k^i(\alpha)=-\nabla_{\alpha_i}\nabla_z b(\alpha,t_{k-1},z(\alpha,t_{k-1}))+\Delta O(1).$$

To study $E_{k,i}$, we use that $\Phi(\alpha,t_k,t_{k-1})-I_p=\Delta\nabla_z b(\alpha,t_{k-1},z(\alpha,t_{k-1}))+\Delta^2O(1)$ and $\nabla_{\alpha_i}(b(\alpha,t,z(\alpha,t)))=\nabla_{\alpha_i}b(\alpha,t,z(\alpha,t))+\nabla_z b(\alpha,t,z(\alpha,t))\nabla_{\alpha_i}z(\alpha,t)$. Therefore $E_{k,i}=-\nabla_{\alpha_i}b(\alpha,t_{k-1},z(\alpha,t_{k-1}))+M_k^i(\alpha)(z(\alpha_0,t_{k-1})-z(\alpha,t_{k-1}))+\Delta O(1)$.

This achieves the proof of (i).

Let us prove (ii). We have $\nabla^2_{\alpha_i\alpha_j}B_k(\alpha,X)=f_k^{ij}(\alpha_0,\alpha,\Delta)+\xi_k^{ij}(\theta_0,\alpha,\varepsilon,\Delta)$ with $\xi_k^{ij}=(\nabla^2_{\alpha_i\alpha_j}\Phi(\alpha,t_k,t_{k-1}))[X(t_{k-1})-z(\alpha_0,t_{k-1})]$ and

$$\begin{aligned}f_k^{ij}(\alpha_0,\alpha,\Delta)=&-\left(\nabla^2_{\alpha_i\alpha_j}z(\alpha,t_k)-\Phi(\alpha,t_k,t_{k-1})\nabla^2_{\alpha_i\alpha_j}z(\alpha,t_{k-1})\right)\\ &+\nabla_{\alpha_i}\Phi(\alpha,t_k,t_{k-1})\nabla_{\alpha_j}z(\alpha,t_{k-1})\end{aligned}$$

$$+\nabla_{\alpha_j}\Phi(\alpha,t_k,t_{k-1})\nabla_{\alpha_i}z(\alpha,t_{k-1})$$
$$-\nabla^2_{\alpha_i\alpha_j}\Phi(\alpha,t_k,t_{k-1})(z(\alpha,t_{k-1})-z(\alpha_0,t_{k-1})).$$

The result is obtained using Proposition 3.3.1 and the property that $\frac{1}{\Delta}\|\nabla_{\alpha_i}\Phi(\cdot)\|$ and $\frac{1}{\Delta}\left\|\nabla^2_{\alpha_i,\alpha_j}\Phi(\cdot)\right\|$ are uniformly bounded. □

3.4 Inference Based on High Frequency Observations on $[0,T]$

We assume that both ε and $\Delta=\Delta_n$ go to 0. The number of observations n goes to infinity. We study the estimation of $\theta=(\alpha,\beta)$ based on $(X(t_k),k=1,\dots,n)$.

Lemmas 3.3.4 and 3.3.5 yield that the random variables $\frac{1}{\varepsilon\sqrt{\Delta}}B_k(\alpha_0,X)$ are approximately conditionally independent centered Gaussian random variables in $\mathbb{R}^p$ with covariance approximated by $\Sigma_{k-1}(\beta_0)$. Analogously to [85] or [56], we introduce a contrast function, using definitions (3.3.7), (3.3.9),

$$\check{U}_{\varepsilon,\Delta}(\alpha,\beta)=\sum_{k=1}^{n}\log\det\Sigma_{k-1}(\beta)+\frac{1}{\varepsilon^2\Delta}\sum_{k=1}^{n}B_k(\alpha,X)^*\,\Sigma_{k-1}^{-1}(\beta)\,B_k(\alpha,X). \quad (3.4.1)$$

The minimum contrast estimators are defined as any solution of

$$(\check{\alpha}_{\varepsilon,\Delta},\check{\beta}_{\varepsilon,\Delta})=\underset{(\alpha,\beta)\in\Theta}{\operatorname{argmin}}\,\check{U}_{\varepsilon,\Delta}(\alpha,\beta). \quad (3.4.2)$$

3.4.1 Properties of the Estimators

In what follows, we use to describe the asymptotics with respect to $\Delta=\Delta_n$ either $\Delta\to 0$ or $n\to\infty$. Indeed, it is more explicit to state results according to the number of observations n rather than in terms of the size of the sampling interval $\Delta=\Delta_n$. Results are obtained when $\varepsilon\to 0$ and $\Delta\to 0$ (or $n\to\infty$) simultaneously.

Define, for $\theta=(\alpha,\beta)\in\Theta$ with Θ a compact subset of $\mathbb{R}^a\times\mathbb{R}^b$, the matrices $I_b(\theta)=(I_b(\theta)_{ij},1\le i,j\le a)$, $I_\sigma(\theta)=(I_\sigma(\theta)_{i,j},1\le i,j\le b)$ and $I(\theta)$ by

$$(I_b(\theta))_{ij}=\int_0^T(\nabla_{\alpha_i}b(\alpha,t,z(\alpha,t)))^*\Sigma^{-1}(\beta,t,z(\alpha,t))\nabla_{\alpha_j}b(\alpha,t,z(\alpha,t))dt, \quad (3.4.3)$$

$$(I_\sigma(\theta))_{i,j}= \quad (3.4.4)$$
$$\frac{1}{2T}\int_0^T\mathrm{Tr}\left(\nabla_{\beta_i}\Sigma(\beta,t,z(\alpha,t))\Sigma^{-1}(\beta,t,z(\alpha,t))\nabla_{\beta_j}\Sigma(\beta,t,z(\alpha,t))\Sigma^{-1}(\beta,t,z(\alpha,t))\right)dt.$$

$$I(\theta) = \begin{pmatrix} I_b(\theta)) & 0 \\ 0 & I_\sigma(\theta) \end{pmatrix}. \tag{3.4.5}$$

Recall that A^* denotes the transpose of a matrix A and $\mathrm{Tr}(A)$ its trace.

Theorem 3.4.1. *Assume that $(X(t))$ satisfying* (3.3.1) *is observed at times $t_k = k\Delta_n$ with $T = n\Delta_n$ fixed. Assume* **(S1)–(S7)** *and that $I_b(\theta_0)$ is non-singular. Then, as $\varepsilon \to 0, \Delta = \Delta_n \to 0$,*

(i) $(\breve{\alpha}_{\varepsilon,\Delta}, \breve{\beta}_{\varepsilon,\Delta}) \to (\alpha_0, \beta_0)$ in $\mathbb{P}_{\theta_0}$-probability.

(ii) If moreover $I_\sigma(\theta_0)$ is non-singular,

$$\begin{pmatrix} \varepsilon^{-1}\left(\breve{\alpha}_{\varepsilon,\Delta} - \alpha_0\right) \\ \sqrt{n}\left(\breve{\beta}_{\varepsilon,\Delta} - \beta_0\right) \end{pmatrix} \to \mathscr{N}_{a+b}\left(0, \begin{pmatrix} I_b^{-1}(\alpha_0,\beta_0) & 0 \\ 0 & I_\sigma^{-1}(\alpha_0,\beta_0) \end{pmatrix}\right)$$

in distribution under $\mathbb{P}_{\theta_0}$.

Note that results are obtained without any condition linking ε and Δ (or n). Indeed, the previous results obtained in [56] require conditions linking ε and Δ that do not fit epidemic data, where generally the orders of magnitude for N and n satisfy $N >> n$ so that Δ is comparatively large with respect to $\varepsilon = 1/\sqrt{N}$. We proposed in [60] another method based on Theorem 3.2.1 which extends results obtained in [46], where the inference in the case $\sigma(\beta,x) \equiv 1$ was investigated for one-dimensional diffusions using expansion (3.2.15).

Since estimators of parameters in the drift (here α) and in the diffusion coefficient (here β) converge at distinct rates, ε^{-1} and $\sqrt{n} = \Delta^{-1/2}$ respectively, the study of asymptotic properties has to be performed according to the successive steps:

Step (1): Consistency of $\breve{\alpha}_{\varepsilon,\Delta}$ (Proposition 3.4.2).
Step (2): Tightness of the sequence $\varepsilon^{-1}(\breve{\alpha}_{\varepsilon,\Delta} - \alpha_0)$ with respect to β (Proposition 3.4.3).
Step (3): Consistency of $\breve{\beta}_{\varepsilon,\Delta}$ (Proposition 3.4.5).
Step (4): Asymptotic normality for both estimators (Theorem 3.4.1,(ii)).

The proof is technical and detailed in a separate section. Before this proof, let us state some comments.

3.4.1.1 Comments

(1) *Efficiency of estimators*: Note that the matrix $I_b(\theta)$ is equal to the Fisher information matrix associated to the estimation of α when $(X(t))$ is continuously observed on $[0,T]$ (see e.g. [91] and Section A.3 in the Appendix). Therefore $\breve{\alpha}_{\varepsilon,\Delta}$ is efficient for this statistical model.

(2) *Comparison with estimation based on complete observation of the jump process* $(\mathscr{Z}^N(t))$: Coming back to epidemics, we can compare the estimation of the parameters of the pure jump process $(\mathscr{Z}^N(t))$ and $(Z^N(t) = \frac{1}{N}\mathscr{Z}^N(t))$ describing the epidemic dynamics in a finite population of size N and the estimators built from its diffusion approximation. Let us stress that there is a main difference between these two approaches. Statistical inference for $(\mathscr{Z}^N(t))$ is based on the observations of all the jumps, which implies here the observation of all the times of infection and recovery for each individual in the population, while for the diffusion $(X(t))$, we consider discrete observations $(X(t_k), k = 1,\dots,n)$.

(3) *Comparison of estimators for the SIR epidemic dynamics*: Assume that the jump process $(\mathscr{Z}^N(t))$ is continuously observed on $[0,T]$. Its dynamics is described by the two parameters (λ,γ). Set $Z^N(t) = (S^N((),I^N(t))^*$, and assume that $Z^N(0) \to x_0 = (s_0,i_0)^*$, with $s_0 > 0, i_0 > 0$. Let $s(t) = s(\lambda_0,\gamma_0,t); i(t) = i(\lambda_0,\gamma_0,t)$ the solution of the corresponding ODE.

The Maximum Likelihood Estimator $(\hat{\lambda},\hat{\gamma})$ is explicit (see [2] or Chapter 4 of this part). Indeed, let (T_i) denote the successive jump times and set $J_i = 0$ if we have an infection and $J_i = 1$ if we have a recovery. Let $K_N(T) = \sum_{i\geq 0} 1_{T_i \leq T}$. Then

$$\hat{\lambda}_N = \frac{1}{N}\frac{\sum_{i=1}^{K_N(T)}(1-J_i)}{\int_0^T S^N(t)I^N(t)dt} = \frac{1}{N}\frac{\text{\# Infections}}{\int_0^T S^N(t)I^N(t)dt},$$

$$\hat{\gamma}_N = \frac{1}{N}\frac{\sum_{i=1}^{K_N(T)} J_i}{\int_0^T I^N(t)dt} = \frac{\text{\# Recoveries}}{\text{“Mean infectious period”}}.$$

As the population size N goes to infinity, $(\hat{\lambda}_N,\hat{\gamma}_N)$ is consistent and

$$\sqrt{N}\begin{pmatrix}\hat{\lambda}_N - \lambda \\ \hat{\gamma}_N - \gamma\end{pmatrix} \to \mathscr{N}_2\left(0, I^{-1}(\lambda,\gamma)\right), \text{ where } I(\lambda,\gamma) = \begin{pmatrix}\frac{\int_0^T s(t)i(t)dt}{\lambda} & 0 \\ 0 & \frac{\int_0^T i(t)dt}{\gamma}\end{pmatrix}.$$

The matrix $I(\lambda,\gamma)$ is the Fisher information matrix of this statistical model.

Consider now the *SIR* diffusion approximation $X(t)$ described in Section 3.2.2.1. We have

$$b(\theta,(s,i)) = \begin{pmatrix}-\lambda si \\ \lambda si - \gamma i\end{pmatrix}; \quad \Sigma(\theta,(s,i)) = \begin{pmatrix}\lambda si & -\lambda si \\ -\lambda si & \lambda si + \gamma i\end{pmatrix}. \tag{3.4.6}$$

Therefore,

$$\nabla_\theta b(\theta,(s,i)) = \begin{pmatrix}-si & 0 \\ si & -i\end{pmatrix}; \Sigma^{-1}(\theta,(s,i)) = \frac{1}{\lambda\gamma si}\begin{pmatrix}\lambda s + \gamma & \lambda s \\ \lambda s & \lambda s\end{pmatrix}.$$

The matrix $I_b(\theta)$ defined in (3.4.3) is

$$I_b(\lambda,\gamma) = \begin{pmatrix}\frac{1}{\lambda}\int_0^T s(t)i(t)dt & 0 \\ 0 & \frac{1}{\gamma}\int_0^T i(t)dt\end{pmatrix}.$$

Therefore, we obtain the same information matrix in both cases.

Consider the *SIRS* model with immunity waning δ. We have $\theta = (\lambda, \gamma, \delta)$ The diffusion approximation satisfies

$$b(\theta,(s,i)) = \begin{pmatrix} -\lambda si + \delta(1-s-i) \\ \lambda si - \gamma i \end{pmatrix}; \quad \Sigma(\theta,(s,i)) = \begin{pmatrix} \lambda si + \delta(1-s-i) & -\lambda si \\ -\lambda si & \lambda si + \gamma i \end{pmatrix}.$$

Hence,

$$\nabla_\theta b(\theta,s,i) = \begin{pmatrix} -si & 0 & (1-s-i) \\ si & -i & 0 \end{pmatrix},$$

$$I_b(\theta) = \int_0^T \nabla_\theta^* b(\theta,s(t),i(t))\Sigma^{-1}(\theta,s(t),i(t))\nabla_\theta b(\theta,s(t),i(t))dt.$$

Then $I_b(\theta)$ can be computed and compare to the Fisher information matrix derived from the statistical model corresponding to complete observation of the *SIRS* jump process.

3.4.2 Proof of Theorem 3.4.1

Recall the notations: for a matrix A, A^* the transposition of A, $\det(A)$ the determinant of A and $\mathrm{Tr}(A)$ the trace of A.

3.4.2.1 Step (1): Consistency of $\check{\alpha}_{\varepsilon,\Delta}$

Let us define, using (3.3.10),

$$K_1(\alpha_0,\alpha,\beta) = \int_0^T \Gamma(\alpha_0,\alpha,t)^*\Sigma^{-1}(\beta,t,z(\alpha_0,t))\Gamma(\alpha_0,\alpha,t)dt. \tag{3.4.7}$$

By Assumption (S4), if $\alpha \neq \alpha_0$, $b(\alpha,t,z(\alpha,t)) \not\equiv b(\alpha_0,t,z(\alpha_0))$, therefore the function $\Gamma(\alpha_0,\alpha,\cdot) \not\equiv 0$, which implies that $K_1(\alpha_0,\alpha,\beta)$ is non-negative and equal to 0 if and only if $\alpha = \alpha_0$.

The contrast function $\check{U}_{\varepsilon,\Delta}(\alpha,\beta)$ defined in (3.4.1) satisfies

Proposition 3.4.2. *Assume (S1)–(S6). Then, as $\varepsilon,\Delta \to 0$, the following convergences hold.*

(i) $\sup_{\theta\in\Theta} |\varepsilon^2 (\check{U}_{\varepsilon,\Delta}(\alpha,\beta) - \check{U}_{\varepsilon,\Delta}(\alpha_0,\beta)) - K_1(\alpha_0,\alpha,\beta)| \to 0$ *in $\mathbb{P}_{\theta_0}$-probability.*
(ii) $\check{\alpha}_{\varepsilon,\Delta} \to \alpha_0$ *in probability under $\mathbb{P}_{\theta_0}$.*

Proof. Let us prove (i). We have, by (3.4.1) and (3.3.9),

$$\varepsilon^2(\check{U}_{\varepsilon,\Delta}(\alpha,\beta) - \check{U}_{\varepsilon,\Delta}(\alpha_0,\beta)) = T_1 + T_2$$

with

$$T_1 = 2\sum_{k=1}^{n} \frac{(B_k(\alpha,X)-B_k(\alpha_0,X))^*}{\Delta}\,\Sigma_{k-1}^{-1}(\beta)\,B_k(\alpha_0,X),$$
$$T_2 = \Delta\sum_{k=1}^{n} \frac{(B_k(\alpha,X)-B_k(\alpha_0,X))^*}{\Delta}\,\Sigma_{k-1}^{-1}(\beta)\,\frac{(B_k(\alpha,X)-B_k(\alpha_0,X))}{\Delta}.$$

By Lemma 3.3.7, $\dfrac{(B_k(\alpha,X)-B_k(\alpha_0,X))}{\Delta}$ is bounded, and (ii) of Lemma 3.3.8 yields that T_1 goes to 0 in $\mathbb{P}_{\theta_0}$-probability. Using now (3.3.10), we have by Lemma 3.3.7, setting $\zeta_k = \Delta r_k + \varepsilon\,\|\alpha-\alpha_0\|\,\eta_k$,

$$\begin{aligned} T_2 &= \Delta\sum_{k=1}^{n}(\Gamma(\alpha_0,\alpha,t_{k-1})+\zeta_{k-1})^*\Sigma_{k-1}^{-1}(\beta)\,(\Gamma(\alpha_0,\alpha,t_{k-1})+\zeta_{k-1})\\ &= \Delta\sum_{k=1}^{n}\left(\Gamma(\alpha_0,\alpha,t_{k-1})^*\Sigma_{k-1}^{-1}(\beta)\Gamma(\alpha_0,\alpha,t_{k-1})+R_k(\theta_0,\theta,\varepsilon,\Delta)\right).\end{aligned}$$

The first term of the above formula as a Riemann sum converges by Lemma 3.3.6 to the function $K_1(\alpha_0,\alpha,\beta)$ defined in (3.4.7) as $\Delta\to 0$. This convergence is uniform with respect to the parameters. The remainder term is

$$\begin{aligned} R_k(\theta_0,\theta,\varepsilon,\Delta) =& \Gamma(\alpha_0,\alpha,t_{k-1})^*(\Sigma_{k-1}^{-1}(\beta)-\Sigma^{-1}(\beta,t_{k-1},z(\alpha_0,t_{k-1})))\Gamma(\alpha_0,\alpha,t_{k-1})\\ &+\Delta R_k^1(\theta_0,\theta,\varepsilon,\Delta)+\varepsilon R_k^2(\theta_0,\theta,\varepsilon,\Delta).\end{aligned}$$

Using Proposition 3.3.1 and Lemma 3.3.7, it is straightforward to get that $\sup_k\|R_k(\theta_0,\theta,\varepsilon,\Delta)\|\to 0$ in $\mathbb{P}_{\theta_0}$-probability uniformly with respect to θ. Hence, T_2 converges to $K_1(\alpha_0,\alpha,\beta)$ in $\mathbb{P}_{\theta_0}$-probability uniformly with respect to θ.
Let us prove (ii). Noting that, for all β, $K_1(\alpha_0,\alpha_0,\beta)=0$, we have

$$\begin{aligned} 0\le& K_1(\alpha_0,\check{\alpha}_{\varepsilon,\Delta},\check{\beta}_{\varepsilon,\Delta})-K_1(\alpha_0,\alpha_0,\check{\beta}_{\varepsilon,\Delta})\\ \le&[\varepsilon^2(\check{U}_{\varepsilon,\Delta}(\alpha,\check{\beta}_{\varepsilon,\Delta})-\check{U}_{\varepsilon,\Delta}(\alpha_0,\check{\beta}_{\varepsilon,\Delta}))-K_1(\alpha_0,\alpha,\check{\beta}_{\varepsilon,\Delta})]\\ &+[K_1(\alpha_0,\check{\alpha}_{\varepsilon,\Delta},\check{\beta}_{\varepsilon,\Delta})-\varepsilon^2(\check{U}_{\varepsilon,\Delta}(\check{\alpha}_{\varepsilon,\Delta},\check{\beta}_{\varepsilon,\Delta})-\check{U}_{\varepsilon,\Delta}(\alpha_0,\check{\beta}_{\varepsilon,\Delta}))]\\ &+\varepsilon^2[\check{U}_{\varepsilon,\Delta}(\check{\alpha}_{\varepsilon,\Delta},\check{\beta}_{\varepsilon,\Delta})-\check{U}_{\varepsilon,\Delta}(\alpha,\check{\beta}_{\varepsilon,\Delta})]\\ \le& 2\sup_{\beta\in K_b}|\varepsilon^2[\check{U}_{\varepsilon,\Delta}(\alpha,\beta)-\check{U}_{\varepsilon,\Delta}(\alpha_0,\beta)]-K_1(\alpha_0,\alpha,\beta)|,\end{aligned}$$

where the last inequality is obtained using that the minimum of $\check{U}_{\varepsilon,\Delta}(\alpha,\beta)$ is attained at $(\check{\alpha}_{\varepsilon,\Delta},\check{\beta}_{\varepsilon,\Delta})$. By Proposition 3.4.2 (i), we finally get that

$$|K_1(\alpha_0,\check{\alpha}_{\varepsilon,\Delta},\check{\beta}_{\varepsilon,\Delta})-K_1(\alpha_0,\alpha_0,\check{\beta}_{\varepsilon,\Delta})|\to 0,$$

which yields by Assumption **(S6)** that $\check{\alpha}_{\varepsilon,\Delta}\to\alpha_0$ in $\mathbb{P}_{\theta_0}$-probability as $\varepsilon,\Delta\to 0$. □

3.4.2.2 Step (2): Tightness of the Sequence $\varepsilon^{-1}(\check{\alpha}_{\varepsilon,\Delta}-\alpha_0)$

This step is crucial in the presence of different rates of convergence for α and β and concerns results that hold for all $\beta \in K_b$.

Proposition 3.4.3. *Assume* **(S1)–(S4)** *and that $I_b(\alpha_0,\beta_0)$ defined in (3.4.3) is non-singular. Then, as $\varepsilon,\Delta \to 0$, $\sup_{\beta\in K_b}\left\|\varepsilon^{-1}\left(\check{\alpha}_{\varepsilon,\Delta}-\alpha_0\right)\right\|$ is bounded in $\mathbb{P}_{\theta_0}$-probability.*

Proof. Recall the notation: for f a twice differentiable real function, $\nabla^2_\alpha f = (\frac{\partial^2 f}{\partial\alpha_i\partial\alpha_j})_{1\le i,j\le a}$.
Under (S5), $\check{U}_{\varepsilon,\Delta}(\alpha,\beta)$ is C^2 and a Taylor expansion of $\nabla_\alpha\check{U}_{\varepsilon,\Delta}$ at point $(\alpha_0,\check{\beta}_{\varepsilon,\Delta})$ w.r.t. α yields,

$$0=\varepsilon\nabla_\alpha\check{U}_{\varepsilon,\Delta}(\check{\alpha}_{\varepsilon,\Delta},\check{\beta}_{\varepsilon,\Delta})=\varepsilon\nabla_\alpha\check{U}_{\varepsilon,\Delta}(\alpha_0,\check{\beta}_{\varepsilon,\Delta})+\varepsilon^2N_{\varepsilon,\Delta}(\check{\alpha}_{\varepsilon,\Delta},\check{\beta}_{\varepsilon,\Delta})\frac{(\check{\alpha}_{\varepsilon,\Delta}-\alpha_0)}{\varepsilon}, \tag{3.4.8}$$

$$\text{with}\quad N_{\varepsilon,\Delta}(\alpha,\beta)=\int_0^1\nabla^2_\alpha\check{U}_{\varepsilon,\Delta}(\alpha_0+t(\alpha-\alpha_0),\beta)dt. \tag{3.4.9}$$

The proof relies on two properties: under $\mathbb{P}_{\theta_0}$, as $\varepsilon,\Delta\to 0$, for all $\beta\in K_b$, $(\varepsilon\nabla_\alpha\check{U}_{\varepsilon,\Delta}(\alpha_0,\beta))$ converges in distribution to a Gaussian law and the sequence $\varepsilon^2\nabla^2_\alpha\check{U}_{\varepsilon,\Delta}(\alpha_0,\beta)$ converges almost surely.

Let us study $-\varepsilon\nabla_\alpha\check{U}_{\varepsilon,\Delta}(\alpha_0,\beta)$. Define the $a\times a$ matrix

$$J(\theta_0,\beta)=\int_0^T(\nabla_\alpha b(\alpha_0,t,z(\alpha_0,t)))^*\Xi(\theta_0,\beta,t)\nabla_\alpha b(\alpha_0,t,z(\alpha_0,t))dt,\ \text{with} \tag{3.4.10}$$

$$\Xi(\theta_0,\beta,t)=\Sigma^{-1}(\beta,t,z(\alpha_0,t))\Sigma(\beta_0,t,z(\alpha_0,t))\Sigma^{-1}(\beta,t,z(\alpha_0,t)). \tag{3.4.11}$$

The following holds.

Lemma 3.4.4. *Assume (S1)–(S5). Then, as $\varepsilon,\Delta\to 0$,*

$$-\varepsilon\nabla_\alpha\check{U}_{\varepsilon,\Delta}(\alpha_0,\beta)\to\mathcal{N}(0,4J(\theta_0,\beta))\ \textit{in distribution under}\ \mathbb{P}_{\theta_0}.$$

Proof. We have, using the notations of Lemma 3.3.9 and setting

$$H^i_k(\alpha_0,\beta)=\Sigma^{-1}(\beta,t_{k-1},z(\alpha_0,t_{k-1}))\nabla_{\alpha_i}b(\alpha_0,t_{k-1},z(\alpha_0,t_{k-1})) \tag{3.4.12}$$

$$-\varepsilon\nabla_{\alpha_i}\check{U}_{\varepsilon,\Delta}(\alpha_0,\beta)=-\frac{2}{\varepsilon\Delta}\sum_{k=1}^n(\nabla_{\alpha_i}B_k(\alpha_0,X))^*\Sigma^{-1}_{k-1}(\beta)B_k(\alpha_0,X)=A^i_n+A'^{,i}_n+A''^{,i}_n,$$

with

$$A^i_n=\frac{2}{\varepsilon}\sum_{k=1}^n H^i_k(\alpha_0,\beta)^*B_k(\alpha_0,X),$$

$$A_n^{\prime,i} = -2\sum_{k=1}^{n}(M_k^i(\alpha_0)Z_{k-1}(\theta_0))^*\Sigma_{k-1}^{-1}(\beta)B_k(\alpha_0,X),$$

$$A_n^{\prime\prime,i} = 2\sum_{k=1}^{n}\frac{\nabla_{\alpha_i}B_k(\alpha_0,X)}{\Delta}^*\frac{\Sigma_{k-1}^{-1}(\beta)-\Sigma^{-1}(\beta,t_{k-1},z(\alpha_0,t_{k-1}))}{\varepsilon}B_k(\alpha_0,X).$$

By Lemma 3.3.8 (ii), Lemma 3.3.9 and Theorem 3.3.1, $A_n^{\prime,i}$ and $A_n^{\prime\prime,i}$ tend to 0 in $\mathbb{P}_{\theta_0}$-probability as $\varepsilon,\Delta\to 0$.
To study A_n^i, we write, using the notations of Lemma 3.3.4,

$$B_k(\alpha_0,X) = \varepsilon\sqrt{\Delta}T_k(\theta_0)+\varepsilon^2(R(\theta_0,t_k)-R(\theta_0,t_{k-1})) + \varepsilon^2(I_p-\Phi(\alpha_0,t_k,t_{k-1}))R(\theta_0,t_{k-1}). \tag{3.4.13}$$

Hence, $A_n^i = D_n^i + C_n^i + C_n^{\prime,i}$ where, using (3.4.12),

$$D_n^i = 2\sqrt{\Delta}\sum_{k=1}^{n}(H_k^i(\alpha_0,\beta))^*T_k(\theta_0), \tag{3.4.14}$$

$$C_n^i = 2\varepsilon\sum_{k=1}^{n}(H_k^i(\alpha_0,\beta))^*(R(\theta_0,t_k)-R(\theta_0,t_{k-1})) \text{ and}$$

$$C_n^{\prime,i} = 2\varepsilon\Delta\sum_{k=1}^{n}(H_k^i(\alpha_0,\beta))^*\frac{1}{\Delta}(I_p-\Phi(\alpha_0,t_k,t_{k-1}))R(\theta_0,t_{k-1}).$$

Let us first study $C_n^{\prime,i}$. Noting that

$$\frac{1}{\Delta}(I_p-\Phi(\alpha_0,t_k,t_{k-1})) = \nabla_z b(\alpha_0,z(\alpha_0,t_{k-1}))+\Delta O(1),$$

we have $|C_n^{\prime,i}|\le \varepsilon n C(\theta_0)$, with $C(\theta_0)$ bounded in probability.

To study C_n^i, we first apply an Abel transform to the sequence and get

$$C_n^i = 2\varepsilon\sum_{k=1}^{n}(H_{k-1}^i(\alpha_0,\beta)-H_k^i(\alpha_0,\beta))^*R(\theta_0,t_{k-1})+\varepsilon H_k^n(\alpha_0,\beta)^*R(\theta_0,t_n).$$

The continuity assumptions ensure that $\sup_{k\le n}\frac{1}{\Delta}\left\|H_{k-1}^i(\alpha_0,\beta)-H_k^i(\alpha_0,\beta))\right\|$ is bounded. Hence $C_n^i\to 0$ since $\|R(\theta_0,t_k)\|$ is uniformly bounded.

It remains to study the main term $D_n = (D_n^i)_{1\le i\le a}$ defined in (3.4.14). Let

$$H_k(\alpha_0,\beta) = \Sigma_{k-1}^{-1}(\beta)\nabla_\alpha b(\alpha_0,t_{k-1},z(\alpha_0,t_{k-1})).$$

Then (D_n) is a multidimensional triangular array which reads as $D_n=\sum_{k=1}^n\zeta_k^n$ with $\zeta_k^n = \sqrt{\Delta}H_k(\alpha_0,\beta)^*T_k(\theta_0)\in\mathbb{R}^a$.
Note that D_n does not depend on ε and convergence results are obtained for $\Delta_n\to 0$. To apply to (D_n) a theorem of convergence in law for triangular arrays (Theorem A.4.2 in the Appendix or [73] Theorem 2.2.14), we have to prove that,

(i) $\sum_{k=1}^n\mathbb{E}_{\theta_0}(\zeta_k^n|\mathscr{G}_{k-1}^n)=0,$

(ii) $\sum_{k=1}^{n} \mathbb{E}_{\theta_0}(\zeta_k^{n,i}\zeta_k^{n,j}|\mathcal{G}_{k-1}^n) \to J_{ij}(\theta_0,\beta)$ (see Definition 3.4.10 below),
(iii) $\sum_{k=1}^{n} \mathbb{E}_{\theta_0}((\zeta_k^{n,i})^4|\mathcal{G}_{k-1}^n) \to 0$.

Since $T_k(\alpha_0)$ is centered, (i) is clearly satisfied. For (ii), consider for $1 \le i,j \le a$,

$$\begin{aligned}\mathbb{E}_{\theta_0}(\zeta_k^{n,i}\zeta_k^{n,j}|\mathcal{G}_{k-1}^n) &= \Delta H_k^i(\alpha_0,\beta)^*\mathbb{E}_{\theta_0}(T_k(\theta_0)T_k^*(\theta_0))H_k^j(\alpha_0,\beta)\\ &= \Delta H_k^i(\alpha_0,\beta)^* S_k(\alpha_0,\beta_0)H_k^j(\alpha_0,\beta).\end{aligned}$$

Noting that $\|S_k(\theta_0) - \Sigma(\beta_0,t_{k-1},z(\alpha_0,t_{k-1}))\| \le C\Delta$ yields, using Definition 3.4.11,

$$\begin{aligned}&\mathbb{E}_{\theta_0}(\zeta_k^{n,i}\zeta_k^{n,j}|\mathcal{G}_{k-1}^n)\\ &= \Delta(\nabla_{\alpha_i}b(\alpha_0,t_{k-1},z(\alpha_0,t_{k-1})))^*\Xi(\theta_0,\beta,t_{k-1})\nabla_{\alpha_j}b(\alpha_0,t_{k-1},z(\alpha_0,t_{k-1}))\\ &\quad +\Delta^2 o(1).\end{aligned}$$

Therefore, as a Riemann sum,

$$\begin{aligned}&\sum_{k=1}^{n}\mathbb{E}_{\theta_0}(\zeta_k^{n,i}\zeta_k^{n,j}|\mathcal{G}_{k-1}^n)\\ &\quad\to \int_0^T (\nabla_{\alpha_i}b(\alpha_0,t,z(\alpha_0,t)))^*\Xi(\theta_0,\beta,t)\nabla_{\alpha_j}b(\alpha_0,t,z(\alpha_0,t))dt.\end{aligned}$$

Checking (iii) is easily obtained since $\mathbb{E}_{\theta_0}((\zeta_k^{n,i})^4|\mathcal{G}_{k-1}^n) \le \Delta^2 \sup_{k,\beta}\|H_k(\alpha_0,\beta)\|$. Joining these results achieves the proof of Lemma 3.4.4. □

Using (3.4.8) and 3.4.9, it remains to study the term

$$\varepsilon^2\nabla_\alpha^2\check{U}_{\varepsilon,\Delta}(\alpha_0+t(\check{\alpha}_{\varepsilon,\Delta}-\alpha_0),\check{\beta}_{\varepsilon,\Delta})$$

We have $\varepsilon^2\nabla^2_{\alpha_i\alpha_j}\check{U}_{\varepsilon,\Delta}(\alpha,\beta) = \sum_{l=1}^4 A_l^{ij}$ with

$$\begin{aligned}A_1^{ij} &= \frac{2}{\Delta}\sum_{k=1}^{n}(\nabla_{\alpha_i}B_k(\alpha_0))^*\Sigma_{k-1}^{-1}(\beta)\nabla_{\alpha_j}B_k(\alpha_0),\\ A_2^{ij} &= \frac{2}{\Delta}\sum_{k=1}^{n}(\nabla_{\alpha_i}B_k(\alpha)-\nabla_{\alpha_i}B_k(\alpha_0))^*\Sigma_{k-1}^{-1}(\beta)(\nabla_{\alpha_j}B_k(\alpha)+\nabla_{\alpha_j}B_k(\alpha_0)),\\ A_3^{ij} &= 2\sum_{k=1}^{n}\frac{1}{\Delta}(\nabla^2_{\alpha_i\alpha_j}B_k(\alpha))^*\Sigma_{k-1}^{-1}(\beta)B_k(\alpha_0),\\ A_4^{ij} &= 2\Delta\sum_{k=1}^{n}\frac{1}{\Delta}(\nabla^2_{\alpha_i\alpha_j}B_k(\alpha,X))^*\Sigma_{k-1}^{-1}(\beta)\frac{1}{\Delta}(B_k(\alpha,X)-B_k(\alpha_0,X)).\end{aligned}$$

By Lemmas 3.3.6, 3.3.9 and 3.3.7, A_2^{ij} and A_4^{ij} satisfy $\left\|A_l^{ij}\right\| \le CT\|\alpha-\alpha_0\|$. Lemma 3.3.9 (ii) and Lemma 3.3.8 (ii) yield that $A_3^{ij} \to 0$.

The main term A_1^{ij} satisfies, by Lemma 3.3.9 (i),

$$A_1^{ij} = 2\Delta \sum_{k=1}^{n} (\nabla_{\alpha_i} b(\alpha_0, t_{k-1}, z(\alpha_0, t_{k-1})))^* \Sigma_{k-1}^{-1}(\beta) \nabla_{\alpha_j} b(\alpha_0, t_{k-1}, z(\alpha_0, t_{k-1}))$$
$$+ \varepsilon O_P(1).$$

Theorem 3.3.1 yields that, under $\mathbb{P}_{\theta_0}$, $\Sigma_{k-1}^{-1}(\beta) = \Sigma^{-1}(\beta, t, z(\alpha_0, t)) + \varepsilon O_P(1)$. Therefore, as a Riemann sum, we get, using (3.4.3), that $A_1^{ij} \to (I_b(\alpha_0, \beta))_{ij}$ in $\mathbb{P}_{\theta_0}$-probability as $\varepsilon, \Delta \to 0$. Joining these results, we get that, under $\mathbb{P}_{\theta_0}$, as $\varepsilon, \Delta \to 0$, for all β, $\varepsilon^2 \nabla_\alpha^2 \check{U}_{\varepsilon,\Delta}(\alpha_0, \beta) \to 2I_b(\alpha_0, \beta)$. Using now the consistency of $\check{\alpha}_{\varepsilon,\Delta}$ yields that

$$\sup_{\beta \in K_b} \left\| \varepsilon^2 \nabla_\alpha^2 \check{U}_{\varepsilon,\Delta}(\alpha_0 + t(\check{\alpha}_{\varepsilon,\Delta} - \alpha_0), \beta) - \varepsilon^2 \nabla_\alpha^2 \check{U}_{\varepsilon,\Delta}(\alpha_0, \beta) \right\| \leq K \left\| \check{\alpha}_{\varepsilon,\Delta} - \alpha_0) \right\|. \tag{3.4.15}$$

Coming back to (3.4.8), it remains to prove that $N_{\varepsilon,\Delta}(\check{\alpha}_{\varepsilon,\Delta}, \beta)$ is non-singular. Under (S3), $\Sigma(\beta, t, z)$ is non-singular. Hence,

$$\inf_{\beta \in K_b} \det \left(\left[\int_0^T \nabla_{\alpha_i} b(\alpha_0, t, z(\alpha_0, t))^* \Sigma^{-1}(\beta, t, z(\alpha_0, t)) \nabla_{\alpha_j} b(\alpha_0, t, z(\alpha_0, t) dt \right]_{1 \leq i,j \leq a} \right)$$
$$\geq \quad c \det \left(\left[\int_0^T \nabla_{\alpha_i} b(\alpha_0, t, z(\alpha_0, t))^* \nabla_{\alpha_j} b(\alpha_0, t, z(\alpha_0, t) dt \right]_{1 \leq i,j \leq a} \right) > 0.$$

Now, the consistency of $\check{\alpha}_{\varepsilon,\Delta}$ implies that, using (3.4.9), $\mathbb{P}_{\theta_0}^{\varepsilon}(\det(\varepsilon^2 N_{\varepsilon,\Delta}(\check{\alpha}, \beta)) > 0)$ tends to 1. Therefore (3.4.8) yields

$$\varepsilon^{-1}(\check{\alpha}_{\varepsilon,\Delta} - \alpha_0) = -(\varepsilon^2 N_{\varepsilon,\Delta}^{-1}(\check{\alpha}_{\varepsilon,\Delta}, \check{\beta}_{\varepsilon,\Delta})(\varepsilon \nabla_\alpha \check{U}_{\varepsilon,\Delta}(\alpha_0, \check{\beta}_{\varepsilon,\Delta}))$$

is tight. □

3.4.2.3 Step (3): Consistency of $\check{\beta}_{\varepsilon,\Delta}$

Let us now study the estimation for the diffusion parameter. Set

$$K_2(\alpha_0, \beta_0, \beta) = \frac{1}{T} \int_0^T \mathrm{Tr}\left(\Sigma^{-1}(\beta, t, z(\alpha_0, t)) \Sigma(\beta_0, t, z(\alpha_0, t))\right) dt$$
$$- \frac{1}{T} \int_0^T \log\det\left(\Sigma^{-1}(\beta, t, z(\alpha_0, t)) \Sigma(\beta_0, t, z(\alpha_0, t))\right) dt \; - p \tag{3.4.16}$$

Using the following inequality for invertible symmetric $p \times p$ matrices A, $\log\det A + p \leq \mathrm{Tr}(A)$, $K_2(\alpha_0, \beta_0, \beta) \geq 0$ and $K_2(\alpha_0, \beta_0, \beta) = 0$ if and only if

$$\{\forall t \in [0,T], \Sigma(\beta_0, t, z(\alpha_0, t)) = \Sigma(\beta, t, z(\alpha_0, t)),$$

which implies $\beta = \beta_0$ by (S7).

Proposition 3.4.5. *Assume* **(S1)–(S7)**. *Then, if* $I_b(\alpha_0,\beta_0)$ *defined in* (3.4.3) *is non-singular, the following holds in* $\mathbb{P}_{\theta_0}$*-probability, using* (3.4.1), (3.4.2) *and* (3.4.16)

(i) $\sup_{\beta\in K_b} |\frac{1}{n}\left(\check{U}_{\Delta,\varepsilon}(\check{\alpha}_{\varepsilon,\Delta},\beta) - \check{U}_{\Delta,\varepsilon}(\check{\alpha}_{\varepsilon,\Delta},\beta_0)\right) - K_2(\alpha_0,\beta_0,\beta)| \to 0$ *as* $\varepsilon,\Delta \to 0$.

(ii) $\check{\beta}_{\varepsilon,\Delta} \to \beta_0$ *as* $\varepsilon,\Delta \to 0$.

Proof. Let us first prove (i). Using (3.4.1) and (3.3.9),we get $\frac{1}{n}\left(\check{U}_{\Delta,\varepsilon}(\alpha,\beta) - \check{U}_{\Delta,\varepsilon}(\alpha,\beta_0)\right) = A_1(\beta_0,\beta) + A_2(\alpha,\beta_0,\beta)$ with

$$A_1(\beta_0,\beta) = \frac{1}{n}\sum_{k=1}^{n} log\det(\Sigma_{k-1}(\beta)\Sigma_{k-1}^{-1}(\beta_0)), \tag{3.4.17}$$

$$A_2(\alpha,\beta_0,\beta) = \frac{1}{n\Delta\varepsilon^2}\sum_{k=1}^{n} B_k(\alpha,X)^*(\Sigma_{k-1}^{-1}(\beta) - \Sigma_{k-1}^{-1}(\beta_0))B_k(\alpha,X). \tag{3.4.18}$$

Using that, under **(S5)**, $z \to \log\left(\det\left[\Sigma(\beta,t,z)\Sigma^{-1}(\beta_0,t,z)\right]\right)$ is differentiable, an application of Proposition 3.3.1 yields that, under $\mathbb{P}_{\theta_0}$,

$$A_1(\beta_0,\beta) = \frac{\Delta}{T}\left(\sum_{k=1}^{n} \log\left(\det\left[\Sigma(\beta,t_{k-1},z(\alpha_0,t_{k-1}))\Sigma^{-1}(\beta_0,t_{k-1},z(\alpha_0,t_{k-1}))\right]\right) + \varepsilon R^{1,\varepsilon}_{\theta_0,\beta}(t_{k-1})\right),$$

with $\left\|R^{1,\varepsilon}_{\alpha_0,\beta,\beta_0}\right\|$ uniformly bounded in probability. Hence, $A_1(\beta_0,\beta)$, as a Riemann sum, converges to $\frac{1}{T}\int_0^T \log\left(\det\left[\Sigma(\beta,t,z(\alpha_0,t))\Sigma^{-1}(\beta_0,t,z(\alpha_0,t))\right]\right)dt$ as $\varepsilon,\Delta \to 0$.

Applying Lemma 3.3.8 to $B_k(\alpha_0,X)$ and the notations therein yields

$$A_2(\theta_0,\theta) = \frac{\Delta}{T}\sum_{k=1}^{n} Z_k^* M_k Z_k + \sum_{i=1}^{4} \Lambda^i(\theta_0,\theta), \tag{3.4.19}$$

with

$$Z_k = \frac{1}{\sqrt{\Delta}}\left(B(t_k) - B(t_{k-1})\right), T_k = \Sigma_{k-1}^{-1}(\beta) - \Sigma_{k-1}^{-1}(\beta_0), M_k = \sigma_{k-1}^*(\beta_0)T_k\,\sigma_{k-1}(\beta_0),$$

and

$$\Lambda_1(\alpha,\theta_0) = \frac{2\sqrt{\Delta}}{\varepsilon}\sum_{k=1}^{n} E_k^* T_k\, Z_k,$$

$$\Lambda_2(\alpha,\theta_0) = \frac{1}{T\varepsilon^2}\sum_{k=1}^{n} E_k^* E_k,$$

$$\Lambda_3(\alpha,\theta_0) = \frac{2}{T\varepsilon^2}\sum_{k=1}^{n} (B_k^*(\alpha,X) - B_k^*(\alpha_0,X))T_k\, B_k(\alpha_0,X), \text{ and}$$

$$\Lambda_4(\alpha,\theta_0) = \frac{1}{T\varepsilon^2}\sum_{k=1}^{n} (B_k^*(\alpha,X) - B_k^*(\alpha_0,X))T_k\,(B_k(\alpha,X) - B_k(\alpha_0,X)).$$

The random vectors Z_k are $\mathcal{N}(0,I_p)$ independent of $\mathcal{G}_{k-1}^n$ and M_k is $\mathcal{G}_{k-1}^n$-measurable. Using that for $Z \sim \mathcal{N}(0,I_p)$, $E(Z^*MZ) = \mathrm{Tr}(M)$, we get

$$\mathbb{E}_{\theta_0}^{\varepsilon}(Z_k^* M_k Z_k|\mathcal{G}_{k-1}^n) = \mathrm{Tr}(M_k) = \mathrm{Tr}\left(\Sigma_{k-1}^{-1}(\beta)\Sigma_{k-1}(\beta_0) - I_p\right).$$

Hence, the first term of $A_2(\alpha_0,\beta_0,\beta)$ converges to

$$\frac{1}{T}\int_0^T \mathrm{Tr}\left(\Sigma^{-1}(\beta,t,z(\alpha_0,t))\Sigma(\beta_0,t,z(\alpha_0,t))\right) dt - p.$$

It remains to study the other terms of $A_2(\alpha_0,\beta_0,\beta)$. To study Λ_1, let $\zeta_k^n = \frac{\sqrt{\Delta}}{\varepsilon} E_k^* T_k Z_k$.

We have, by Lemma 3.3.8 that, in $\mathbb{P}_{\theta_0}$-probability,

$$\mathbb{E}(\zeta_k^n|\mathcal{G}_{k-1}^n) \leq \frac{\sqrt{\Delta}}{\varepsilon} \sup\|T_k\| \left(\mathbb{E}(\|E_k\|^2|\mathcal{G}_{k-1}^n)\right)^{1/2} \leq C\Delta^{3/2}, \text{ and}$$
$$\mathbb{E}((\zeta_k^n)^2|\mathcal{G}_{k-1}^n) \leq \frac{\Delta}{\varepsilon^2} \sup\|T_k\|^2 \Delta^2\varepsilon^2 \leq C\Delta^3.$$

Therefore, by Lemma A.4.3, $\Lambda_1(\alpha,\theta_0) \to 0$ in $\mathbb{P}_{\theta_0}$-probability as $\varepsilon,\Delta \to 0$. Similar arguments yield that $\Lambda_2(\alpha,\theta_0) \to 0$ in $\mathbb{P}_{\theta_0}$-probability.
For $\Lambda_3(\alpha,\theta_0)$, set $\zeta_k^n = \frac{1}{\varepsilon^2}(B_k^*(\alpha,X) - B_k^*(\alpha_0,X))T_k B_k(\alpha_0,X)$ Using Lemma 3.3.7 yields that

$$E(\zeta_k^n|\mathcal{G}_{k-1}^n) \leq \frac{\|\alpha-\alpha_0)\|}{\varepsilon}\Delta^2 O_P(1), \text{ and}$$
$$\mathbb{E}((\zeta_k^n)^2|\mathcal{G}_{k-1}^n) \leq \frac{\|\alpha-\alpha_0\|^2}{\varepsilon^2}\Delta^3 O_P(1),$$

so that $\sum \mathbb{E}(\zeta_k^n|\mathcal{G}_{k-1}^n) \leq \Delta\frac{\|\breve{\alpha}_{\varepsilon,\Delta}-\alpha_0)\|}{\varepsilon}$. By Proposition 3.4.3, the sequence $(\varepsilon^{-1}\|\breve{\alpha}_{\varepsilon,\Delta}-\alpha_0\|)$ is uniformly bounded in probability, so that $\sum \mathbb{E}(\zeta_k^n|\mathcal{G}_{k-1}^n) \to 0$ and $\sum \mathbb{E}((\zeta_k^n)^2|\mathcal{G}_{k-1}^n) \to 0$.

Another application of Lemma A.4.3 yields that $\Lambda_3(\breve{\alpha}_{\varepsilon,\Delta},\theta_0) \to 0$. For Λ_4, the result is straightforward since $|\Lambda_4| \leq n\Delta^2(\frac{\|\breve{\alpha}_{\varepsilon,\Delta}-\alpha_0\|}{\varepsilon})^2$. This achieves the proof of (i).
Let us study (ii). We have, using (3.4.16),

$$0 \leq K_2(\alpha_0,\beta_0,\breve{\beta}_{\varepsilon,\Delta}) \leq [K_2(\alpha_0,\beta_0,\breve{\beta}_{\varepsilon,\Delta}) - \frac{1}{n}(\breve{U}_{\Delta,\varepsilon}(\breve{\alpha}_{\varepsilon,\Delta},\breve{\beta}_{\varepsilon,\Delta}) - \breve{U}_{\Delta,\varepsilon}(\breve{\alpha}_{\varepsilon,\Delta},\beta_0))]$$
$$+ \frac{1}{n}(\breve{U}_{\Delta,\varepsilon}(\breve{\alpha}_{\varepsilon,\Delta},\breve{\beta}_{\varepsilon,\Delta}) - \breve{U}_{\Delta,\varepsilon}(\breve{\alpha}_{\varepsilon,\Delta},\beta_0)).$$

Noting that the last term of the above inequality is non-negative, (i) yields that $K_2(\alpha_0,\beta_0,\check{\beta}_{\varepsilon,\Delta}) \to 0$, which ensures, by Assumption (S5), that $\check{\beta}_{\varepsilon,\Delta} \to \beta_0$ in $\mathbb{P}_{\theta_0}$-probability. □

3.4.2.4 Step (4): Asymptotic Normality

Let us now study the asymptotic properties of these estimators and achieve the proof of Theorem 3.4.1. Let us define for $\theta = (\alpha,\beta)$,

$$\Lambda_{\varepsilon,n}(\theta) = \begin{pmatrix} \varepsilon \nabla_\alpha \check{U}_{\varepsilon,\Delta}(\alpha,\beta) \\ \frac{1}{\sqrt{n}} \nabla_\beta \check{U}_{\varepsilon,\Delta}(\alpha,\beta) \end{pmatrix} \quad \text{and} \tag{3.4.20}$$

$$D_{\varepsilon,n}(\theta) = \begin{pmatrix} \varepsilon^2 \left(\nabla^2_{\alpha_i,\alpha_j} \check{U}_{\varepsilon,\Delta}(\theta)\right)_{1\le i,j\le a} & \frac{\varepsilon}{\sqrt{n}} \left(\nabla^2_{\alpha_i\beta_j} \check{U}_{\varepsilon,\Delta}(\theta)\right)_{1\le i\le a, 1\le j\le b} \\ \frac{\varepsilon}{\sqrt{n}} \left(\nabla^2_{\alpha_i\beta_j} \check{U}_{\varepsilon,\Delta}(\theta)\right)_{1\le i\le a, 1\le j\le b} & \frac{1}{n} \left(\nabla^2_{\beta_i\beta_j} \check{U}_{\varepsilon,\Delta}(\theta)\right)_{1\le i,j\le b} \end{pmatrix}. \tag{3.4.21}$$

A Taylor expansion at point θ_0 yields,

$$\begin{aligned} \begin{pmatrix} 0 \\ 0 \end{pmatrix} &= \Lambda_{\varepsilon,n}(\check{\alpha}_{\varepsilon,\Delta},\check{\beta}_{\varepsilon,\Delta}) \qquad (3.4.22) \\ &= \Lambda_{\varepsilon,n}(\theta_0) + \int_0^1 D_{\varepsilon,n}(\theta_0 + t(\check{\theta}_{\varepsilon,\Delta} - \theta_0))dt \begin{pmatrix} \varepsilon^{-1}(\check{\alpha}_{\varepsilon,\Delta} - \alpha_0) \\ \sqrt{n}(\check{\beta}_{\varepsilon,\Delta} - \beta_0) \end{pmatrix}. \end{aligned}$$

Therefore, we have to prove that, under $\mathbb{P}_{\theta_0}$, as $\varepsilon,\Delta \to 0$ (or $n = \Delta^{-1/2} \to \infty$),

(i) $-\Lambda_{\varepsilon,n}(\theta_0) \to \mathcal{N}(0, 4I(\theta_0))$ in distribution,
(ii) $\sup_{t\in[0,1]} \left\| D_{\varepsilon,n}(\theta_0 + t(\check{\theta}_{\varepsilon,\Delta} - \theta_0)) - 2I(\theta_0) \right\| \to 0$ in probability.

Proof. Let us prove (i). We have that, for $1 \le i \le a$,

$$-\varepsilon \nabla_{\alpha_i} \check{U}_{\varepsilon,\Delta}(\alpha_0,\beta_0) = \sum_{k=1}^n \xi_k^i(\theta_0) \ \text{ with } \ \xi_k^i(\theta_0) = -\frac{2}{\varepsilon\Delta} B_k^*(\alpha) \Sigma_{k-1}^{-1}(\beta_0) \nabla_{\alpha_i} B_k(\alpha_0). \tag{3.4.23}$$

Using that, for a positive symmetric matrix $M(x)$,

$$\frac{d}{dx}(\log \det M(x)) = \mathrm{Tr}\left(M^{-1}(x) \frac{d}{dx} M(x) \right)$$

and (3.3.9), set

$$M_k^j(\beta) = \Sigma_k^{-1}(\beta) \nabla_{\beta_j} \Sigma_k(\beta). \tag{3.4.24}$$

Then $\frac{1}{\sqrt{n}} \nabla_{\beta_j} \check{U}_{\varepsilon,\Delta}(\alpha_0,\beta_0) = \sum_{k=1}^n \eta_k^i(\theta_0)$ with

$$\eta_k^j(\theta_0) = \frac{1}{\sqrt{n}} [\mathrm{Tr}(M_{k-1}^j(\beta_0)) - \frac{1}{\varepsilon^2\Delta} B_k^*(\alpha_0) M_{k-1}^j(\beta_0) \Sigma_{k-1}^{-1}(\beta_0) B_k(\alpha_0, X)]. \tag{3.4.25}$$

The proof that $-\varepsilon\nabla_\alpha \check{U}_{\varepsilon,\Delta}(\alpha_0,\beta_0)$ converges to the Gaussian distribution $\mathscr{N}(0,I_b(\theta_0))$ is obtained by substituting β with β_0 in the proof of Proposition 3.4.3.

Let us study $-\frac{1}{\sqrt{n}}\nabla_\beta \check{U}_{\varepsilon,\Delta}(\alpha_0,\beta_0)$. Let us first prove

Lemma 3.4.6. *If M is a $\mathscr{G}^n_{k-1}$-measurable random matrix, then*

$$\frac{1}{\varepsilon^2\Delta}\mathbb{E}\left(B_k^*(\alpha_0)M\Sigma_{k-1}^{-1}(\beta_0)B_k(\alpha_0,X)|\mathscr{G}^n_{k-1}\right)=\mathrm{Tr}(M)+\Delta R_k(\varepsilon,\Delta) \qquad (3.4.26)$$

with $\sup_k|R_k(\varepsilon,\Delta)|$ *uniformly bounded in $\mathbb{P}_{\theta_0}$-probability.*

Proof. Using Lemma 3.3.8,

$$\mathbb{E}(B_k^*(\alpha_0)M\Sigma_{k-1}^{-1}(\beta_0)B_k(\alpha_0)|\mathscr{G}^n_{k-1})=\sum_{l,l'=1}^{p}\left(M\Sigma_{k-1}^{-1}(\beta_0)\right)_{ll'}\mathbb{E}(B_k^l(\alpha_0)B_k^{l'}(\alpha_0)|\mathscr{G}^n_{k-1})$$
$$=\varepsilon^2\Delta\sum_{l,l'=1}^{p}\left(M\Sigma_{k-1}^{-1}(\beta_0)\right)_{ll'}(\Sigma_{k-1}(\beta_0))_{l'l}+\sum_{l,l'=1}^{p}\left(M\Sigma_{k-1}^{-1}(\beta_0)\right)_{ll'}\mathbb{E}(E_k^lE_k^{l'}|\mathscr{G}^n_{k-1})$$
$$=\varepsilon^2\Delta\,\mathrm{Tr}(M)+R_k(\varepsilon,\Delta)$$

with $|R_k(\varepsilon,\Delta)|\le C\varepsilon^2\Delta^2$ in probability. □

Let us study the convergence of the triangular array $\sum_{k=1}^n\mathbb{E}(\xi_k^i(\theta_0))$. By Lemma 3.4.6, we have for $j\le b$,

$$\sum_{k=1}^n\mathbb{E}(\eta_k^j(\theta_0)|\mathscr{G}^n_{k-1})=\frac{1}{\varepsilon^2\Delta\sqrt{n}}\sum_{k=1}^nR_k(\varepsilon,\Delta)\le\frac{CT}{\sqrt{n}}\to 0.$$

Consider now, for $j_1,j_2\le b$, $\sum_{k=1}^n\mathbb{E}(\eta_k^{j_1}(\theta_0)\eta_k^{j_2}(\theta_0)|\mathscr{G}^n_{k-1})$.

We have

$$\mathbb{E}(\eta_k^{j_1}(\theta_0)\eta_k^{j_2}(\theta_0)|\mathscr{G}^n_{k-1})$$
$$=\frac{1}{n}[\mathrm{Tr}(M^{j_1}_{k-1}(\beta_0)M^{j_2}_{k-1}(\beta_0))-2\mathrm{Tr}M^{j_1}_{k-1}(\beta_0))\mathrm{Tr}M^{j_2}_{k-1}(\beta_0)+C_k^{j_1,j_2}(\varepsilon,\Delta)+\Delta O_P(1)],$$

with

$$C_k^{j_1j_2}(\varepsilon,\Delta)$$
$$=\frac{1}{\varepsilon^4\Delta^2}\mathbb{E}\left(B_k^*(\alpha_0)M^{j_1}_{k-1}(\beta_0)\Sigma_{k-1}^{-1}(\beta_0)B_k(\alpha_0)B_k^*(\alpha_0)M^{j_2}_{k-1}(\beta_0)\Sigma_{k-1}^{-1}(\beta_0)B_k(\alpha_0)|\mathscr{G}^n_{k-1}\right).$$

Therefore, omitting the parameters when there is no ambiguity,

$$C_k^{j_1j_2}(\varepsilon,\Delta)$$
$$=\sum_{l_1,l_2,l_3,l_4}(M^{j_1}_{k-1}\Sigma_{k-1}^{-1})_{l_1l_2}(M^{j_2}_{k-1}\Sigma_{k-1}^{-1})_{l_3l_4}\mathbb{E}\left(B_k^{l_1}(\alpha_0)B_k^{l_2}(\alpha_0)B_k^{l_3}(\alpha_0)B_k^{l_4}(\alpha_0)|\mathscr{G}^n_{k-1}\right).$$

Based on the property that, if Z is a p-dimensional Gaussian random variable $\mathcal{N}(0,\Sigma)$, $E(Z_{l_1}Z_{l_2}Z_{l_3}Z_{l_4}) = \Sigma_{l_1l_2}\Sigma_{l_3l_4} + \Sigma_{l_1l_3}\Sigma_{l_2l_4} + \Sigma_{l_1l_4}\Sigma_{l_2l_3}$, we get that

$$C_k^{j_1j_2}(\varepsilon,\Delta) = \left(\mathrm{Tr}(M_{k-1}^{j_1}M_{k-1}^{j_2}) + 2\mathrm{Tr}M_{k-1}^{j_1}\mathrm{Tr}M_{k-1}^{j_2} + \Delta O_P(1)\right).$$

Therefore $\sum_{k=1}^n \mathbb{E}(\eta_k^{j_1}(\theta_0)\eta_k^{j_2}(\theta_0)|\mathscr{G}_{k-1}^n) = \frac{2}{n}\sum_{k=1}^n \mathrm{Tr}(M_{k-1}^{j_1}M_{k-1}^{j_2}) + \Delta O_P(1)$. Now, under $\mathbb{P}_{\theta_0}$, $M_k^j(\beta_0) = \Sigma^{-1}(\beta_0,t_k,z(\alpha_0,t_k))\nabla_{\beta_j}\Sigma(\beta_0,t_k,z(\alpha_0,t_k)) + \varepsilon O_P(1)$ so that, using (3.4.4), as $\varepsilon,\Delta \to 0$,

$$\sum_{k=1}^n \mathbb{E}(\eta_k^{j_1}(\theta_0)\eta_k^{j_2}(\theta_0)|\mathscr{G}_{k-1}^n) \to 4(I_\sigma(\theta_0))_{j_1j_2}.$$

The proofs that $\sum_{k=1}^n \mathbb{E}(\|\eta_k^i(\theta_0)\|^4|\mathscr{G}_{k-1}^n) \to 0$, $\sum_{k=1}^n \mathbb{E}(\xi_k^i(\theta_0)\eta_k^j(\theta_0)|\mathscr{G}_{k-1}^n) \to 0$ are similar and omitted. Finally, applying the theorem of convergence in law for triangular arrays recalled in Section A.4 yields that $\sum_{k=1}^n \eta_k^i(\theta_0) \to \mathcal{N}(0,4I_\sigma(\theta_0))$. Joining these results achieves the proof of (i). □

It remains to study $D_{\varepsilon,n}(\theta)$ defined in (3.4.21).

Proof. We have already proved that

$$\sup_{t\in[0,1]} \left\|\varepsilon^2(\nabla^2_{\alpha_i,\alpha_j}\check{U}_{\varepsilon,\Delta}(\theta_0 + t(\check{\theta}_{\varepsilon,\Delta} - \theta_0)) - 2(I_b(\theta_0))_{ij}\right\| \to 0$$

in probability. Consider now the term $\frac{1}{n}\nabla^2_{\beta_i,\beta_j}\check{U}_{\varepsilon,\Delta}(\alpha,\beta)$. It reads as

$$\begin{aligned}
&\nabla^2_{\beta_i\beta_j}\check{U}_{\varepsilon,\Delta}(\alpha,\beta)\\
&= \sum_{k=1}^n \left(\mathrm{Tr}\left(\nabla_{\beta_i}M_{k-1}^j(\beta)\right) - \frac{1}{\varepsilon^2\Delta}B_k(\alpha)^*(\nabla_{\beta_i}M_{k-1}^j(\beta))\Sigma_{k-1}^{-1}(\beta)B_k(\alpha)\right)\\
&+ \frac{1}{\varepsilon^2\Delta}\sum_{k=1}^n B_k(\alpha)^*M_{k-1}^j(\beta)M_{k-1}^i(\beta)\Sigma_{k-1}^{-1}(\beta)B_k(\alpha).
\end{aligned}$$

Let us define the matrices, for $1 \le i,j \le b$,

$$M^i(\alpha,\beta,t) = \Sigma^{-1}(\beta,t,z(\alpha,t))\nabla_{\beta_i}\Sigma(\beta,t,z(\alpha,t)), \quad \text{and} \tag{3.4.27}$$

$$T_k^{ij}(\beta) = [M_k^j(\beta)M_k^i(\beta) - \nabla_{\beta_i}M_k^j(\beta)]\Sigma_{k-1}^{-1}(\beta). \tag{3.4.28}$$

Using (3.4.26) yields that the first term of $\nabla^2_{\beta_i\beta_j}\check{U}_{\varepsilon,\Delta}(\alpha_0,\beta_0)$ is uniformly bounded in probability and that the second term satisfies $\sum_{k=1}^n(\mathrm{Tr}\left(M_{k-1}^j(\beta_0)M_{k-1}^i(\beta_0)\right) + \Delta O_P(1))$. Hence,

$$\frac{1}{n}\nabla^2_{\beta_i\beta_j}\check{U}_{\varepsilon,\Delta}(\alpha_0,\beta_0) \to -\frac{1}{T}\int_0^T \mathrm{Tr}(M^j(\alpha_0,\beta_0,t)M^i(\alpha_0,\beta_0,t))dt.$$

It remains to prove that, under $\mathbb{P}_{\theta_0}$,

$$\sup_{t\in[0,1]} \frac{1}{n} \left\| \nabla^2_{\beta_i\beta_j} \check{U}_{\varepsilon,\Delta}(\theta_t) - \nabla^2_{\beta_i\beta_j} \check{U}_{\varepsilon,\Delta}(\theta_0) \right\| \to 0$$

with $\theta_t = \theta_0 + t(\check{\theta}_{\varepsilon,\Delta} - \theta_0)$ and that the terms

$$\frac{\varepsilon}{\sqrt{n}} (\nabla^2_{\alpha_i\beta_j} \check{U}_{\varepsilon,\Delta}(\alpha,\beta) - \nabla^2_{\alpha_i\beta_j} \check{U}_{\varepsilon,\Delta}(\alpha_0,\beta_0)) \to 0.$$

These two proofs rely on similar tools and are omitted. □

3.5 Inference Based on Low Frequency Observations

Consider now the case where the sampling interval Δ is fixed and the time interval for observations is fixed. It follows that the number of observation points $n = T/\Delta$ is finite. We prove that only parameters in the drift function can be consistently estimated. This agrees with the previous results where the rate of estimation of parameter β in the diffusion coefficient is $\sqrt{n}$ in the high frequency set-up. Sometimes, when modeling epidemic dynamics, a parameter is added in the *SIR* model to take account of larger fluctuations, substituting the term $\sqrt{SI}$ by $(S(t)I(t))^a$ in the diffusion term. While in the "High frequency" set-up, this parameter a can be consistently estimated, this is no longer true for a fixed sampling interval.

In order to illustrate that β cannot be consistently estimated in this set-up, we study the inference on a simple example, the one-dimensional Brownian motion with drift on $[0,T]$.

3.5.1 Preliminary Result on a Simple Example

Let us consider the estimation of (α,β) as $\varepsilon \to 0$ and $n = T/\Delta$ finite, for the process

$$dX(t) = \alpha dt + \varepsilon\beta dB(t); \quad X(0) = 0. \tag{3.5.1}$$

The observations are $(X(t_k), k = 1,\dots,n)$. The n random variables $(X(t_k) - X(t_{k-1}))$ are independent Gaussian with distribution $\mathcal{N}(\alpha\Delta, \varepsilon^2\beta^2\Delta)$. The likelihood is explicit and the maximum likelihood estimators are

$$\hat{\alpha}_\varepsilon = \frac{X(T)}{T}; \quad \hat{\beta}^2_\varepsilon = \frac{1}{n\Delta\varepsilon^2} \sum_{k=1}^{n} (X(t_k) - X(t_{k-1}) - \Delta\hat{\alpha}_{\varepsilon,\Delta})^2. \tag{3.5.2}$$

Under $\mathbb{P}_{\theta_0}$, $\hat{\alpha}_\varepsilon = \alpha_0 + \varepsilon\beta_0 \frac{B(T)}{T}$. Therefore, as $\varepsilon \to 0$, $\hat{\alpha}_\varepsilon \to \alpha_0$ and $\varepsilon^{-1}(\hat{\alpha}_\varepsilon - \alpha_0) = \beta_0 \frac{B(T)}{T}$ is a Gaussian random variable $\mathcal{N}(0, \frac{\beta_0^2}{T})$.

The MLE of β_0^2 is $\hat{\beta}_\varepsilon^2 = \beta_0^2(\frac{1}{n}\sum_{k=1}^{n} Z_k^2 - \frac{1}{n}\frac{B(T)^2}{T})$, where $(Z_k, k = 1,\dots,n)$ are i.i.d. $\mathcal{N}(0,1)$.
Hence, since n is fixed, $\hat{\beta}_\varepsilon^2$ is a fixed random variable which does not depend on ε with expectation $\beta_0^2(1 - \frac{1}{n}) \neq \beta_0^2$, implying that it is a biased estimator of β_0^2.

This simple example shows that parameters in the diffusion coefficient cannot be estimated as $\varepsilon \to 0$.

3.5.2 Inference for Diffusion Approximations of Epidemics

Considering equation (3.3.1), three cases might occur: β unknown; β known or $\Sigma(\beta,x) = \phi(\beta)\Sigma(x)$ (with $\phi(\beta)$ a known real function on $\mathbb{R}^+$); β present in the drift coefficient (e.g. $\beta = \varphi(\alpha)$ with φ a known function). This last case systematically occurs for the diffusion approximation of epidemic dynamics: the parameters ruling the jump process modeling the epidemic dynamics are both present in the drift and in the diffusion coefficients, i.e. $\beta \equiv \alpha$. For example, the diffusion approximation of the *SIR*, we have, setting $\alpha = (\lambda,\gamma)$, that the drift term is $b(\alpha,z)$ and the diffusion term is $\Sigma(\alpha,z)$

Having in mind epidemics, we study here this case and assume that, under $\mathbb{P}_\alpha$,

$$dX(t) = b(\alpha,t,X(t))dt + \varepsilon\sigma(\alpha,t,X(t))dB(t), \quad X(0) = x. \tag{3.5.3}$$

The time interval is $[0,T]$, the sampling interval is Δ with $T = n\Delta$, and both T,Δ,n are fixed.

The observations consist of the n random variables $(X(t_k), k = 1,\dots,n)$ with $t_k = k\Delta$. As in the previous section, the inference is based on the random variables $B_k(\alpha,X)$ defined in (3.3.7), which satisfy using Lemma 3.3.4

$$B_k(\alpha,X) = \varepsilon\sqrt{\Delta}T_k(\alpha) + \varepsilon^2 D_k^\varepsilon(\alpha), \text{ with } D_k^\varepsilon = R^\varepsilon(\alpha,t_k) - \Phi(\alpha,t_k,t_{k-1})R^\varepsilon(\alpha,t_{k-1}). \tag{3.5.4}$$

$$T_k(\alpha) = \frac{1}{\sqrt{\Delta}}\int_{t_{k-1}}^{t_k} \Phi(\alpha,t_k,u)\sigma(\alpha,u,z(\alpha,u))dB(u), \tag{3.5.5}$$

$$S_k(\alpha) = \frac{1}{\Delta}\int_{t_{k-1}}^{t_k} \Phi(\alpha,t_k,u)\Sigma(\alpha,u,z(\alpha,u))\Phi^*(\alpha,t_k,u)du. \tag{3.5.6}$$

This leads to define the contrast function depending now on $(X(t_1),\dots,X(t_n))$,

$$\bar{U}_\varepsilon\left(\alpha,(X_{t_k})\right) = \bar{U}_\varepsilon(\alpha) = \sum_{k=1}^{n} \log\det S_k(\alpha) + \frac{1}{\varepsilon^2\Delta}\sum_{k=1}^{n} B_k^*(\alpha,X)S_k^{-1}(\alpha)B_k(\alpha,X). \tag{3.5.7}$$

Denote by α_0 the true value of the parameter and Θ the parameter set. We assume

(S4b): Θ a compact set of $\mathbb{R}^a$; $\alpha \in \mathrm{Int}(\Theta)$.
(S5b): Assumption (S5) on $b(\alpha,t,z)$ and $\sigma(\alpha,t,z)$.

(S6b): $\alpha \neq \alpha_0 \Rightarrow \{\exists k,\ 1 \leq k \leq n,\ z(\alpha, t_k) \neq z(\alpha_0, t_k)\}$.

The estimator is defined as any solution of

$$\bar{\alpha}_\varepsilon = \underset{\alpha \in K_a}{\operatorname{argmin}}\, \bar{U}_\varepsilon\left(\alpha, (X_{t_k})\right). \tag{3.5.8}$$

Let us study the properties of $\bar{\alpha}_\varepsilon$. For this, define, using (3.5.6), the $p \times a$ matrix $G_k(\alpha) = (G_k^1, \ldots, G_k^a)$ and the $a \times a$ matrix $M(\alpha)$,

$$M(\alpha) = \Delta \sum_{k=1}^{n} G_k(\alpha)^* S_k(\alpha)^{-1} G_k(\alpha), \text{ with} \tag{3.5.9}$$

$$G_k^i(\alpha) = \frac{1}{\Delta}(-\nabla_{\alpha_i} z(\alpha, t_k) + \Phi(\alpha, t_k, t_{k-1})\nabla_{\alpha_i} z(\alpha, t_{k-1})). \tag{3.5.10}$$

Then, the following holds

Theorem 3.5.1. *Assume (S1)–(S3), (S4b)–(S6b). Then, as $\varepsilon \to 0$, under $\mathbb{P}_{\alpha_0}$,*

(i) $\bar{\alpha}_\varepsilon \to \alpha_0$ in probability.
(ii) If moreover $M(\alpha_0)$ defined in (3.5.9) *is non-singular, then*

$$\varepsilon^{-1}(\bar{\alpha}_\varepsilon - \alpha_0) \to \mathcal{N}_a(0, M^{-1}(\alpha_0))$$

in distribution.

Proof. Let us first prove (i). Define, using (3.5.4), (3.5.6),

$$\bar{K}_\Delta(\alpha_0, \alpha) = \frac{1}{\Delta} \sum_{k=1}^{n} B_k^*(\alpha, z(\alpha_0, \cdot)) S_k^{-1}(\alpha) B_k(\alpha, z(\alpha_0, \cdot)). \tag{3.5.11}$$

Since $B_k(\alpha_0, z(\alpha_0, \cdot)) = 0$, $\bar{K}_\Delta(\alpha_0, \alpha) \geq 0$ and $\bar{K}_\Delta(\alpha_0, \alpha_0) = 0$. Assume now that $\bar{K}_\Delta(\alpha_0, \alpha) = 0$. Then, for all $k \in \{1, ..n\}$,

$$z(\alpha, t_k) - z(\alpha_0, t_k) = \Phi(\alpha, t_k, t_{k-1})(z(\alpha, t_{k-1}) - z(\alpha_0, t_{k-1})).$$

The matrix $\Phi(\alpha, t_k, t_{k-1})$ being non-singular, the identifiability Assumption **(S6b)** implies that $\alpha = \alpha_0$.
Since the sum in (3.5.7) is finite, we get, using (3.3.7) and Proposition 3.3.1, that $\sup_{\alpha \in K_a} |\varepsilon^2 \bar{U}_\varepsilon(\alpha) - \bar{K}_\Delta(\alpha_0, \alpha)| \to 0$ in $\mathbb{P}_{\theta_0}$-probability as $\varepsilon \to 0$. Therefore, we have

$$\begin{aligned} 0 &\leq \bar{K}_\Delta(\alpha_0, \bar{\alpha}_\varepsilon) - \bar{K}_\Delta(\alpha_0, \alpha_0) \\ &\leq 2 \sup_{\alpha \in K_a} |\varepsilon^2 U_\varepsilon(\alpha) - \bar{K}_\Delta(\alpha_0, \alpha)| + \varepsilon^2 |U_\varepsilon(\bar{\alpha}) - U_\varepsilon(\alpha_0)| \\ &\leq 2 \sup_{\alpha \in K_a} |\varepsilon^2 U_\varepsilon(\alpha) - \bar{K}_\Delta(\alpha_0, \alpha)|. \end{aligned}$$

Then the proof of (i) is achieved by means of the identifiability Assumption **(S6b)**.

Let us now prove (ii). To study the asymptotic properties of $\bar{\alpha}_\varepsilon$ as $\varepsilon \to 0$, we write, for $i, j \leq a$,

$$
\begin{aligned}
0 &= \varepsilon \nabla_{\alpha_i} \bar{U}_\varepsilon(\bar{\alpha}_\varepsilon) \\
&= \varepsilon \nabla_{\alpha_i} \bar{U}_\varepsilon(\alpha_0) + \varepsilon^2 \sum_{j=1}^{a} \Big(\int_0^1 (\nabla^2_{\alpha_j \alpha_i} \bar{U}_\varepsilon(\alpha_0 + t(\bar{\alpha}_\varepsilon - \alpha_0)) dt \Big) \Big(\frac{\bar{\alpha}^j_\varepsilon - \alpha^j_0}{\varepsilon} \Big).
\end{aligned}
$$

Consider first $\varepsilon \nabla_\alpha \bar{U}_\varepsilon(\alpha_0)$. Using (3.3.7) and (3.5.6), for $i = 1, \dots, a$, it reads as

$$
\begin{aligned}
\varepsilon \nabla_{\alpha_i} \bar{U}_\varepsilon(\alpha_0) &= \varepsilon \sum_{k=1}^{n} \nabla_{\alpha_i} \log \det S_k(\alpha_0) + \frac{1}{\varepsilon \Delta} \sum_{k=1}^{n} B_k^*(\alpha_0) \nabla_{\alpha_i} S_k^{-1}(\alpha_0) B_k(\alpha_0) \\
&+ \frac{2}{\varepsilon \Delta} \sum_{k=1}^{n} (\nabla_{\alpha_i} B_k^*(\alpha_0)) \, S_k^{-1}(\alpha_0) B_k(\alpha_0) = A_1^i(\alpha_0) + A_2^i(\alpha_0) + A_3^i(\alpha_0).
\end{aligned}
$$

Since $\nabla_{\alpha_i} \log(\det S_k(\alpha_0)) = \mathrm{Tr}(S_k^{-1}(\alpha_0) \nabla_{\alpha_i} S_k(\alpha_0))$, $A_1^i(\alpha_0)$ is well defined and, under the regularity assumptions, $A_1^i(\alpha_0) = n\varepsilon O(1)$, which goes to 0 as $\varepsilon \to 0$, n being fixed.

Applying Lemma 3.3.4 for the variables $T_k(\alpha_0)$, $D_k^\varepsilon(\alpha_0)$ yields that

$$
\begin{aligned}
A_2^i(\alpha_0) &= \varepsilon \sum_{k=1}^{n} T_k^*(\alpha_0) \nabla_{\alpha_i} S_k^{-1}(\alpha_0) T_k(\alpha_0) \\
&+ 2 \frac{\varepsilon}{\sqrt{\Delta}} \sum_{k=1}^{n} T_k^*(\alpha_0) \nabla_{\alpha_i} S_k^{-1}(\alpha_0) (\varepsilon D_k^\varepsilon(\alpha_0)) \\
&+ \frac{\varepsilon}{\Delta} \sum_{k=1}^{n} (\varepsilon D_k^\varepsilon(\alpha_0))^* \nabla_{\alpha_i} S_k^{-1}(\alpha_0) (\varepsilon D_k^\varepsilon(\alpha_0)).
\end{aligned}
$$

It follows from Lemma 3.3.4, that $\sup_k \left\| \varepsilon D_k^\varepsilon(\alpha_0) \right\|$ is bounded. Therefore, $A_2^i(\alpha_0) \to 0$ in $\mathbb{P}_{\alpha_0}$-probability.

Let us study the main term $(A_3^i(\alpha)$ of $\varepsilon \nabla_{\alpha_i} \bar{U}_\varepsilon(\alpha_0)$.
Using Proposition 3.3.1 and (3.3.7), (3.5.10) yields that, under $\mathbb{P}_{\alpha_0}$,

$$
\nabla_{\alpha_i} B_k(\alpha_0) = \Delta G_k^i(\alpha_0) - \varepsilon (\nabla_{\alpha_i} \Phi(\alpha_0, t_k, t_{k-1})(g(\alpha_0, t_{k-1}) + \varepsilon R^\varepsilon(\alpha_0, t_{k-1}))), \tag{3.5.12}
$$

where $\sup_k \|\varepsilon R(\alpha, t_k)\|$ is uniformly bounded in probability. Therefore,

$$
A_3^i(\alpha_0) = 2\sqrt{\Delta} \sum_{k=1}^{n} ((G_k^i(\alpha_0))^* S_k^{-1}(\alpha_0) T_k(\alpha_0) + \varepsilon R_k'(\alpha_0)),
$$

with $R_k'(\alpha_0)$ uniformly bounded in probability. By Lemma 3.3.4, $(T_k(\alpha_0)), k = 1, \dots, n)$ are independent centered Gaussian random variables with covariance matrix $S_k(\alpha_0)$. We that $A_3(\alpha_0) = (A_3^1(\alpha_0), \dots, A_3(\alpha_0))^*$ converges to the Gaussian random variable $\mathcal{N}_a(0, 4M(\alpha_0))$. Joining all these results yields that

$$
-\varepsilon \nabla_\alpha \bar{U}_\varepsilon(\alpha_0) \to \mathcal{N}_a(0, 4M(\alpha_0)) \text{ with}
$$

$$
M(\alpha_0) = (M(\alpha_0))_{ij} = \Delta \sum_{k=1}^{n} (G_k^i(\alpha_0))^* S_k^{-1}(\alpha_0) G_k^j(\alpha_0).
$$

Consider $\varepsilon^2\nabla^2_{\alpha_j\alpha_i}\bar{U}_\varepsilon(\alpha)$. Similar computations yield that

$$\varepsilon^2\nabla^2_{\alpha_j\alpha_i}\bar{U}_\varepsilon(\alpha_0) = 2\Delta\sum_{k=1}^{n}(G^i_k(\alpha_0))^* S_k^{-1}(\alpha_0)G^j_k(\alpha_0) + n\varepsilon O_P(1).$$

Therefore, for all $1 \le i, j \le a$,

$$\varepsilon^2\nabla^2_{\alpha_i\alpha_j}\bar{U}_\varepsilon(\alpha_0) \to 2M_{ij}(\alpha_0) \quad \mathbb{P}_{\alpha_0}\text{a.s. as } \varepsilon \to 0.$$

It remains to study $\sup_{t\in[0,1]}|\varepsilon^2\nabla^2_{\alpha_j\alpha_i}\bar{U}_\varepsilon(\alpha_0+t(\bar{\alpha}_\varepsilon-\alpha_0)) - \varepsilon^2\nabla^2_{\alpha_j\alpha_j}\bar{U}_\varepsilon(\alpha_0)|$. We have $\varepsilon^2\nabla^2_{\alpha_j\alpha_i}\bar{U}_\varepsilon(\alpha) = \frac{1}{\Delta}(A^{ij}_1(\alpha)+A^{ij}_2(\alpha))$, where

$$A^{ij}_1(\alpha) = 2\sum_{k=1}^{n}\nabla_{\alpha_i}B^*_k(\alpha)S_k^{-1}(\alpha)\nabla_{\alpha_j}B_k(\alpha), \quad A^{ij}_2(\alpha) = \sum_{k=1}^{n}Z^*_k(\alpha)B_k(\alpha)$$

with

$$\begin{aligned}Z^*_k(\alpha) = {} & 2\nabla_{\alpha_j}B^*_k(\alpha)\nabla_{\alpha_i}S_k^{-1}(\alpha) + B^*_k(\alpha)\nabla^2_{\alpha_i\alpha_j}S_k^{-1}(\alpha) + 2\nabla_{\alpha_i}B^*_k(\alpha)\nabla_{\alpha_j}S_k^{-1}(\alpha)\\ & + 2\nabla^2_{\alpha_i\alpha_j}B^*_k(\alpha)S_k^{-1}(\alpha).\end{aligned}$$

Similarly to the previous section, we need that, under $\mathbb{P}_{\alpha_0}$, the properties stated below hold.

$$\|B_k(\alpha) - B_k(\alpha_0)\| \le \|\alpha-\alpha_0\|(C_1 + C_2 O_P(1)) \text{ uniformly with respect to } k, \alpha; \tag{3.5.13}$$

$$\left\|\frac{1}{\varepsilon}B_k(\alpha_0)\right\| \text{ are uniformly bounded random variables;} \tag{3.5.14}$$

$$\cdot\sup_{k\le n,\alpha\in\Theta}\|\nabla_{\alpha_i}B_k(\alpha)\| = O_P(1); \quad \text{and } \|\nabla_{\alpha_i}B_k(\alpha) - \nabla_{\alpha_i}B_k(\alpha_0\| \le C_1\|\alpha-\alpha_0\|. \tag{3.5.15}$$

The proofs of these properties are similar to the previous section and omitted.

Therefore,

$$A^{ij}_2(\alpha) - A^{ij}_2(\alpha_0) = \sum_{k=1}^{n}(Z^*_k(\alpha)-Z^*_k(\alpha_0))B_k(\alpha_0) + \sum_{k=1}^{n}Z^*_k(\alpha)(B_k(\alpha)-B_k(\alpha_0)).$$

Using (3.5.13), (3.5.14) we get

$$|A^{ij}_2(\alpha) - A^{ij}_2(\alpha_0)| \le \sup\|Z_k(\alpha)\|\,(2n\varepsilon\sup\left\|\frac{B_k(\alpha_0)}{\varepsilon}\right\| + \|\alpha-\alpha_0\|(C_1+C_2O_P(1)).$$

Consider now $A^{ij}_1(\alpha) - A^{ij}_1(\alpha_0)$. It reads as

$$A_1^{ij}(\alpha) - A_1^{ij}(\alpha_0) = 2\sum_{k=1}^{n} [\nabla_{\alpha_i} B_k^*(\alpha) S_k^{-1}(\alpha)(\nabla_{\alpha_j} B_k(\alpha) - \nabla_{\alpha_j} B_k(\alpha_0))]$$
$$+ [\nabla_{\alpha_j} B_k^*(\alpha) S_k^{-1}(\alpha)(\nabla_{\alpha_i} B_k(\alpha) - \nabla_{\alpha_i} B_k(\alpha_0))]$$
$$+ [\nabla_{\alpha_i} B_k^*(\alpha)(S_k^{-1}(\alpha) - S_k^{-1}(\alpha_0))\nabla_{\alpha_j} B_k(\alpha_0)].$$

Hence, $\left\| A_1 ij(\alpha) - A_1^{ij}(\alpha_0) \right\| \leq 2nC \|\alpha - \alpha_0\|$.

Using the consistency $\bar{\alpha}_\varepsilon$, we get that

$$\sup_{t\in[0,1]} |\varepsilon^2 \nabla^2_{\alpha_j\alpha_i)} \bar{U}_\varepsilon(\alpha_0 + t(\bar{\alpha}_\varepsilon - \alpha_0)) - \varepsilon^2 \nabla^2_{\alpha_j\alpha_j} \bar{U}_\varepsilon(\alpha_0)| \to 0.$$

This achieves the proof of (ii) and of Theorem 3.5.1. □

3.5.2.1 Comments

(1) The term $\sum_{k=1}^n \log\det S_k(\alpha)$ could have been omitted in the definition of $\bar{U}_\varepsilon(\alpha)$. It has no influence on the asymptotic properties of $\bar{\alpha}_\varepsilon$. However, we have observed in the simulation results that it yields better estimators (less biased). An explanation lies in the fact that in practice ε is small, but probably not enough to compensate this first term. the observations of less biased estimators non-asymptotically.

(2) In [60], we considered the case of an unknown parameter β in the diffusion coefficient and therefore used a Conditional Least Square estimator based on $U_\varepsilon(\alpha) = \sum_{k=1}^n B_k^*(\alpha) B_k(\alpha)$. The CLS estimator obtained is consistent. It converges at the same rate, but with a larger covariance matrix $J_\Delta^{-1}(\alpha) I_\Delta(\alpha) J_\Delta^{-1}(\alpha)$ with $J_\Delta^{ij} = \sum_{k=1}^n (G_k^i(\alpha))^* G_k^j(\alpha)$ and $I_\Delta(\alpha) = \sum_{k=1}^n (G_k^i(\alpha))^* S_k(\alpha) G_k^j(\alpha)$.

(3) We can compare the result of Theorem 3.5.1 to the inference of an unknown parameter in the drift coefficient for a continuously observed diffusion on $[0,T]$ in the asymptotics $\varepsilon \to 0$. According to [91], assuming a known diffusion coefficient $\varepsilon\sigma(x)$, the Maximum Likelihood Estimator is consistent and the Fisher information matrix is

$$(I_b(\alpha_0,\beta_0))_{ij} = \int_0^T (\nabla_{\alpha_i} b(\alpha_0, z(\alpha_0,s)))^* \Sigma^{-1}(z(\alpha_0,s)) \nabla_{\alpha_j} b(\alpha_0, z(\alpha_0,s)) ds. \tag{3.5.16}$$

To compare the estimator $\bar{\alpha}_{\varepsilon,\Delta}$ with the CLS estimator, we can study the limits of the two Information matrices when Δ goes to zero. Using that $z(\alpha,\cdot)$ satisfies the ODE (3.2.8), we have,

$$G_k(\alpha_0) = -\nabla_\alpha b(\alpha_0, z(\alpha_0, t_{k-1})) + o_\Delta(1), \text{ as } \Delta \text{ goes to zero.} \tag{3.5.17}$$

This result together with Lemma 3.3.5 implies that $I_\Delta(\alpha_0,\beta_0) \to I_b(\alpha_0,\beta_0)$ as $\Delta \to 0$. Since $I_b(\alpha_0,\beta_0)$ is the optimal information matrix for continuous time observation, this convergence provides some kind of optimality result for fixed Δ.

Consider now the covariance matrix of the CLS estimator. We have, $\varepsilon \to 0$,

$$(J_\Delta(\alpha))_{ij} \to \int_0^T \nabla_{\alpha_i} b(\alpha_0, z(\alpha_0,t))^* \nabla_{\alpha_j} b(\alpha_0, z(\alpha_0,t))dt, \text{ and}$$

$$(I_\Delta(\alpha))_{ij} \to \int_0^T \nabla_{\alpha_i} b(\alpha_0, z(\alpha_0,t))^* \Sigma(\beta_0, z(\alpha_0,t)) \nabla_{\alpha_j} b(\alpha_0, z(\alpha_0,t))dt.$$

This clearly differs from the optimal asymptotic variance and confirms that the CLS estimator is not efficient. However, it might be easier to minimize the CLS function $\sum_{k=1}^n G_k(\alpha)^* G_k(\alpha)$ than the actual contrast function $\sum_{k=1}^n G_k(\alpha)^* S_{k-1}^{-1}(\alpha) G_k(\alpha)$. Therefore this CLS estimator can be useful to serve as an initialization for other computations or algorithms.

3.6 Assessment of Estimators on Simulated Data Sets

We consider two examples of epidemic dynamics, the *SIR* and the *SIRS* presented in the first part of these notes and recalled in Section 3.2.2 for the diffusion approximation. We used the Gillespie algorithm (see Part I of these notes) to simulate the *SIR* epidemic dynamics $(\mathscr{Z}^N(t), 0 \le t \le T)$ and, for the *SIRS* model, the τ-leaping method ([21]), which is more efficient for large populations.

As pointed in the introduction, diffusion approximations are relevant in case of a major outbreak in a large community. Therefore, we keep only in the analysis what we called "non-extinct trajectories", chosen according to a frequently used empirical criterion: we keep epidemic trajectories such that the final epidemic size is larger than the observed empirical size minus the standard empirical error of the final epidemic size.

The inference is based only on non-extinct trajectories . Since we possess, for each simulation, the whole sample path of the epidemic process, we can compute the maximum likelihood estimator (see Chapter 4 of this part) which depends on the whole path of the jump process. For instance, for the *SIR* case, the MLE is

$$\hat{\lambda}_N = \frac{1}{N} \frac{\#\,\text{Infections}}{\int_0^T S^N(t) I^N(t) dt}; \quad \hat{\gamma}_N = \frac{1}{N} \frac{\#\,\text{Recoveries}}{\int_0^T I^N(t) dt}. \tag{3.6.1}$$

We call this MLE based on complete epidemic data **the reference estimator**. This is the best result that can be achieved from these epidemic data.

In order to investigate the influence of various parameters, we consider various scenarios. Each scenario corresponds to the choice of the model, the parameters θ, the population size N, the time interval of observation $[0, T]$ and the sampling interval Δ. We proceeded to 1000 repetitions for each scenario.
Hence, we varied the total size of the population N, the parameters ruling the *SIR*, *SIRS* epidemics, the time interval for observations $[0, T]$. Then, we sampled with sampling Δ each path of the Markov jump process. This sampling interval also

varies. Therefore the observations coming from the simulations are

$$\frac{\mathscr{Z}^N(k\Delta)}{N} = Z^N(k\Delta)\ k = 1,\dots,n \text{ with } T = n\Delta.$$

Each scenario corresponds to the choice of the model, the parameters θ, the population size N, the time interval of observation $[0,T]$ and the sampling interval Δ.

We compare the estimators obtained with the method described in the two previous sections with the MLE (3.6.1). The properties of our minimum contrast estimators are assessed and compared to reference estimators.
For parameters with dimension greater than two, confidence ellipsoids are projected on planes, by considering all pairs of parameters. Theoretical confidence ellipsoids are built as follows. Let $V(\theta_0)$ denote the covariance matrix of the asymptotic normal distribution of parameters estimation in drift term (i.e. $I_b^{-1}(\theta_0)$ defined in (3.4.3) and $M^{-1}(\theta_0)$ defined in (3.5.9). Since $\varepsilon^{-1}V(\theta_0)^{-1/2}(\hat{\theta}_{\varepsilon,\Delta} - \theta_0) \to_{\mathscr{L}} \mathscr{N}(0,I_k)$ (where $\hat{\theta}_{\varepsilon,\Delta}$ represents $\check{\alpha}_{\varepsilon,\Delta}$ obtained minimizing (3.4.1) or $\bar{\eta}_{\varepsilon,\Delta}$ in (3.5.8) Then, for $k = a$ (dimension of α), we have,

$$\frac{1}{\varepsilon^2}(\hat{\theta}_{\varepsilon,\Delta} - \theta_0)^* V(\theta_0)^{-1}(\hat{\theta}_{\varepsilon,\Delta} - \theta_0) \to_{\mathscr{L}} \chi_2(k). \tag{3.6.2}$$

The matrix $V(\theta_0)^{-1}$ being positive, the quantity $(\hat{\theta}_{\varepsilon,\Delta} - \theta_0)^* V(\theta_0)^{-1}(\hat{\theta}_{\varepsilon,\Delta} - \theta_0)$ is the squared norm of vector $\hat{\theta}_{\varepsilon,\Delta} - \theta_0$ for the scalar product associated to $V(\theta_0)^{-1}$. If we denote by $\chi_k^2(0.95)$ the 95% quantile of the χ_k^2 distribution, the relation (3.6.2) could be rewritten as $||(\hat{\theta}_{\varepsilon,\Delta} - \theta_0)^2 M(\theta_0)^{-1}|| \leq \varepsilon^2 \chi_k^2(0.95)$ and define an ellipsoid in $\mathbb{R}^k$.
Empirical confidence ellipsoids are based on the variance-covariance matrix of centered estimators (based on 1000 independent estimations), whose eigenvalues define the axes of ellipsoids.
In the two epidemic models detailed below, we assume both components of $Z^N(t) = S^N(t), I^N(t)$ are observed with sampling interval Δ, $((S^N(k\Delta), I^N(k\Delta)), k = 1,\dots n)$ with $T = n\Delta$.

3.6.1 The SIR Model

The parameters of interest for epidemics are considered following a reparameterization: the basic reproduction number, $R_0 = \frac{\lambda}{\gamma}$, which represents the average number of secondary cases generated by one infectious in a completely susceptible population, and the average infectious duration, $d = \frac{1}{\gamma}$. Two values were tested for $R_0 = \{1.5, 5\}$ and d was set to 3 (in days, an average value consistent with influenza infection). Three values for the population size $N = \{400, 1000, 10000\}$ and of the number of observations $n = \{5, 10, 40\}$ were considered, along with two values for the final time of observation, $T = \{20, 40\}$ (in days). For each scenario defined by a combination of parameters, the analytical maximum likelihood estimator (*MLE*), calculated from the observation of all the jumps of the Markov process (see 4), was taken as reference.

Effect of the parameter values $\{R_0, d\}$ *and of the number of observations n*
The accuracy of the two estimators $\breve{\alpha}_{\varepsilon,\Delta}$ and $\bar{\alpha}_{\varepsilon}$, for $N = 1000$ and from trajectories with weak ($R_0 = 5$) and strong ($R_0 = 1.5$) stochasticity is illustrated in Figure 3.6.1. We observe that R_0 and d are moderately correlated (ellipsoids are deviated with respect to the x-axis and y- axis). The shape of confidence ellipsoids depends on parameter values: for $R_0 = 5$, the 95% confidence interval is larger for R_0 than for d, whereas the opposite occurs for $R_0 = 1.5$. For $R_0 = 5$, all these confidence intervals are almost superimposed, which suggests that the estimation accuracy is not altered by the fact that all the jumps are not observed. However, for $R_0 = 1.5$ the shape of ellipsoids varies with n. Point estimates for *MLE* derived for complete observation of $(\mathscr{Z}^N(t)$ of the original jump process and the estimators $\breve{\alpha}_{\varepsilon,\Delta}$, $\bar{\alpha}_{\varepsilon}$ are very similar for different values of n, which confirms the interest of using these estimators when small number of observations is available.

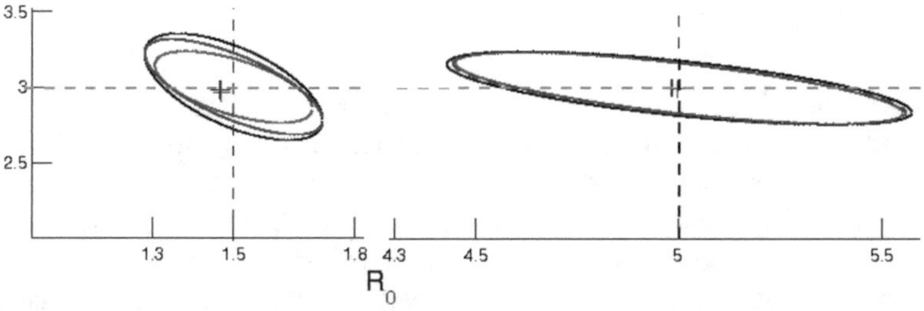

Fig. 3.6.1 Point estimators (+) are computed by averaging over 1000 independent simulated trajectories of the *SIR* stochastic model (completely observed) together with their associated theoretical confidence ellipses centered on the true value: *MLE* with complete observations (red), *CE* for one observation/day, $n = 40$ (blue) and *CE* for $n = 10$ (black). Two scenarios are illustrated: $(R_0, d, T) = \{(1.5, 3, 40); (5, 3, 20)\}$, with $N = 1000$. For both scenarios $(S(0), I(0)) = (0.99, 0.01)$.The value of d is reported on the y-axis. Horizontal and vertical dotted lines cross at the true value

.

Effect of the parameter values $\{R_0, d\}$ *and of the population size N* From Figure 3.6.2, we can notice that $\sqrt{N}$ has an impact on estimation accuracy (the width of the confidence intervals decreases with $\sqrt{N}$). The case of very few observations ($n = 5$) leads to the largest confidence intervals. The *MLE* appears biased for $N = 400$. This could be due to the fact that the *MLE* is optimal when data represent a 'typical' realization (i.e. a trajectory that emerges leading to a non-negligible number of infected individuals) of the Markov process, but could yield a bias when observations are far from the average behaviour. Our *CE*s seem robust to the departure from the 'typical' behaviour (i.e. for noisy trajectories obtained either for small N or small R_0).

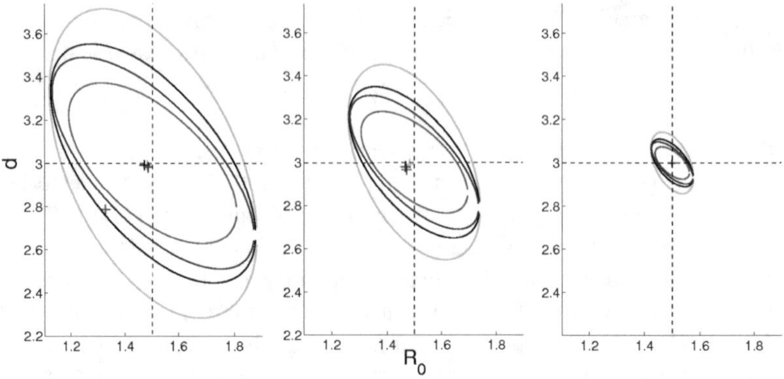

Fig. 3.6.2 Point estimators (+) computed by averaging over 1000 independent simulated trajectories of the *SIR* stochastic model completely observed and their associated theoretical confidence ellipses centered on the true value: *MLE* with complete observations (red), *CE* for one observation/day, $n = 40$ (blue), *CE* for $n = 10$ (black) and *CE* for $n = 5$ (green) for $(S(0), I(0)) = (0.99, 0.01)$, $(R_0, d) = (1.5, 3)$ and $N = \{400, 1000, 10000\}$ (from left to right). Horizontal and vertical dotted lines cross at the true value.

3.6.2 The SIRS Model

For the *SIRS* model introduced in Section 3.2.2.2, four parameters were estimated: R, d, λ_1 and δ. Concerning the remaining parameters,μ was set to $1/50$ years^{-1} (a value usually considered in epidemic models), T_{per} was set to 365 days (corresponding to annual epidemics) and η was taken equal to 10^{-6} (which corresponds to 10 individuals in a population size of $N = 10^7$). We should notice that instead of estimating the real R_0 (more complicated to calculate for periodical dynamics), we prefer to estimate a parameter combination similar to the R_0 for *SIR* model, λ_0/γ, which was called here R.The performances of *CE*s were assessed on parameter combinations: $(R, d, \lambda_1, \delta) = \{(1.5, 3, 0.05, 2)$ and $(1.5, 3, 0.15, 2)\}$ and $T = 20$ years, with $\lambda_1 = 0.05$ leading to annual cycles and $\lambda_1 = 0.15$ to biennial dynamics (Figure 3.2.2). Numerically, the scenarios considered are consistent with influenza seasonal outbreaks. The accuracy of estimation is relatively high, as illustrated in Figure 3.6.3, regardless of the parameter. For one observation per day (which can be assimilated to a limit of data availability), the accuracy is very similar to the one based on a complete observation of the epidemic process (blue and red ellipsoids respectively). Estimations based on one observation per week are less but still reasonably accurate.

3.7 Inference for Partially Observed Epidemic Dynamics

In the case of epidemics, numbers of susceptible and infected individuals over time are generally not observed. In practice, (sometimes noisy) observations are often assumed to correspond to cumulated numbers, over the sampling interval Δ, of newly

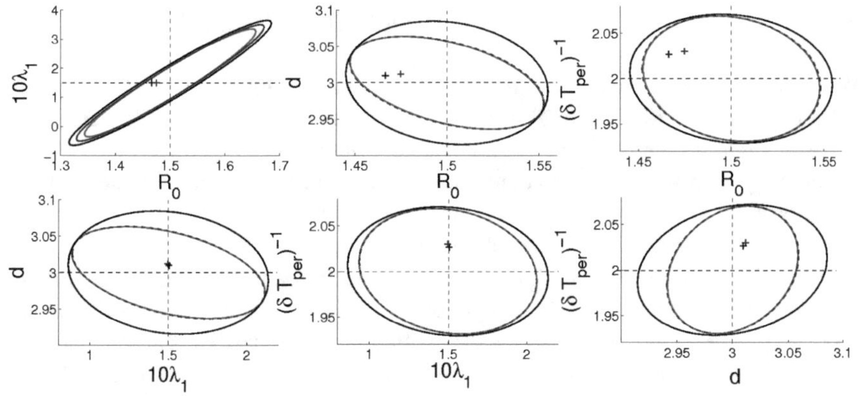

Fig. 3.6.3 Point estimators (+) computed by averaging over 1000 independent simulated trajectories of the *SIRS* stochastic model with demography and seasonal forcing in transmission, completely observed (red), and their associated planar projections of theoretical confidence ellipsoids centered on the true value: *CE* for one observation/day (blue) and for one observation/week (black) for $(R,d,\lambda_1,\delta) = (1.5,3,0.15,2)$, $T = 20$ years and $N = 10^7$. Asymptotic confidence ellipsoids ($n \to \infty$) are also represented (red,blue,black). Horizontal and vertical dotted lines cross at the true value.

infected individuals (i.e. $\int_{t_{k-1}}^{t_k} \lambda S(s)I(s)ds$). In the *SIR* diffusion model, this corresponds to the recovered individuals $\{(R(t_k) - R(t_{k-1})), k = 1,\dots n\}$ for diseases with short duration of the infected period. Hence, this situation can be assimilated, as a first attempt, to the case where only one coordinate can be observed.

In this section, we consider the case of a two-dimensional diffusion process $X(t) = (X_1(t), X_2(t))^*$

$$dX(t) = b(\alpha, X(t))dt + \varepsilon\sigma(\beta, X(t)dB(t))dt; \quad X(0) = x, \tag{3.7.1}$$

where $B(t)$ is a Brownian motion on $\mathbb{R}^2$ and x non-random.

We assume that only the first coordinate $X_1(t)$ is observed on a fixed time interval $[0,T]$ with sampling Δ. We consider the diffusion on $\mathbb{R}^2$ satisfying the stochastic differential equation Therefore, the observations are now

$$X_1(t_k),\ k = 1,\dots n, \quad \text{with } t_k = k\Delta, \quad T = n\Delta. \tag{3.7.2}$$

For continuous observations of $(X_1(t))$ on a finite time interval $[0,T]$, two studies [79], [92] are concerned with parametric inference in this statistical framework. Both studied the maximum likelihood estimator of parameters in the drift function for a diffusion matrix equal to $\varepsilon^2 I_p$. This likelihood is difficult to compute since it relies on integration on the unobserved coordinate. [79], [92] proposed filtering approaches to compute this likelihood, as it is done for general Hidden Markov Models (see e.g. [22] , [37]). Here, we can take advantage of the presence of ε and extend to partial observations the method by contrast processes and M- estimators that had been developed for complete observations ([46], [56], [60]), [118]).

We study the case of small (or high frequency) sampling interval, $\Delta = \Delta_n \to 0$, on a fixed time interval $[0,T]$ with $T = n\Delta$, which yields explicit results. This allows us to disentangle problems coming from discrete observations and those coming from the missing observation of one coordinate and hence provides a better understanding of the problems rising in this context. The case of Δ fixed could be studied similarly, with more cumbersome notations and no such insights .

First, the notations required are introduced, results are then stated, and finally, to illustrate this approach, the example of a two-dimensional Ornstein–Uhlenbeck process, where all the computations are explicit is developed. The consequences on diffusion approximations of Epidemic models where computations are no longer explicit are detailed later.

3.7.1 *Inference for High Frequency Sampling of Partial Observations*

Some specific notations need to be introduced.
For $x \in \mathbb{R}^2$, $X^\varepsilon(t)$, the diffusion process, $B(t)$ the Brownian motion, and M a 2×2 matrix, we write

$$x = \begin{pmatrix} x_1 \\ x_2 \end{pmatrix}; \; X(t) = \begin{pmatrix} X_1(t) \\ X_2(t) \end{pmatrix}; \; B(t) = \begin{pmatrix} B_1(t) \\ B_2(t) \end{pmatrix}; \; M = \begin{pmatrix} M_{11} & M_{12} \\ M_{21} & M_{22} \end{pmatrix}. \tag{3.7.3}$$

For functions $f(\theta,x)$ defined for $x \in \mathbb{R}^2$, we use (3.3.3) for differentiating with respect to x and (3.3.3), (3.3.4) for differentiation with respect to θ.
The observations are $(X_1(k\Delta), k = 0,\dots n)$. Since x_2 is not observed and unknown, we add it to the parameters. Therefore, setting $x_2 = \xi$, define using (S4),

$$\eta = (\alpha,\xi) \in \mathbb{R}^{a+1}; \quad \theta = (\alpha,\xi,\beta) = (\eta,\beta) \in \mathbb{R}^{a+b+1}. \tag{3.7.4}$$

The quantities introduced in (3.2.15) depend on α, η or θ and can be written, using (3.7.3), The expansion of $X(t)$ stated in (3.2.15) yields that $X_1(t)$ satisfies, using notations (3.7.3),

$$X_1(t) = z_1(\eta,t) + \varepsilon g_1(\theta,t) + \varepsilon^2 R_1^\varepsilon(\theta,t) \text{ with} \tag{3.7.5}$$

$$\begin{aligned} g_1(\theta,t) = \int_0^t & (\Phi(\eta,t,u)\sigma(\beta,z(\eta,u)))_{11}\, dB_1(u) \\ & + (\Phi(\eta,t,u)\sigma(\beta,z(\eta,u)))_{12}\, dB_2(u). \end{aligned} \tag{3.7.6}$$

Using that $\Phi(t,u) = \Phi(t,s)\Phi(s,u)$ yields another expression for $g_1(\theta,t_k)$,

$$g_1(\theta,t_k) = (\Phi(\eta,t_k,t_{k-1})g(\theta,t_{k-1}))_1$$

$$+\int_{t_{k-1}}^{t_k} (\Phi(\eta,t,u)\sigma(\beta,z(\eta,u)))_{11}\, dB_1(u)$$
$$+ (\Phi(\eta,t,u)\sigma(\beta,z(\eta,u)))_{12}\, dB_2(u). \tag{3.7.7}$$

For estimating the unknown parameters, we use, instead of a filtering approach, the stochastic expansion of $X(t)$, where the unobserved component $X_2(t)$ is substituted by its deterministic counterpart $z_2(\eta,t)$. For building a tractable estimation function, we also simplify the expression of $B_k(\alpha,X)$ (see (3.3.7)) by replacing $\Phi(\eta;t_k,t_{k-1})$ by its first-order approximation $I_2+\Delta\nabla_x b(\alpha,z(\eta,t_{k-1}))$, so that $\Phi_{11}(\eta,t_k,t_{k-1}) \simeq 1+\Delta\nabla_{x_1} b_1(\alpha,z(\eta,t_{k-1}))$.

The path used in (3.3.7) is $\begin{pmatrix} X_1(t) \\ z_2(\eta,t) \end{pmatrix}$ leading, instead of $B_k(\alpha,X)$ to $\begin{pmatrix} A_k(\eta,X_1) \\ 0 \end{pmatrix}$, with

$$A_k(\eta,X_1) = X_1(t_k) - z_1(\eta,t_k) - (1+\Delta\nabla_{x_1} b_1(\alpha,z(\eta,t_{k-1})))\,(X_1(t_{k-1}) - z_1(\eta,t_{k-1})). \tag{3.7.8}$$

For a first approach, we consider an estimation method based on the Conditional Least Squares built on the $A_k(\eta,X_1)$'s defined in (3.7.8).

$$\bar{U}_{\varepsilon,\Delta}(\eta,X_1) = \frac{1}{\varepsilon^2\Delta}\sum_{k=1}^{n} A_k(\eta,X_1)^2. \tag{3.7.9}$$

This CLS functional does not depend on β, and therefore β cannot be estimated using $\bar{U}_{\varepsilon,\Delta}$. estimated. The associated estimators are then defined as

$$\bar{\eta}_{\varepsilon,\Delta} = \underset{\eta\in K_a\times K_z}{\operatorname{argmin}}\ \bar{U}_{\varepsilon,\Delta}(\eta,X_1). \tag{3.7.10}$$

Note that this process could also be used for estimating η for fixed Δ and low frequency data, using $\Phi_{11}(t_k,t_{k-1})$ instead of its approximation.

Assume that $\eta = (\alpha,\xi) \in \Theta$, with Θ compact set of $\mathbb{R}^a \times \mathbb{R}$. Denote by $\eta_0 = (\alpha_0,\xi_0)$ the true parameter value and consider the estimation of η. The distribution of $(X(t))$ satisfying (3.7.1) depends on $\theta = (\eta,\beta)$. Set $\theta_0 = (\eta_0,\beta_0)$ and $\mathbb{P}_{\theta_0}$ the distribution of $(X(t))$ on $(C([0,T],\mathbb{R}^2),\mathscr{C}_T)$.

Let us first study $\bar{U}_{\varepsilon,\Delta}(\eta,X_1)$.

Lemma 3.7.1. *Assume (S1)–(S5). Then, the process $\bar{U}_{\varepsilon,\Delta}(\eta,X_1)$ defined in (3.7.9) satisfies that, under $\mathbb{P}_{\theta_0}$, as $\varepsilon,\Delta \to 0$,*

$$\varepsilon^2\bar{U}_{\varepsilon,\Delta}(\eta,X_1) \to J_T(\eta_0,\eta) = \int_0^T (\Gamma_1(\eta_0,\eta;t))^2 dt \quad \textit{a.s. where} \tag{3.7.11}$$

$$\begin{aligned}\Gamma_1(\eta_0,\eta;t) = {} & b_1(\alpha_0,z(\eta_0,t)) - b_1(\alpha,z(\eta,t)) \\ & - \nabla_{x_1} b_1(\alpha,z(\eta,t))(z_1(\eta_0,t) - z_1(\eta,t)).\end{aligned} \tag{3.7.12}$$

So, to get that $\bar{U}_{\varepsilon,\Delta}(\eta,Y)$ is a contrast function for estimating $\eta = (\alpha,\xi)$, we need an assumption that ensures that $\{\eta \neq \eta_0 \Rightarrow J_T(\eta_0,\eta) > 0\}$. This leads to the additional identifiability assumption,

(S8): $\eta \neq \eta_0 \Rightarrow \{t \to \Gamma_1(\eta_0, \eta; t) \not\equiv 0\}$.

For deterministic systems, the notion of observability is used in the case of partial observations (see e.g. [107], [112]), which sums up to $\{\eta \neq \eta_0 \Rightarrow z(\eta, \cdot) \not\equiv z(\eta_0, \cdot)\}$. If the underlying deterministic system is not observable, Assumption (S8) which makes reference to the identifiability of the model with respect to the parameters is not satisfied. But the converse is not true, Assumption (S8) being a bit stronger.

Proof. The proof of Lemma 3.7.1 is a repetition of the proof of Lemma 3.3.7. First, an application of the stochastic Taylor expansion yields that, as $\varepsilon \to 0$, $(X_1(t), 0 \leq t \leq T) \to (z_1(\eta_0, t), 0 \leq t \leq T)$ almost surely under $\mathbb{P}_{\theta_0}$. Second, letting $\Delta \to 0$, we get that, there exists a constant $C > 0$ such that

$$\frac{1}{\Delta} A_k(\alpha, z_1(\eta_0, \cdot)) = \Gamma_1(\eta_0, \eta, t_{k-1}) + \Delta \|\eta - \eta_0\| r_k(\eta_0, \eta), \tag{3.7.13}$$

with $\sup_k \sup_{\eta \in \Theta} \|r_k(\eta_0, \eta)\| \leq C$. □

To study the asymptotic behaviour of $\bar{\eta}_{\varepsilon,\Delta}$, we have to introduce additional quantities. First, we define the vector $D(\eta, t) \in \mathbb{R}^{a+1}$, using the notations defined in (3.3.3),

$$\begin{aligned} D_i(\eta, t) &= -(\nabla_{\alpha_i} b_1)(\alpha, z(\eta, t)) - \nabla_{x_2} b_1(\alpha, z(\eta, t)) \nabla_{\alpha_i} z_2(\eta, t) \quad \text{for } i = 1, \ldots, a, \\ D_i(t) &= -\nabla_{x_2} b_1(\alpha, z(\eta, t)) \nabla_{\xi} z_2(\eta, t) \quad \text{if } i = a+1, \end{aligned} \tag{3.7.14}$$

Then, built on the D_i's, define the matrix $\Lambda(\eta) = (\Lambda_{ij}(\eta))$ by

$$\Lambda_{ij}(\eta) = 2 \int_0^T D_i(\eta, t) D_j(\eta, t)\, dt. \tag{3.7.15}$$

Finally, define the three functions for $\theta = (\alpha, \xi, \beta)$,

$$\begin{aligned} v_1(\theta; t) &= \sigma_{11}^2(\beta, z(\eta, t)) + \sigma_{12}^2(\beta, z(\eta, t)) \\ &= \Sigma_{11}(\beta, z(\eta, t)), \\ v_2(\theta; t, s) &= \sigma_{11}(\beta, z(\eta, s))\, (\Phi(\eta, t, s)\sigma(\beta, z(\eta, s)))_{21} \\ &\quad + \sigma_{12}(\beta, z(\eta, s))\, (\Phi(\eta, t, s)\sigma(\beta, z(\eta, s)))_{22} \\ &= (\Phi(\eta; t, s)\Sigma(\beta, x(\eta, s)))_{21}, \\ v_3(\theta, t, s) &= \int_0^{t \wedge s} (\Phi(\eta, t, u)\sigma(\beta, z(\eta, u)))_{11}\, (\Phi(\eta, s, u)\sigma(\beta, z(\eta, u)))_{11}\, du \\ &\quad + \int_0^{t \wedge s} (\Phi(\eta, t, u)\sigma(\beta, z(\eta, u)))_{22}\, (\Phi(\eta, s, u)\sigma(\beta, z(\beta, u)))_{22}\, du. \end{aligned} \tag{3.7.16}$$

We can now state the main result of this section.

Theorem 3.7.2. *Assume (S1)–(S8). Then under* $\mathbb{P}_{\theta_0}$*, as* $\varepsilon, \Delta \to 0$*,*

(i) $\bar{\eta}_{\varepsilon,\Delta} \to \eta_0$ *in probability .*

(ii) If moreover $\varepsilon^2\Delta^{-1} = n\varepsilon^2 \to 0$ *and* $\Lambda(\eta_0)$ *defined in (3.7.15) is invertible, then*

$$\varepsilon^{-1}(\bar{\eta}_{\varepsilon,\Delta} - \eta_0) \to \mathcal{N}(0, \Lambda(\eta_0)^{-1}V(\theta_0)\Lambda(\eta_0)^{-1}) \quad \text{in distribution}, \tag{3.7.17}$$

where $V(\theta) = V^{(1)}(\theta) + V^{(2)}(\theta) + V^{(3)}(\theta)$ *with, using (3.7.14), (3.7.16),*

$$V_{ij}^{(1)}(\theta) = \int_0^T D_i(\eta,t)D_j(\eta,t)v_1(\theta,t)\,dt, \tag{3.7.18}$$

$$V_{ij}^{(2)}(\theta) = \int\int_{0\le s\le t\le T} D_i(\eta,s)D_j(\eta,t)\nabla_{x_2}b_1(\alpha,z(\eta,s))v_2(\theta,t,s))ds\,dt, \tag{3.7.19}$$

$$V_{ij}^{(3)}(\theta) = \tag{3.7.20}$$

$$\int_0^T\int_0^T D_i(\eta,s)D_j(\eta,t)\nabla_{x_2}b_1(\alpha,z(\eta,s))\nabla_{x_2}b_1(\alpha,z(\eta,t))v_3(\theta,t,s)ds\,dt.$$

Based on (3.7.11) and Assumption (S8), the proof of the consistency of $\bar{\eta}_{\varepsilon,\Delta}$ is obtained by standard tools and omitted.

For the proof of (ii), the main difficulty lies in a precise study of $\varepsilon\nabla_i\bar{U}_{\varepsilon,\Delta}(\eta_0, X_1)$, which is the sum of n terms that are no longer conditionally independent. The three terms in the matrix $V(\theta_0)$ come from this expansion. Indeed,

$$\varepsilon(\nabla_i\bar{U}(\eta_0,Y))_i, \to \mathcal{N}_{a+1}(0, V(\theta_0)) \quad \text{in distribution under } \mathbb{P}_{\theta_0}. \tag{3.7.21}$$

Then, studying $\varepsilon^2\nabla_{ij}\bar{U}(\eta, Y)$ yields, using (3.7.9), (3.7.14), as $\varepsilon, \Delta \to 0$,

$$\varepsilon^2\nabla_{ij}\bar{U}(\eta_0,Y) \to \Lambda_{ij}(\eta_0) = 2\int_0^T D_i(\eta_0,t)D_j(\eta_0,t)dt \quad \text{a.s. under } \mathbb{P}_{\theta_0}. \tag{3.7.22}$$

The proof is quite technical and is omitted.

Let us describe our method on a partially observed two-dimensional Ornstein–Uhlenbeck diffusion process $X(t) = (X_1(t), X_2(t))^*$ where all the computations are explicit. Let

$$dX(t) = AX(t)dt + \varepsilon\varsigma dB(t), \quad X(0) = \begin{pmatrix} x_1 \\ x_2 \end{pmatrix}, \tag{3.7.23}$$

with $A = \begin{pmatrix} a & b \\ 0 & a+h \end{pmatrix}, \varsigma = \sigma\begin{pmatrix} 1 & 0 \\ 0 & 1 \end{pmatrix}$.

We assume that $h \neq 0$, $\sigma > 0$. The parameter in the drift is $\alpha = (a, b, h)$. For partial observations, we also need introducing $\eta = (a, b, h, \xi)$ and $\theta = (a, b, h, \xi, \sigma)$. The observations are $(X_1(t_k), k = 1, \ldots, n)$ with $t_k = k\Delta$, $T = n\Delta$ and $\Delta = \Delta_n \to 0$.

The solution of the ODE (3.2.8) applied to the drift of diffusion process (3.7.23) is

$$z_1(\eta,t) = (z_1 - \frac{\xi b}{h})e^{at} + \frac{\xi b}{h}e^{(a+h)t}; \quad z_2(\eta,t) = \xi e^{(a+h)t}. \tag{3.7.24}$$

Let us compute the matrix $\Phi(\alpha,t,u) = e^{(t-u)A}$, we have $A = PDP^{-1}$, with

$$P = \begin{pmatrix} 1 & b/h \\ 0 & 1 \end{pmatrix}, \; D = \begin{pmatrix} a & 0 \\ 0 & a+h \end{pmatrix}, \text{ so that}$$

$$\Phi(\alpha,t,s) = \begin{pmatrix} e^{a(t-s)} & \frac{b}{h}\left(e^{(a+h)(t-s)} - e^{a(t-s)}\right) \\ 0 & e^{(a+h)(t-s)} \end{pmatrix}.$$

The solution of (3.7.23) is therefore $X(t) = Pe^{tD}P^{-1}X(0) + \varepsilon\sigma \int_0^t Pe^{(t-s)D}P^{-1}dB(s)$. Hence,

$$X_1(t) = z_1(\eta,t) + \varepsilon\sigma\left(\int_0^t e^{a(t-s)}dB_1(s) + \frac{b}{h}\int_0^t \left(e^{(a+h)(t-s)} - e^{a(t-s)}\right)dB_2(s)\right). \tag{3.7.25}$$

Using that $\nabla_{x_1} b_1(\alpha, z(\eta,t)) = a$ and (3.7.24) yields that

$$A_k(\eta,X_1) = X_1(t_k) - z_1(\eta,t_k) - (1+a\Delta)(X_1(t_{k-1}) - z_1(\eta,t_{k-1})). \tag{3.7.26}$$

$$\Gamma_1(\eta_0,\eta,t) = (a_0 - a)z_1(\eta_0,t) + b_0\xi_0 e^{(a_0+h_0)t} - b\xi e^{(a+h)t}.$$

Assumptions (S1)–(S7) are satisfied. Looking at the analytical expression of $z_1(\eta,t)$, we have that $b\xi = \tilde{b}\tilde{\xi}$ leads to identical solutions $z_1(\eta,t)$. Therefore, Assumption (S8) is not satisfied and b, ξ cannot be estimated separately when observing one coordinate only. This is also true for the deterministic ODE and the non-identifiability is here an intrinsic problem to this partial observation example.

Therefore, we define a new parameter $b' = b\xi$ and consider that the parameter to estimate is now $\eta = (a,b',h)$. Then, checking (S8) is straightforward.
The various quantities introduced in the previous section have a closed expression. Indeed, the functions $D_i(\eta,t)$ defined in (3.7.14) write, using (3.7.22), (3.7.24) with $\eta = (a,b',h)$,

$$\begin{aligned} D_1(\eta,t) &= -(z_1 - \frac{b'}{h})e^{at} - (\frac{b'}{h} + b't)e^{(a+h)t}, \\ D_2(\eta,t) &= -e^{(a+h)t}, \\ D_3(\eta,t) &= -b'te^{(a+h)t}. \end{aligned}$$

The matrix $\Lambda(\eta)$ is defined as $\Lambda(\eta) = (\Lambda_{ij}(\eta))$ with $\Lambda_{ij}(\eta) = \int_0^T D_i(\eta,t)D_j(\eta,t)dt$ $(= \int_0^T D(\eta,t)D^*(\eta,t)dt$. The functions defined in (3.7.16) are, with $\theta = (a,b,h,\sigma)$,

$$v_1(\theta,t) = \sigma^2; \quad v_2(\theta,t,s) = 0; \quad v_3(\theta,t,s) = \sigma^2\left(\frac{e^{a|t-s|}}{2a} + \frac{e^{(a+h)|t-s|}}{2(a+h)}\right).$$

Therefore,

$$V_{ij}(\theta) = \sigma^2 \int_0^T D_i(\eta,t)D_j(\eta,t)dt$$
$$+ \frac{\sigma^2 b^2}{2} \int_0^T \int_0^T D_i(\eta,s)D_j(\eta,t) \left(\frac{e^{a|t-s|}}{a} + \frac{e^{(a+h)|t-s|}}{(a+h)} \right) dsdt.$$

The estimator $\bar{\eta}_{\varepsilon,\Delta}$ defined by (3.7.10) is a consistent estimator of $\eta_0 = (a_0, b'_0, h_0)$ and satisfies (3.7.17) with the matrices $\Lambda(\eta_0)$ and $V(\theta_0)$ obtained above. The asymptotic covariance matrix is therefore

$$\sigma^2 \Lambda^{-1}(\eta) + \tag{3.7.27}$$
$$\frac{\sigma^2 b^2}{2} \Lambda^{-1}(\eta) \left(\int_0^T \int_0^T D_i(\eta,t)D_j(\eta,s) \left(\frac{e^{a|t-s|}}{a} + \frac{e^{(a+h)|t-s|}}{a+h} \right) dsdt \right)_{ij} \Lambda^{-1}(\eta).$$

In the case of complete discrete observations, the first term of (3.7.27) is the asymptotic variance obtained with conditional least squares. Therefore, the loss of information coming from partial observations is measured by the second term of (3.7.27) (added to the fact that only bz_0 is identifiable).

3.7.2 Assessment of Estimators on Simulated and Real Data Sets

We first present the results on the *SIR* studied in the previous section but assuming partial observations. Then we investigate the inference on the real data set of Influenza dynamics modeled with the *SIRS* studied in the previous section.

3.7.2.1 Inference for Partial Observation of the *SIR* Model with Sampling Interval Δ

In this section, we consider the case where one component of the epidemic process $X^N(t) = (S^N(t), I^N(t))$ is observed on $[0,T]$. The observations are the successive numbers of infected individuals

$$(I^N(k\Delta), k = 1, \dots n) \text{ with sampling } \Delta; T = n\Delta.$$

According to the notations of Section 3.7, we have to interchange the coordinates of S, I and set $X(t) = (I(t), S(t))^*$; the drift term can be written as

$$X(t) = \begin{pmatrix} I(t) \\ S(t) \end{pmatrix}; \quad b((\lambda,\gamma),(i,s)) = \begin{pmatrix} \lambda si - \gamma i \\ -\lambda si \end{pmatrix}; \quad \Sigma(i,s) = \begin{pmatrix} \lambda si + \gamma i & -\lambda si \\ -\lambda si & \lambda si \end{pmatrix}.$$

We assume that $I(0) = i_0, S(0) = s_0$. Setting $\xi = s_0$, then the parameter defined in the previous section is $\eta = (\lambda, \gamma, \xi)$. Denote by $z(\eta,t) = (i(\eta,t), s(\eta,t))$ the solution of the ODE

$$di/dt = \lambda si - \gamma i; i(0) = i_0, \quad ds/dt = \lambda si; s(0) = \xi.$$

Then, the conditional least square method now reads as

$$\bar{U}_{\varepsilon,\delta}(\eta, I) = \frac{1}{\varepsilon^2 \Delta} \sum_{k=1}^{n} (I(t_k) - i(\eta, t_k) - (1 + \lambda s(\eta, t_{k-1}) - \gamma)(I(t_{k-1}) - i(\eta, t_{k-1}))^2.$$

Using definition 3.7.12, the function $\Gamma_1(\eta_0, \eta, t)$ reads as

$$\Gamma_1(\eta_0, \eta, t) = i(\eta_0, t)(\lambda_0 s(\eta_0, t) - \lambda s(\eta, t) - \gamma_0 + \gamma).$$

To investigate the identifiability assumption, let us check **(S8)**. It reads as $\eta \neq \eta_0 \Rightarrow \{t \to \Gamma(\eta_0, \eta, t)\} \not\equiv 0$.

Assume that we have observed that the epidemic spreads, so that we have $\forall t \in [0, T], i(\eta_0, t) > 0$. Therefore, we have to prove that

$$\{t \to (\lambda_0 s(\eta_0, t) - \lambda s(\eta, t) - \gamma_0 + \gamma) \equiv 0\} \Rightarrow \{\eta = \eta_0\}. \tag{3.7.28}$$

Differentiating this relation with respect to t yields

$$\forall t, \lambda_0^2 s(\eta_0, t) i(\eta_0, t) - \lambda^2 s(\eta, t) i(\eta, t) = 0. \tag{3.7.29}$$

Using (3.7.28), we get the second relation

$$\forall t, \frac{s(\eta, t)}{i(\eta_0, t)} (\lambda i(\eta, t) - \lambda_0 i(\eta_0, t)) = \frac{\lambda_0(\gamma_0 - \gamma)}{\lambda}.$$

Differentiating this relation with respect to t yields that

$$\lambda \frac{s(\eta, t) i(\eta, t)}{i(\eta_0, t)} (\lambda_0 i(\eta_0, t) - \lambda i(\eta, t)) \equiv 0.$$

Since at time 0, $i(\eta, 0) = i(\eta_0, 0) = i_0$, we get that $\lambda = \lambda_0$. Using now (3.7.29) yields that, at time 0, $s(\eta, 0) = s(\eta_0, 0)$ so that $\xi = \xi_0$. Finally, by relation (3.7.28), we get $\gamma = \gamma_0$.

We conclude that the two parameters λ, γ as well as the initial state s_0 are identifiable when observing $(I(t_k), k = 0, \ldots n)$. The same holds true for $R_0 = \lambda/\gamma$, $d = 1/\gamma$ and s_0.

Performances of estimators in the case of partially observed *SIR* model are assessed on simulations obtained with the following parameters: $N = 10000$, $R_0 = 1.5$, $d = 3$, $s_0 = 0.97$, $T = 40$. Observations are represented by vector $I^N(k\Delta)$. Estimations of parameters (R_0, d, s_0) are performed on 1000 simulated trajectories. Theoretical and empirical confidence ellipses are built as detailed in the introduction of Section 3.6.

As shown in Figure 3.7.1, confidence ellipsoids are quite large in the case of partial data. However, they do not include unreasonable values from the epidemiological point of view. Quantile based empirical 95% confidence intervals are still quite large.

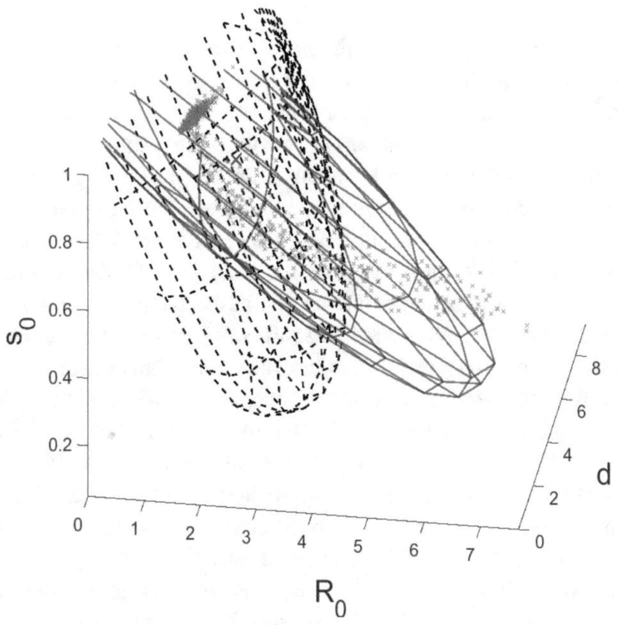

Fig. 3.7.1 Point estimators (green) computed by averaging over 1000 independent simulated trajectories of the *SIR* stochastic model, partially observed ($I(k\Delta)$ only) for $(R_0, d, s_0) = (1.5, 3, 0.15, 0.97)$, $T = 40$ days and $N = 10000$. Theoretical confidence ellipsoid (black), centered on the true value and empirical confidence ellipsoid (blue), centered on mean estimated value are provided. Both ellipsoids are truncated at plausible limits on each direction. Mean and median point estimator are $(R_0, d, s_0) = (1.89, 3.43, 0.88)$ (red cross) and $(1.54, 3.24, 0.99)$ (purple cross), respectively.

The relatively unexpected large volume of confidence ellipsoids, obtained despite theoretical identifiability of model parameters when observing only one component of the system (here $I_N(k\Delta)$) is probably due to the fact that the numerical variance-covariance matrix is ill-conditioned (the order of magnitude of the third eigenvalue is 100 times smaller than that of the first two eigenvalues. It probably corresponds to the notion of "Numerical Identifiability", which does not necessarily coincide with "Theoretical Identifiability".

Concerning point estimators, we successively considered the mean and the median of the estimators obtained for the 1000 simulation experiments. Assuming the complete observation of both coordinates of the *SIR* jump process yields, as expected, accurate values for R_0, d. Assuming that only $I(k\Delta), k = 1, \ldots n$ with $n = 40$, we obtain for a true parameter value $(1.5,3,0.97)$ that the mean point estimator is $(1.89,3.43,0.88)$ and for the median estimator $(1.54,3.24,0.99)$.

3.7.2.2 Partial Observations: *SIRS* Model, Real Data on Influenza Epidemics

The performances of the contrast estimators for the case where only one coordinate of a diffusion process is observed are evaluated on data related to influenza outbreaks in France, collected by the French Sentinel Network (FSN), providing surveillance for several health indicators (www.sentiweb.org). These data are represented by numbers of individuals seeing a doctor during a given time interval, for symptoms related to influenza infection and are reported by a group of general practitioners (GP) voluntarily enrolled into the FSN. Several levels of errors of observation are associated to these data: (i) the state of individuals consulting a GP from the FSN is not exactly known: it can be assimilated to a new infection or to a new recovery, given that symptoms and infectiousness are not necessarily simultaneous and that a certain delay occurs between symptoms onset and consultation time (more correctly, the observed state is probably "infected" but not "newly infected"); (ii) not all infected individuals go and see a GP; (iii) the GP's supplying the FSN database represent only a proportion of all French GP's; (iv) the exact dates of consultations are not known, data are aggregated over two-week time periods; (v) data are preprocessed by the FSN to produce observations with a daily time step.
Here, we account partly for (i) on one hand and jointly for (ii) and (iii) on the other hand and assume that observations $Y(t_k)$ represent a proportion of daily (observation times $t_k = k\Delta$, with $\Delta = 1$ day) numbers of newly recovered individuals: $Y(t_k) = \rho\gamma I(t_k)$, where ρ can be interpreted as the reporting rate. Since data are available over several seasons of influenza outbreaks (data from 1990 to 2011, hence $[0,T] = [0,21.5]$ years), an appropriate model allowing to reproduce periodic dynamics is the *SIRS* model described in Section 3.2.2.2.

$$(S,I) \xrightarrow{\frac{\lambda(t)}{N}S(I+N\eta)} (S-1,I+1)\ ; \quad (S,I) \xrightarrow{\mu S} (S-1,I);$$
$$(S,I) \xrightarrow{(\gamma+\mu)I} (S,I-1)\ ; \quad (S,I) \xrightarrow{\mu N+\delta(N-S-I)} (S+1,I).$$

The seasonality in transmission is modeled via $\lambda(t) = \lambda_0(1+\lambda_1 sin(2\pi t/T_{per}))$.

The parameter is $\theta = (\lambda_0, \lambda_1, \gamma, \delta, \eta, \mu)$, the associated drift function $b(\theta,t,(s,i))$ and diffusion matrix $\Sigma(\theta,t,(s,i))$ are

$$b(\theta,t,(s,i)) = \begin{pmatrix} -\lambda(t)s(i+\eta)+\delta(1-s-i)+\mu(1-s) \\ \lambda(t)s(i+\eta)-(\gamma+\mu)i \end{pmatrix}, \tag{3.7.30}$$

$$\Sigma(\theta,t,(s,i)) = \begin{pmatrix} \lambda(t)s(i+\eta)+\delta(1-s-i)+\mu(1+s) & -\lambda(t)s(i+\eta) \\ -\lambda(t)s(i+\eta) & \lambda(t)s(i+\eta)+(\gamma+\mu)i \end{pmatrix}. \tag{3.7.31}$$

In summary, the data used are assumed to be discrete high frequency observations of one coordinate of the following two-dimensional diffusion with small variance:

$$\begin{cases} dS(t) = -\lambda(t)S(t)(I(t)+\eta)+\delta(1-S(t)-I(t)+\mu(1-S(t)))dt \\ \qquad\qquad +\frac{1}{\sqrt{N}}(\sigma_{11}dB_1(t)+\sigma_{12}dB_2(t)) \\ dI(t) = (\lambda(t)S(t)(I(t)+\eta)-(\gamma+\mu)I(t)dt+\frac{1}{\sqrt{N}}(\sigma_{21}dB_1(t)+\sigma_{22}dB_2(t)). \end{cases}$$

The vector of parameters to be estimated is $\alpha = (R=\lambda_0/\gamma, 10\lambda_1, d=1/\gamma, \delta_{per} = 1/\delta T_{per}, 10\rho)$, where parameters are defined in equation (3.2.19) and more generally in the entire Section 3.2.2.2. Parameters η, μ and T_{per} are fixed at plausible values: $\eta = 10^{-6}$, $\mu = \frac{1}{50}$ (years^{-1}) and $T_{per} = 365$ days. The starting point of the ODE system is unknown, but since we are interested in the stationary behaviour of this process, we fix ($r_{-20T_{per}} = 0.27, i_{-20T_{per}} = 0.0001$, see [26] for example) and let the system evolve until $t = 0$ for the tested set of parameter α to obtain our initial starting point.

Estimation results are summarized in Figure 3.7.2, which represents multi-annual dynamics of influenza cases: observed dynamics (blue curve) and simulated ones (using the ODE version of the *SIRS* model based on estimated parameter values; red curve). Estimators are associated to contrast process defined in (3.7.9). Point estimates of parameters are: $(R, 10\lambda_1, d, \delta_{per}, 10\rho) = (1.47, 1.94, 2.20, 5.66, 0.87)$. These values are in agreement with independent estimation based on data from the same database but using a different inference method, the maximum iterating filtering proposed by [18] (personal communication S. Ballesteros). As shown in Figure 3.7.1 for the *SIR* model, widths of theoretical confidence intervals for each parameter should be larger than those corresponding to complete observations of the *SIRS* model (drawn in Figure 3.6.3). In particular, for λ_1, the width of the confidence interval for partial observations will be larger than $0.35 * \sqrt{(10^7/6*10^7)} = 0.14$ (after correction for the population size, which is $N = 10^7$ in Figure 3.6.3 and $N = 6*10^7$ in Figure 3.7.2).
We can notice from Figure 3.7.2 that predicted trajectories correspond to a regime with bi-annual cycles, composed of two different peaks (red curve). The bifurcation diagram with respect to λ_1 (similar to Figure 3.2.2), when the remaining parameters are either set to fixed values (defined in this section) or to estimated values, exhibits the bifurcation from one annual cycle to bi-annual cycle at $\lambda_1 = 0.035$. This value is likely to belong to the confidence interval of estimated $\lambda_1 = 0.19$, since the width of this interval should be greater than 0.14. Hence, this can have some influence on estimation, influence which is not well characterized in the literature for models exhibiting bifurcation profiles, especially for trajectories corresponding to parameter values close to the bifurcation point. We also observe that the smaller peak in the bi-annual cycles is underestimated, leading to almost no epidemic burst every other year. The presence of a bifurcation in the *SIRS* ODE model probably requires a better approximation of the original jump point process.

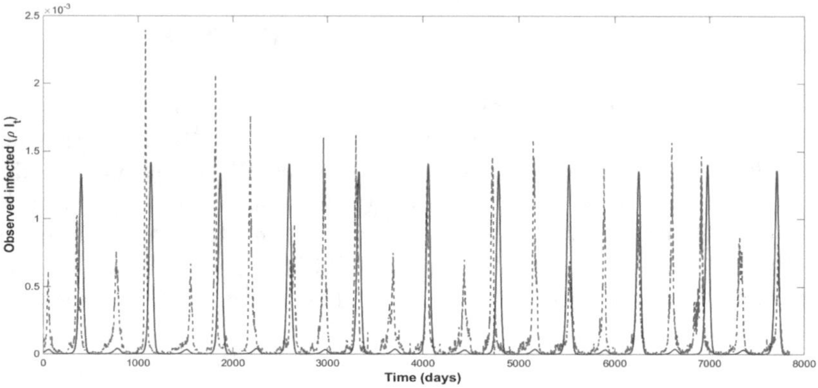

Fig. 3.7.2 Time series of reported cases (expressed as a fraction of the total population in France) of influenza-like illness provided by the FSN (www.sentiweb.org) (blue curve) and deterministic trajectories (mean behaviour) predicted by the *SIRS* model based on estimated parameters using contrast (3.7.9) (red curve).

3.7.2.3 Discussion and Concluding Remarks

Several extensions of this study are possible for partial observations. First, we have chosen to detail the case of high sampling interval. The study in the case of a fixed sampling interval Δ should be obtained with similar tools, leading to similar results. Another extension concerns our choice of a Conditional Least squares for $\bar{U}_{\varepsilon,\Delta}$. An estimation criterium similar to the one used in Section 3.4 could be studied, using $S_k(\alpha,\beta)$ (see (3.3.8)) or substituting $\Sigma(\beta,X(t_k))$ by $\Sigma(\beta,x(\eta,t_k))$ for small sampling. This yields the new process, using (3.7.8),

$$\bar{U}_{\varepsilon,n}(\eta,(Y(t_k))) = \sum_{k=1}^{n} log\, \Sigma(\beta,x(\eta,t_k)) + \frac{1}{\varepsilon^2\Delta}\Sigma(\beta,x(\eta,t_k))^{-1}(A_k(\eta,Y))^2. \tag{3.7.32}$$

The study of this process should yield estimators in the diffusion coefficient β with probably additional assumptions linking ε and Δ. Finally for fixed Δ, $S_k(\alpha,\beta)$ defined in (3.3.8) could be substituted by $(S_k(\alpha,\beta))_{11}$ in the case of two distinct parameters in the drift and diffusion coefficient, and $(S_k(\alpha)_{11}$ in the case corresponding to epidemics where the same parameters are present in the drift and diffusion coefficients. Another extension of the method described in Section 3.7 is the case of a p-dimensional diffusion process where only the first l-coordinates are observed (for instance the *SEIR* model with only Infected observed).

Chapter 4

Inference for Continuous Time SIR models

by Catherine Larédo and Viet Chi Tran

4.1 Introduction

Consider the SIR epidemic model with exponential times in a finite population of size N where $S(t), I(t), R(t)$ denote the number of Susceptible, infected/infectious and Removed individuals at time t with infection rate λ and recovery rate γ ($S(t) + I(t) + R(t) = N$ for all t). There are various ways of describing this process using pure jump Markov processes. We refer to Chapter 2 of Part I of these notes and to Section A.5 of the Appendix for a recap on these processes.

This description now belongs to the domain of event time data, which are conveniently studied by the use of counting processes. We refer to Section A.5 of the Appendix for a short introduction to counting processes in continuous time.

At this point, we need an asymptotic framework to study the properties of these estimators. Two frameworks have been proposed.
Case (1): Assume that the number of initially infected $I(0) = a$ remains fixed and that the number of initial Susceptible is $S(0) = n := N - a$. We also assume for the sake of simplicity that $R(0) = 0$. This leads to a total population size $N = n + a$ that goes to infinity.
Case (2): Assume that the population size $N \to \infty$ and that both $S(0), I(0)$ tend to infinity with N such that $S(0)/N \to s_0 > 0; I(0)/N \to i_0 > 0$ as $N \to \infty$.

Case (1) has been studied by Rida [108], to which we refer for a detailed presentation. We focus here mainly on Case (2).

T. Britton, E. Pardoux (eds.), *Stochastic Epidemic Models with Inference*,
Lecture Notes in Mathematics 2255, https://doi.org/10.1007/978-3-030-30900-8_15

4.2 Maximum Likelihood in the SIR Case

To ease notation, we work here on a simplification of the SEIR process studied in Part I of these notes. We omit the state E and consider an SIR model (corresponding to the limiting case when $\nu \to +\infty$). Recall that the population size is N, that the infection rate is λ and the removal rate γ. We assume that we observe the whole trajectory on a time window $[0,T]$ with $T > 0$: $(S_t^N, I_t^N, R_t^N)_{t\in[0,T]}$. The successive times of events are $(T_i)_{1\leq i\leq K_N(T)}$, where $K_N(T) = \sum_{i\geq 0} \mathbf{1}_{T_i\leq T}$ is the number of events. At each event, $J_i = 0$ if we have an infection and $J_i = 1$ if we have a recovery. Notice that we are here in the case where we have knowledge of all recovery and infection events, i.e. that we have *complete epidemic data*. The case where some data are missing is treated in the next subsections.

Writing the likelihood of our data is important to calibrate the parameters of the model, $\theta = (\lambda, \gamma) \in \mathbb{R}_+^2$ in the case of the SIR model, but also because this is also useful for designing EM or MCMC procedures.

Definition 4.2.1. We define the likelihood $\mathscr{L}_T^N(\theta)$ of the observations as the density, in $\mathbb{D}([0,T],[0,1]^3)$ of the process $(S_t^N, I_t^N, R_t^N)_{t\in[0,T]}$ with respect to the SIR process where intervals between events follow independent exponential distributions of parameter $2N$ and where each event is an infection with probability $1/2$ and a recovery with probability $1/2$. The likelihood is of course a function of $\theta \in \mathbb{R}_+^2$ and of the observations $(S_t^N, I_t^N, R_t^N)_{t\in[0,T]}$ which are omitted in the notation for the sake of notation.

This definition has been proposed in [30] for example. The dominating measure with respect to which the distribution of $(S_t^N, I_t^N, R_t^N)_{t\in[0,T]}$ is written is here the distribution of the process corresponding to the sequence (J_i, T_i)'s where the J_i's are i.i.d. Bernoulli random variables with parameter $1/2$, and where the intervals $\Delta T_i = T_i - T_{i-1}$ are i.i.d. exponential random variables with expectation $1/(2N)$. With the notation above:

$$\begin{aligned}\mathscr{L}_T^N(\theta) &= \mathscr{L}_T^N\big((S_t^N, I_t^N, R_t^N)_{t\in[0,T]}; \lambda, \gamma\big)\\ &= \exp\Big(NT - \int_0^T (\lambda S_s^N I_s^N - \gamma I_s^N) ds\Big) \prod_{i=1}^{K_N(T)} (\lambda S_{T_i-}^N I_{T_i-}^N)^{1-J_i} (\gamma I_{T_i-}^N)^{J_i}. \quad (4.2.1)\end{aligned}$$

Taking the log, and using the formulation of the processes (S_t, I_t, R_t) by means of Poisson point processes Q^1 and Q^2 as in Part I, Chapter 2 of these notes,

$$\begin{aligned}\log \mathscr{L}_T^N(\theta) &= NT - \int_0^T (\lambda S_s^N I_s^N - \gamma I_s^N) ds\\ &\quad + \sum_{i=1}^{K_N(T)} \Big[(1-J_i)\log(\lambda S_{s-}^N I_{s-}^N) + J_i \log(\gamma I_{s-}^N)\Big]\\ &= NT - \int_0^T (\lambda S_s^N I_s^N - \gamma I_s^N) ds + \int_0^T \log(\lambda S_{s-}^N I_{s-}^N) \mathbf{1}_{u\leq \lambda N S_{s-}^N I_{s-}^N} Q^1(ds, du)\end{aligned}$$

$$+\int_0^T \log\left(\gamma I_{s_-}^N\right) \mathbf{1}_{u \le \gamma N I_{s_-}^N} Q^2(ds,du).$$

The above function is concave in λ and γ, for a given observations $(S_t^N, I_t^N)_{t\in[0,T]}$, and maximizing it, we obtain:

Proposition 4.2.2. *The maximum likelihood estimator* $\widehat{\theta}_N = (\widehat{\lambda}_N, \widehat{\gamma}_N)$ *of* θ *(MLE) is then given by:*

$$\widehat{\lambda}_N = \frac{1}{N} \frac{\sum_{i=1}^{K_N(T)} (1-J_i)}{\int_0^T S_s^N I_s^N ds}, \qquad \widehat{\gamma}_N = \frac{1}{N} \frac{\sum_{i=1}^{K_N(T)} J_i}{\int_0^T I_s^N ds}. \tag{4.2.2}$$

These estimators have already been mentioned in (3.6.1) and it had been noticed that the numerators of $\widehat{\lambda}_N$ and $\widehat{\gamma}_N$ are respectively the numbers of infections and recoveries on the period $[0,T]$. Remark also that the estimators (4.2.2) are the same for the Cases (1) and (2) presented in Section 4.1. In what follows, we concentrate on the Case (2).

Using the Law of Large Numbers and the Central Limit Theorem stated in Part I, Section 2.3 of these notes we obtain that

Proposition 4.2.3. *The estimator* $\widehat{\theta}_N$ *is convergent and asymptotically Gaussian when* $N \to +\infty$*:*

$$\sqrt{N}(\widehat{\theta}_N - \theta) = \sqrt{N}\begin{pmatrix} \widehat{\lambda}_N - \lambda \\ \widehat{\gamma}_N - \gamma \end{pmatrix} \Rightarrow \mathscr{N}\left(0_{\mathbb{R}^2}, I^{-1}(\lambda,\gamma)\right),$$

where the Fisher information matrix is:

$$I(\lambda,\gamma) = \begin{pmatrix} V_{11}(t) & 0 \\ 0 & V_{22}(t) \end{pmatrix}$$

with $(s(t),i(t))_{t\in[0,T]}$ *the solution of the limiting ODE that approximates* $(S_t^N, I_t^N)_{t\in[0,T]}$ *when* $N \to +\infty$ *(see Example 2.2.10 in Part I) and with*

$$V_{11}(t) = \frac{\int_0^T s(t)i(t)dt}{\lambda} = \frac{1-s(T)}{\lambda^2};\ V_{22}(t) = \frac{\int_0^T i(t)dt}{\gamma} = \frac{1+\mu-s(T)-i(T)}{\gamma^2}. \tag{4.2.3}$$

Proof. Notice that the estimator $\widehat{\lambda}$ given in Proposition 4.2.2 can be rewritten, with the notations of Example 2.2.1 of Part I of these notes, as

$$\widehat{\lambda}_N = \frac{1}{N} \frac{P_1\left(\lambda N \int_0^T S_s^N I_s^N ds\right)}{\int_0^T S_s^N I_s^N ds}.$$

Using the Law of Large Numbers given in Part I, Section 2.2, the process $(S_t^N, I_t^N)_{t\in[0,T]}$ converges uniformly when $N \to +\infty$ to the unique solution of the ODE

$$s'(t) = -\lambda s(t)i(t),$$

$$i'(t) = \lambda s(t)i(t) - \gamma i(t).$$

Moreover,

$$\lim_{N\to+\infty} \widehat{\lambda}_N = \lambda \frac{\int_0^T s(t)i(t)dt}{\int_0^T s(t)i(t)dt} = \lambda.$$

Now,

$$\sqrt{N}(\widehat{\lambda}_N - \lambda) = \frac{1}{\int_0^T S_s^N I_s^N ds}\left[\frac{1}{\sqrt{N}}P_1\Big(\lambda N\int_0^T S_s^N I_s^N ds\Big) - \sqrt{N}\lambda\int_0^T S_s^N I_s^N ds\right].$$

From Part I, Section 2.3, we have the following convergence in distribution

$$\frac{1}{\sqrt{N}}P_1\Big(\lambda N\int_0^T s(t)i(t)dt\Big) - \sqrt{N}\lambda\int_0^T s(t)i(t)dt \Rightarrow B_1\Big(\lambda\int_0^T s(t)i(t)dt\Big)$$

where B_1 is a standard real Brownian motion. As in the proof of Proposition 2.3.1, the bracket in the right term is then shown to converge to the same limit $B_1(\lambda\int_0^T s(t)i(t)dt)$. Since the denominator of the right-hand side converges in probability to $\int_0^T s(t)i(t)dt$, we obtain the asymptotic normality of $\widehat{\lambda}_N$ with asymptotic variance

$$\frac{\lambda}{\int_0^T s(t)i(t)dt}.$$

Proceeding similarly for $\widehat{\gamma}_N$ and using the asymptotic independence between the two estimators provides the result. Notice that the Fisher information matrix can also be computed from the log-likelihood, and that all regularity assumptions of generic asymptotic normality results are satisfied (see e.g. Chapter 4 of [95]). □

Corollary 4.2.4. *An estimator of $R_0 = \lambda/\gamma$ is $\widehat{R}_0^{(t)} = \frac{\hat{\lambda}_t}{\hat{\gamma}_t}$. Applying the functional delta-theorem (e.g. [123]), it converges in distribution to*

$$\sqrt{n}(\widehat{R}_0^{(t)} - R_0) \to \mathcal{N}(0,\sigma^2(t)) \quad \textit{with} \quad \sigma^2(t) = \frac{V_{11}^{-1}(t) + R_0^2 V_{22}^{-1}(t)}{\gamma^2}. \tag{4.2.4}$$

Remark 4.2.5 (Maximum likelihood estimators in the Case (1)). Let us denote by $(N_t)_{t\in\mathbb{R}_+}$ the counting processes associated to the infection process:

$$N_t = P_1\Big(\int_0^t \lambda N S_s^N I_s^N ds\Big),$$

and by τ_N the extinction time, when there is no infective individual left. Because the population is finite, $\tau_N < +\infty$ almost surely and $N(\tau_N) \le N$. Let

$$A = \{\omega; N(\tau_N,\omega) \to \infty \text{ as } N \to \infty\}$$

be the event on which a major outbreak occurs. Ball [8] proved that $\mathbb{P}(A) = 1 - \min\{1,(\gamma/\lambda)^a\}$. Moreover if $R_0 = \lambda/\gamma > 1$, then $\mathbb{P}(A) > 0$ and as $n\to\infty$,

$$\frac{N(\tau_N)}{N} \to \pi 1_A \text{ where } \pi \text{ is such that } \frac{\lambda}{\gamma} = -\frac{\log(1-\pi)}{\pi}.$$

Asymptotic results for the estimators are obtained on A and A^c. The maximum likelihood estimator satisfies that

$$\hat{\lambda}_N \to \lambda 1_A + Z 1_{A^c}$$

in distribution where Z is a positive explicit random variable such that $\mathbb{E}(Z) < 1/\lambda$ if $\lambda/\gamma > 1$. Note that in this case, $\hat{\lambda}_N$ is not a consistent estimator. We refer to [108] for a detailed presentation of the results.

These methods can be extended to other epidemic models. We will detail later for the SEIR and SIRS epidemic models. The main drawback of this approach is that the epidemic process is rarely observed in such details, which prevents this kind of statistical approach. However, this study sums up the best statistical results that can be obtained when complete observations are available. When incomplete observations are available, the loss of information will be measured with respect to this general reference.

4.2.1 MCMC Estimation

The preceding subsection treated the case of complete observation. In practice, parameter estimation for SIR models is usually a difficult task because of missing observations, which is a recurrent issue in epidemiology. O'Neill Roberts [106] developed a Markov chain Monte Carlo method (MCMC) to make inferences about the missing data and the unknown parameters in a Bayesian framework.

We consider an SIR model as in Section 4.2. Instead of observing the sequence $(J_i, T_i)_{i\in\{1\dots K_T^N\}}$ (type – infection or recovery – and time of occurrence of the successive events, as described in the beginning of Section 4.2), we observe only the T_i's such that $J_i = 1$ (recovery events, that can also be detection events in some applications) and the total number of events K_T^N is unknown. In this section, we adopt the following notation. Let us assume that there are m infections at times $\sigma = (\sigma_1 < 0, \dots \sigma_m)$ that are unobserved and n removals at times $\tau = (\tau_1 = 0, \dots \tau_n)$ which constitute our observations. For later purposes, we will denote by $\sigma_{-1} = (\sigma_2, \dots \sigma_m)$ the vector of infection times starting from the second infection. We observe the total size of the population N, the number n of removal times and the vector τ of these removal times. The parameter of interest is $(\lambda, \gamma, \sigma_1)$ and the vector σ_{-1} is the vector of nuisance parameters.

The MCMC algorithm proposed by O'Neill and Roberts [106] take place in a Bayesian framework. Given λ, γ and the first infection time σ_1, the likelihood of $(\sigma_{-1}, \tau) = (\sigma_2 \dots \sigma_m, \tau_1, \dots \tau_m)$ is obtained from adapting (4.2.1):

$$\mathscr{L}_T^N(\sigma_{-1},\tau|\lambda,\gamma,\sigma_1) = \exp\left(NT - \int_{\sigma_1}^T (\lambda S_s^N I_s^N - \gamma I_s^N)ds\right)\prod_{i=1}^n(\lambda S_{\sigma_i-}^N I_{\sigma_i-}^N)\prod_{i=1}^m(\gamma I_{\tau_i-}^N). \tag{4.2.5}$$

4.2.1.1 A Priori Distributions

We suppose that λ and γ have *a priori* Gamma distribution with parameters $(\alpha_\lambda, \beta_\lambda)$ and $(\alpha_\gamma, \beta_\gamma)$ respectively, where we recall that the density of a Gamma distribution with parameter (α, β) is:

$$\frac{\beta^\alpha}{\Gamma(\alpha)} x^{\alpha-1} e^{-\beta x} \mathbf{1}_{(0,+\infty)}(x)$$

where $\Gamma(x)$ is the gamma function such that for any positive integer k, $\Gamma(k) = (k-1)!$. Following [106], we also chose for the *a priori* distribution of σ_1 the 'exponential' distribution with density (on $\mathbb{R}_-$) with $\rho > 0$:

$$\rho e^{\rho\sigma_1}\mathbf{1}_{(-\infty,0)}(\sigma_1).$$

4.2.1.2 A Posteriori Distributions

The purpose is now to generate a sample from the *a posteriori* distribution $\pi(\sigma, \lambda, \beta|\tau)$. For this, O'Neill and Roberts propose a Metropolis–Hastings algorithm.

Recall the principle of the Metropolis–Hastings algorithm used to obtain a sample $\mathbf{x}$ in a distribution with a density $\pi(x)$ that is proportional to some $f(x)$. Consider a transition kernel with a density $q(y|x)$ from which it is easy to simulate. Starting from a first point x_0, construct a sequence of points $(x_k)_{k\in N}$ with f and q as follows. Assume that x_k has been constructed, then:

- draw y from $q(y|x_k)$.
- With probability

$$\phi(x_k, y) = \min\left(\frac{f(y)q(x_k|y)}{f(x_k)q(y|x_k)}, 1\right)$$

  define $x_{k+1} = y$.
  With probability $1 - \phi(x_k, y)$, define $x_{k+1} = x_k$.

This defines a reversible Markov chain whose stationary distribution is π.

We apply the above idea to sample σ, λ, β from the *a posteriori* distribution. To choose the transition kernels, notice first that with direct computation, we obtain:

$$\pi(\sigma_1|\tau,\sigma_{-1},\lambda,\gamma) \sim (\rho + \lambda N + \gamma)e^{-(\theta+\lambda N+\gamma)(\sigma_2 - y)}\mathbf{1}_{y<\sigma_2}$$

$$\pi(\lambda|\tau,\sigma,\gamma) \sim \Gamma\left(\alpha_\lambda + \int_{\sigma_1}^T S_s^N I_s^N ds, m-1+\beta_\lambda\right)$$

$$\pi(\gamma|\tau,\sigma,\lambda) \sim \Gamma\left(\alpha_\gamma + \int_{\sigma_1}^{T} I_s^N ds, n+\beta_\gamma\right).$$

Hence, it is natural to choose the above distributions for the proposals of σ_1, λ and β. It remains to propose a transition kernel for σ_{-1}. O'Neill and Roberts propose a Hasting algorithm with the three following moves:

- Move an infection time chosen at random by sampling the candidate uniformly in $[0,T]$. If the infection time chosen at random was at time s and the proposal time drawn uniformly in $[0,T]$ is t, the move is accepted with probability

$$\begin{aligned}\phi(\sigma,\sigma\cup\{t\}\setminus\{s\}) &= \frac{\mathscr{L}_T^N(\sigma\cup\{t\}\setminus\{s\},\tau|\lambda,\gamma,\sigma_1)\frac{1}{|\sigma|-1}\frac{1}{T}}{\mathscr{L}_T^N(\sigma,\tau|\lambda,\gamma,\sigma_1)\frac{1}{|\sigma|-1}\frac{1}{T}} \wedge 1\\ &= \frac{\mathscr{L}_T^N(\sigma\cup\{t\}\setminus\{s\},\tau|\lambda,\gamma,\sigma_1)}{\mathscr{L}_T^N(\sigma,\tau|\lambda,\gamma,\sigma_1)} \vee 1.\end{aligned}$$

- Remove an infection time chosen at random. If the chosen infection time was at time s, the acceptation probability is then:

$$\frac{\mathscr{L}_T^N(\sigma\setminus\{s\},\tau|\lambda,\gamma,\sigma_1)\frac{1}{T-\sigma_1}}{\mathscr{L}_T^N(\sigma,\tau|\lambda,\gamma,\sigma_1)\frac{1}{|\sigma|-1}} \wedge 1 = \frac{\mathscr{L}_T^N(\sigma\setminus\{s\},\tau|\lambda,\gamma,\sigma_1)(|\sigma|-1)}{\mathscr{L}_T^N(\sigma,\tau|\lambda,\gamma,\sigma_1)(T-\sigma_1)} \wedge 1.$$

- Add a new infection at a time t drawn uniformly on $[0,T]$:

$$\frac{\mathscr{L}_T^N(\sigma\cup\{t\},\tau|\lambda,\gamma,\sigma_1)\frac{1}{|\sigma|}}{\mathscr{L}_T^N(\sigma,\tau|\lambda,\gamma,\sigma_1)\frac{1}{(T-\sigma_1)}} \wedge 1 = \frac{\mathscr{L}(\sigma+\{t\})(T-\sigma_1)}{\mathscr{L}(\sigma)|\sigma|} \wedge 1.$$

A numerical application is performed in [106] for small epidemics. This algorithm is simulated and compared with other ones in Section 4.3.2.

4.2.2 EM Algorithm for Discretely Observed Markov Jump Processes

We consider now the situation where the Markov jump process is only observed at discrete time points. This has been considered by Bladt and Sorensen [14]. We study the maximum likelihood estimation of the Q-matrix based on a discretely sampled Markov jump process. The problem of identifiability and of existence and uniqueness of the MLE is related to the following problem in probability: can a given discrete time Markov chain be obtained as a discrete time sampling of a continuous time Markov jump process?

4.2.2.1 Likelihood Function

Let $X = (X(s), s \geq 0)$ be a Markov jump process with finite state space $E = \{1, \ldots, N\}$ and Q-matrix $\mathbf{Q} = (q_{kl})$. If X is continuously observed on the time interval $[0, T]$, the likelihood function is given by,

$$L_T(\mathbf{Q}) = \prod_{k=1}^{N} \prod_{l \neq k} q_{kl}^{N_{kl}(T)} \exp(-q_{kl} R_k(T)), \text{ where} \tag{4.2.6}$$

the process $N_{kl}(t)$ is the number of transitions from state k to state l in the time interval $[0, t]$ and $R_k(t)$ is the time spent in state k before time t.

$$R_k(t) = \int_0^t \delta_{\{X(s)=k\}}\, ds. \tag{4.2.7}$$

For details see e.g. [72] .
Therefore, if the process is continuously observed on $[0, T]$, the maximum likelihood estimator of its $\mathbf{Q}$- matrix is easily obtained:

$$\hat{\mathbf{Q}}_{kl} = \frac{N_{kl}(T)}{R_k(T)}. \tag{4.2.8}$$

Assume now that the process is observed with a sampling interval Δ with $T = n\Delta$. Then, setting $X_i = X(t_i)$ is a discrete time Markov chain with transition matrix

$$P^{\Delta}(\mathbf{Q}) \quad \text{where } P^t(\mathbf{Q}) = \exp(t\mathbf{Q}), \quad t > 0,$$

with $\exp(\cdot)$ denoting the matrix exponential function.

Hence the likelihood for the discrete observations $(x_0, \ldots, x_n)$ is

$$L_{n,\Delta}(\mathbf{Q}) = \prod_{i=1}^{n} P^{\Delta}(\mathbf{Q})_{x_{i-1} x_i},$$

with the notation that the ij entry of a matrix A is denoted A_{ij}. Since it is a discrete time Markov chain, it satisfies,

$$L_{n,\Delta}(\mathbf{Q}) = \prod_{k=1}^{N} \prod_{l=1}^{N} (P^{\Delta}(\mathbf{Q})_{kl}^{N^{kl}(n)},$$

$$N^{kl}(n) = \sum_{i=1}^{n} \delta_{\{X_{i-1}=k, X_i=l\}}.$$

The random variables $(N^{kl}(n))$ are the number of transitions from state k to state l before n. We have proved in Section 2.1) that the associated MLE of the transition matrix $\hat{\mathbf{P}}$ is explicit. But building an estimator of Q from $\hat{\mathbf{P}}$ is not straightforward.

Indeed, let $\mathscr{P}_0 = \{\exp \mathbf{Q} \mid \mathbf{Q} \in \mathscr{Q}\}$ denote the set of transition matrices that correspond to discrete time observation of a continuous time Markov jump process. If $\hat{\mathbf{P}} \in \mathscr{P}_0$, there exists a $\hat{\mathbf{Q}} \in \mathscr{Q}$ such that $P^{\Delta}(\hat{\mathbf{Q}}) = \hat{\mathbf{P}}$. This raises two distinct problems. First the set $\mathscr{P}_0$ is quite complex, and second the matrix exponential function is not an injection on its domain, so $\hat{\mathbf{Q}}$ may not be unique leading to identifiability questions for the statistical model. Additional assumptions are thus required in order to ensure the convergence of stochastic algorithms such as *EM*, *MCMC*. We refer to Bladt and Sorensen [14] for details.

4.2.2.2 The Expectation-Maximization (EM) Algorithm

This is a broadly used method for optimizing the likelihood function in cases where only partial information is available (see e.g. [33, 34, 122, 126]). A discretely observed Markov jump process is such an example where only data $Y_i = X(t_i); i = 1, \ldots, n$ are available. Let $X = \{X(t); 0 \leq t \leq T\}$ and $Y = \{Y_i; i = 1 \ldots, n\}$. The EM-algorithm aimed at estimating the Q-matrix $Q = (q_{ij},; i, j \in E)$ iterating the two steps:
E-step: replace the unobserved parts by their conditional expected values given the data $Y = y$
M-step: perform maximum likelihood on the complete data.

The difficult part in the EM algorithm here is the **E-step**:
i.e. compute $\mathbb{E}_{Q_0}[\log L_T(\mathbf{Q})|Y = y]$ where Q_0 is an arbitrary Q-matrix.
Indeed, consider the **M-step**. From equation (4.2.6), we have

$$\begin{aligned}\mathbb{E}_{\mathbf{Q}_0}(\log L_T(\mathbf{Q})|Y = y) &= \sum_{k=1}^{N} \sum_{l \neq k} \log(q_{kl}) \mathbb{E}_{\mathbf{Q}_0}(N_{kl}(T)|Y = y) \\ &\quad - \sum_{k=1}^{N} \sum_{l \neq k} q_{kl} \mathbb{E}_{\mathbf{Q}_0}(N_k(T)|Y = y).\end{aligned}$$

This is the likelihood of a continuous time process with observed statistics $\mathbb{E}_{\mathbf{Q}_0}(N_{kl}(T)|Y = y), \mathbb{E}_{\mathbf{Q}_0}(N_k(T)|Y = y)$. It is maximized, as a function of Q, according to (4.2.8) by

$$\hat{Q}_{kl} = \frac{\mathbb{E}_{\mathbf{Q}_0}(N_{kl}(T)|Y = y)}{\mathbb{E}_{\mathbf{Q}_0}(N_k(T)|Y = y)}. \tag{4.2.9}$$

Therefore, to perform the algorithm, we have to compute the two quantities $\mathbb{E}_{\mathbf{Q}_0}(N_{kl}(T)|Y = y)$ and $\mathbb{E}_{\mathbf{Q}_0}(N_k(T)|Y = y)$.
For this, let us consider a fixed intensity matrix $\mathbf{Q}$ and omit the index $\mathbf{Q}$. Denote by e_i the unit vector with i^{th} coordinate equal to 1, and for U a vector or a matrix, let U^* the transpose of U.

Noting that $N^k(T) = \sum_{p=1}^{n}(N^k(t_p) - N^k(t_{p-1}))$, we get by the Markov property and the time homogeneity of $X = X(t)$,

$$\begin{aligned}\mathbb{E}(N^k(t_p) - N^k(t_{p-1})/Y = y) &= \mathbb{E}(N^k(t_p) - N^k(t_{p-1})|X(t_p) = y_p, X(t_{p-1}) = y_{p-1}) \\ &= \mathbb{E}(N^k(t_p - t_{p-1})|X(t_p - t_{p-1}) = y_p, X(0) = y_{p-1}).\end{aligned}$$

Similarly $N^{kl}(T) = \sum_{p=1}^{n}(N^{kl}(t_p) - N^{kl}(t_{p-1}))$, and

$$\mathbb{E}(N^{kl}(t_p)-N^{kl}(t_{p-1})/Y=y)=\mathbb{E}(N^{kl}(t_p-t_{p-1})|X(t_p-t_{p-1})=y_p,X(0)=y_{p-1}).$$

Hence,

$$\mathbb{E}(N^k(T)|Y=y)=\sum_{p=1}^{n}E^k_{y_{p-1}y_p}(t_p-t_{p-1});\quad \mathbb{E}^{kl}(T)|Y=y)=\sum_{p=1}^{n}F^{kl}_{y_{p-1}y_p}(t_p-t_{p-1});\tag{4.2.10}$$

where if (i,j) and $(k,l)\in E$, and $t>0$,

$$\begin{aligned}E^k_{ij}(t)&=\mathbb{E}_{\mathbf{Q}_0}(N^k(t)|X(t)=j,X(0)=i),\\ F^{kl}_{ij}(t)&=\mathbb{E}_{\mathbf{Q}_0}(N^{kl}(t)|X(t)=j,X(0)=i).\end{aligned}$$

Fix $k\in E$ and define the matrix $M^k(t)$ by

$$M^k_{ij}(t)=\mathbb{E}(N_k(t)1_{X(t)=j}|X(0)=i).\tag{4.2.11}$$

Then, according to [13],

$$\frac{d}{dt}M^k_{ij}(t)=\sum_{l=1}^{N}M^k_{il}(t)q_{lj}+\exp(t\mathbf{Q})_{ij}\delta_{jk};\quad M^k_{ij}(t_0)=0.$$

This equation has an explicit solution which reads as $\mathbf{M}^k(t)=(M^k_{ij}(t),i,j\in E)$,

$$\mathbf{M}^k(t)=\int_0^t\exp(s\mathbf{Q})(e_ke_k^*)\exp((t-s)\mathbf{Q})\,ds.\tag{4.2.12}$$

Fix now $k,l\in E$ and define the matrix $\mathbf{f}^{kl}_{ij}(t)=\mathbb{E}(N^{kl}(t)1_{X(t)=j}|X(0)=i)$. Similarly

$$\mathbf{f}^{kl}(t)=q_{kl}\int_0^t\exp(s\mathbf{Q})(e_ke_l^*)\exp((t-s)\mathbf{Q})ds.\tag{4.2.13}$$

Hence, using that $\mathbb{P}(X(t)=j|X(0)=i)=e_i^*\exp(\mathbf{Q}t)e_j$ yields that

$$E^k_{ij}(t)=\frac{M^k_{ij}(t)}{e_i^*\exp(t\mathbf{Q})e_j};\quad F^{kl}_{ij}(t)=\frac{\mathbf{f}^{kl}_{ij}(t)}{e_i^*\exp(t\mathbf{Q})e_j}.\tag{4.2.14}$$

So the EM-algorithm works along the successive iterations. Start from an initial Q-matrix $\mathbf{Q}_0$. Let $\mathbf{Q}_m$ denote the Q-matrix of iteration m. Then

- For all $k,l\in E$, compute using (4.2.12), (4.2.13), (4.2.14) the matrices $E_{y_iy_{i+1}}(t_{i+1}-t_i)$, and $F^{kl}_{y_iy_{i+1}}(t_{i+1}-t_i)$ associated to $Q=\mathbf{Q}_m$
- Compute the two quantities $\mathbb{E}(N^k(T)|Y=y)$, $\mathbb{E}(N^{kl}(T)|Y=y)$ using (4.2.10)
- Define $\mathbf{Q}_{m+1}$ by (4.2.9).

Let $\mathbf{Q}_0,\mathbf{Q}_1,\ldots,\mathbf{Q}_p,\ldots$ a sequence a Q- matrices obtained by the EM algorithm. Then $L_{n,\Delta}(\mathbf{Q}_{p+1})\geq L_{n,\Delta}(\mathbf{Q}_p)$ for $p=0,1,2,\ldots$ (see e.g. [34]). Under additional regularity conditions, one can prove (cf [14], Theorem 4) that,
If $\mathbf{Q}_0$ satisfies that, for all $k,l\in E$, $(\mathbf{Q}_0)_{kl}>0$, then the sequence $(\mathbf{Q}_p)$ converge to a stationary point of the likelihood function $L_{n,\Delta}$ or $det\{exp(\mathbf{Q}_p)\}\to 0$.

4.3 ABC Estimation

Markov Chain Monte Carlo (MCMC) methods that treat the missing data as extra parameters, have become increasingly popular for calibrating stochastic epidemiological models with missing data [25, 104, 106]. However, MCMC may be computationally prohibitive for high-dimensional missing observations [26, 119] and fine tuning of the proposal distribution is required for efficient algorithms [52]. The computation of the likelihood can sometimes be numerically infeasible because it involves integration over the unobserved events. In discrete time, or when the total population size is known and small as in [106], this is possible. But in (4.2.1) for example, because we are in continuous time, the likelihood of removal times, when the infection times and K_t^N are unknown, involves a summation over all possibilities which is impossible: the sum is over all the possible numbers of infections between each successive removal times, plus on the possible times of these infections. An alternative is given by Approximate Bayesian Computation (ABC), which was originally proposed for making inference in population genetics [10]. This approach is not based on the likelihood function but relies on numerical simulations and comparisons between simulated and observed summary statistics. We detail here the ABC procedure and its application to epidemiology. For more information on ABC methods, the interested reader is referred to [99, 113]. In particular, there have been many refinements of the ABC method presented here, for instance using simulations to modify the sampling distributions (e.g. [9, 115, 120]).

In [17], the development of ABC estimation techniques for SIR models is motivated by the study of the Cuban HIV-AIDS database. In this case, the population is separated into the following compartments: 1) susceptible individuals who can be infected by HIV, 2) non-detected HIV positive infectious individuals who can propagate the disease, and 3) detected HIV positive individuals. When an individual is detected as HIV positive, we assume that the transmission of the disease ceases. So detection corresponds here to 'recovery' events in the classical SIR model presented in Part I of this book. The Cuban database contains the dates of detection of the 8,662 individuals that have been found to be HIV positive in Cuba between 1986 and 2007 [4]. The database contains additional covariates including the manner by which an individual has been found to be HIV positive. The individuals can be detected either by *random screening* (individuals 'spontaneously' take a detection test) or *contact-tracing*. The total number of infectious individuals as well as the infection times are unknown. Blum and Tran [17] proposed an ABC estimation procedure when all detection times are known, which they then extend to noisy or binned detection times. They also propose an extension of ABC to path-valued summary statistics consisting of the cumulated number of detections through time. They introduce a finite-dimensional vector of summary statistics and compare the statistical properties of point estimates and credibility intervals obtained with full and binned detection times. We present here these methods for a simple SIR model and compare numerically the posterior distributions obtained with ABC and MCMC. We refer the reader to [17] for more details and treatment of Cuban HIV data. Other use of ABC estimation techniques in public health can be found in [38, 102] for example.

4.3.1 Main Principles of ABC

For simplicity, we deal here with densities and not general probability measures. Let $\mathbf{x}$ be the available data and $\pi(\theta)$ be the prior where θ is the parameter. Two approximations are at the core of ABC.

Replacing observations with summary statistics Instead of focusing on the posterior density $p(\theta\,|\,\mathbf{x})$, ABC aims at a possibly less informative *target* density $p(\theta\,|\,S(\mathbf{x}) = s_{obs}) \propto \Pr(s_{obs}|\theta)\pi(\theta)$ where S is a summary statistic that takes its values in a normed space, and s_{obs} denotes the observed summary statistic. The summary statistic S can be a d-dimensional vector or an infinite-dimensional variable such as a L^1 function. Of course, if S is sufficient, then the two conditional densities are the same. The target distribution will also be coined as the *partial posterior distribution.*

Simulation-based approximations of the posterior Once the summary statistics have been chosen, the second approximation arises when estimating the partial posterior density $p(\theta\,|\,S(\mathbf{x}) = s_{obs})$ and sampling from this distribution. This step involves nonparametric kernel estimation and possibly correction refinements.

4.3.1.1 Sampling from the Posterior

The ABC method with smooth rejection generates random draws from the target distribution as follows (see e.g. [10])

1. Generate N random draws (θ_i, s_i), $i = 1,\dots,N$. The parameter θ_i is generated from the prior distribution π and the vector of summary statistics s_i is calculated for the ith data set that is simulated from the generative model with parameter θ_i.
2. Associate to the ith simulation the weight $W_i = K_\delta(s_i - s_{obs})$, where δ is a tolerance threshold and K_δ a (possibly multivariate) smoothing kernel.
3. The distribution $(\sum_{i=1}^N W_i \delta_{\theta_i})/(\sum_{i=1}^N W_i)$, in which δ_θ denotes the Dirac mass at θ, approximates the target distribution.

4.3.1.2 Point Estimation and Credibility Intervals

Assume here that $\theta = (\theta_1, \dots \theta_d)$ is a d-dimensional vector. We denote by $\theta_i = (\theta_{1,i}, \dots \theta_{d,i})$ the simulated vectors of parameters in the previous paragraph. Once a sample from the target distribution has been obtained, several estimators may be considered for point estimation of each one-dimensional component θ_j, $j \in$

$\{1,\ldots d\}$. Using the weighted sample $(\theta_{j,i}, W_i)$, $i = 1,\ldots,N$, the *mean* of the target distribution $p(\theta_j | s_{obs})$ is estimated by

$$\hat{\theta}_j = \frac{\sum_{i=1}^{N} \theta_{j,i} W_i}{\sum_{i=1}^{N} W_i} = \frac{\sum_{i=1}^{N} \theta_{j,i} K_\delta(s_i - s_{obs})}{\sum_{i=1}^{N} K_\delta(s_i - s_{obs})}, \quad j = 1,2,3 \tag{4.3.1}$$

which is the well-known Nadaraya–Watson regression estimator of the conditional expectation $\mathbb{E}(\theta_j \,|\, s_{obs})$ (see e.g. [121, Chapter 1]). We also compute the *medians*, *modes*, and 95% credibility intervals (CI) of the marginal posterior distribution (see Section 3 of the supplementary material).

4.3.1.3 Summary Statistics

We are here interested in estimating the parameter $\theta = (\lambda, \gamma)$ of a SIR model (see Part I of this book). Two different sets of summary statistics are considered.

First, we consider the (infinite-dimensional) statistics $(R_t, t \in [0,T])$ consisting of the cumulated number of recoveries at time t since the beginning of the epidemic. Because the data consist of the recovery times this curve $(R_t, t \in [0,T])$ can simply be viewed as a particular coding of the whole dataset. It is thus a sufficient statistic implying that the partial posterior distribution $p(\theta \,|\, R^1, R^2)$ is equal to the posterior distribution $p(\theta \,|\, \mathbf{x})$.
The L^1-norm between the ith simulated path R_i and the observed one R_{obs} is

$$\|R_{obs} - R_i\|_1 = \int_0^T |R_{obs,s} - R_{i,s}|\, ds \quad , i = 1,\ldots,N. \tag{4.3.2}$$

The weights W_i are then computed as $W_i = K_\delta(\|R_{obs} - R_i\|_1)$ where δ is a tolerance threshold found by accepting a given percentage P_δ of the simulations and where an Epanechnikov kernel is chosen for K.

Second, when there is noise or when the recovery times have been binned, the full observations $(R_t, t \in [0,T])$ are unavailable. Then, we replace these summary statistics by a vector of summary statistics such as the numbers of recoveries per year during the observation period. We consider a d-dimensional vector of summary statistics of three different types: 1) number R_T of individuals detected by the end of the observation period, 2) for each year j, numbers of removed individuals $R_{j+1} - R_j$, 3) numbers of new infectious in the first years (assuming for instance that all of them have been detected since) $I_{j+1} - I_j$ for $j = 0,\ldots,J_0$, where J_0 is a small number of years where the information is supposed to be known, 4) mean time during which an individual is infected but has not been detected in the J_0 first years. This mean time corresponds to the mean sojourn time in the class I for the J_0 first years. Since these new summary statistics are not sufficient anymore, the new partial posterior distribution may be different from the posterior $p(\theta \,|\, \mathbf{x})$.
In order to compute the weights W_i, we consider the following spherical kernel $K_\delta(x) \propto K(\|\mathbf{H}^{-1}x\|/\delta)$. Here K denotes the one-dimensional Epanechnikov kernel,

$\|\cdot\|$ is the Euclidean norm of $\mathbb{R}^d$ and $\mathbf{H}^{-1}$ a matrix. Because the summary statistics may span different scales, $\mathbf{H}$ is taken equal to the diagonal matrix with the standard deviation of each one-dimensional summary statistic on the diagonal.

4.3.2 Comparisons Between ABC and MCMC Methods for a Standard SIR Model

Following [10] a performance indicator for ABC techniques consists in their ability to replicate likelihood-based results given by MCMC. Here the situation is particularly favourable for comparing the two methods since the partial and the full posterior are the same. In the following examples, we choose samples of small sizes ($n = 3$ and $n = 29$) so that the dimension of the missing data is reasonable and MCMC achieves fast convergence. For large sample sizes with high-dimensional missing data, MCMC convergence might indeed be a serious issue and more thorough updating scheme shall be implemented [26, 119].

We consider the standard SIR model with infection rate λ and recovery rate γ. The data consist of the recovery times and we assume that the infection times are not observed. We implement the MCMC algorithm of [106]. A total of $10,000$ steps are considered for MCMC with an initial burn-in of $5,000$ steps. For ABC, the summary statistic consists of the cumulative number of recoveries as a function of time. A total of $100,000$ simulations are performed for ABC.

The first example was previously considered by [106]. They simulated recovery times by considering one initial infectious individual and by setting $S_0 = 9$, $\lambda = 0.12$, and $\gamma = 1$. We choose gamma distributions for the priors of λ and γ with a shape parameters of 0.1 and rate parameters of 1 and 0.1. As displayed by Figure 4.3.1, the posterior distributions obtained with ABC are extremely close to the ones obtained with MCMC provided that the tolerance rate is sufficiently small. We see that the tolerance rate changes importantly the posterior distribution obtained with ABC (see the posterior distributions for λ).

In a second example, we simulate a standard SIR trajectory with $\lambda = 0.12$, $\gamma = 1$, $S_0 = 30$ and $I_0 = 1$. The data now consist of 29 recovery times (and are given in the supplementary material of [17]). Once again, Figure 4.3.1 shows that the ABC and MCMC posteriors are close provided that the tolerance rate is small enough. ABC produces posterior distributions with larger tails compared to MCMC, even with the lowest tolerance rate of 0.1%. This can be explained by considering the extreme scenario in which the tolerance threshold δ goes to infinity: every simulation has a weight of 1 so that ABC targets the prior instead of the posterior. As the prior has typically larger tails than the posterior, ABC inflates the posterior tails.

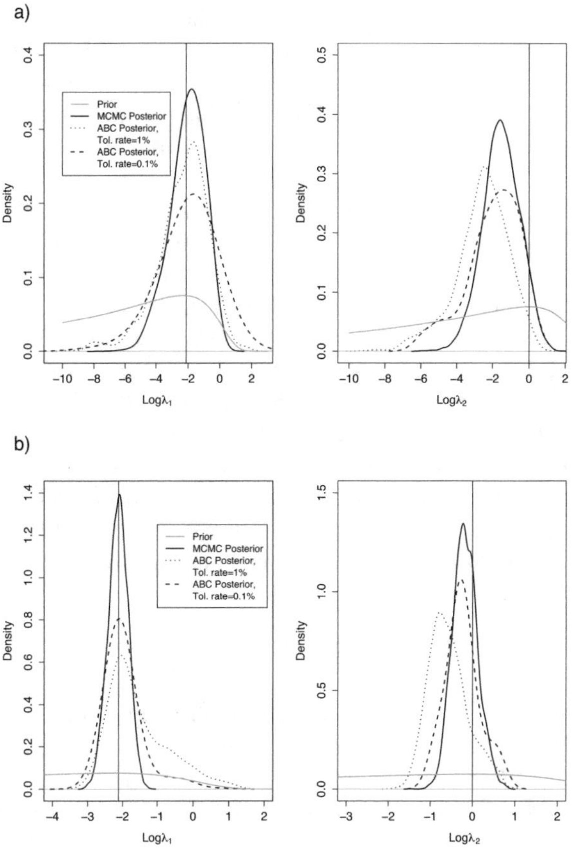

Fig. 4.3.1 *Comparison of the posterior densities obtained with MCMC and ABC. The vertical lines correspond to the values of the parameters used for generating the synthetic data. Left: the data consist of 3 recovery times that have been simulated by [106]. Right: The data consist of 29 recovery times that we simulated by setting* $\lambda = 0.12$, $\gamma = 1$, $S_0 = 30$, $I_0 = 1$, *and* $T = 5$ *(see the supplementary material of [17] for the 29 recovery times).*

4.3.3 Comparison Between ABC with Full and Binned Recovery Times

4.3.3.1 The Curse of Dimensionality and Regression Adjustments

In this case, the first set of summary statistics presented in Section 4.3.1 can not be used any more and we have to use the second set of summary statistics, which constitute a vector of descriptive statistics as is much often encountered in the literature. In the case of a d-dimensional vector of summary statistics, the estimator of the conditional mean (4.3.1) is convergent if the tolerance rate satisfies $\lim_{N\to+\infty} \delta_N = 0$, so that its bias converges to 0, and $\lim_{N\to+\infty} N\delta_N^d = +\infty$, so that its variance converges to 0 [40]. As d increases, a larger tolerance threshold shall be chosen to keep the variance small. As a consequence, the bias may increase with the number of summary statistics. This phenomenon known as the *curse of dimensionality* may be an issue for the ABC-rejection approach. The following paragraph presents regression-based adjustments that cope with the curse of dimensionality.

The adjustment principle is presented in a general setting within which the corrections of [10] and [16] can be derived. Correction adjustments aim at obtaining from a random couple (θ_i, s_i) a random variable distributed according to $p(\theta \mid s_{obs})$. The idea is to construct a coupling between the distributions $p(\theta|s_i)$ and $p(\theta|s_{obs})$, through which we can shrink the θ_i's to a sample of i.i.d. draws from $p(\theta|s_{obs})$. In the remaining of this subsection, we describe how to perform the corrections for each of the one-dimensional components separately. For $\theta \in \mathbb{R}$, correction adjustments are obtained by assuming a relationship $\theta = G(s, \varepsilon) =: G_s(\varepsilon)$ between the parameter and the summary statistics. Here G is a (possibly complicated) function and ε is a random variable with a distribution that does not depend on s. A possibility is to choose $G_s = F_s^{-1}$, the (generalized) inverse of the cumulative distribution function of $p(\theta|s)$. In this case, $\varepsilon = F_s(\theta)$ is a uniform random variable on $[0, 1]$. The formula for adjustment is given by

$$\theta_i^* = G_{s_{obs}}^{-1}(G_{s_i}(\theta_i)) \quad i = 1, \ldots, N. \tag{4.3.3}$$

For $G_s = F_s^{-1}$, the fact that the θ_i^*'s are i.i.d. with density $p(\theta|s_{obs})$ arises from the standard inversion algorithm. Of course, the function G shall be approximated in practice. As a consequence, the adjusted simulations θ_i^*, $i = 1, \ldots, N$, constitute an approximate sample of $p(\theta \mid s_{obs})$. The ABC algorithm with regression adjustment can be described as follows

1. Simulate, as in the rejection algorithm, a sample (θ_i, s_i), $i = 1, \ldots, N$.
2. By making use of the sample of the (θ_i, s_i)'s weighted by the W_i's, approximate the function G such that $\theta_i = G(s_i, \varepsilon_i)$ in the vicinity of s_{obs}.
3. Replace the θ_i's by the adjusted θ_i^*'s. The resulting weighted sample (θ_i^*, W_i), $i = 1, \ldots, N$, form a sample from the target distribution.

Local linear regression (LOCL) The case where G is approximated by a linear model $G(s, \varepsilon) = \alpha + s^t\beta + \varepsilon$, was considered by [10]. The parameters α and β are inferred by minimizing the weighted squared error

$$\sum_{i=1}^{N} K_\delta(s_i - s_{obs})(\theta_i - (\alpha + (s_i - s_{obs})^T \beta))^2.$$

Using (4.3.3), the correction of [10] is derived as

$$\theta_i^* = \theta_i - (s_i - s_{obs})^T \hat{\beta}, \; i = 1, \ldots, N. \tag{4.3.4}$$

Asymptotic consistency of the estimators of the partial posterior distribution with the correction (4.3.4) is obtained by [15].

Nonlinear conditional heteroscedastic regressions (NCH) To relax the assumptions of homoscedasticity and linearity inherent to local linear regression, Blum and Francois [16] approximated G by $G(s,\varepsilon) = m(s) + \sigma(s) \times \varepsilon$ where $m(s)$ denotes the conditional expectation, and $\sigma^2(s)$ the conditional variance. The estimators $\hat{m}$ and $\log\hat{\sigma}^2$ are found by adjusting two feed-forward neural networks using a regularized weighted squared error. For the NCH model, parameter adjustment is performed as follows

$$\theta_i^* = \hat{m}(s_{obs}) + (\theta_i - \hat{m}(s_i)) \times \frac{\hat{\sigma}(s_{obs})}{\hat{\sigma}(s_i)},\ i = 1,\ldots,N.$$

In practical applications of the NCH model, we train $L = 10$ neural networks for each conditional regression (expectation and variance) and we average the results of the L neural networks to provide the estimates $\hat{m}$ and $\log\hat{\sigma}^2$.

Reparameterization In both regression adjustment approaches, the regressions can be performed on transformations of the responses θ_i rather that on the responses themselves. Parameters whose prior distributions have finite supports are transformed via the logit function and non-negative parameters are transformed via the logarithm function. These transformations guarantee that the θ_i^*'s lie in the support of the prior distribution and have the additional advantage of stabilizing the variance.

Comparison between the first and second set of summary statistics A simulation study is carried to compare the ABC methods based on the two different sets of summary statistics presented in Section 4.3.1 has been carried in [17] using a slightly more elaborate SIR model with contact-tracing introduced in [30]. Blum and Tran simulated $M = 200$ synthetic data sets epidemic. When using the finite-dimensional vector of summary statistics, they perform the smooth rejection approach as well as the LOCL and NCH corrections with a total of 21 summary statistics. Each of the $M = 200$ estimations of the partial posterior distributions are performed using a total of $N = 5000$ simulations.

Figure 4.3.2 displays the boxplots of the 200 estimated modes, medians, 2.5% and 97.5% quantiles of the posterior distribution for λ as a function of the tolerance rate P_δ. First, the medians and modes are found to be equivalent except for the rejection method with 21 summary statistics for which the mode is less biased. For the lowest tolerance rates, the point estimates obtained with the four possible methods are close to the value λ used in the simulations, with smaller CI for the LOCL and NCH variants. When increasing the tolerance rate, the bias of the point estimates obtained with the rejection method with 21 summary statistics slightly increases. By contrast, up to tolerance rates smaller than 50%, the biases of the point estimates obtained with the three other methods remain small. As can be expected, the widths of the CI obtained with the rejection methods increase with the tolerance rate while they remain considerably less variable for the methods with regression adjustment.

For further comparison of the different methods, we can compute the rescaled mean square errors (ReMSEs):

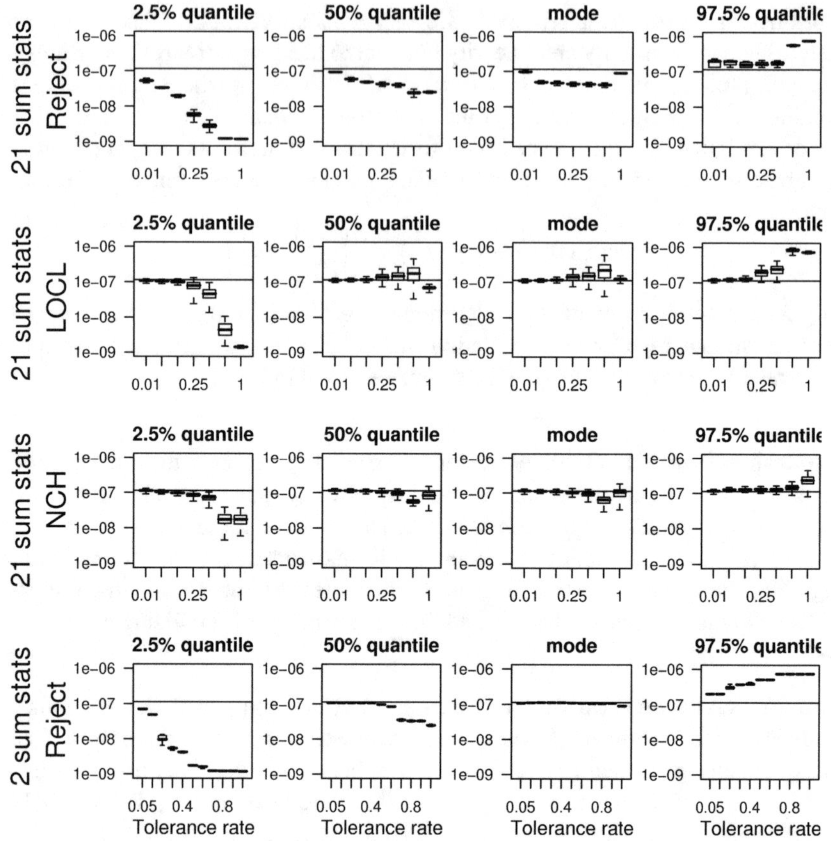

Fig. 4.3.2 *Boxplots of the* $M = 200$ *estimated modes and quantiles (2.5%, 50%, and 97.5%) of the partial posterior distributions of* λ *in a model presented in Blum and Tran [17]. For each ABC method and each value of the tolerance rate,* 200 *posterior distributions are computed for each of the 200 synthetic data sets. The horizontal lines correspond to the true value* $\lambda = 1.14 \times 10^{-7}$ *used when simulating the 200 synthetic data sets. The different tolerance rates are 0.01, 0.05, 0.10, 0.25, 0.50, 0.50, 0.75, and 1 for all the ABC methods except the rejection scheme with the two summary statistics. For the latter method, the tolerance rates are* 0.007, 0.02, 0.06, 0.13, 0.27, 0.37, 0.45, 0.53, 0.66, 0.80, 1.

$$\text{ReMSE}(\lambda) = \frac{1}{M} \sum_{k=1}^{M} \frac{(\log(\hat{\lambda}^k) - \log(\lambda))^2}{\text{Range}(\text{prior}(\lambda))^2}, \tag{4.3.5}$$

where $\hat{\lambda}^k$ is a point estimate obtained with the kth synthetic data set.

To compare the whole posterior distributions obtained with the four different methods, we can also compute the different CIs. The rescaled mean CI (RMCI) is defined as follows

$$\text{RMCI} = \frac{1}{M} \sum_{k=1}^{M} \frac{|IC^k|}{\text{Range}(\text{prior}(\lambda))}, \tag{4.3.6}$$

where $|IC^k|$ is the length of the kth estimated 95% CI for the parameter λ. As displayed by Figure 4.3.2, the CIs obtained with smooth rejection increase importantly with the tolerance rate whereas such an important increase is not observed with regression adjustment.

4.4 Sensitivity Analysis

Epidemiological models designed in order to test public health scenarios by simulations or disentangle various factors for a better understanding of the disease propagation are often over-parameterized. Input parameters are the rates describing the times that individuals stay in each compartment, for example. The sources that are used to calibrate the model can also be numerous: some parameters are for example obtained from epidemiological studies or clinical trials, but there can be uncertainty on their values due to various reasons. The restricted size of the sample in these studies brings uncertainty on the estimates, which are given with uncertainty intervals (classically, a 95% confidence interval). Different studies can provide different estimates for the same parameters. The study populations can be subject to selection biases. In the case of clinical trials where the efficacy of a treatment is estimated, the estimates can be optimistic compared with what will be the effectiveness in real-life, due to the protocol of the trials. It is important to quantify how theses uncertainties on the input parameters can impact the results and the conclusion of an epidemiological modelling study. To check the robustness of some output with respect to the parameters, sensitivity analyses are often performed.

In a mathematical model where the output $y \in \mathbb{R}$ depends on a set of $p \in \mathbb{N}$ input parameters $x = (x_1, ...x_p) \in \mathbb{R}^p$ through the relation $y = f(x)$, there are various ways to measure the influence of the input x_ℓ, for $\ell \in \{1, \ldots, p\}$, on y. In this article, we are interested in Sobol indices [116], which are based on an ANOVA decomposition (see [111, 76, 77] for a review). These indices have been proposed to take into account the uncertainty on the input parameters that are here considered as a realisation of a set of independent random variables $X = (X_1, ...X_p)$, with a known distribution and with possibly correlated components. Denoting by $Y = f(X)$ the random response, the first-order Sobol indices can be defined for $\ell \in \{1, \ldots, p\}$ by

$$S_\ell = \frac{\text{Var}\big(\mathbb{E}[Y \mid X_\ell]\big)}{\text{Var}(Y)}. \tag{4.4.1}$$

This first-order index S_ℓ corresponds to the sensitivity of the model to X_ℓ alone. Higher order indices can also be defined using ANOVA decomposition: considering $(\ell, \ell') \in \{1, \ldots, p\}$, we can define the second order sensitivity, corresponding to the sensitivity of the model to the interaction between X_ℓ and $X_{\ell'}$ index by

$$S_{\ell\ell'} = \frac{\text{Var}\big(\mathbb{E}[Y \mid X_\ell, X_{\ell'}]\big)}{\text{Var}(Y)} - S_\ell - S_{\ell'} \tag{4.4.2}$$

We can also define the total sensitivity indices by

$$S_{T_\ell} = \sum_{L \subset \{1,\dots,p\} \,|\, \ell \in L} S_L. \tag{4.4.3}$$

As the estimation of the Sobol indices can be computer time consuming, a usual practice consists in estimating the first-order and total indices, to assess 1) the sensitivity of the model to each parameter taken separately and 2) the possible interactions, which are quantified by the difference between the total order and the first-order index for each parameter. Several numerical procedures to estimate the Sobol indices have been proposed, in particular by Jansen [81] (see also [110, 111]). These estimators, that we recall in the sequel, are based on Monte Carlo simulations of $(Y, X_1 \dots X_p)$.

The literature focuses on deterministic relations between the input and output parameters. In a stochastic framework where the model response Y is not unique for given input parameters, few works have been done, randomness being usually limited to input variables. Assume that:

$$Y = f(X, \varepsilon), \tag{4.4.4}$$

where $X = (X_1, \dots X_p)$ still denotes the random variables modelling the uncertainty of the input parameters and where ε is a noise variable. When noise is added in the model, the classical estimators do not always work: Y can be very sensitive to the addition of ε. Moreover, this variable is not always controllable by the user.

When the function f is linear, we can refer to [43]. In the literature, meta-models are used: approximating the mean and the dispersion of the response by deterministic functions allows us to come back to the classical deterministic framework (e.g. Janon et al. [80], Marrel et al. [100]). We study here another point of view, which is based on the non-parametric statistical estimation of the term $\mathrm{Var}\big(\mathbb{E}[Y \mid X_\ell]\big)$ appearing in the numerator of (4.4.1).

Approaches based on the Nadaraya–Watson kernel estimator have been proposed by Da Veiga and Gamboa [125] or Solís [117] while an approach based on warped wavelet decompositions is proposed by Castellan et al. [24]. An advantage of these non-parametric estimators is that their computation requires less simulations of the model. For Jansen estimators, the number of calls of f required to compute the sensitivity indices is $n(p+1)$, where n is the number of independent random vectors $(Y^i, X_1^i, \dots X_p^i)$ $(i \in \{1, \dots n\})$ that are sampled for the Monte Carlo procedure, making the estimation of the sensitivity indices time-consuming for sophisticated models with many parameters. In addition, for the non-parametric estimators, the convergence of the mean square error to zero may be faster than for Monte Carlo estimators, depending on the regularity of the model.

4.4.1 A Non-parametric Estimator of the Sobol Indices of Order 1

Denoting by $V_\ell = \mathbb{E}\big(\mathbb{E}^2(Y \mid X_\ell)\big)$ the expectation of the square conditional expectation of Y knowing X_ℓ, we have:

$$S_\ell = \frac{V_\ell - \mathbb{E}(Y)^2}{\mathrm{Var}(Y)}, \tag{4.4.5}$$

which can be approximated by

$$\widehat{S}_\ell = \frac{\widehat{V}_\ell - \bar{Y}^2}{\widehat{\sigma}_Y^2} \tag{4.4.6}$$

where

$$\bar{Y} = \frac{1}{n}\sum_{j=1}^{n} Y_j \text{ and } \widehat{\sigma}_Y^2 = \frac{1}{n}\sum_{j=1}^{n}(Y_j - \bar{Y})^2$$

are the empirical mean and variance of Y. We consider here two approximations $\widehat{V}_\ell$ of V_ℓ, based on Nadaraya–Watson and on warped wavelet estimators.

Assume that we have n independent couples $(Y^i, X_1^i, \ldots X_p^i)$ in $\mathbb{R} \times \mathbb{R}^p$, for $i \in \{1, \ldots, n\}$, generated by (4.4.4). Let us start with the kernel-based estimator:

Definition 4.4.1. Let $K : \mathbb{R} \mapsto \mathbb{R}$ be a kernel such that $\int_{\mathbb{R}} K(u)du = 1$. Let $h > 0$ be a window and let us denote $K_h(x) = K(x/h)/h$. An estimator of S_ℓ for $\ell \in \{1, \ldots p\}$ is:

$$\widehat{S}_\ell^{(NW)} = \frac{\frac{1}{n}\sum_{i=1}^{n}\left(\frac{\sum_{j=1}^{n} Y_j K_h(X_\ell^j - X_\ell^i)}{\sum_{j=1}^{n} K_h(X_\ell^j - X_\ell^i)}\right)^2 - \bar{Y}^2}{\widehat{\sigma}_Y^2}. \tag{4.4.7}$$

This estimator is based on the Nadaraya–Watson estimator of $\mathbb{E}(Y \mid X_\ell = x)$ given by (e.g. [121])

$$\frac{\sum_{j=1}^{n} Y_j K_h(X_\ell^j - x)}{\sum_{j=1}^{n} K_h(X_\ell^j - x)}.$$

Replacing this expression in (4.4.6) provides $\widehat{S}_\ell^{(NW)}$. This estimator and the rates of convergence have been studied by Solís [117]. If we instead use a warped wavelet decomposition of $\mathbb{E}(Y \mid X_\ell = x)$ (see e.g. [28, 84]), this provides an estimator studied by Castellan et al. [24]. Let us present this second estimator.

Let us denote by G_ℓ the cumulative distribution function of X_ℓ. Let $(\psi_{jk})_{j \geq -1, k \in \mathbb{Z}}$ be a Hilbert wavelet basis of L^2, the space of real functions that are square integrable with respect to the Lebesgue measure on $\mathbb{R}$. In the sequel, we denote by $\langle f, g \rangle = \int_{\mathbb{R}} f(u)g(u)du$, for $f, g \in L^2$, the usual scalar product of L^2. The wavelet ψ_{-10} is the father wavelet, and for $k \in \mathbb{Z}$, $\psi_{-1k}(x) = \psi_{-10}(x-k)$. The wavelet ψ_{00} is the mother wavelet, and for $j \geq 0$, $k \in \mathbb{Z}$, $\psi_{jk}(x) = 2^{j/2}\psi_{00}(2^j x - k)$.

Definition 4.4.2. Let us define for $j \geq -1$, $k \in \mathbb{Z}$,

$$\widehat{\beta}^{\ell}_{jk} = \frac{1}{n}\sum_{i=1}^{n} Y_i \psi_{jk}(G_\ell(X^i_\ell)). \tag{4.4.8}$$

Then, we define the (block thresholding) estimator of S_ℓ as

$$\widehat{S}^{(WW)}_\ell = \frac{\widehat{V}_\ell - \bar{Y}^2}{\widehat{\sigma}^2_Y}, \tag{4.4.9}$$

where $\widehat{V}_\ell$ is an estimator of the variance V_ℓ given by:

$$\widehat{V}_\ell = \sum_{j=-1}^{J_n} \Big[\sum_{k\in\mathbb{Z}} \big(\widehat{\beta}^{\ell}_{jk}\big)^2 - w(j)\Big] \mathbf{1}_{\sum_{k\in\mathbb{Z}}\left(\widehat{\beta}^{\ell}_{jk}\right)^2 \geq w(j)} \tag{4.4.10}$$

with $w(j) = K\left(\frac{2^j + \log 2}{n}\right)$ and $J_n := \left[\log_2\left(\frac{\sqrt{n}}{\log(n)}\right)\right]$ (where $[\cdot]$ denotes the integer part) and K a positive constant.

Let us present the idea explaining the estimator proposed in Definition 4.4.2. Let us introduce centered random variables η_ℓ such that

$$Y = f(X,\varepsilon) = \mathbb{E}(Y \,|\, X_\ell) + \eta_\ell. \tag{4.4.11}$$

Let $g_\ell(x) = \mathbb{E}(Y \,|\, X_\ell = x)$ and $h_\ell(u) = g_\ell \circ G_\ell^{-1}(u)$. h_ℓ is a function from $[0,1] \mapsto \mathbb{R}$ that belong to L^2 since $Y \in L^2$. Then

$$h_\ell(u) = \sum_{j\geq -1}\sum_{k\in\mathbb{Z}} \beta^{\ell}_{jk}\psi_{jk}(u), \quad \text{with} \tag{4.4.12}$$

$$\beta^{\ell}_{jk} = \int_0^1 h_\ell(u)\psi_{jk}(u)du = \int_{\mathbb{R}} g_\ell(x)\psi_{jk}(G_\ell(x))G_\ell(dx). \tag{4.4.13}$$

Notice that the sum in k is finite because the function h_ℓ has compact support in $[0,1]$. It is then natural to estimate $h_\ell(u)$ by

$$\widehat{h}_\ell = \sum_{j\geq -1}\sum_{k\in\mathbb{Z}} \widehat{\beta}^{\ell}_{jk}\psi_{jk}(u), \tag{4.4.14}$$

and we then have:

$$\begin{aligned} V_\ell &= \mathbb{E}\big(\mathbb{E}^2(Y \,|\, X_\ell)\big) \\ &= \int_{\mathbb{R}} G_\ell(dx)\Big(\sum_{j\geq -1}\sum_{k\in\mathbb{Z}} \beta^{\ell}_{jk}\psi_{jk}(G_\ell(x))\Big)^2 \\ &= \int_0^1 \Big(\sum_{j\geq -1}\sum_{k\in\mathbb{Z}} \beta^{\ell}_{jk}\psi_{jk}(u)\Big)^2 du \\ &= \sum_{j\geq -1}\sum_{k\in\mathbb{Z}} (\beta^{\ell}_{jk})^2 = \|h_\ell\|_2^2. \end{aligned} \tag{4.4.15}$$

Adaptive estimation of $\|h_\ell\|_2^2$ has been studied in [94], which provides the block thresholding estimator $\widehat{V}_\ell$ in Definition 4.4.2. The idea is: 1) to sum the terms $\left(\beta_{jk}^\ell\right)^2$, for $j \geq 0$, by blocks $\{(j,k),\ k \in \mathbb{Z}\}$ for $j \in \{-1,\ldots,J_n\}$ with a penalty $w(j)$ for each block to avoid choosing too large j's, 2) to cut the blocks that do not sufficiently contribute to the sum, in order to obtain statistical adaptation.

Notice that $\widehat{V}_\ell$ can be seen as an estimator of V_ℓ resulting from a model selection on the choice of the blocks $\{(j,k),\ k \in \mathbb{Z}\}$, $j \in \{-1,\ldots,J_n\}$ that are kept, with the penalty function $\mathrm{pen}(\mathscr{J}) = \sum_{j\in\mathscr{J}} w(j)$, for $\mathscr{J} \subset \{-1,\ldots,J_n\}$. Indeed:

$$\begin{aligned}
\widehat{V}_\ell = & \sup_{\mathscr{J}\subset\{-1,0,\ldots,J_n\}} \sum_{j\in\mathscr{J}} \Big[\sum_{k\in\mathbb{N}} \big(\widehat{\beta}_{jk}^\ell\big)^2 - w(j)\Big] \\
= & \sup_{\mathscr{J}\subset\{-1,0,\ldots,J_n\}} \sum_{j\in\mathscr{J}} \sum_{k\in\mathbb{N}} \big(\widehat{\beta}_{jk}^\ell\big)^2 - \mathrm{pen}(\mathscr{J}).
\end{aligned} \tag{4.4.16}$$

Note that the definition of the estimator and the penalization depend on a constant K through the definition of $w(j)$. The value of this constant is chosen in order to obtain oracle inequalities. In practice, this constant is hard to compute, and can be chosen by a slope heuristic approach (see e.g. [5]).

4.4.2 Statistical Properties

In this Section, we are interested in the rate of convergence to zero of the mean square error (MSE) $\mathbb{E}\big((S_\ell - \widehat{S}_\ell)^2\big)$. Let us consider the generic estimator $\widehat{S}_\ell$ defined in (4.4.6), where $\widehat{V}_\ell$ is an estimator of $V_\ell = \mathbb{E}(\mathbb{E}^2(Y \mid X_\ell))$ (not necessarily (4.4.10)). We first start with a Lemma stating that the MSE can be obtained from the rate of convergence of $\widehat{V}_\ell$ to V_ℓ.

Lemma 4.4.3. *Consider the generic estimator $\widehat{S}_\ell$ defined in* (4.4.6) *and $\widehat{V}_\ell$ an estimator of V_ℓ (not necessarily* (4.4.10)*). Then there is a constant C such that:*

$$\mathbb{E}\big((S_\ell - \widehat{S}_\ell)^2\big) \leq \frac{C}{n} + \frac{4}{\mathrm{Var}(Y)^2}\mathbb{E}\Big[\big(\widehat{V}_\ell - V_\ell\big)^2\Big]. \tag{4.4.17}$$

Proof. From (4.4.5) and (4.4.6),

$$\begin{aligned}
\mathbb{E}\big((S_\ell - \widehat{S}_\ell)^2\big) = & \mathbb{E}\Big[\Big(\frac{V_\ell - \mathbb{E}(Y)^2}{\mathrm{Var}(Y)} - \frac{\widehat{V}_\ell - \bar{Y}^2}{\widehat{\sigma}_Y^2}\Big)^2\Big] \\
\leq & 2\mathbb{E}\Big[\Big(\frac{\mathbb{E}(Y)^2}{\mathrm{Var}(Y)} - \frac{\bar{Y}^2}{\widehat{\sigma}_Y^2}\Big)^2\Big] + 2\mathbb{E}\Big[\Big(\frac{V_\ell}{\mathrm{Var}(Y)} - \frac{\widehat{V}_\ell}{\widehat{\sigma}_Y^2}\Big)^2\Big].
\end{aligned} \tag{4.4.18}$$

The first term in the right-hand side (r.h.s.) is in C/n. For the second term in the right-hand side of (4.4.18):

$$\mathbb{E}\Big[\Big(\frac{V_\ell}{\mathrm{Var}(Y)}-\frac{\widehat{V}_\ell}{\widehat{\sigma}_Y^2}\Big)^2\Big] \leq 2\mathbb{E}\Big[\widehat{V}_\ell^2\Big(\frac{1}{\mathrm{Var}(Y)}-\frac{1}{\widehat{\sigma}_Y^2}\Big)^2\Big]+\frac{2}{\mathrm{Var}(Y)^2}\mathbb{E}\Big[\big(\widehat{V}_\ell-V_\ell\big)^2\Big]. \tag{4.4.19}$$

The first term in the r.h.s. is also in C/n, which concludes the proof. □

The preceding lemma implies that the rate of convergence of $\widehat{V}_\ell$ to V_ℓ is determinant for the rate of convergence of $\widehat{S}_\ell$. We recall the result of Solís [117], where an elbow effect for the MSE is shown when the regularity of the density of (X_ℓ,Y) varies. The case of the warped wavelet estimator introduced by Castellan et al [24] is studied at the end of the section and the rate of convergence is stated in Corollary 4.4.8.

4.4.2.1 MSE for the Nadaraya–Watson Estimator

Using the preceding Lemma, Loubes Marteau and Solís prove an elbow effect for the estimator $\widehat{S}_\ell^{(NW)}$. Let us introduce $\mathscr{H}(\alpha,L)$, for $\alpha,L>0$, the set of functions ϕ of class $[\alpha]$, whose derivative $\phi^{([\alpha])}$ is $\alpha-[\alpha]$ Hölder continuous with constant L.

Proposition 4.4.4 (Loubes Marteau and Solís [98, 117]). *Assume that* $\mathbb{E}(X_\ell^4)<+\infty$, *that the joint density* $\phi(x,y)$ *of* (X_ℓ,Y) *belongs to* $\mathscr{H}(\alpha,L)$, *for* $\alpha,L>0$ *and that the marginal density of* X_ℓ, ϕ_ℓ *belongs to* $\mathscr{H}(\alpha',L')$ *for* $\alpha'>\alpha$ *and* $L'>0$. *Then:*
If $\alpha\geq 2$, *there exists a constant* $C>0$ *such that*

$$\mathbb{E}\big((S_\ell-\widehat{S}_\ell)^2\big)\leq\frac{C}{n}.$$

If $\alpha<2$, *there exists a constant* $C>0$ *such that*

$$\mathbb{E}\big((S_\ell-\widehat{S}_\ell)^2\big)\leq C\Big(\frac{\log^2 n}{n}\Big)^{\frac{2\alpha}{\alpha+2}}.$$

For smooth functions ($\alpha\geq 2$), Loubes et al. recover a parametric rate, while they still have a nonparametric one when $\alpha<2$. Their result is based on (4.4.17) and a bound for $\mathbb{E}\Big[\big(\widehat{V}_\ell-V_\ell\big)^2\Big]$ given by [98, Th. 1], whose proof is technical. Since their result is not adaptive, they require the knowledge of the window h for numerical implementation. Our purpose is to provide a similar result for the warped wavelet adaptive estimator, with a shorter proof.

4.4.2.2 MSE for the Warped Wavelet Estimator

Let us introduce first some additional notation. We define, for $\mathscr{J}\subset\{-1,\dots,J_n\}$, the projection $h_{\mathscr{J},\ell}$ of h on the subspace spanned by $\{\psi_{jk}$, with $j\in\mathscr{J}, k\in\mathbb{Z}\}$ and its estimator $\widehat{h}_{\mathscr{J},\ell}$:

$$h_{\mathscr{J},\ell}(u) = \sum_{j\in\mathscr{J}}\sum_{k\in\mathbb{Z}} \beta_{jk}^{\ell}\psi_{jk}(u) \tag{4.4.20}$$

$$\widehat{h}_{\mathscr{J},\ell}(u) = \sum_{j\in\mathscr{J}}\sum_{k\in\mathbb{Z}} \widehat{\beta}_{jk}^{\ell}\psi_{jk}(u). \tag{4.4.21}$$

We also introduce the estimator of V_ℓ for a fixed subset of resolutions $\mathscr{J}$:

$$\widehat{V}_{\mathscr{J},\ell} = \|\widehat{h}_{\mathscr{J},\ell}\|_2^2 = \sum_{j\in\mathscr{J}}\sum_{k\in\mathbb{Z}} (\widehat{\beta}_{jk}^{\ell})^2. \tag{4.4.22}$$

Note that $\widehat{V}_{\mathscr{J},\ell}$ is one possible estimator $\widehat{V}_\ell$ in Lemma 4.4.3.

The estimators $\widehat{\beta}_{jk}$ and $\widehat{V}_{\mathscr{J},\ell}$ have natural expressions in term of the empirical process $\gamma_n(dx)$ defined as follows:

Definition 4.4.5. The empirical measure associated with our problem is:

$$\gamma_n(dx) = \frac{1}{n}\sum_{i=1}^{n} Y_i\delta_{G_\ell(X_\ell^i)}(dx) \tag{4.4.23}$$

where $\delta_a(dx)$ denotes the Dirac mass in a.
For a measurable function f, $\gamma_n(f) = \frac{1}{n}\sum_{i=1}^n Y_i f\big(G_\ell(X_\ell^i)\big)$. We also define the centered integral of f with respect to $\gamma_n(dx)$ as:

$$\bar{\gamma}_n(f) = \gamma_n(f) - \mathbb{E}\big(\gamma_n(f)\big) \tag{4.4.24}$$

$$= \frac{1}{n}\sum_{i=1}^{n}\Big(Y_i f(G_\ell(X_\ell^i)) - \mathbb{E}\big[Y_i f(G_\ell(X_\ell^i))\big]\Big). \tag{4.4.25}$$

Using the empirical measure $\gamma_n(dx)$, we have:

$$\widehat{\beta}_{jk}^{\ell} = \gamma_n\big(\psi_{jk}\big) = \beta_{jk}^{\ell} + \bar{\gamma}_n\big(\psi_{jk}\big).$$

Let us introduce the correction term

$$\zeta_n = 2\bar{\gamma}_n\big(h_\ell\big) \tag{4.4.26}$$

$$= 2\Big[\frac{1}{n}\sum_{i=1}^{n} Y_i h_\ell\big(G_\ell(X_\ell^i)\big) - \mathbb{E}\Big(Y_1 h_\ell\big(G_\ell(X_\ell^1)\big)\Big)\Big]$$

$$= 2\Big[\frac{1}{n}\sum_{i=1}^{n} h_\ell^2\big(G_\ell(X_\ell^i)\big) - \|h_\ell\|_2^2\Big] + \frac{2}{n}\sum_{i=1}^{n}\eta_\ell^i h_\ell\big(G_\ell(X_\ell^i)\big). \tag{4.4.27}$$

The rate of convergence of the estimator (4.4.10) is obtained in [24] based on the estimate presented in the next theorem. This result is derived using ideas due to Laurent and Massart [94] who considered estimation of quadratic functionals in a Gaussian setting. Because we are not necessarily in a Gaussian setting here, we rely on empirical processes and use sophisticated technology developed by Castellan [23].

Theorem 4.4.6 (Castellan, Cousien, Tran [24]). *Let us assume that the random variables Y are bounded by a constant M, and let us choose a father and a mother wavelets ψ_{-10} and ψ_{00} that are continuous with compact support (and thus bounded). The estimator $\widehat{V}_\ell$ defined in* (4.4.10) *is almost surely finite, and:*

$$\mathbb{E}\Big[\big(\widehat{V}_\ell - V_\ell - \zeta_n\big)^2\Big] \leq C \inf_{\mathscr{J}\subset\{-1,\dots,J_n\}} \Big(\|h_\ell - h_{\mathscr{J},\ell}\|_2^4 + \frac{2^{J_{max}}}{n^2}\Big) + \frac{C'}{n\log^2(n)}, \tag{4.4.28}$$

for constants C and $C' > 0$.

We deduce the following corollary from the estimate obtained above. Let us consider the Besov space $\mathscr{B}(\alpha,2,\infty)$ of functions $h = \sum_{j\geq -1}\sum_{k\in\mathbb{Z}} \beta_{jk}\psi_{jk}$ of L^2 such that

$$|h|_{\alpha,2,\infty} := \sum_{j\geq 0} 2^{j\alpha}\sqrt{\sup_{0<v\leq 2^{-j}} \int_0^{1-v} |h(u+v)-h(u)|^2 du} < +\infty.$$

For a $h \in \mathscr{B}(\alpha,2,\infty)$ and $h_{\mathscr{J}}$ its projection on

$$\mathrm{Vect}\{\psi_{jk},\ j\in\mathscr{J} = \{-1,\dots J_{\max}\},\ k\in\mathbb{Z}\},$$

we have the following approximation result from [65, Th. 9.4].

Proposition 4.4.7 (Härdle, Kerkyacharian, Picard and Tsybakov). *Assume that the wavelet function ψ_{-10} has compact support and is of class $\mathscr{C}^N$ for an integer $N > 0$. Then, if $h \in \mathscr{B}(\alpha,2,\infty)$ with $\alpha < N+1$,*

$$\sup_{\mathscr{J}\subset\mathbb{N}\cup\{-1\}} 2^{\alpha J_{max}}\|h - h_{\mathscr{J}}\|_2 = \sup_{\mathscr{J}\subset\mathbb{N}\cup\{-1\}} 2^{\alpha J_{max}}\Big(\sum_{j\geq J_{max}}\sum_{k\in\mathbb{Z}}\beta_{jk}^2\Big)^{1/2} < +\infty. \tag{4.4.29}$$

Notice that Theorem 9.4 of [65] requires assumptions that are fulfilled when ψ_{-10} has compact support and is smooth enough (see the comment after the Corol. 8.2 of [65]).

Corollary 4.4.8. *If ψ_{-10} has compact support and is of class $\mathscr{C}^N$ for an integer $N > 0$ and if h_ℓ belongs to a ball of radius $R > 0$ of $\mathscr{B}(\alpha,2,\infty)$ for $0 < \alpha < N+1$, then*

$$\sup_{h\in\mathscr{B}(\alpha,2,\infty)} \mathbb{E}\Big[\big(\widehat{V}_\ell - V_\ell\big)^2\Big] \leq C\Big(n^{-\frac{8\alpha}{4\alpha+1}} + \frac{1}{n}\Big). \tag{4.4.30}$$

As a consequence, we obtain the following elbow effect:
If $\alpha \geq \frac{1}{4}$, there exists a constant $C > 0$ such that

$$\mathbb{E}\big((S_\ell - \widehat{S}_\ell)^2\big) \leq \frac{C}{n}.$$

If $\alpha < \frac{1}{4}$, there exists a constant $C > 0$ such that

$$\mathbb{E}\big((S_\ell - \widehat{S}_\ell)^2\big) \le Cn^{-\frac{8\alpha}{4\alpha+1}}.$$

Proof. Using (4.4.28) and the fact that

$$\mathbb{E}(\zeta_n^2) = \frac{4}{n}\mathrm{Var}\Big(Y_1 h_\ell\big(G_\ell(X_\ell^1)\big)\Big) \le \frac{2M^2\|h_\ell\|_2^2}{n}, \tag{4.4.31}$$

we obtain:

$$\mathbb{E}\Big[\big(\widehat{\theta}_\ell - V_\ell\big)^2\Big] \le C\Big[\inf_{\mathscr{J}\subset\{-1,\dots,J_n\}}\Big(\|h_\ell - h_{\mathscr{J},\ell}\|_2^4 + \frac{2^{J_{\max}}}{n^2}\Big) + \frac{1+\|h_\ell\|_2^2}{n}\Big]. \tag{4.4.32}$$

If $h_\ell \in \mathscr{B}(\alpha, 2, \infty)$, then from Proposition 4.4.7, we have for $\mathscr{J} = \{-1,\dots,J_{\max}\}$ that $\|h_\ell - h_{\mathscr{J},\ell}\|_2^4 \le 2^{-4\alpha\, J_{\max}}$. Thus, for subsets $\mathscr{J}$ of the form considered, the infimum is attained when choosing $J_{\max} = \frac{2}{4\alpha+1}\log_2(n)$, which yield an upper bound in $n^{8\alpha/(4\alpha+1)}$.

For h_ℓ in a ball of radius R, $\|h_\ell\|_2^2 \le R^2$, and we can find an upper bound that does not depend on h. Because the last term in (4.4.32) is in $1/n$, the elbow effect is obtained by comparing the order of the first term in the r.h.s. ($n^{8\alpha/(4\alpha+1)}$) with $1/n$ when α varies. □

□

Let us remark that in comparison with the result of Loubes et al. [98], the regularity assumption here is on the function h_ℓ rather than on the joint density $\phi(x,y)$ of (X_ℓ, Y). The adaptivity of the estimator is then welcomed since the function h_ℓ is *a priori* unknown. Note that in applications, the joint density $\phi(x,y)$ also has to be estimated and hence has an unknown regularity.

When $\alpha < 1/4$ and $\alpha \to 1/4$, the exponent $8\alpha/(4\alpha+1) \to 1$. In the case when $\alpha > 1/4$, we can show from the estimate of Th. 4.4.6 that:

$$\lim_{n\to+\infty} n\mathbb{E}\Big[\big(\widehat{V}_\ell - V_\ell - \zeta_n\big)^2\Big] = 0, \tag{4.4.33}$$

which yields that $\sqrt{n}\big(\widehat{V}_\ell - V_\ell - \zeta_n\big)$ converges to 0 in L^2. Since $\sqrt{n}\zeta_n$ converges in distribution to $\mathscr{N}\Big(0, 4\mathrm{Var}\big(Y_1 h_\ell(G_\ell(X_\ell^1))\big)\Big)$ by the central limit theorem, we obtain that:

$$\lim_{n\to+\infty} \sqrt{n}\big(\widehat{V}_\ell - V_\ell\big) = \mathscr{N}\Big(0, 4\mathrm{Var}\big(Y_1 h_\ell(G_\ell(X_\ell^1))\big)\Big), \tag{4.4.34}$$

in distribution.

4.4.2.3 Numerical Illustration on an SIR Model

Let us consider an SIR model. The input parameters are the rates λ and γ. The output parameter is the final size of the epidemic, i.e. at a time $T > 0$ where $I_T^N = 0$, $Y = R_T^N$.

Recall from Chapter 2 that the fractions $(S_t^N/N, I_t^N/N, R_t^N/N)_{t\in[0,T]}$ can be approximated by the unique solution $(s(t), i(t), r(t))_{t\in[0,T]}$ of a system of ODE (see Example 2.2.2 of Chapter 2 in Part I of this volume). These limiting equations provide a natural deterministic approximating meta-model (recall [100]) for which sensitivity indices can be computed.

For the numerical experiment, we consider a close population of 1200 individuals, starting with $S_0 = 1190$, $I_0 = 10$ and $R_0 = 0$. The parameters distributions are uniformly distributed with $\lambda/N \in [1/15000, 3/15000]$ and $\gamma \in [1/15, 3/15]$. Here the randomness associated with the Poisson point measures is treated as the nuisance random factor in (4.4.4).
We compute the Jansen estimators of S_λ and S_γ for the deterministic meta-model constituted by the Kermack–McKendrick ODEs of Chapter 2 in Part I of this volume, with $n = 30,000$ simulations. For the estimators of S_λ and S_γ in the SDE, we compute the Jansen estimators with $n = 10,000$ (i.e. $n(p+1) = 30,000$ calls to the function f), and the estimators based on Nadaraya–Watson and on wavelet regressions with $n = 30,000$ simulations.

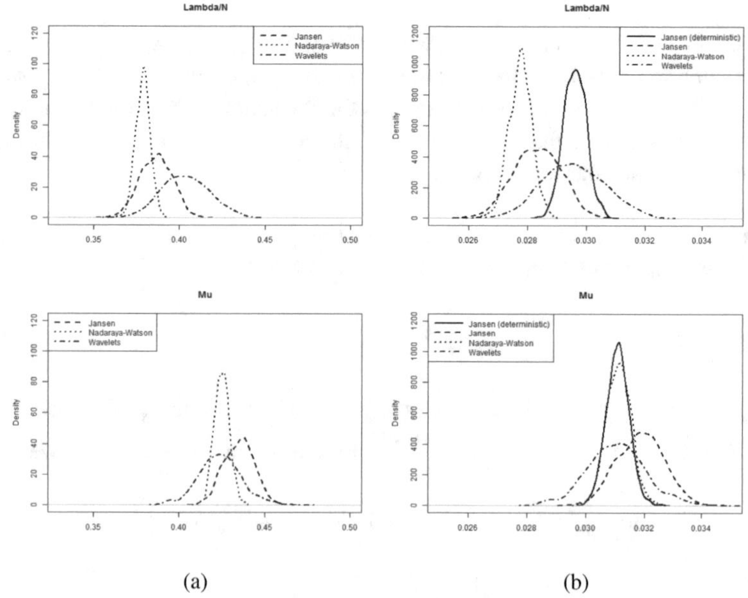

Fig. 4.4.1 *Estimations of the first-order Sobol indices, using Jansen estimators on the meta-model with $n = 10,000$ and the non-parametric estimations based on Nadaraya–Watson and wavelet regressions. (a): the distributions of the estimators of S_λ and S_γ is approximated by Monte-carlo simulations. (b): the distributions of $\mathbb{E}(Y \mid \lambda)$ and $\mathbb{E}(Y \mid \gamma)$ are approximated by Monte Carlo simulations.*

Let us comment on the results. First, the comparison of the different estimation methods is presented in Fig. 4.4.1. Since the variances in the meta-model and in the stochastic model differ, we start with comparing the distributions of $\mathbb{E}(Y \mid \lambda)$ and $\mathbb{E}(Y \mid \gamma)$ that are centered around the same value, independently of whether the meta-model or the stochastic model is used. These distributions are obtained from 1,000 Monte-carlo simulations. In Fig. 4.4.1(b), taking the meta-model as a benchmark, we see that the wavelet estimator performs well for both λ and γ while Nadaraya–Watson regression estimator performs well only for γ and exhibit biases for λ. Jansen estimator on the stochastic model exhibit biases for both λ and γ.

In a second time, we focus on the estimation of the Sobol indices for the stochastic model. The smoothed distributions of the estimators of S_λ and S_γ, for 1,000 Monte Carlo replications, are presented in Fig. 4.4.1 (a); the means and standard deviations of these distributions are given in Table 4.4.1. Although there is no theoretical values for S_λ and S_γ, we can see (Table 4.4.1) that the estimators of the Sobol indices with non-parametric regressions all give similar estimates in expectation for γ. For λ, the estimators are relatively different, with the Nadaraya–Watson showing the lower estimate. This is linked with the bias seen on Fig. 4.4.1 (b) and discussed below. In term of variance, the Nadaraya–Watson estimator gives the tightest distribution, while the wavelet estimator gives the highest variance.

	Jansen	Nadaraya–Watson	Wavelet
$\widehat{S_\lambda}$	0.39	0.38	0.40
s.d.	(9.2e-3)	(4.3e-3)	(1.4e-2)
$\widehat{S_\gamma}$	0.44	0.42	0.42
s.d.	(9.0e-3)	(4.4e-3)	(1.2e-2)

Table 4.4.1 *Estimators of the Sobol indices for λ and γ and their standard deviations using n =10,000 Monte Carlo replications of the stochastic SIR model.*

The advantage of using the estimators with wavelets lies in their robustness to the inclusion of high frequencies and in the fact that they can overcome some smoothing biases that the Nadaraya–Watson regressions exhibit (Fig. 4.4.1 (b)). This can be understood when looking at Fig. 4.4.2: the simulations can give very noisy Y's. For example, extinctions of the epidemics can be seen in very short time in simulations, due to the initial randomness of the trajectories. This produces distributions for Y's that are not unimodal or with peaks at 0, which makes the estimation of $\mathbb{E}(Y \mid \lambda)$ or $\mathbb{E}(Y \mid \gamma)$ more difficult. The variance of the estimator with wavelets is however the widest and in practice, finding the thresholding constants for the wavelet coefficients can be somewhat tricky when the number of input parameters is large.

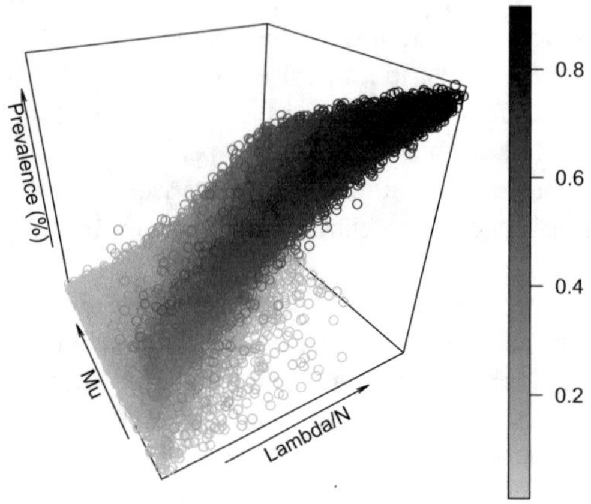

Fig. 4.4.2 *Prevalence (Y) simulated from the* $n(p+1) = 30,000$ *simulations of* λ *and* γ*, for the SIR model.*

Appendix

A.1 Some Classical Results in Statistical Inference

In this section, we have gathered results on inference useful for this part of these notes.

A.1.1 Heuristics on Maximum Likelihood Methods

As a guide for statistical inference for epidemic dynamics, we first describe the heuristics for getting properties of Maximum likelihood Estimators, each family of statistical models having to be studied specifically (see [22] for more details).

Definitions and properties are given for general discrete time stochastic processes. Consider a sequence $(X_1,\ldots,X_n)$ of random variables with values in E, and let P_θ^n denote the distribution of $(X_1,\ldots,X_n)$ on $(E^n,\mathscr{E}^n)$. Assume that the parameter set Θ is included in $\mathbb{R}^q$ and that θ_0 the true value of the parameter belongs to $\mathrm{Int}(\Theta)$.

The properties on the MLE relies on three basic results that hold as $n\rightarrow\infty$ under $\mathbb{P}_{\theta_0}^n$:

(i) a law of large numbers for the log-likelihood $\ell_n(\theta)$,
(ii) a central limit theorem for the score function $\nabla_\theta\ell_n(\theta_0)$
(iii) a law of large numbers for the observed information $\nabla_\theta^2\ell_n(\theta_0)$ under $\mathbb{P}_{\theta_0}^n$.

For a regular statistical model with a standard rate of convergence $\sqrt{n}$,

(i) For all $\theta\in\Theta$, $n^{-1}\ell_n(\theta)\rightarrow J(\theta_0,\theta)$ in $P_{\theta_0}^n$-probability. uniformly w.r.t. θ, $\theta\rightarrow J(\theta_0,\theta)$ is a continuous function with a global unique maximum at θ_0.
(ii) $n^{-1/2}\nabla_\theta\ell_n(\theta_0)\rightarrow\mathscr{N}(0,\mathscr{I}(\theta_0))$ in distribution under $P_{\theta_0}^n$,
(iii) $-\frac{1}{n}\nabla_\theta^2\ell_n(\theta_0)\rightarrow\mathscr{I}(\theta_0)$ in $P_{\theta_0}^n$-probability.

Condition (i) ensures consistency of the MLE $\hat{\theta}_n$.

Assuming that $\mathscr{I}(\theta_0)$ is non-singular, a Taylor expansion of the score function $\nabla_\theta\ell_n$ at point θ_0 leads, using that $\nabla_\theta\ell_n(\hat{\theta}_n)=0$,

$$0 = \nabla_\theta \ell_n(\hat{\theta}_n) = \nabla_\theta \ell_n(\theta_0) + \left(\int_0^1 \nabla^2_\theta \ell_n(\theta_0 + t(\hat{\theta}_n - \theta_0))dt \right) (\hat{\theta}_n - \theta_0). \quad \text{(A.1.1)}$$

From this expansion, we get, using that $\mathscr{I}(\theta_0)$ is non-singular,

$$\sqrt{n}(\hat{\theta}_n - \theta_0) = \left(-\frac{1}{n} \int_0^1 \nabla^2_\theta \ell_n(\theta_0 + t(\hat{\theta}_n - \theta_0))dt \right)^{-1} \left(\frac{1}{\sqrt{n}} \nabla_\theta \ell_n(\theta_0) \right). \quad \text{(A.1.2)}$$

Since $\hat{\theta}_n \to \theta_0$ in $P^n_{\theta_0}$-probability we get, using (iii), that

- the first factor of the r.h.s. of the equation above converges to $\mathscr{I}(\theta_0)^{-1}$ P_{θ_0} a.s.
- the second factor converges in distribution under P_{θ_0} to $\mathscr{N}(0, \mathscr{I}(\theta_0))$.

Finally, Slutsky's Lemma yields that $\sqrt{n}(\hat{\theta}_n - \theta_0) \to_{\mathscr{L}} \mathscr{N}(0, \mathscr{I}(\theta_0)^{-1})$ under P_{θ_0}.

A.1.2 Miscellaneous Results

We first state a theorem concerning the properties of the $\phi(\theta)$.

Theorem A.1.1. *Let (X_n) be a sequence of random variables with values in $\mathbb{R}^p$ and $a_n > 0$ such that $a_n \to \infty$ as $n \to \infty$. Assume that $a_n(X_n - m)$ converges in distribution to a random variable Z. Let $\phi : \mathbb{R}^p \to \mathbb{R}^q$ a continuously differentiable application. Then $a_n(\phi(X_n) - \phi(m))$ converges in distribution to the random variable $\nabla_x \phi(m) Z$, where $\nabla_x \phi$ is the Jacobian matrix of ϕ: $\nabla_x \phi = (\frac{\partial \phi_k}{\partial x_l})_{1 \le k \le q, 1 \le l \le p}$.*

We refer to [123] for the proof.

For sake of clarity, we also give a recap on Exponential families of distributions (see e.g. [11] or [123]). Indeed, among parametric families of distributions, exponential families of distributions, widely used in statistics, provide here a nice framework to study the likelihood.

Let X be a random variable in $\mathbb{R}^k$ (or $\mathbb{Z}^k$) with distribution P_θ and density $p(\theta, x)$, with $\theta \in \Theta$, subset of $\mathbb{R}^q$.

Definition A.1.2. The family $\{P_\theta, \theta \in \Theta\}$ is an exponential family if there exist q functions $(\eta_1, \ldots, \eta_q)$ and ϕ defined on Θ, q real functions $T_1, \ldots, T_q$ and a function $h(\cdot)$ defined on $\mathbb{R}^k$ such that

$$p(\theta, x) = h(x) \exp\{\sum_{j=1}^q \eta_j(\theta) T_j(x) - \phi(\theta)\} \,; x \in \mathbb{R}^k \quad \text{(A.1.3)}$$

Then $T(X) = (T_1(X), \ldots, T_q(X))$ is a sufficient statistic in the i.i.d. case. The random variable X satisfies

$$m(\theta) := \mathbb{E}_\theta(X) = \nabla_\theta \phi(\theta); \quad \sigma^2(\theta) := \mathrm{Var}_\theta(X) = \nabla^2_\theta \phi(\theta). \quad \text{(A.1.4)}$$

A.2 Inference for Markov Chains

In order to present a good overview of the statistical problems, we detail the statistical inference for Markov chains. We have rather focus here on parametric inference since epidemic models always include in their dynamics parameters that need to be estimated in order to derive predictions.

A.2.1 Recap on Markov Chains

We first begin setting the notations used throughout this chapter and introducing the basic definitions.

Let $(X_n, n \geq 0)$ a Markov chain on a probability space $(\Omega, \mathbb{F}, \mathbb{P})$ with state space $(E, \mathscr{E})$, transition kernel Q and initial distribution μ on $(E, \mathscr{E})$.

The space of observations: $(E^{\mathbb{N}}, \mathscr{E}^{\otimes \mathbb{N}})$. Based on a classical theorem of probability, there exists a unique probability measure on $(E^{\mathbb{N}}, \mathscr{E}^{\otimes \mathbb{N}})$, denoted $P_{\mu,Q}$ such that the coordinate process $(X_n, n \geq 0)$ is a Markov chain (with respect to its natural filtration) with initial distribution μ and transition kernel Q. Then, based on a classical theorem in probability, there exists a unique probability measure on $(E^{\mathbb{N}}, \mathscr{E}^{\otimes \mathbb{N}})$, denoted $P_{\mu,Q}$ such that the coordinate process $(X_n, n \geq 0)$ is a Markov chain (with respect to its natural filtration) with initial distribution μ and transition kernel Q.

The probability $P_{\mu,Q}$ has the property:

- if $A_0, A_1, \ldots, A_n$ are measurable sets in E, then

$$P_{\mu,Q}(X_i \in A_i; i = 0, \ldots, n) = \int_{A_0} \mu(dx_0) \int_{A_1} Q(x_0, dx_1) \ldots \int_{A_n} Q(x_{n-1}, dx_n).$$

Let Θ denote some subset of "probability measures $\times$ transition kernels on $(E, \mathscr{E})$". The canonical statistical model is $(E^{\mathbb{N}}, \mathscr{E}^{\mathbb{N}}, (P_{\mu,Q}, (\mu, Q) \in \Theta))$. Let us denote by $P^n_{\mu,Q}$ the distribution of $(X_0, \ldots, X_n)$ on E^{n+1}. The successive observations of (X_i) allow to estimate μ, Q.

Let α be a σ-finite positive measure on $(E, \mathscr{E})$ dominating all the distributions $\{\mu(dy), (Q(x, dy), x \in E)\}$ and assume that $\mu(dy) = \mu(y)\alpha(dy), Q(x, dy) = Q(x, y)\alpha(dy)$. Then, the likelihood of the observations $(x_0, \ldots, x_n)$ is the probability density function of $(X_0, \ldots, X_n)$, $P^n_{\mu,Q}$, with respect to the measure $\alpha_n = \otimes_{i=0}^n \alpha^i(dy)$ on E^{n+1}, with $\alpha^i(\cdot)$ copies of $\alpha(\cdot)$.

$$\frac{dP^n_{\mu,Q}}{d\alpha_n}(x_i, i = 0, \ldots, n) = \mu(x_0) Q(x_0, x_1) \ldots Q(x_{n-1}, x_n).$$

Then, the likelihood function at time n is

$$L_n(\mu, Q) = \frac{dP^n_{\mu,Q}}{d\alpha_n}(X_0, \ldots, X_n) = \mu(X_0) Q(X_0, X_1) \ldots Q(X_{n-1}, X_n). \tag{A.2.1}$$

The associated Loglikelihood is

$$\ell_n(\mu, Q) = \log L_n(\mu, Q). \tag{A.2.2}$$

A.2.1.1 Maximum Likelihood Method for Markov Chains

Let us consider the case of positive recurrent Markov chains. We follow the sketch detailed above to study the properties of MLE estimators.

Assume that the parameter set Θ is is a compact subset of $\mathbb{R}^q$.

Definition A.2.1. A family $(Q_\theta(x,dy), \theta \in \Theta)$ of transition probability kernels on $(E, \mathscr{E}) \to [0,1]$ is dominated by the transition kernel $Q(x,dy)$ if $\forall x \in E, Q_\theta(x,dy) = f_\theta(x,y)Q(x,dy)$, with $f_\theta : (E \times E, \mathscr{E} \times \mathscr{E}) \to \mathbb{R}^+$ measurable.

Assume that the initial distribution μ is known and let $\mathbb{P}_\theta$ (resp. $\mathbb{Q}$ denote the distribution of the Markov chain (X_n) with initial distribution μ and transition kernel Q_θ (resp. $Q(x,dy)$. Then the likelihood function and loglikelihood write

$$L_n(\theta) = \frac{d\mathbb{P}_\theta}{d\mathbb{Q}}(X_0, \ldots, X_n) = \Pi_{i=1}^n f_\theta(X_{i-1}, X_i), \quad \ell_n(\theta) = \sum_{i=1}^n \log f_\theta(X_{i-1}, X_i). \tag{A.2.3}$$

The maximum likelihood estimator is defined as: $\hat{\theta}_n = \mathrm{argsup}_{\theta \in \Theta} L_n(\theta)$.

A.2.1.2 Consistency

Denote by θ_0 the true value of the parameter. In order to study the properties of t$\hat{\theta}_n$ as $n \to \infty$, we introduce some assumptions.

(H0): The family $(Q_\theta(x,dy), \theta \in \Theta)$ is dominated by the transition kernel $Q(x,dy)$.
(H1): The Markov chain (X_n) with transition kernel Q_{θ_0} is irreducible, positive recurrent and aperiodic, with stationary measure $\lambda_{\theta_0}(dx)$ on E.
(H2): $\lambda_{\theta_0}(\{x, Q_\theta(x,\cdot) \neq Q_{\theta_0}(x,\cdot)\}) > 0$.
(H3): $\forall \theta, \log f_\theta(x,y)$ is integrable with respect to $\lambda_{\theta_0}(dx)Q_{\theta_0}(x,dy) := \lambda_{\theta_0} \otimes Q_{\theta_0}$.
(H4): $\forall (x,y) \in E^2$, $\theta \to f_\theta(x,y)$ is continuous w.r.t. θ.
(H5): There exists a function $h(x,y)$ integrable w.r.t. $\lambda_{\theta_0} \otimes Q_{\theta_0}$ and such that

$$\forall \theta \in \Theta, |\log f_\theta(x,y)| \leq h(x,y).$$

Assumption (H0) ensures the existence of the likelihood, (H1) is analogous for Markov chains to repetitions in a n sample of i.i.d. random variables, (H2) corresponds to an identifiability assumption, which ensures that different parameter values lead to distinct distributions for the observations. Assumptions (H3)–(H5) are regularity assumptions.

Theorem A.2.2. *Assume (H0)–(H5) and that Θ is a compact subset of $\mathbb{R}^q$. Then the MLE $\hat{\theta}_n$ is consistent: it converges in $\mathbb{P}_{\theta_0}$-probability to θ_0 as $n \to \infty$.*

Proof. Using that, under (H0),(H1), the sequence $(Y_n = (X_{n-1}, X_n), n \geq 1)$ is a positive recurrent Markov chain on $(E \times E, \mathscr{E} \times \mathscr{E})$ with stationary distribution $\lambda_{\theta_0}(dx)Q_{\theta_0}(x,dy)$, the ergodic theorem applies to (Y_n) and yields that, under (H3),

$$\frac{1}{n}\sum_{i=1}^{n} \log f_\theta(X_{i-1}, X_i) \to J(\theta_0, \theta) := \int\int_{E\times E} \log f_\theta(x,y)\lambda_{\theta_0}(dx)Q_{\theta_0}(x,dy) \quad P_{\theta_0}\text{-a.s.} \tag{A.2.4}$$

Rewriting this equation yields that $J(\theta_0, \theta)$ defined in (A.2.4),

$$J(\theta_0,\theta) = \int\int \log \frac{f_\theta(x,y)}{f_{\theta_0}(x,y)} \lambda_{\theta_0}(dx)Q_{\theta_0}(x,dy) + A(\theta_0),$$

with $A(\theta_0) = \int\int \log f_{\theta_0}(x,y)\lambda_{\theta_0}(dx)Q_{\theta_0}(x,dy)$. Under (H0),

$$Q_\theta(x,dy) = f_\theta(x,dy)Q(x,dy),$$

so that

$$\begin{aligned} J(\theta_0,\theta) &= \int \lambda_{\theta_0}(dx) \int \log \frac{Q_\theta(x,dy)}{Q_{\theta_0}(x,dy)} Q_{\theta_0}(x,dy) + A(\theta_0) \\ &= -\int K(Q_{\theta_0}(x,\cdot), Q_\theta(x,\cdot))\, \lambda_{\theta_0}(dx) + A(\theta_0), \end{aligned}$$

where $K(P,Q)$ denotes the Kullback–Leibler divergence between two probabilities. Recall that it satisfies

- if $P << Q$, then $K(P,Q) = \mathbb{E}_P(\log \frac{dP}{dQ}) = \int \log \frac{dP}{dQ} dP = E_Q(\phi(\frac{dP}{dQ}))$ with $\phi(x) = x\log(x) + 1 - x$.
- $K(P,Q) = +\infty$ otherwise.

A well-known property is that $K(P,Q) \geq 0$ and $K(P,Q) = 0$ if and only if $P = Q$ a.s. Assumption (H2) ensures that $\theta \to J(\theta_0, \theta)$ possesses a global unique maximum at $\theta = \theta_0$.

The MLE $\hat{\theta}_n$ satisfies that $\hat{\theta}_n = \text{Argsup}_\theta(\frac{1}{n}\ell_n(\theta))$. The maximum of the right-hand side of (A.2.4) is θ_0. Hence to get consistency, we have to prove that "lim Argsup $\frac{1}{n}\ell_n(\theta)$" is equal to "Argsup lim $\frac{1}{n}\ell_n(\theta)$", which is θ_0. Note that, for all $\theta \in \Theta$, $\ell_n(\hat{\theta}_n) \geq \ell_n(\theta)$ and $J(\theta_0,\theta_0) \geq J(\theta_0,\hat{\theta}_n)$. Combining these two inequalities we get,

$$\begin{aligned} 0 \leq J(\theta_0,\theta_0) - J(\theta_0,\hat{\theta}_n) &\leq J(\theta_0,\theta_0) - \frac{1}{n}\ell_n(\theta_0) + \frac{1}{n}\ell_n(\theta_0) - \frac{1}{n}\ell_n(\hat{\theta}_n) \\ &\quad + \frac{1}{n}\ell_n(\hat{\theta}_n) - J(\theta_0,\hat{\theta}_n) \\ &\leq 2\sup_{\theta\in\Theta} |J(\theta_0,\theta) - \frac{1}{n}\ell_n(\theta)|. \end{aligned}$$

Therefore, by taking Θ a compact subset of $\mathbb{R}^q$, we get that $J(\theta_0,\hat{\theta}_n) \to J(\theta_0,\theta_0)$ $\mathbb{P}_{\theta_0}$- a.s. as $n \to \infty$. Assumptions (H4),(H5) ensure that $J(\theta_0,\cdot)$ is continuous with a unique global maximum at θ_0 so that the MLE converges to θ_0 in $\mathbb{P}_{\theta_0}$-probability. □

A.2.1.3 Limit Distribution

This section is based on general results presented in [63]. For V a vector or a matrix, let V^* denote its transposition. Define the $q \times q$ matrix

$$\mathscr{I}(\theta_0) = \int\int \frac{\nabla_\theta f_{\theta_0}(x,y)\, \nabla^*_\theta f_{\theta_0}(x,y)}{f_{\theta_0}(x,y)^2} \lambda_{\theta_0}(dx) Q_{\theta_0}(x,dy). \tag{A.2.5}$$

Let us introduce the additional assumptions.

(H6) $\theta \to \ell_n(\theta)$ is $C^2(\Theta)$ $\mathbb{P}_{\theta_0}$ -a.s.
(H7) $\mathscr{I}(\theta_0)$ defined in (A.2.5) is non-singular.
(H8) $\int \phi_{\theta_0}(r,x,y)\lambda_{\theta_0}(dx)Q_{\theta_0}(x,dy) \to 0$ as $r \to 0$ where

$$\phi_{\theta_0}(r,x,y) = \sup\{\| \nabla^2_\theta \log f_\theta(x,y) - \nabla^2_\theta \log f_{\theta_0}(x,y) \| \cdot \| \theta - \theta_0 \| \leq r\}.$$

We can state the result on the asymptotic normality of the MLE

Theorem A.2.3. *Assume (H0)–(H8). Then the MLE $\hat{\theta}_n$ is asymptotically Gaussian: under P_{θ_0},*

$$\sqrt{n}(\hat{\theta}_n - \theta_0) \to_{\mathscr{L}} \mathscr{N}_q(0, \mathscr{I}(\theta_0)^{-1}).$$

Proof. Under (H6), the score function is well defined and reads as

$$\nabla_\theta \ell_n(\theta) = \sum_{i=1}^{n} \nabla_\theta \log f_\theta(X_{i-1}, X_i) = \sum_{i=1}^{n} v_i(\theta). \tag{A.2.6}$$

The score function satisfies

Proposition A.2.4. *Under assumptions (H0)–(H5), $\nabla_\theta \ell_n(\theta_0)$ is a q-dimensional $\mathbb{P}_{\theta_0}$-martingale w.r.t. $(\mathscr{F}_n)_{n\geq 0}$, which is centered and square integrable.*

Proof: By (A.2.6), we have, $\nabla_\theta \ell_n(\theta_0) = \nabla_\theta \ell_{n-1}(\theta_0) + v_n(\theta_0)$. We get, using that, under (H5), $\int \nabla_\theta f = \nabla_\theta(\int f)$ holds true,

$$\begin{aligned}
\mathbb{E}_{\theta_0}(v_i(\theta_0)|\mathscr{F}_{i-1}) &= \mathbb{E}_{\mathbb{Q}}(\,\nabla_\theta \log f_{\theta_0}(X_{i-1}, X_i) f_{\theta_0}(X_{i-1}, X_i)|\mathscr{F}_{i-1}) \\
&= \mathbb{E}_{\mathbb{Q}}(\nabla_\theta f_{\theta_0}(X_{i-1}, X_i)|\mathscr{F}_{i-1}) \\
&= \nabla_\theta\, \mathbb{E}_{\mathbb{Q}}(f_{\theta_0}(X_{i-1}, X_i)|\mathscr{F}_{i-1}) = \nabla_\theta 1 = 0.
\end{aligned}$$

Noting that $E_{\theta_0}(\nabla_\theta \ell_1(\theta_0)) = \nabla_\theta(E_{\theta_0} 1) = 0$, $\nabla_\theta \ell_n(\theta_0)$ is a centered martingale.

Consider now the increasing process associated with this martingale. We have $\langle \nabla_\theta \ell_n(\theta_0) \rangle = \sum_{i=1}^n E_{\theta_0}(v_i(\theta_0)\, v_i^*(\theta_0)|\mathscr{F}_{i-1})$.
An application of the ergodic theorem yields $\frac{1}{n}\sum v_i(\theta_0)\, v_i^*(\theta_0) \to \mathscr{I}(\theta_0)$ $\mathbb{P}_{\theta_0}$ a.s. Therefore for $j = 1, \ldots q$, $E_{\theta_0}\langle \nabla_\theta \ell_n(\theta_0) \rangle_{jj} \to \infty$ as $n \to \infty$. Applying a central limit theorem, we get that

$$\frac{1}{\sqrt{n}}\nabla_\theta \ell_n(\theta_0) \to \mathscr{N}_q(0, \mathscr{I}(\theta_0)).$$

The matrix $\mathscr{I}(\theta_0)$ is the Fisher information matrix .

A Taylor expansion of the score function $\nabla_\theta \ell_n$ at point θ_0 leads, using that $\nabla_\theta \ell_n(\hat{\theta}_n) = 0$, to

$$0 = \frac{1}{\sqrt{n}}\nabla_\theta \ell_n(\hat{\theta}_n) = \frac{1}{\sqrt{n}}\nabla_\theta \ell_n(\theta_0) + \frac{1}{n}\Big(\int_0^1 \nabla^2_\theta \ell_n(\theta_0 + t(\hat{\theta}_n - \theta_0))dt\Big)\,\frac{\hat{\theta}_n - \theta_0}{\sqrt{n}}. \tag{A.2.7}$$

Now, (A.2.4) yields, using (A.2.1),

$$\frac{1}{n}\nabla^2_\theta \ell_n(\theta_0) \to \int \lambda_{\theta_0}(dx) \int \nabla^2_\theta(\log f_{\theta_0}(x,y))Q_{\theta_0}(x,dy) = -\mathscr{I}(\theta_0),$$

Indeed, the last equality is obtained using Assumptions (H3)–(H6) and

$$\int \frac{\nabla^2_\theta f_{\theta_0}(x,y)}{f_{\theta_0}(x,y)} Q_{\theta_0}(x,dy) = \nabla^2_\theta\Big(\int f_{\theta_0}(x,y)Q(x,dy)\Big) = 0.$$

Therefore, from expansion (A.2.7), we get,

$$\sqrt{n}(\hat{\theta}_n - \theta_0) = \Big(-\frac{1}{n}\int_0^1 \nabla^2_\theta \ell_n(\theta_0 + t(\hat{\theta}_n - \theta_0))dt\Big)^{-1}\Big(\frac{1}{\sqrt{n}}\nabla_\theta \ell_n(\theta_0)\Big). \tag{A.2.8}$$

Since $\hat{\theta}_n \to \theta_0$ in $P^n_{\theta_0}$-probability we get that the first factor of the r.h.s. of (A.2.8) converges to $\mathscr{I}(\theta_0)^{-1}$ under $\mathbb{P}_{\theta_0}$ a.s., and that the second factor converges in distribution under P_{θ_0} to $\mathscr{N}(0, \mathscr{I}(\theta_0))$. Finally, Slutsky's Lemma yields that $\sqrt{n}(\hat{\theta}_n - \theta_0)$ converges to $\mathscr{N}(0, \mathscr{I}(\theta_0)^{-1}\mathscr{I}(\theta_0)\mathscr{I}(\theta_0)^{-1}) = \mathscr{N}(0, \mathscr{I}(\theta_0)^{-1})$ in distribution. □

A.2.2 Other Approaches than the Likelihood

It often occurs in practice that the likelihood is difficult to compute. One way to overcome this problem relies on stochastic algorithms. However, another way round is to build other processes than the likelihood to derive estimators. These methods include for the i.i.d. case the M-estimators ([123]) and, for stochastic processes, Estimating equations, approximate likelihoods, pseudolikelihoods. ([87]), Generalized Moment Methods ([64]), Contrast functions ([31]).

A.2.2.1 Minimum Contrast Approaches

What if, instead of the likelihood, another process (contrast process) $U_n(\theta)$ is used as for instance the C.L.S. method (in essence think of $U_n \simeq -\ell_n$))

Let us assume that $U_n(\theta) = U_n(\theta, X_0, \ldots, X_n)$ satisfies

(H1b) For all $\theta \in \Theta$, $U_n(\theta)$ is $\mathscr{F}_n$-measurable and $\theta \to U_n(\theta)$ is under $\mathbb{P}_{\theta_0}$ a.s. continuous and twice continuously differentiable on a subset $V(\theta_0)$.

(H2b) For all θ, $n^{-1}U_n(\theta) \to K(\theta_0, \theta)$ in P_{θ_0}-probability uniformly over compacts subsets of Θ, where $\theta \to K(\theta_0, \theta)$ is continuous with a unique global minimum at θ_0.

(H3b) $n^{-1/2}\nabla_\theta U_n(\theta_0) \to \mathscr{N}_q(0, I_U(\theta_0))$ in distribution under $\mathbb{P}_{\theta_0}$.

(H4b) There exists a symmetric positive matrix $J_U(\theta_0)$ such that

$$\lim_{n\to\infty} \sup_{|\theta-\theta_0|\leq\delta} \| \frac{1}{n}\nabla^2_\theta U_n(\theta) - J_U(\theta_0) \| \to 0 \text{ as } \delta \to 0 \quad P_{\theta_0}\text{-a.s.}$$

Define the MCE estimator $\tilde{\theta}_n$ associated with $U_n(\theta)$ as any solution of

$$U_n(\tilde{\theta}_n) = \inf_{\theta\in\Theta} U_n(\theta). \tag{A.2.9}$$

Then, using similar proofs than in Section A.2.1.1 yields that

Theorem A.2.5. *Assume that (H1b)–(H4b) hold. Then, the MCE defined in* (A.2.9)

(1) $\tilde{\theta}_n \to \theta_0$ *in* $P_{\theta_0}-$ *probability.*
(2) $\sqrt{n}(\tilde{\theta}_n - \theta_0) \to_{\mathscr{L}} \mathscr{N}_q(0, J_U(\theta_0)^{-1}I_U(\theta_0)J_U^{-1}(\theta_0))$ *under* P_{θ_0}.

Note that contrary to the MLE where $J_U(\theta_0) = I_U(\theta_0)$, the asymptotic covariance matrix of $\tilde{\theta}_n$ is no longer $I_U(\theta_0)^{-1}$. Analytic properties of matrices yield that $J_U(\theta_0)^{-1}I_U(\theta_0)J_U^{-1}(\theta_0))$ is always greater (as a linear form) than $I_U(\theta_0)^{-1}$.

A.2.2.2 Conditional Least Squares

A classical approach associated to this method is the Conditional Least Squares method.
Let (X_n) be an Markov chain on $\mathbb{R}^p$ with transition kernel $Q_\theta(x, dy)$ on $\mathbb{R}^p$ and initial distribution μ. Assume that it is positive recurrent with stationary distribution $\lambda_\theta(dx)$.

Define the two functions

$$g(\theta, x) = \int y Q_\theta(x, dy) \text{ and}$$
$$V(\theta, x) = \int {}^t(y - g(\theta, x))\,(y - g(\theta, x))Q_\theta(x, dy).$$

Clearly, $E_\theta(X_i|X_{i-1}) = g(\theta, X_{i-1})$ and $\mathrm{Var}_\theta(X_i|X_{i-1}) = V(\theta, X_{i-1})$. We assume
The CLS method is associated with the process

$$U_n(\theta) = \frac{1}{2}\sum_{i=1}^{n} (X_i - E_\theta(X_i|X_{i-1}))^* \, (X_i - E_\theta(X_i|X_{i-1})). \tag{A.2.10}$$

Applying the ergodic theorem to $((X_{i-1}, X_i), i \geq 1)$ yields that, under $\mathbb{P}_{\theta_0}$

$$\frac{1}{n}U_n(\theta) \to K(\theta_0, \theta) = \frac{1}{2}\int\int (y - g(\theta,x))^*(y - g(\theta,x))\lambda_{\theta_0}(dx)Q_{\theta_0}(x,dy) \text{ a.s.}$$

Rewriting this limit yields that

$$K(\theta_0,\theta) = \frac{1}{2}\int\int (g(\theta,x) - g(\theta_0,x))^*(g(\theta,x) - g(\theta_0,x))\lambda_{\theta_0}(dx)Q_{\theta_0}(x,dy) + A(\theta_0)$$

with

$$A(\theta_0) = \frac{1}{2}\int\int (y - g(\theta,x))^*(y - g(\theta,x))\lambda_{\theta_0}(dx)Q_{\theta_0}(x,dy).$$

To study the MCE $\tilde{\theta}_n = \text{Argmin}\{U_n(\theta), \theta \in \Theta\}$, we assume

(A1) For all $x \in \mathbb{R}^p$, $g(\theta,x)$ and $V(\theta,x)$ are finite and C^2 with respect to θ.
(A2) $\theta \to K(\theta_0,\theta)$ continuous and $\lambda_{\theta_0}(\{x, g(\theta,x) \neq g(\theta_0,x)\}) > 0$.
(A3) The matrix $J_U(\theta) = \int (\nabla_\theta g(\theta,x) \, \nabla^*_\theta g(\theta,x)\lambda_\theta(dx)$ is non-singular at θ_0.
(A4) The function $\phi(\delta,x) = \sup_{||\theta-\theta_0|| \leq \delta} ||\nabla^2_\theta g(\theta,x) - \nabla^2_\theta g(\theta_0,x)||$ satisfies

$$\int \phi(\delta,x)\lambda_{\theta_0}(dx) \to 0 \text{ as } \delta \to 0.$$

Assumption (A1) ensures that U_n is well defined, (A2) that $\theta \to K(\theta_0,\theta)$ has a global unique minimum at θ_0. Assumption (A3),(A4) ensure that (H3b), (H4b) hold.

Let us study $\nabla_\theta U_n(\theta)$. We have that

$$0 = \nabla_\theta U_n(\tilde{\theta}_n) = \nabla_\theta U_n(\theta_0) + \left(\int_0^1 \nabla^2_\theta U_n(\theta_0 + t(\hat{\theta}_n - \theta_0))dt\right)(\hat{\theta}_n - \theta_0). \tag{A.2.11}$$

The first term of the r.h.s. of (A.2.11) reads as

$$\nabla_\theta U_n(\theta_0) = -\sum_{i=1}^{n} (\nabla_\theta g(\theta_0, X_{i-1}))^* \, (X_i - g(\theta_0, X_{i-1})).$$

Hence, under (A1), $\nabla_\theta U_n(\theta_0)$ is a centered L^2-martingale under P_{θ_0} with

$$\langle \nabla_\theta U_n(\theta_0) \rangle = \sum_{i=1}^{n} E_{\theta_0}\Big((\nabla_\theta g(\theta_0, X_{i-1}))^* \, V(\theta_0, X_{i-1}) \nabla_\theta g(\theta_0, X_{i-1})\Big).$$

Applying the ergodic theorem yields

$$\frac{1}{n}\langle \nabla_\theta U_n(\theta_0)\rangle_n \to \int (\nabla_\theta g_{\theta_0}(x)^*) \, V(\theta_0,x) \, \nabla_\theta g_{\theta_0}(x)\lambda_{\theta_0}(dx) := I_U(\theta_0) \text{ a.s.}$$

Therefore, we can apply the central limit theorem for martingales (see Theorem A.4.2) and obtain,

$$\frac{1}{\sqrt{n}}\nabla_\theta U_n(\theta_0) \to_{\mathscr{L}} \mathscr{N}_q(0, I_U(\theta_0)) \text{ under } P_{\theta_0}.$$

For the second term, we get $\nabla^2_\theta U_n(\theta_0) = \sum_{i=1}^n \nabla_\theta g(\theta_0, X_{i-1})^* \nabla_\theta g(\theta_0, X_{i-1})$ which satisfies

$$\frac{1}{n}\nabla^2_\theta U_n(\theta_0) \to J_U(\theta_0) := \int \nabla_\theta g(\theta_0, x)^* \, \nabla_\theta g(\theta_0, x) \, \lambda_{\theta_0}(dx) \quad P_{\theta_0} \text{ a.s.}$$

Therefore under (A3), (A4), $J_U(\theta_0)$ is invertible. Therefore, $\tilde{\theta}_n$ is consistent and $\sqrt{n}(\tilde{\theta}_n - \theta_0) \to \mathscr{N}(0, \Sigma(\theta_0))$ with $\Sigma(\theta_0) = J_U^{-1}(\theta_0) I_U(\theta_0) J_U^{-1}(\theta_0)$.

A.2.3 Hidden Markov Models

A Hidden Markov Model is, roughly speaking, a Markov chain observed with noise. This raises new problems for the statistical inference of parameters ruling the Markov chain model (X_n).
Consider a Markov chain $(X_n, n \geq 0))$ with state space E. The term "hidden " corresponds to the situation where the Markov chain cannot be directly observable, Instead of (X_n) , the observations consists in another stochastic process (Y_n) whose distribution is ruled by (X_n). The simplest case is for instance the case of measurements errors $Y_n = X_n + \varepsilon_n$, with (ε_i) i.i.d. random variables. All the statistical inference for (X_n) has to be done in terms of (Y_n) only, since (X_n) cannot be observed.

For epidemic data, this situation occurs when the exact status of individuals cannot be observed or when there is a systematic error in the reporting rate of Infected individuals.

The precise definition of a Hidden Markov Model (HMM) is:

Definition A.2.6. A Hidden Markov Model (HMM) is a bivariate discrete time process $((X_n, Y_n), n \geq 0)$ with state space $\mathscr{X} \times \mathscr{Y}$ such that
(i) (X_n) is a Markov chain with state space $\mathscr{X}$.
(ii) For all $i \leq n$, the conditional distribution of Y_i given $(X_0, \ldots, X_n)$ only depends on X_i.

A classical example of Hidden Markov models is obtained as follows:
Let (ε_n) is a sequence of i.i.d. random variables on E and $F(.,.) : \mathscr{X} \times E \to \mathscr{Y}$ a given measurable function. Then, if $Y_n = F(X_n, \varepsilon_n)$, the bivariate sequence (X_n, Y_n) is a Hidden Markov Model.

It follows from this definition that (X_n, Y_n) is a Markov chain on $\mathscr{X} \times \mathscr{Y}$, while the sequence (Y_n) is no longer Markov:
$\mathscr{L}(Y_n|Y_0, \ldots, Y_{n-1})$ effectively depends on all the past observations.

This is why the inference for parameters ruling (X_n) is difficult and rely on specific tools (see e.g. [22], [124]).

A.3 Results for Statistics of Diffusions Processes

Inference for diffusion processes observed on a finite time-interval presents some specific properties. For sake of comprehensiveness, a short recap of classical results for diffusion processes inference is then given.We first present the general framework required for time-dependent diffusions and then detail these results. (see [87] for a presentation of available results).

On a probability space $(\Omega, \mathscr{F}, (\mathscr{F}_t, t \geq 0), \mathbb{P})$, consider the stochastic differential equation

$$d\xi_t = b(t, \xi_t)dt + \sigma(t, \xi_t)dB_t, \xi_0 = \eta. \tag{A.3.1}$$

We assume that (B_t) is a p-dimensional Brownian motion, that b and σ satisfy regularity assumptions which ensure the existence and uniqueness of solutions of (A.3.1) and that η is $\mathscr{F}_0$-measurable and that

We detail results on the inference on parameters in the drift and diffusion coefficient depending on various kinds of observations of $(\xi_t, t \in [0,T])$. For this, let us recall some basic definitions concerning these processes. The state space of $(\xi_t, t \leq T)$ is $C_T = \{x = (x(t)) : [0,T] \to \mathbb{R}^p \text{ continuous}, \mathscr{C}_T\}$, where $\mathscr{C}_T$ denote the Borel filtration associated with the uniform topology. Denote by $X_t : C_T \to \mathbb{R}^p,\ X_t(x) = x(t)$. the coordinate functions defined for $0 \leq t \leq T$. The distribution of $\xi^T : (\xi_t, t \in [0,T])$ on $(C_T, \mathscr{C}_T)$ is denoted by $P^T_{b,\sigma}$.

A.3.1 Continuously Observed Diffusions on [0,T]

The distributions $P_{b,\sigma} P_{b',\sigma'}$ of two diffusion processes having distinct diffusion coefficients are singular. Therefore, we assume that $\sigma(\cdot) = \sigma'(\cdot)$. From a statistical point of view, this means that $\sigma(\cdot)$ can be identified from the continuous observation of (ξ_t). Consider the parametric model associated to the diffusion (ξ_t) in $\mathbb{R}^p$:

$$d\xi_t = b(\theta, t, \xi_t)dt + \sigma(t, \xi_t)dB_t, \xi_0 = x_0. \tag{A.3.2}$$

Define the diffusion matrix $\Sigma(t,x) = \sigma(t,x)\sigma^*(t,x)$.

Consider the estimation of a q-dimensional parameter $\theta \in \Theta$, with Θ a subset of $\mathbb{R}^q$. Then, under conditions ensuring existence and uniqueness of solutions (see e.g. [82]) and additional assumptions for the Girsanov formula (cf. [67], [96]) on $C([0,T], \mathbb{R}^p), \mathscr{C}_T)$,

$$L_T(\theta) = \frac{dP_\theta^T}{dP_0^T}(X) \tag{A.3.3}$$
$$= \exp\left[\int_0^T \Sigma^{-1}(t,X_t)b(\theta;t,X_t)dX_t - \frac{1}{2}\int_0^T b^*(\theta;t,X_t)\Sigma^{-1}(t,X_t)b(\theta,t,X_t)dt\right].$$

The statistical model is $(C_T, \mathscr{C}_T, (P^T_{\theta,\sigma}, \theta \in \Theta))$. The loglikelihood is $\ell_T(\theta) = \log L_T(\theta)$. The Maximum Likelihood Estimator is $\hat{\theta}_T$ s.t.

$$\ell_T(\hat{\theta}_T) = \sup\{\ell_T(\theta), \theta \in \Theta\}. \tag{A.3.4}$$

There is no general theory for the properties of the MLE as $T \to \infty$, except in the case of ergodic diffusions.

Consider the case of an autonomous diffusion ξ_t satisfying the stochastic differential equation on $\mathbb{R}^p$:

$$d\xi_t = b(\theta, \xi_t)dt + \sigma(\xi_t)dB_t;\ \xi_0 \simeq \eta.$$

Assume that, for $\theta \in \Theta \in \mathbb{R}^q$, (ξ_t) positive recurrent diffusion process with stationary distribution $\lambda(\theta, x)dx$ on $\mathbb{R}^p$. Then, under assumptions ensuring that the statistical model is regular (see [68] for general results and [93] for ergodic diffusions), then, as $T \to \infty$, the MLE $\hat{\theta}_T$ is consistent and

$$\sqrt{T}(\hat{\theta}_T - \theta_0) \xrightarrow{\mathscr{L}} \mathscr{N}_k(0, I^{-1}(\theta_0)) \text{ under } \mathbb{P}_{\theta_0}, \text{ with}$$
$$I(\theta) = I(\theta) = \int_{\mathbb{R}^p} \nabla_\theta b^*(\theta,x)\Sigma^{-1}(x)\nabla_\theta b(\theta,x)\lambda(\theta,x)dx.$$

A.3.2 Discrete Observations with Sampling Δ on a Time Interval [0,T]

Consider the stochastic differential equation (A.3.2), where parameters in the drift are α and in the diffusion coefficient β.

$$d\xi_t = b(\alpha, t, \xi_t)dt + \sigma(\beta, t, \xi_t)dB_t, \xi_0 = x_0. \tag{A.3.5}$$

Let $T = n\Delta$ and assume that the observations are obtained at times $(t_i^n = i\Delta; i = 0, \ldots n)$.
The space of observations is $((\mathbb{R}^p)^n, (\mathscr{B}(\mathbb{R}^p))^n$. Let $\mathbb{P}^n_{\alpha,\beta}$ denote the distribution of the n-tuple. Contrary to continuous observations, the probabilities $\mathbb{P}^n_{\alpha,\beta}, \mathbb{P}^n_{\alpha',\beta'}$ are absolutely continuous, leading to a likelihood $L_n(\alpha,\beta)$ for the n-tuple. However, it depends on the transition probabilities $\mathbb{P}_\theta(X(t_{i+1}) \in A | X(t_i) = x)$ of the underlying Markov chain. The main difficulty here lies in the intractable likelihood. This is a well known problem for discrete observations of diffusion processes. Alternative approaches based on M-estimators or contrast processes (see [123] for i.i.d. observations, [87] for SDE) have to be investigated.

Several cases can be considered according to T and Δ with $T = n\Delta$.

(a) $T \to \infty$. Results are obtained for ergodic diffusions.

1- Δ fixed: Both parameters in the drift coefficient α and in the diffusion coefficient β can be consistently estimated and ([85]),

$$\sqrt{n}\begin{pmatrix} \hat{\alpha}_n - \alpha_0 \\ \hat{\beta}_n - \beta_0 \end{pmatrix} \xrightarrow{\mathscr{L}} \mathscr{N}(0, I_\Delta^{-1}(\alpha_0, \beta_0). \tag{A.3.6}$$

2- $\Delta = \Delta_n \to 0$ and $T = n\Delta_n \to \infty$ as $n \to \infty$. As $n \to \infty$, there is a double asymptotics $\Delta_n \to 0$ and $T = n\Delta_n \to \infty$.
Both parameters in the drift coefficient α and in the diffusion coefficient β can be consistently estimated and the following holds (see [85] and [86]

- Parameters in the drift coefficient α are estimated at rate $\sqrt{n\Delta_n}$.
- Parameters in the diffusion coefficient β are estimated at rate $\sqrt{n}$.

$$\begin{pmatrix} \sqrt{n\Delta_n}(\hat{\alpha}_n - \alpha_0) \\ \sqrt{n}(\hat{\beta}_n - \beta_0) \end{pmatrix} \xrightarrow{\mathscr{L}} \mathscr{N}(0, I^{-1}(\alpha_0, \beta_0).) \tag{A.3.7}$$

(b) $T = n\Delta_n$ fixed and $\Delta = \Delta_n \to 0$ as $n \to \infty$.
It presents the following properties.

- Except for specific models, there is no consistent estimators for parameters in the drift.
- Parameters in the diffusion coefficient can be consistently estimated and satisfy

  $$\sqrt{n}(\hat{\beta}_n - \beta_0) \xrightarrow{\mathscr{L}} Z = \eta\, U, \text{ with } \eta, U \text{ independent, } U \sim \mathscr{N}(0, I).$$

  The random variable Z is not normally distributed but Gaussian but has Mixed variance Gaussian law. It corresponds to a Local Asymptotic Mixed Normal statistical model (see [123], [67] for general references on LAMN; [36], [48] and [57] for diffusion processes).

A.3.3 Inference for Diffusions with Small Diffusion Matrix on $[0, T]$

The asymptotic properties of estimators are now studied with respect to the asymptotic framework "$\varepsilon \to 0$". Consider the SDE

$$d\xi_t = b(\alpha, \xi_t)dt + \varepsilon\sigma(\xi_t)dB_t, \xi_0 = x_0.$$

Contrary to the previous section, it is possible to estimate parameters in the drift α. For continuous observations on $[0,T]$, Kutoyants ([91]) has studied the estimation of α using the likelihood and proved that the MLE is consistent and satisfies

$$\varepsilon^{-1}(\hat{\alpha}_\varepsilon - \alpha_0) \to \mathcal{N}(0, I_b^{-1}(\alpha_0)) \text{ with} \tag{A.3.8}$$
$$I_b(\alpha) = \int_0^T (\nabla_\alpha b)^*(\alpha, z(\alpha,t))\Sigma^{-1}(z(\alpha,t))\nabla_\alpha b(\alpha, z(\alpha,t))dt.$$

The Fisher information of this statistical model is $I_b(\alpha)$.

The statistical inference based on discrete observations of the sample path with sampling interval $\Delta = \Delta_n \to 0$ has first been studied for one-dimensional diffusions with $\sigma \equiv 1$ ([46]), and [118], [56] assuming a parameter β in the diffusion coefficient $\sigma(\beta,x)$. Under assumptions linking the two asymptotics ε and n, [56] proved the existence of consistent and asymptotically Gaussian estimators $(\tilde{\alpha}_{\varepsilon,n}, \tilde{\beta}_{\varepsilon,n})$ of (α_0, β_0), which converge at different rates, parameters in the drift function being estimated at rate ε^{-1} and parameters in the diffusion coefficient at rate $\sqrt{n} = \Delta_n^{-1/2}$.

$$\begin{pmatrix} \varepsilon^{-1}(\hat{\alpha}_{\varepsilon,n} - \alpha_0) \\ \sqrt{n}(\hat{\beta}_{\varepsilon,n} - \beta_0) \end{pmatrix} \underset{n\to\infty,\varepsilon\to 0}{\longrightarrow} \mathcal{N}\left(0, \begin{pmatrix} I_b^{-1}(\alpha_0,\beta_0) & 0 \\ 0 & I_\sigma^{-1}(\alpha_0,\beta_0) \end{pmatrix}\right). \tag{A.3.9}$$

The matrix I_b is the matrix (A.3.8) and the matrix I_σ is

$$I_\sigma(\alpha,\beta)_{ij} = \tag{A.3.10}$$
$$\left(\frac{1}{2T}\int_0^T \mathrm{Tr}(\nabla_{\beta_i}\Sigma(\beta,s,z(\alpha,s))\Sigma^{-1}(\beta,s,z(\alpha,s))\nabla_{\beta_j}\Sigma(\beta,s,z(\alpha,s))ds\right),$$

where $I_b(\alpha_0,\beta_0)$ and $I_\sigma(\alpha_0,\beta_0)$ are assumed invertible.

A.4 Some Limit Theorems for Martingales and Triangular Arrays

A.4.1 Central Limit Theorems for Martingales

This Central Limit Theorem for martingales in $\mathbb{R}$ is stated in [63].

Let $M_n = \sum_{i=1}^n X_i$ and $\langle M\rangle_n = \sum_{i=1}^n E(X_i^2/\mathcal{F}_{i-1})$. Set $s_n^2 = EM_n^2 = E\langle M\rangle_n$.

Theorem A.4.1. *Assume that the sequence (M_n) of L^2 centered martingales satisfy that, as $n\to\infty$, $s_n^2 \to \infty$ and*

(H1): *$\forall\varepsilon > 0$, $\frac{1}{s_n^2}\sum_{i=1}^n E(X_i^2 \mathbf{1}_{|X_i|\geq s_n\varepsilon}|\mathcal{F}_{i-1}) \to 0$ in probability.*

(H2): *$\frac{1}{s_n^2}\langle M\rangle_n \to \eta^2$ in probability (η is an r.v. such that, if $\eta^2 < \infty$, $E\eta^2 = 1$).*

Then $(\frac{M_n}{s_n}, \frac{\langle M\rangle_n}{s_n^2}) \to_{\mathcal{L}} (\eta N, \eta^2)$ with η, N independent r.v.s, $N \sim \mathcal{N}(0,1)$.

Note that $Z = \eta N$ satisfies $E(\exp(iuZ)) = E(\exp(-u^2\eta^2/2))$.

The Lindberg condition (H1) is often replaced by the stronger assumption:

(H1b): $\exists\, \delta > 0,\ \frac{1}{s_n^{2+\delta}} \sum_{i=1}^n E(|X_i|^{2+\delta}|\mathscr{F}_{i-1}) \to 0$ in probability.

If the dimension of the parameter is q, the score function $\nabla_\theta \ell_n(\theta_0)$ is a $\mathbb{P}_{\theta_0}$-martingale in $\mathbb{R}^q$. So we need theorems for multidimensional martingales in $\mathbb{R}^q$.

Let (M_n) be a sequence of random variables in $\mathbb{R}^q$ with $M_n^* = (M_n^1, \ldots, M_n^q)$. Then (M_n) is a $\mathscr{F}_n$-martingale if (M_n^p) is a $\mathscr{F}_n$-martingale for $p = 1, \ldots q$.

Assume that (M_n) is a centered L^2-martingale in $\mathbb{R}^q$ and set $X_i = M_i - M_{i-1}$ with $X_i^* = (X_i^1, \ldots, X_i^q)$.
Then the increasing process $\langle M \rangle_n$ is the $q \times q$ random matrix defined by $\langle M \rangle_0 = 0$ and $\langle M \rangle_n - \langle M \rangle_{n-1} = E(X_n\, X_n^* | \mathscr{F}_{n-1}) = \left(E(X_n^p X_n^l | \mathscr{F}_{n-1})\right)_{1 \le p,l \le q}$.
Hence, for $1 \le p, l \le q$, $\langle M \rangle_n^{pl} = \sum_{i=1}^n E(X_i^p\, X_i^l | \mathscr{F}_{i-1})$.

This theorem is derived from a convergence theorem for triangular arrays stated in [73].
For each p, assume that $\mathbb{E}(\langle M_n^p \rangle) = (s_n^p)^2 \to \infty$ and define

$$\zeta_i^{n,p} = \frac{X_i^p}{s_n^p} \quad \text{and } (\zeta_i^n)^* = (\zeta_i^{n,1}, \ldots \zeta_i^{n,q}).$$

Theorem A.4.2. *Assume that there exists a positive random matrix Γ such that, as $n \to \infty$,*

(H1): $\sum_{i=1}^n \mathbb{E}(\zeta_i^n (\zeta_i^n)^* | \mathscr{F}_{i-1}) \to \Gamma$ *in probability.*
(H2): *There exists $\delta > 0$, $\sum_{i=1}^n E(\|\zeta_i^n\|^{2+\delta}\, |\mathscr{F}_{i-1}) \to 0$ in probability.*

Then the following holds

$$\left(\sum_{i=1}^n \zeta_i^n, \sum_{i=1}^n \mathbb{E}(\zeta_i^n (\zeta_i^n)^* | \mathscr{F}_{i-1}\right) \xrightarrow{\mathscr{L}} \left(\Gamma^{1/2} N_q\,, \Gamma\right)$$

with $N_q \sim \mathscr{N}_q(0, I)$ and Γ, N_q independent.

Here again, if $Z = \Gamma^{1/2} N_q$, then, for $u \in \mathbb{R}^q$, $E(\exp(iuZ)) = E(\exp(-\frac{u^*\Gamma u}{2}))$.

A.4.2 Limit Theorems for Triangular Arrays

When dealing with discrete observations with small sampling interval, classical limit theorems for martingales can no longer be used since the σ-algebras $\mathscr{G}_k^n =$

$\sigma(Z(s), s \leq k/n)$ do not satisfy the nesting property. We need general theorems for triangular arrays as stated in [73].

A.4.2.1 Recap on Triangular Arrays

Let $(\Omega, \mathscr{F}, (\mathscr{F}_t, t \geq 0), \mathbb{P})$ be a filtered probability space satisfying the usual conditions. Assume that for each n, there is a strictly increasing sequence $(T(n,k), k \geq 0)$ of finite $(\mathscr{F}_t)$-stopping times with limit $+\infty$ and $T(n,0) = 0$. The stopping rule is defined as

$$N_n(t) = \sup\{k, T(n,k) \leq t\} = \sum_{k \geq 1} 1_{T(n,k) \leq t}.$$

A q-dimensional triangular array is a double sequence $(\zeta_k^n), n, k \geq 1)$ of q-dimensional variables $\zeta_k^n = (\zeta_k^{n,j})_{1 \leq j \leq q}$. such that each ζ_k^n is $\mathscr{F}_{T(n,k)}$-measurable.

We consider the behavior of the sums

$$S_t^n = \sum_{k=1}^{N_n(t)} \zeta_k^n.$$

The triangular array is asymptotically negligible (A.N.) if

$$\sum_{k=1}^{N_n(t)} \zeta_k^n \overset{u.c.p.}{\to} 0 \quad \text{i.e. } \sup_{s \leq t} |\sum_{k=1}^{N_n(s)} \zeta_k^n| \overset{\mathbb{P}}{\to} 0.$$

In the sequel, we assume that the $T(n,k)$ are non-random and set $\mathscr{G}_k^n = \mathscr{F}_{T(n,k)}$. The example we have in mind consists in the deterministic times

$$T(n,k) = \inf\{t, [nt] \geq k\Delta\} \Rightarrow N_n(t) = \sup\{k, \frac{k\Delta}{n} \leq t\}. \tag{A.4.1}$$

Triangular arrays often occur as follows: ζ_k^n may be a function of the increment $Y_{T(n,k)} - Y_{T(n,k-1)}$ for some underlying adapted càdlàg process Y. For discretely observed diffusion processs, we have $\zeta_k^n = X(k\Delta/n) - X((k-1)\Delta/n)$. We first state a lemma proved in [48].

Lemma A.4.3. *Let ζ_k^n, U be random variables with ζ_k^n being $\mathscr{G}_k^n$-measurable. Assume that*

(i) $\sum_{k=1}^n \mathbb{E}(\zeta_k^n | \mathscr{G}_{k-1}^n) \to U$ *in $\mathbb{P}$-probability,*
(ii) $\sum_{k=1}^n \mathbb{E}[(\zeta_k^n)^2 | \mathscr{G}_{k-1}^n)] \to 0$ *in $\mathbb{P}$-probability,*

Then

$$\sum_{k=1}^n \zeta_k^n \to U \quad \textit{in } \mathbb{P}\textit{-probability}.$$

Corollary A.4.4. *Let ζ_k^n, U be d-dimensional random variables with ζ_k^n being $\mathscr{G}_k^n$-measurable. Assume*

(i) $\sum_{k=1}^n \mathbb{E}(\zeta_k^n|\mathscr{G}_{k-1}^n) \to U$ *in $\mathbb{P}$-probability,*
(ii) $\sum_{k=1}^n \mathbb{E}[\|\zeta_k^n\|^2 |\mathscr{G}_{k-1}^n)] \to 0$ *in $\mathbb{P}$-probability,*

Then

$$\sum_{k=1}^n \zeta_k^n \to U \quad \text{in } \mathbb{P}\text{-probability.}$$

A.4.2.2 Convergence in Law of Triangular Arrays

Let (ζ_k^n) be a triangular array of d-dimensional random variables such that ζ_k^n is $\mathscr{G}_k^n$-measurable.

Theorem A.4.5. *Assume that (ζ_k^n) satisfy for $N_n(t)$ defined in* (A.4.1)

(i) $\sum_{k=1}^{N_n(t)} \mathbb{E}(\zeta_k^n|\mathscr{G}_{k-1}^n) \overset{u.c.p.}{\to} A_t$ *with A an $\mathbb{R}^d$-valued deterministic function.*
(ii) $\sum_{k=1}^{N_n(t)} \mathbb{E}(\zeta_k^{n,i}\zeta_k^{n,j}|\mathscr{G}_{k-1}^n) - \mathbb{E}(\zeta_k^{n,i}|\mathscr{G}_{k-1}^n)\mathbb{E}(\zeta_k^{n,j}|\mathscr{G}_{k-1}^n) \overset{\mathbb{P}}{\to} C_t^{ij}$ *for $1 \le i,j \le d$ and for all $t \ge 0$, where $C = (C^{ij})$ is a deterministic continuous $\mathscr{M}_{d\times d}^+$-valued function.*
(iii) For some $p > 2$, $\sum_{k=1}^{N_n(t)} \mathbb{E}(\|\zeta_k^n\|^p |\mathscr{G}_{k-1}^n) \overset{\mathbb{P}}{\to} 0.$

Then, we have

$$\sum_{k=1}^{N_n(t)} \zeta_k^n \overset{\mathscr{L}}{\to} A + Y, \text{ w.r.t. the Skorokhod topology,} \tag{A.4.2}$$

where Y is a continuous centered Gaussian process on $\mathbb{R}^d$ with independent increments s.t. $\mathbb{E}(Y_t^i Y_t^j) = C_t^{ij}$.

Remark: If (ii) holds for a single time t, the convergence $\sum_{k=1}^{N_n(t)} \zeta_k^n \overset{\mathscr{L}}{\to} A_t + Y_t$ for this particular t fails in general. There is an exception detailed below (Theorem VII-2-36 of [75]).

Theorem A.4.6. *Assume that for each n, the variables $(\zeta_k^n, k \ge 1)$ are independent and let l_n be integers, or ∞. Assume that, for all $i,j = 1,\dots,d$ and for some $p > 2$,*

$$\sum_{k=1}^{l_n} \mathbb{E}(\zeta_k^{n,i}) \overset{\mathbb{P}}{\to} A_i,$$
$$\sum_{k=1}^{l_n} \left(\mathbb{E}(\zeta_k^{n,i}\zeta_k^{n,j}) - \mathbb{E}(\zeta_k^{n,i})\mathbb{E}(\zeta_k^{n,j})\right) \overset{\mathbb{P}}{\to} C^{ij},$$
$$\sum_{k=1}^{l_n} \mathbb{E}(\|\zeta_k^n\|^p) \overset{\mathbb{P}}{\to} 0,$$

where C^{ij} and A_i are deterministic numbers. Then the variables $\sum_{k=1}^{l_n} \zeta_k^n$ converge in distribution to a Gaussian vector with mean $A = (A^i)$ and covariance matrix $C = (C^{ij})$.

A.5 Inference for Pure Jump Processes

In statistical applications, we study likelihood ratios formed by taking Radon–Nikodym derivatives of members of the family of probability measures $(P_\theta, \theta \in \Theta \subset \mathbb{R}^q)$ with respect to one fixed reference distribution.

A.5.1 Girsanov Type Formula for Counting Processes

Rather than giving the general expression of the Girsanov formula for semi-martingales (see [75]), we state it first for the case of a counting process on $\mathbb{N}$ and then for multivariate counting processes.

Let X be a stochastic process such that the predictable compensator Λ of X satisfies $\Lambda(t) = \int_0^t \lambda(s)ds)$. assume that, under $\mathbb{P}_\theta$, it is a counting process with intensity $\lambda^\theta(t)$ where $\lambda^\theta(t) > 0$ for all $t > 0$. Denote by $T_1, T_2, \ldots$ the sequence of jump times of X and let $N(t)$ denotes the number of jumps up to time t. Then

$$\frac{d\mathbb{P}_\theta}{d\mathbb{P}_{\theta_0}}|\mathscr{F}_t = \exp\{\sum_{i=1}^{N(t)}[\log(\lambda^\theta(T_i)) - \log(\lambda^{\theta_0}(T_i))] - \int_0^t [\lambda^\theta(s) - \lambda^{\theta_0}(s)]ds.\} \tag{A.5.1}$$

Consider now multivariate counting processes $N(t) = (N_1(t), \ldots, N_k(t))$. We refer to Jacod's formula (see e.g. Andersen [1, II.7]) for a general expression of two probability measures $\mathbb{P}, \tilde{\mathbb{P}}$ on a filtered probability space under which $\mathbf{N}$ has compensators $\boldsymbol{\Lambda}, \tilde{\boldsymbol{\Lambda}}$ respectively. Usually, we will have continuous or absolutely continuous compensators with intensities $\lambda_l(t), \tilde{\lambda}_l(t)$. Since no jumps can occur simultaneously, the sequence of jump times T_i is well defined, together with the mark $J_i \in \{1, \ldots, k\}$ ($J_i = l$ if the jump T_i occurs in N_l ($\Delta N_l(T_i) = 1$). The process $N_.(t) = \sum_{l=1}^k N_l(t)$ is a counting process with compensator $\Lambda_.(t) = \sum_{l=1}^k \Lambda_l(t)$. Assume $\tilde{\mathbb{P}}$ is absolutely continuous with respect to $\mathbb{P}$ (written $\tilde{\mathbb{P}} << \mathbb{P}$).

Theorem A.5.1. *Assume that $\tilde{\mathbb{P}} << \mathbb{P}$. Then*

$$\tilde{\Lambda}_l << \Lambda_l \textit{ for all } l = 1, \ldots, k, \quad P\text{- a.s.}$$

$$\Delta\Lambda_.(t) = 1 \textit{ for any time } t \textit{ implies } \Delta\tilde{\Lambda}_.(t) = 1, \quad P\text{-a.s.}$$

$$\frac{d\tilde{\mathbb{P}}}{d\mathbb{P}}|\mathscr{F}_t = \frac{d\tilde{P}}{dP}|\mathscr{F}_0 \frac{\prod_{l=1}^k \prod_{s\le t} \tilde{\lambda}_l(t)^{\Delta N_l(t)} \exp(-\int_0^t \tilde{\lambda}_.(s)ds)}{\prod_{l=1}^k \prod_{s\le t} \lambda_l(t)^{\Delta N_l(t)} \exp(-\int_0^t \lambda_.(s)ds)}$$

$$= \frac{d\tilde{\mathbb{P}}}{d\mathbb{P}}|\mathscr{F}_0 \exp\left\{\sum_{l=1}^k \sum_{i=1}^{N(t)} [\log\tilde{\lambda}_l(T_i) - \log\lambda_l(T_i)]\Delta N_l(T_i) - \sum_{l=1}^k \int_0^t [\tilde{\lambda}_l(s) - \lambda_l(s)]ds\right\}.$$

Note that the products in the above formula are just $\prod_n \tilde{\lambda}_{J_n}(T_n)$, $\prod_n \lambda_{J_n}(T_n)$.

A.5.2 Likelihood for Markov Pure Jump Processes

Let us consider a pure jump process with state space $E = \{0,\dots,N\}$ and Q-matrix $\mathbf{Q} = (q_{ij})$ observed up to time T. The likelihood is

$$L_T(\mathbf{Q}) = \prod_{i=0}^{N}\prod_{j\neq i} q_{ij}^{N_{ij}(T)} \exp(-q_{ij}N_i(T)), \tag{A.5.2}$$

where the process $N_{ij}(t)$ counts the number of transitions from state i to state j on the time interval $[0,t]$ and $N_i(t)$ is the time spent in state i before time t:

$$N_i(t) = \int_0^t \delta_{\{X(s)=i\}} ds.$$

We refer to [72] for a complete study of Marked point processes.
This yields that the maximum likelihood estimator of $\mathbf{Q}$ is

$$\hat{q}_{ij}(T) = \frac{N_{ij}(T)}{N_i(T)}, \quad \text{for } j \neq i \quad \text{and } N_i(T) > 0. \tag{A.5.3}$$

If $N_T(i) = 0$, the process has not been in state i: there is no information about q_{ij} in the observations and the MLE of q_{ij} does not exist. As for Markov chains with countable state space, $\hat{q}_{ij}(T)$ is the empirical estimate of q_{ij}.

A.5.3 Martingale Properties of Likelihood Processes

In statistical applications, we want to consider a whole family of probability measures $\mathbb{P}$, not necessarily mutually absolutely continuous and therefore cannot apply the above theorem to obtain $\frac{d\tilde{\mathbb{P}}}{d\mathbb{P}}|_{\mathscr{F}_t}$ for each $\tilde{\mathbb{P}}, \mathbb{P}$ considered. However, for any two probability measures $\tilde{\mathbb{P}}, \mathbb{P}$, the measure $\mathbf{Q} = \frac{1}{2}(\tilde{\mathbb{P}} + \mathbb{P})$ dominates both $\tilde{\mathbb{P}}$ and $\mathbb{P}$. We can therefore calculate $d\mathbb{P}/d\mathbf{Q}$ and $d\tilde{\mathbb{P}}/d\mathbf{Q}$ and finally set,

$$\frac{d\tilde{\mathbb{P}}}{d\mathbb{P}} = \frac{d\tilde{\mathbb{P}}}{d\mathbf{Q}} / \frac{d\mathbb{P}}{d\mathbf{Q}} \text{ where } \frac{d\mathbb{P}}{d\mathbf{Q}} > 0,$$
$$\frac{d\tilde{\mathbb{P}}}{d\mathbb{P}} = \infty \text{ where } \frac{d\mathbb{P}}{d\mathbf{Q}} = 0.$$

Suppose now that we have a statistical model $(\mathbb{P}_\theta, \theta \in \Theta)$ for some subset $\Theta \in \mathbb{R}^q$. Suppose that all $\mathbb{P}_\theta$ are dominated by a fixed probability measure $\mathbf{Q}$. For simplicity, we assume that all the $\mathbb{P}_\theta$'s coincide on $\mathscr{F}_0$ and consider only the absolute continuous case:
under $\mathbb{P}_\theta$, $\mathbf{N} = (N_1,\dots,N_k)$ has compensator $\boldsymbol{\Lambda}^\theta = (\int \lambda_l^\theta), l = 1,\dots,k)$ for certain intensity process λ^θ. We consider the likelihood function as depending on both $t \in \mathbb{R}^+$ and $\theta \in \Theta$. Dropping the denominator in Theorem A.5.1 (which does not

depend on θ), we have that the likelihood at time t as a function of θ is proportional to

$$L(\theta,t) = \exp(-\sum_{l=1}^{k} \int_0^t \lambda_l^\theta(s)ds) \prod_{T_n \le t} \lambda_{J_n}^\theta(T_n),$$
$$= \exp\{\sum_{l=1}^{k} \int_0^t [\log \lambda_l^\theta(s)dN_l(s) - \lambda_l^\theta(s)ds]\}.$$

Remark A.5.2. This is another expression of the general Girsanov formula given in the appendix of Part I of these notes.

The likelihood process $L(\theta,t)$ is a $(\mathbf{Q}, (\mathscr{F}_t))$-martingale. Indeed, let Y a $\mathscr{F}_s$ measurable random variable. We have $E_{\mathbf{Q}}(YL(\theta,t)) = E_{\mathbf{Q}}(Y\frac{d\mathbb{P}_\theta}{dQ}) = \mathbb{E}_\theta(Y) = E_{\mathbf{Q}}(YL(\theta,s))$ since $Y \in \mathscr{F}_s$.
Hence $E_{\mathbf{Q}}(L(\theta,t)|\mathscr{F}_s) = L(\theta,s)$.

Consider now the log-likelihood

$$\log L(\theta,t) = \sum_{l=1}^{k} \int_0^t (\log \lambda_l^\theta(s)dN_l(s) - \lambda_l^\theta(s)ds). \tag{A.5.4}$$

The score process is defined as $\nabla_\theta \log L(\theta,t)$. Assuming that differentiation may be taken under the integral sign, we get

$$\nabla_{\theta_j} \log L(\theta,t) = \frac{\partial}{\partial \theta_j} \log L(\theta,t) \tag{A.5.5}$$
$$= \sum_{l=1}^{k} \int_0^t \nabla_{\theta_j} \log \lambda_l^\theta(s)\ (dN_l(s) - \lambda_l^\theta(s)ds),\ j = 1,\ldots,q.$$

Hence the score process is a $(P_\theta,(\mathscr{F}_t))$- local martingale in $\mathbb{R}^q$. It is a centered L^2-martingale with associated predictable $q \times q$ matrix variation process

$$\langle \nabla_\theta \log L(\theta;\cdot)\rangle_{r,j} = \sum_{l=1}^{k} \int_0^t \nabla_{\theta_r} \log \lambda_l^\theta(s) \nabla_{\theta_j} \log \lambda_l^\theta(s)\ \lambda_l^\theta(s)ds. \tag{A.5.6}$$

The "observed information" at θ is obtained by differentiating again with respect to θ. If differentiation can be taken under the integral sign, we get

$$\nabla^2_{\theta_r \theta_j} \log L(\theta;t) = \sum_{l=1}^{k} \int_0^t \nabla^2_{\theta_r \theta_j j} \lambda_l^\theta(s)(dN_l(s) - \lambda_l(s)ds)$$
$$- \int_0^t \nabla_{\theta_r} \log \lambda_l^\theta(s) \nabla_{\theta_j} \log \lambda_l^\theta(s) \lambda_l^\theta(s)ds. \tag{A.5.7}$$

Using (A.5.6) yields that the compensator of the process $-\nabla^2 \log L(\theta;\cdot)$ is $\langle \nabla_\theta \log L(\theta;\cdot)\rangle$. This is a version of a well-known result: the variance matrix of the score coincides with the expected information matrix.

References for Part IV

1. P.K. Andersen, O. Borgan, R.D. Gill and N. Keiding, *Statistical Models Based on Counting Processes*, Springer Series in Statistics. Springer, New York, 1993.
2. H. Andersson and T. Britton, *Stochastic Epidemic Models and their Statistical Analysis*, Lecture Notes in Statistics Series. Springer, 2000.
3. C. Andrieu, A. Doucet and R. Holenstein, Particle Markov Chain Monte Carlo Methods, *Journal of the Royal Statistical Society: Series B*, 72:269–342, 2010.
4. H. De Arazoza, J. Joanes, R. Lounes, C. Legeai, S. Clémencon, J. Perez and B. Auvert, The HIV/AIDS epidemic in Cuba: description and tentative explanation of its low prevalence, *BMC Infectious Disease*, 7:130, 2007.
5. S. Arlot and P. Massart, Data-driven calibration of penalties for least-squares regression, *Journal of Machine Learning Research*, 10:245–279, 2009.
6. K.B. Athreya and P. Ney, *Branching Processes*, Springer Series in Probability. Springer, 1972.
7. R. Azencott, Formule de Taylor stochastique et développement asymptotique integrales de Feynmann, *Séminaire de Probabilités XVI*, pages 237–285, 1982.
8. F. Ball, The threshold behaviour of epidemic models, *Journal of Applied Probability*, 20(2):227–241, 1983.
9. M.A. Beaumont, J.M. Marin, J.M. Cornuet and C.P. Roberts, Adaptive Approximate Bayesian Computation, *Biometrika*, 96(4):983–990, 2009.
10. M.A. Beaumont, W. Zhang and D.J. Balding, Approximate Bayesian Computation in population genetics, *Genetics*, 162:2025–2035, 2002.
11. P.J. Bickel and K.A. Doksum, *Mathematical Statistics: Basic Ideas and Selected Topics, Volume I*, Chapman and Hall/CRC, 2nd edition, 2015.
12. O.N. Bjørnstad, B.F. Finkenstadt and B.T. Grenfell, Dynamics of Measles Epidemics: Estimating Scaling of Transmission Rates Using a Time Series SIR Model, *Ecological Monographs*, 72(2):169–184, 2002.
13. M. Bladt, B. Meini, M.F. Neuts and B. Sericola, Distributions of reward functions on continuous-time Markov chains, *Matrix-Analytic Methods: Theory and Applications*, pages 39–62, 2002.
14. M. Bladt and M. Sørensen, Statistical inference for discretely observed Markov jump processes, *Journal of the Royal Statistical Society, Series B*, 67(3):395–410, 2005.
15. M.G. Blum, Approximate Bayesian Computation: a non-parametric perspective, *Journal of the American Statistical Association*, 105:1178–1187, 2010.
16. M.G. Blum and O. Francois, Non-linear regression models for Approximate Bayesian Computation, *Statistics and Computing*, 20:63–73, 2010.
17. M.G. Blum and V.C. Tran, HIV with contact-tracing: a case study in Approximate Bayesian Computation, *Biostatistics*, 11(4):644–660, 2010.
18. C. Bretó, E.L. He, D. Ionides and A.A. King, Time series analysis via mechanistic models, *Annals of Applied Statistics*, 3(1):319–348, 2009.

19. T. Britton and F. Giardina, Introduction to statistical inference for infectious diseases. *Journal de la Société Francaise de Statistiques*, 157(1):53–70, 2016.
20. A. Camacho, A. Kucharski, Y. Aki-Sawyerr, M.A. White, S. Flasche, M. Baguelin, T. Pollington, J.R. Carney, R. Glover, E. Smout, A. Tiffany, W.J. Edmunds, and S. Funk, Temporal changes in ebola transmission in sierra leone and implications for control requirements: a real-time modelling study, *PLOS Currents Outbreaks*, Edition 1(10.1371), 2015.
21. Y. Cao, D.T. Gillespie and L.R. Petzold, Avoiding negative populations in explicit Poisson tau-leaping. *Journal of Chemical Physics*, 123:054–104, 2005.
22. O. Cappé, E. Moulines and T. Ryden, *Inference in Hidden Markov Models*, Springer Series in Statistics. Springer, 2005.
23. G. Castellan, *Sélection d'histogrammes ou de modèles exponentiels de polynômes par morceaux à l'aide d'un critère de type Akaike*, PhD thesis, Université d'Orsay, 2000.
24. G. Castellan, A. Cousien and V.C. Tran, Nonparametric adaptive estimation of order 1 Sobol indices in stochastic models, with an application to epidemiology, Submitted, 2017.
25. S. Cauchemez, F. Carrat, C. Viboud, A.J. Valleron and P.Y. Boelle, A Bayesian MCMC approach to study transmission of influenza: application to household longitudinal data, *Statistics in Medicine*, 23(22):3469–3487, 2004.
26. S. Cauchemez and N.M. Ferguson, Likelihood-based estimation of continuous-time epidemic models from time-series data: application to measles transmission in London, *Journal of The Royal Society Interface*, 5(25):885–897, 2008.
27. S. Cauchemez and N.M. Ferguson, Methods to infer risk factors in complex outbreak data, *Journal of The Royal Society Interface*, 9(68):456–469, 2012.
28. G. Chagny, Penalization versus Goldenshluger-lepski strategies in warped bases regression, *ESAIM: P&S*, 17:328–358, 2013.
29. A. Chatzilena, E. van Leeuwen, O. Ratmann, M. Baguelin and N. Demiris, Contemporary statistical inference for infectious disease models using Stan, *arXiv: 1903.00423*, 2019.
30. S. Clémencon, V.C. Tran and H. De Arazoza, A stochastic SIR model with contact-tracing: large population limits and statistical inference, *Journal of Biological Dynamics*, 2(4):391–414, 2008.
31. D. Dacunha-Castelle and M. Duflo, *Probabilités et Statistiques: 2. Problèmes à Temps Mobile*, Masson, Paris, 1993.
32. D.J. Daley and J. Gani, *Epidemic Modelling: an Introduction*, Cambridge University Press, 2001.
33. B. Delyon, M. Lavielle and E. Moulines, Convergence of a stochastic approximation version of the EM algorithm, *The Annals of Statistics*, 27(1):94–128, 1999.
34. A.P. Dempster, N.M. Laird and D.B. Rubin, Maximum likelihood from incomplete data via the EM algorithm, *Journal of the Royal Statistical Society. Series B*, 39(1):1–38, 1977.
35. O. Diekmann, H. Heesterbeek and T. Britton, *Mathematical Tools for Understanding Infectious Disease Dynamics*, Princeton University Press, 2013.
36. G. Dohnal, On estimating the diffusion coefficient, *Journal of Applied Probability*, 24:105–114, 1987.
37. A. Doucet, N. De Freitas and N. Gordon, *Sequential Monte Carlo Methods in Practice*, Springer, 2001.
38. C.C. Drovandi and A.N. Pettitt, Using approximate bayesian computation to estimate transmission rates of nosocomial pathogens, *Statistical Communications in Infectious Diseases*, 3(1):online, 2011.
39. S.N. Ethier and T.G. Kurtz, *Markov Processes: Characterization and Convergence*, Wiley, 2nd edition, 2005.
40. J. Fan, Design-adaptive nonparametric regression, *Journal of the American Statistical Association*, 87(420):998–1004, 1992.
41. P. Fearnhead, O. Papaspiliopoulos and G.O. Roberts, Particle filters for partially observed diffusions, *Journal of the Royal Statistical Society: Series B*, 70(4):755–777, 2008.
42. P. Fearnhead and D. Prangle, Constructing Summary Statistics for Approximate Bayesian Computation: Semi-automatic ABC, *Journal of the Royal Statistical Society*, 74(3):419–474, 2012.

43. J.C. Fort, T. Klein, A. Lagnoux and B. Laurent, Estimation of the Sobol indices in a linear functional multidimensional model, *Journal of Statistical Planning and Inference*, 143(9):1590–1605, 2013.
44. M.I. Freidlin and A.D. Wentzell, *Random Perturbations of Dynamical Systems*, Springer, 1978.
45. C. Fuchs, *Inference for diffusion processes*, Springer, 2013.
46. V. Genon-Catalot, Maximum contrast estimation for diffusion processes from discrete observations, *Statistics*, 21(1):99–116, 1990.
47. V. Genon-Catalot, *Cours de Statistique des diffusions*, Preprint, 2018.
48. V. Genon-Catalot and J. Jacod, On the estimation of the diffusion coefficient for multidimensional diffusion processes, *Annales de l'I.H.P. Probabilités et statistiques*, 29(1):119–151, 1993.
49. V. Genon-Catalot, T. Jeantheau and C. Larédo, Stochastic volatility models as hidden markov models and statistical applications, *Bernoulli*, 6(6):105, 2000.
50. V. Genon-Catalot and C. Larédo, Leroux's method for general Hidden Markov Models, *Stochastic Processes and their Applications*, 116(2):222–243, 2006.
51. W.R. Gilks, S. Richardson and D.J. Spieghalter, *Markov Chain Monte Carlo in practice*, Chapman and Hall, 1996.
52. W.R. Gilks and G.O. Roberts, Strategies for improving mcmc, In W.R. Gilks, S. Richardson and D.J. Spiegelhalter, editors, *Markov chain Monte Carlo in Practice*, pages 89–114, Boca Raton, Chapman and Hall/CRC, 1996.
53. D.T. Gillespie, Exact stochastic simulation of coupled chemical reactions, *Journal of Physical Chemistry*, 81(25):2340–2361, 1977.
54. A. Gloter. Parameter estimation for a discrete sampling of an integrated Ornstein–Uhlenbeck process, *Statistics*, 35(3):225–243, 2001.
55. A. Gloter, Discrete sampling of an integrated diffusion process and parameter estimation of the diffusion coefficient, *ESAIM: Probability and Statistics*, 4:205–227, 2010.
56. A. Gloter and M. Sørensen, Estimation for stochastic differential equations with a small diffusion coefficient, *Stochastic Processes and their Applications*, 119(3):679–699, 2009.
57. E. Gobet, Local asymptotic normality property for elliptic diffusion: a malliavin calculus approach, *Bernoulli*, 7(6):899–912, 2001.
58. M. Greenwood, On the statistical measure of infectiousness, *J. Hyg.*, 31:336–351, 1931.
59. P. Guttorp, *Statistical Inference for Branching Processes*, Wiley Series in Probability and Mathematical Statistics. Wiley, 1991.
60. R. Guy, C. Larédo and E. Vergu, Parametric inference for discretely observed multidimensional diffusions with small diffusion coefficient, *Stochastic Processes and their Applications*, 124:51–80, 2014.
61. R. Guy, C. Larédo and E. Vergu, Approximation of epidemic models by diffusion processes and their statistical inference, *Journal of Mathematical Biology*, 70:621–646, 2015.
62. R. Guy, C. Larédo and E. Vergu, Approximation and inference of epidemic dynamics by diffusion processes, *Journal de la Société Francaise de Statistiques*, 157(1):71–100, 2016.
63. P. Hall and C.C. Heyde, *Martingale Limit Theory and its Application*, Probability and Mathematical Statistics. Academic Press, 1980.
64. L.P. Hansen and J.A. Scheinkman, Back to the Future: Generating Moment Implications for Continuous-Time Markov Processes, *Econometrica*, 63:767–804, 1995.
65. W. Härdle, G. Kerkyacharian, D. Picard and A. Tsybakov, *Wavelets, Approximation and Statistical Applications*, volume 129 of *Lecture Notes in Statistics*, Springer, New York, 1987.
66. M. Høhle, E. Jørgensen and P.D. O'Neill, Inference in disease transmission experiments by using stochastic epidemic models, *Journal of the Royal Statistical Society: Series C*, 54(2):349–366, 2005.
67. R. Hopfner, *Asymptotic Statistics with a View to Stochastic Processes*, Graduate. Walter de Gruyter GmbH, Berlin/Boston, 2014.
68. I.A. Ibragimov and R.Z. Has'minskii, *Statistical Estimation. Asymptotic Theory*, Applications of Mathematics. Springer, 1981.
69. N. Ikeda and S. Watanabe, *Stochastic Differential Equations and Diffusion Processes*, volume 24, North-Holland Publishing Company, 1989, Second Edition.

70. E.L. Ionides, A. Bhadra and A. King, Iterated filtering, *Annals of Statistics*, 39:1776–1802, 2011.
71. E.L. Ionides, C. Bretó and A.A. King, Inference for nonlinear dynamical systems, *Proceedings of the National Academy of Sciences*, 103(49):18438–18443, 2006.
72. M. Jacobsen, *Marked Point and Piecewise Deterministic Processes*, Applied Mathematics. Probability and Its Applications. Birkhäuser, Berlin, 2006.
73. J. Jacod and P. Protter, *Discretization of Processes*, volume 67 of *Stochastic Modelling and Applied Probability*, Springer, 2012.
74. J. Jacod and A.N. Shiryaev, *Limit Theorems for Stochastic Processes*, Springer-Verlag, Berlin, 1987.
75. J. Jacod and A.N. Shiryaev, *Limit Theorems for Stochastic Processes*, volume 288 of *A series of Comprehensive Studies in Mathematics*, Springer, 2003.
76. J. Jacques, *Contributions à l'analyse de sensibilité et à l'analyse discriminante*, PhD thesis, Université Joseph Fourier, Grenoble, 12, 2005.
77. J. Jacques, Pratique de l'analyse de sensibilité : comment évaluer l'impact des entrées aléatoires sur la sortie d'un modèle mathématique, *IRMA Lille*, 71(III), 2011.
78. P. Jagers, *Branching Processes with Biological Applications*, Wiley, 1975.
79. M.R. James and F. Le Gland, Consistent parameter estimation for partially observed diffusions with small noise, *Applied Mathematics and Optimization*, 32(1):47–72, 1995.
80. A. Janon, M. Nodet and C. Prieur, Uncertainties assessment in global sensitivity indices estimation from metamodels, *International Journal for Uncertainty Quantification*, 4(1):21–36, 2014.
81. M.J.W. Jansen, Analysis of variance designs for model output, *Computer Physics Communications*, 117:35–43, 1999.
82. I. Karatzas and S.E. Shreve, *Brownian Motion and Stochastic Calculus*, volume Second Edition of *Graduate Texts in Mathematics*, Springer, 2000.
83. M.J. Keeling and P. Rohani, *Modeling Infectious Diseases in Humans and Animals*, Princeton University Press, 2011.
84. G. Kerkyacharian and D. Picard, Regression in random design and warped wavelets, *Bernoulli*, 10(6):1053–1105, 2004.
85. M. Kessler, Estimation of an ergodic diffusion from discrete observations, *Scandinavian Journal of Statistics*, 24:221–229, 1997.
86. M. Kessler, Simple and explicit estimating functions for a discretely observed diffusion process, *Scandinavian Journal of Statistics*, 27(1):65–82, 2000.
87. M. Kessler, A. Lindner and M. Sørensen, *Statistical Methods for Stochastic Differential Equations*, volume 124 of *Monographs on Statistics and Applied Probability*, CRC Press, 2012.
88. A.A. King, E.L. Ionides, M. Pascual and M.J. Bouma, Inapparent infections and cholera dynamics, *Nature*, 454(7206):877–880, 2008.
89. A.A. King, D. Nguyen and E.L. Ionides, Statistical inference for partially observed markov processes via the r package pomp, *Journal of Statistical Software*, 69(12):1–43, 2016.
90. E. Kuhn and M. Lavielle, Coupling a stochastic approximation version of em with an mcmc procedure, *ESAIM: Probability and Statistics*, 8:115–131, 2004.
91. Y.A. Kutoyants, *Parameter Estimation for Stochastic Processes*, volume 6 of *Research and Exposition in Mathematics*, Heldermann, 1984.
92. Y.A. Kutoyants, *Identification of Dynamical Systems with Small Noise*, Springer, 1994.
93. Y.A. Kutoyants, *Statistical Inference for Ergodic Diffusion Processes*, Springer, 2004.
94. B. Laurent and P. Massart, Adaptive estimation of a quadratic functional by model selection, *The Annals of Statistics*, 28(5):1302–1338, 2000.
95. Y.N. Linkov, *Asymptotic Statistical Methods for Stochastic Processes*, volume 196 of *Translations of Mathematical Monographs*, American Mathematical Society, Providence, 2001, translated from the 1993 Russian original by V. Kotov.
96. R.S. Liptser and A.N. Shiryaev, *Statistics of Random Processes. I. General Theory*, volume Second Edition, Springer, 2001.
97. R.S. Liptser and A.N. Shiryaev, *Statistics of Random Processes .II. Applications*, volume Second Edition, Springer, 2001.

98. J.-M. Loubes, C. Marteau and M. Solís, Rates of convergence in conditional covariance matrix estimation, `ArXiv:1310.8244`, 2014.
99. J.-M. Marin, P. Pudlo, C.P. Robert and R. Ryder, Approximate Bayesian computation methods, *Statistics and Computing*, 22(6):1167–1180, 2012.
100. A. Marrel, B. Iooss, S. Da Veiga and M. Ribatet, Global sensitivity analysis of stochastic computer models with joint metamodels, *Statistics and Computing*, 22(3):833–847, 2012.
101. T.J. McKinley, A.R. Cook and R. Deardon, Inference in epidemic models without likelihoods, *International Journal of Biostatistics*, 5(1), 2009.
102. T.J. McKinley, J.V. Ross, R. Deardon and A.R. Cook, Simulation-based Bayesian inference for epidemic models, *Computational Statistics & Data Analysis*, 71:434–447, 2014.
103. S. Méléard, *Modèles aléatoires en Ecologie et Evolution*, Springer, 2016.
104. P.D. O'Neill, A tutorial introduction to Bayesian inference for stochastic epidemic models using Markov Chain Monte Carlo methods , *Mathematical Biosciences*, 180:103–114, 2002.
105. P.D. O'Neill, Introduction and snapshot review: Relating infectious disease transmission models to data, *Statistics in medicine*, 29(20):2069–2077, 2010.
106. P.D. O'Neill and G.O. Roberts, Bayesian inference for partially observed stochastic epidemics, *Journal of the Royal Statistical Society: Series A* 162:121–129, 1999.
107. H. Pohjanpalo, System identifiability based on the power series expansion of the solution, *Mathematical Biosciences*, 41(1-2):21–33, September 1978.
108. W.N. Rida, Asymptotic properties of some estimators for the infection rate in the general stochastic epidemic model, *Journal of the Royal Statistical Society. Series B*, 53(1):269–283, 1991.
109. J.V. Ross, D.E. Pagendam and P.K. Polett, On parameter estimation in population models II: Multi-dimensional processes and transient dynamics, *Theoretical Population Biology*, 75(2-3):123–132, 2009.
110. A. Saltelli, K. Chan and E.M. Scott, *Sensitivity analysis*, Wiley Series in Probability and Statistics. John Wiley & Sons, Chichester, 2000.
111. A. Saltelli, M. Ratto, T. Andres, F. Campolongo, J. Cariboni, D. Gatelli, M. Saisana and S. Tarantola, *Global sensitivity analysis*, John Wiley & Sons, Chichester, 2008.
112. A. Sedoglavic, A probabilistic algorithm to test local algebraic observability in polynomial time, *Journal of Symbolic Computation*, 33(5):735–755, 2002.
113. S.A. Sisson, M.A. Beaumont and Y. Fan, editors, *Handbook fo Approximate Bayesian Computation*, Handbooks of Modern Statistical Methods. Chapman & Hall/CRC Press, 2018.
114. S.A. Sisson, Y. Fan and M. Beaumont, *Handbook of Approximate Bayesian Computation*, Handbooks of Modern Statistical Methods. Chapman and Hall /CRC, 2018.
115. S.A. Sisson, Y. Fan and M. Tanaka, Sequential Monte Carlo without likelihoods, *Proc. Nat. Acad. Sci. USA*, 104:1760–1765, 2007.
116. I.M. Sobol, Sensitivity estimates for nonlinear mathematical models, *Math. Modeling Comput. Experiment*, 1(4):407–414, 1993.
117. M. Solís, *Conditional covariance estimation for dimension reduction and sensivity analysis*, Phd thesis, Université de Toulouse, Université Toulouse III-Paul Sabatier, Toulouse, France, 2014.
118. M. Sørensen and M. Uchida, Small-diffusion asymptotics for discretely sampled stochastic differential equations, *Bernoulli*, 9(6):1051–1069, 2003.
119. I. Chis Ster, B.K. Singh and N.M. Ferguson, Epidemiological inference for partially observed epidemics: the example of the 2001 foot and mouth epidemic in Great Britain, *Epidemics*, 1:21–34, 2009.
120. T. Toni, D. Welch, N. Strelkowa, A. Ipsen and M.P. Stumpf, Approximate Bayesian computation scheme for parameter inference and model selection in dynamical systems, *Journal of The Royal Society Interface*, 6:187–202, 2009.
121. A.B. Tsybakov, *Introduction à l'estimation non-paramétrique*, volume 41 of *Mathématiques & Applications*, Springer, 2004.
122. F. Vaida, Parameter convergence for EM and MM algorithms, *Statistica Sinica*, 15:831–840, 2005.
123. A.W. van der Vaart, *Asymptotic Statistics*, Cambridge Series in Statistical and Probabilistic Mathematics. Cambridge University Press, 2000.

124. R. van Handel, *Lecture Notes on Hidden Markov Models*, Princeton University, 2008.
125. S. Da Veiga and F. Gamboa, Efficient estimation of sensitivity indices, *Journal of Nonparametric Statistics*, 25(3):573–595, 2013.
126. C.F.J. Wu, On the convergence properties of the EM algorithm, *Annals of Statistics*, 11(1):95–103, 1983.

LECTURE NOTES IN MATHEMATICS Springer

Editors in Chief: J.-M. Morel, B. Teissier;

Editorial Policy

1. Lecture Notes aim to report new developments in all areas of mathematics and their applications – quickly, informally and at a high level. Mathematical texts analysing new developments in modelling and numerical simulation are welcome.

   Manuscripts should be reasonably self-contained and rounded off. Thus they may, and often will, present not only results of the author but also related work by other people. They may be based on specialised lecture courses. Furthermore, the manuscripts should provide sufficient motivation, examples and applications. This clearly distinguishes Lecture Notes from journal articles or technical reports which normally are very concise. Articles intended for a journal but too long to be accepted by most journals, usually do not have this "lecture notes" character. For similar reasons it is unusual for doctoral theses to be accepted for the Lecture Notes series, though habilitation theses may be appropriate.

2. Besides monographs, multi-author manuscripts resulting from SUMMER SCHOOLS or similar INTENSIVE COURSES are welcome, provided their objective was held to present an active mathematical topic to an audience at the beginning or intermediate graduate level (a list of participants should be provided).

   The resulting manuscript should not be just a collection of course notes, but should require advance planning and coordination among the main lecturers. The subject matter should dictate the structure of the book. This structure should be motivated and explained in a scientific introduction, and the notation, references, index and formulation of results should be, if possible, unified by the editors. Each contribution should have an abstract and an introduction referring to the other contributions. In other words, more preparatory work must go into a multi-authored volume than simply assembling a disparate collection of papers, communicated at the event.

3. Manuscripts should be submitted either online at www.editorialmanager.com/lnm to Springer's mathematics editorial in Heidelberg, or electronically to one of the series editors. Authors should be aware that incomplete or insufficiently close-to-final manuscripts almost always result in longer refereeing times and nevertheless unclear referees' recommendations, making further refereeing of a final draft necessary. The strict minimum amount of material that will be considered should include a detailed outline describing the planned contents of each chapter, a bibliography and several sample chapters. Parallel submission of a manuscript to another publisher while under consideration for LNM is not acceptable and can lead to rejection.

4. In general, **monographs** will be sent out to at least 2 external referees for evaluation.

   A final decision to publish can be made only on the basis of the complete manuscript, however a refereeing process leading to a preliminary decision can be based on a pre-final or incomplete manuscript.

   Volume Editors of **multi-author works** are expected to arrange for the refereeing, to the usual scientific standards, of the individual contributions. If the resulting reports can be forwarded to the LNM Editorial Board, this is very helpful. If no reports are forwarded or if other questions remain unclear in respect of homogeneity etc, the series editors may wish to consult external referees for an overall evaluation of the volume.

5. Manuscripts should in general be submitted in English. Final manuscripts should contain at least 100 pages of mathematical text and should always include

   - a table of contents;
   - an informative introduction, with adequate motivation and perhaps some historical remarks: it should be accessible to a reader not intimately familiar with the topic treated;
   - a subject index: as a rule this is genuinely helpful for the reader.
   - For evaluation purposes, manuscripts should be submitted as pdf files.

6. Careful preparation of the manuscripts will help keep production time short besides ensuring satisfactory appearance of the finished book in print and online. After acceptance of the manuscript authors will be asked to prepare the final LaTeX source files (see LaTeX templates online: https://www.springer.com/gb/authors-editors/book-authors-editors/manuscriptpreparation/5636) plus the corresponding pdf- or zipped ps-file. The LaTeX source files are essential for producing the full-text online version of the book, see http://link.springer.com/bookseries/304 for the existing online volumes of LNM). The technical production of a Lecture Notes volume takes approximately 12 weeks. Additional instructions, if necessary, are available on request from lnm@springer.com.

7. Authors receive a total of 30 free copies of their volume and free access to their book on SpringerLink, but no royalties. They are entitled to a discount of 33.3 % on the price of Springer books purchased for their personal use, if ordering directly from Springer.

8. Commitment to publish is made by a *Publishing Agreement*; contributing authors of multiauthor books are requested to sign a *Consent to Publish form*. Springer-Verlag registers the copyright for each volume. Authors are free to reuse material contained in their LNM volumes in later publications: a brief written (or e-mail) request for formal permission is sufficient.

Addresses:

Professor Jean-Michel Morel, CMLA, École Normale Supérieure de Cachan, France
E-mail: moreljeanmichel@gmail.com

Professor Bernard Teissier, Equipe Géométrie et Dynamique,
Institut de Mathématiques de Jussieu – Paris Rive Gauche, Paris, France
E-mail: bernard.teissier@imj-prg.fr

Springer: Ute McCrory, Mathematics, Heidelberg, Germany,
E-mail: lnm@springer.com